PATIENT-BASED APPROACHES TO COGNITIVE NEUROSCIENCE

NOTICE

PATIENT-BASED APPROACHES TO COGNITIVE NEUROSCIENCE

EDITED BY

Martha J. Farah and Todd E. Feinberg

The MIT Press
Cambridge, Massachusetts
London, England

This book was set in Times Ten and Helvetica by Graphic Composition, Inc., Athens, Georgia.

Printed and bound in the United States of America.

Library of Congress Cataloging-in-Publication Data

Patient-based approaches to cognitive neuroscience / edited by Martha J. Farah and Todd E. Feinberg.
    p. cm.—(Issues in clinical and cognitive neuropsychology)
    Abridged ed. of: Behavioral neurology and neuropsychology, ©1997.
    Originally published: New York : McGraw-Hill. Health Professions
Division, ©1997.
    Includes bibliographical references and index.
    ISBN 0-262-56123-9 (pbk. : alk. paper)
    1. Clinical neuropsychology. 2. Neuropsychiatry. 3. Cognitive
neuroscience. I. Feinberg, Todd E. II. Farah, Martha J. III. Series. IV.
Series: Behavioral neurology and neuropsychology.
    [DNLM: 1. Nervous System Diseases. 2. Neuropsychology. WL 140
P2977 1997a]
RC341.B424 2000
616.8—dc21
DNLM/DLC
for Library of Congress
                                       99-34052
                                          CIP

CONTENTS

PREFACE

Fifteen years ago, a behavioral neurology fellow in Gainesville called a cognitive science postdoc in Cambridge, Massachusetts, to discuss mental imagery in neurologic patients. The conversation lasted well over an hour—or perhaps we should say it lasted fifteen years, with the parties on each end of the line moving from Gainesville to New York, and from Cambridge to Pittsburgh to Philadelphia. Throughout this time we have each learned about the other's fields, collaborated on occasional research projects, and significantly bolstered the value of AT&T stock.

It was during one of these long-distance explorations of mind and brain that Todd raised the possibility of a joint book. An editor at McGraw-Hill had approached him with the idea of editing a textbook on behavioral neurology, to complement Adams and Victor's classic *Principles of Neurology*. He was interested, but made a counteroffer—a book that would combine traditional behavioral neurology with current developments in cognitive neuropsychology. McGraw-Hill approved of the idea. So did Martha, who joined as coeditor.

The book, entitled *Behavioral Neurology and Neuropsychology*, covered a broad range of issues, from purely clinical concerns (when should you shunt for hydrocephalus in the elderly?) to purely theoretical (is there a conscious awareness module in the brain?). Thanks to the tremendous talents and efforts of our contributing authors and the guiding wisdom of our McGraw-Hill editor, Joe Hefta, the book covered this long and varied agenda without seeming disjointed. We have been gratified by the responses from our colleagues, as well as the appreciative reviews in medical journals, which invariably praise the integration of clinical neurology with cognitive neuroscience.

Nevertheless we felt that within this book there was another book of a more focused nature. About a third of the chapters taken together make a complete survey of the current state of patient-based cognitive neuroscience. We suspected that there would be many readers who would like an up-to-date review of theory and evidence in neurological disorders of perception, attention, language, and executive functions, but who have never pondered when to shunt. When McGraw-Hill's sales reports showed almost every buyer of our book had an M.D. after his or her name, this clinched the decision: We needed to reach more of the cognitive neuroscience community with an abridged edition of the book. Joe Hefta and McGraw-Hill agreed with us the best person to make this happen was Michael Rutter of The MIT Press.

It is a pleasure to thank our contributing authors again, as well as Michael Rutter and the excellent editorial and production staff with whom he works. We also thank Irene Kan for her help with all manner of paper and electronic communications during the preparation of this book, and Norma Kamen for additional secretarial support. Finally, even though the preparation of this book was a short and pleasant task, not requiring of much intellectual or moral support, we can't pass up the oportunity to thank our teachers, colleagues, families, and friends again for all they have given us over the years.

PATIENT-BASED APPROACHES TO COGNITIVE NEUROSCIENCE

Part I
HISTORY, METHODS, PRINCIPLES

Chapter 1

A HISTORICAL PERSPECTIVE ON COGNITIVE NEUROSCIENCE

Todd E. Feinberg
Martha J. Farah

ANTIQUITY THROUGH THE EIGHTEENTH CENTURY

The most fundamental fact of cognitive neuroscience was established in ancient times, when the Greeks first determined that the brain was the physical seat of the mind. Alcamaeon of Croton, who may have been a student of Pythagoras, is credited with making this basic advance in the fifth century B.C. on the basis of his observations of human patients with brain damage. The alternative hypothesis held the heart to be the organ responsible for sensation and thought. This was the accepted view among Egyptian writers and continued to attract adherents in ancient Greece centuries after Alcamaeon. Although Hippocrates and Plato held a cerebrocentric view of the mind, no less a thinker than Aristotle remained in the cardiocentric camp.

Among the ancient cerebrocentrists, the nature of the mind-brain relation was poorly understood. The brain itself was considered by many to be a mere package for the real substance of thought, the cerebrospinal fluid, and the most important anatomical features of the brain were therefore the ventricles. Although brain tissue itself was considered important by some writers, including Galen, for many centuries the mind was predominantly identified with cerebrospinal fluid. The present-day use of the word *spirit* to refer both to certain fluids and to the soul is vestige of this idea.

For the entire period of the middle ages in Europe (approximately the fourth to fourteenth centuries), the ventricles continued to be the focus of theories relating mind and brain.[1] For example, according to fourth-century church fathers, the anterior ventricles were associated with perception (later to be known as the *sensorium commune*), the middle with reason, and the posterior with memory.[2] It has been suggested that this focus on the ventricles accorded better with the dualism of Christian theology, as the hollow cavities could be said to contain the soul without hypothesizing an identity between mind and the physical substrate of brain tissue.[1] Figure 1-1 shows an early illustration of the ventricular system.

During the Renaissance, the ventricular doctrine and the role of the *rete mirabile* began to lose their influence on theories of mind-brain relations.[2,3,4] The seventeenth-century writings of René Descartes mark a transitional phase, in which the interaction between fluid in the ventricles and brain tissue itself was hypothesized to explain intelligent action, as shown in Fig. 1-2. For reflexive action, Descartes proposed a simple loop, in which stimulated nerves caused the release of animal spirits in the ventricles, which, in turn, caused efferent nerves and muscles to act. For intelligent human action, this loop was modulated by the soul via its effects on the pineal gland. The pineal gland was chosen in part because it is unpaired and centrally located and also because it is surrounded by cerebrospinal fluid. It was also mistakenly thought to be uniquely human. Of course, the pineal gland was just the vehicle for the mind's influence on the body; Descartes' theory still denied any form of identity between the mind and neural tissue.[3,5-8]

Descartes' theory was formulated at a time when neuroanatomic knowledge was quite primitive. This situation began to change with the work of such figures as Thomas Willis later in the seventeenth century[3,10] and Malpighi Pacchioni and Albrecht von Haller in the eighteenth.[11,12] For example, Von Haller stimulated the nerves of live animals in an effort to discover the pathways for perception and motor action, thus establishing the experimental method in neurophysiology. This work set the stage for the explosion of experimental and clinical research of the nineteenth century, in which the brain organization underlying perception, action, language, and many other cognitive functions was revealed.

THE LOCALISM/HOLISM DEBATE OF THE NINETEENTH CENTURY

One of the more notorious figures in the history of behavioral neurology is Franz Josef Gall, shown in Fig. 1-3. In the late eighteenth and early nineteenth centuries, he and his collaborator Johann Spurzheim made a number of important contributions to functional neuroanatomy, including proving by dissection the crossing of the pyramids and establishing the distinction between gray and white matter.[13-15] Gall is also credited with one of the earliest descriptions of aphasia linked to a lesion of the frontal lobes.[16] He is most famous, however, for his general theory of cerebral localization, known today as phrenology. At the age of 9, Gall had noted that his schoolmates who excelled at rote memory tasks had quite prominent eyes, *"les yeux à fleur de tête"* (cow's eyes). He reasoned that this was the result of the overdevelopment of the subjacent regions of the brain, and speculated that these regions of the brain might be particularly involved in language functions and especially verbal memory.

Gall identified 27 basic human faculties and associated them with particular brain centers that could affect the shape of the skull, as shown in Fig.

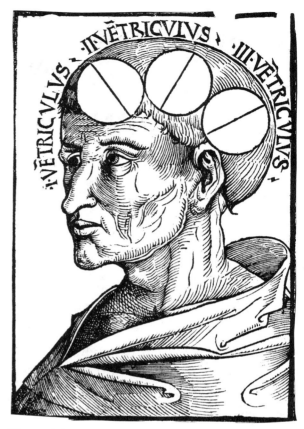

Figure 1-1
The ventricular system according to Albertus Magnus from his Philosophia naturalis (1506).[2]

1–4. These included memory of things and facts, sense of spatial relations, vanity, God and religion, and love for one's offspring.[15] His theory was based on hundreds of skulls and casts of humans and beasts. For instance, the disposition to murder and cruelty was based on a bump above the ear possessed by carnivorous animals. He located the same feature in sadistic persons whom he had examined personally,[3] skulls of famous criminals, and the busts and paintings of famous murderers.[12] Gall taught and practiced medicine in Vienna from 1781 to around 1802, until Emperor Francis I banned Gall's public lectures because they were materialistic and thus opposed to morality and religion.[12] Gall then took to the road,

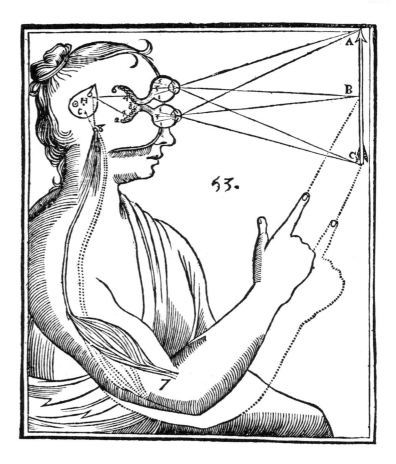

Figure 1-2
Descartes' conception of sensation and action as conceived in his De homine *(1662). Light was transferred from the retina to the ventricles, causing the release of animal spirits. The pineal gland modulated this mechanism for voluntary action.*[9]

lecturing across Europe to enthusiastic popular audiences. By the time he settled in Paris in 1807, he was hugely popular and internationally known. However, phrenology continued to create controversy in scientific circles.

The best-known critic of Gall was Marie-Jean-Pierre Flourens. Flourens mounted a scientific research program to disprove Gall's theory, but it appears to have been motivated at least as much by religious discomfort with the implications of Gall's straightforward mind-brain equivalences as by scientific considerations. Flourens viewed Gall's theory as tantamount to denying the existence of the soul, because it divided the mind and brain into functionally distinct parts and Flourens believed the soul to be unitary.[12,17–19] He carried out extensive lesion experiments on a variety of animal species to demonstrate the equipotentiality of cortex.

Gall's status as a popularizer, and Flourens's empirical attacks, helped to push localism out of the mainstream of contemporary scientific thought in the early nineteenth century. When, in 1825, Jean-Baptiste Bouillaud, shown in Fig. 1-5, presented a large series of clinical cases of loss of speech following frontal lesions,[12,18,19] his work was largely ignored. This landmark work, in which speech per se was distinguished from nonspeech movements of the mouth and tongue, is still relatively unknown.

Bouillaud was not the only one to suggest a frontal location for language functions. During this period and lasting up to the 1860s, numerous clinical reports of patients with frontal lobe

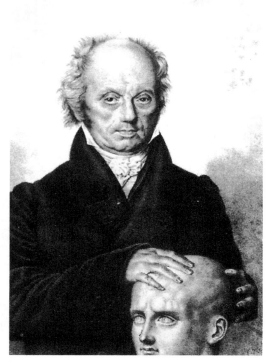

Figure 1-3
Franz Josef Gall (1758–1828).

reported his clinical observations of a patient whose frontal bone was removed following a suicide attempt. He reported that when the blade of a spatula was applied to the "anterior lobes," there was complete cessation of speech without loss of consciousness.[3,12,25] Aubertin went on to describe a patient of Bouillaud's who had a speech disturbance and was near death. Aubertin boldly vowed if this patient lacked a frontal lesion he would renounce his views.[12,24–27]

The 1861 debate is best known not for the presentations of Gratiolet and Aubertin but for the eventual participation of the society's founder and secretary, Paul Broca, shown in Fig. 1-7. Although Broca did not initially take a strong position, his observations of a patient then under his care led him to play a pivotal role in the debate. His patient, Leborgne, suffered from epilepsy,

Figure 1-4
An example of a porcelain phrenology bust with demarcations that demonstrate the reflection of the human faculties on the skull. (Photograph courtesy of Joseph A. Hefta.)

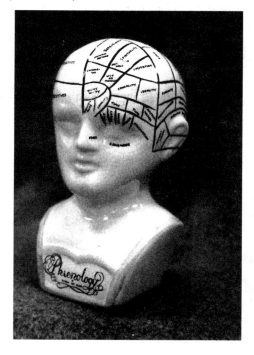

damage and loss of speech were recorded in Europe and America. Indeed, this idea had considerable historical precedence throughout antiquity.[20–22] However, intense interest in localization of brain functions, particularly language, was now developing. It was during this time that Marc Dax noted the association between left-hemispheric damage, right hemiplegia, and aphasia, based upon his examination of 40 patients over a 20-year period. This paper was handwritten in 1836 and not published at the time,[23] but copies may have been distributed to friends and colleagues.[3]

It was not until 1861 that the field reconsidered localism with a more open mind. That year the Société d'Anthropologie in Paris held a series of debates between Pierre Gratiolet, arguing in favor of holism or equipotentiality, and Ernest Aubertin, the son-in-law of Bouillaud, arguing in favor of localism.[12,24,25] Aubertin, shown in Fig. 1-6,

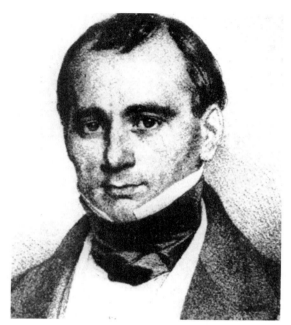

Figure 1-5
Jean-Baptiste Bouillaud (1796–1881).

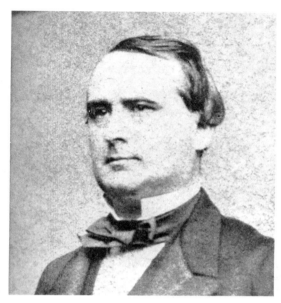

Figure 1-6
Ernest Aubertin (1825–1865).

Figure 1-7
Paul Broca (1824–1880).

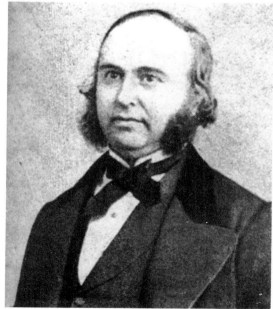

right hemiplegia, and loss of speech, the last for a period of over 20 years. Leborgne had been institutionalized for some 31 years and throughout the hospital was known by the name "Tan," as this was his only utterance along with a few obscenities.[3,9] In light of Aubertin's declaration, Broca invited him to examine Tan, which Aubertin did and afterward concluded that indeed the patient met the critieria of his prior challenge. Six days later Leborgne died; the following day, April 18, 1961, Broca presented the brain to the society along with a brief statement but without firm conclusions.[25] Figure 1-8 shows the brain of Leborgne.

Four months later, at a meeting of the Société Anatomique de Paris in August, Broca made a more extensive report. The brain of Leborgne had demonstrated an egg-sized fluid-filled cavity located in the posterior second and third frontal convolutions, with involvement of adjacent structures as well, including the corpus striatum.[36] In this report, Broca claimed that his findings would "support the ideas of M. Bouillaud on the seat of

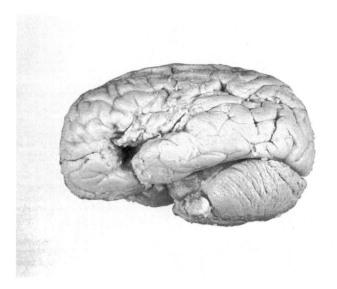

Figure 1-8
Photograph of the brain of Broca's first patient, Leborgne ("Tan"). It is now housed in the Musée Dupuytren.

the faculty for language";[25,28] he later suggested a possible localization of speech functions to the second or more probably third frontal convolution. Later the same year, Broca presented another patient with speech disturbance, an 84-year-old laborer whose lesion also involved the left second and third frontal convolutions. The lesion was more circumscribed than that found in Leborgne and strengthened the association of those structures with speech localization.

In the mid-1860s the issue of hemispheric asymmetry entered the debate on localization. The previous cases strongly suggested that speech is localized to the left hemisphere, and an additional series of eight cases published by Broca in 1863 were exclusively left-sided.[3,23,29] In spite of the strong lateralization of lesion locus in these cases, Broca made note of this "remarkable" observation but made no further claims.[23] In this same year and shortly before Broca's paper was presented,[3] Gustave Dax, son of Marc Dax, sent a handwritten copy of his father's manuscript to the Académie de Médecine in Paris. In this document, Marc Dax had previously described his view on the relation between speech and the left hemisphere. The paper was read before the Académie in December 1864 and published in 1865.[30,31] By

1865, Broca clearly expressed the opinion that the left hemisphere played a dominant role in speech production.[32,33] As far as the issue of priority of discovery is concerned (a matter of controversy among historians), most writers agree that the Dax paper in its original form in 1836 had no influence on Broca or the scientific community when first written. This paper did, however, make clear the association of language functions and the left hemisphere. While Broca alone clarified the role of the second and third frontal convolutions, he apparently did not take a firm position on the specific role of the left hemisphere until after the Dax paper was read before the Académie de Médecine in Paris in December 1964.[3] It appears that the reemergence of the Dax manuscript and Broca's discovery were nearly simultaneous events.

THE AFTERMATH OF 1861: THE EMERGENCE OF MODERN NEUROPSYCHOLOGY

The events in Paris in the 1860s constituted a turning point in the history of ideas regarding brain function. The concepts and methods developed in the course of debating the localization of speech were extended to a variety of different higher functions, experimental work on animals also developed apace. From this period onward, it is impossible to trace a single line of scientific development. Here we simply present a summary of some of the major advances seen in the behavioral neurology and neuropsychology of the late nineteenth and early twentieth centuries.

In the decade following Broca's contributions, two important developments took place in Germany. First, Edward Hitzig and Gustav Fritsch performed a series of experiments in which the cortex of a dog was stimulated while the dog lay on a dressing table in Hitzig's Berlin home.[4,9,34,42] These experiments established that motor functions are localized to anterior cortex and demonstrated experimentally the somatotopic organization of motor cortex inferred indirectly from previous clinical-anatomic correlations in humans. In their report, the investigators specifically noted that their results refuted the holism of Flourens. Following their work, Sir David Ferrier in England confirmed the findings of Hitzig and Fritsch and improved upon their method of stimulation to discover more detailed structure-function relationships.[11]

About the same time, the German neurologist Carl Wernicke began to investigate language functions other than speech. Wernicke, shown in Fig. 1-9, documented a form of aphasia different from the nonfluent variety that followed frontal damage. In what he called sensory aphasia, a posterior lesion in the region of the first temporal gyrus caused a disturbance in auditory comprehension, inappropriate word selection in spontaneous speech, and impaired naming and writing. In his landmark monograph *Der aphasische Symptomen-complex,* Wernicke reasoned that Broca's area was the center for the motor representation of speech, and the posterior first temporal gyrus was the center for "sound images." Wernicke also described global aphasia and explained it as a result of destruction of both anterior and posterior language areas. He also made a prediction that a disturbance of the pathways between these two areas would produce another variety of

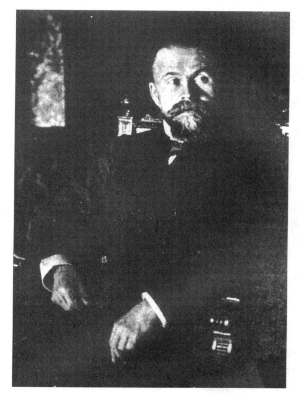

Figure 1-9
Carl Wernicke (1848–1904).

aphasia he called "conduction aphasia," in which comprehension would be preserved but output would be as impaired as in sensory aphasia.[35–38] Wernicke had, in effect, proposed a model that could explain a number of different aphasic syndromes by lesions to different combination of centers and connections between centers. This type of theorizing came to be known as "associationism," because language use was viewed in terms of associating representations in different brain centers, or as "connectionism," because of the emphasis that view put on the connections between centers, as shown in Fig. 1-10.

The connectionist paradigm was quickly extended to explain other disorders. Ludwig Lichtheim placed pure word deafness in this framework, predicting the critical lesion site as well as noting that, given the connectionist explanation

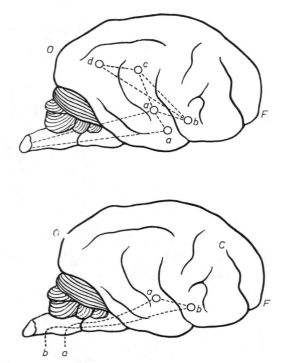

Figure 1-10
Wernicke's model of the speech mechanism.[36] *The auditory areas (a) project to centers subserving vocal output (b) and areas which contain tactile (c) and visual (d) images.*

for this syndrome, a disturbance in repetition should accompany conduction aphasia.[38,39] Hugo Liepmann described the apraxias, including ideomotor apraxia,[40] and, with Maas, callosal apraxia,[41] explaining them in terms of connectionist principles. Joseph Jules Déjerine, shown in Fig. 1-11, also used the framework of centers and connections in his explanation of alexia without agraphia.[42]

The nineteenth-century connectionist framework proved to have both parsimony and explanatory power. Rather than hypothesizing a new center for every ability or every observed deficit, after the fashion of Gall, a relatively small number of basic centers (vision, sound images, motor outputs) could be combined through connections to explain a wide variety of higher functions and

their deficits. Connectionist explanations of aphasia, apraxia, alexia, and other disorders survived well into the twentieth century; indeed, Norman Geschwind, one of the most influential behavioral neurologists of our time, championed them throughout his career.[43] Despite the current proliferation of theories and approaches in our field, the theories of Déjerine, Liepmann, Lichtheim, and Wernicke are still held to be correct by many.

Nevertheless, as successful as the connectionist framework was in late nineteenth century in explaining a variety of disorders, skeptics continued to reject the localism implicit in it. One of the most influential of these was the English neurologist John Hughlings Jackson, shown in Fig. 1-12. He viewed the nervous system not as a series of centers connected by pathways but rather as a hierarchically organized and highly interactive whole that could not be understood piecemeal.[24] Figure 1-13 shows Pierre Marie, a Parisian student of Broca and Charcot, who also took issue with the connectionist theorizing of the late nineteenth

Figure 1-11
Joseph Jules Déjerine (1849–1917).

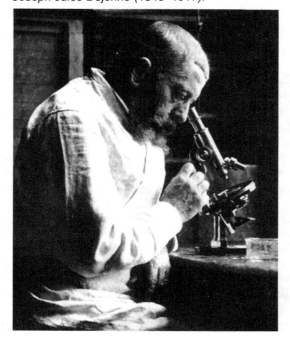

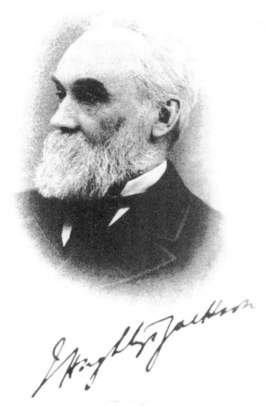

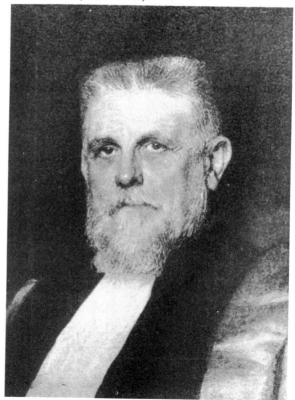

toward holism continued into the early twentieth century, with Jackson and Marie followed by a number of influential neurologists and psychologists, including Henry Head in England,[24] shown in Fig. 1-14, Kurt Goldstein in Germany,[45–47] shown in Fig. 1-15, and Karl Lashley in the United States.[48–51] This swing of the pendulum back toward holism has been explained by the waning of German influence following World War I[60] and the growing influence of Gestalt psychology.[61]

While these workers emphasized the brain's unity, other researchers had pointed out the difference between brain regions in cellular morphology, cell densities, and lamination and produced the first cytoarchitectonic maps. Oskar and Cécile Vogt[62,63] and Alfred W. Campbell[64,65] produced some of the earliest examples of these

Figure 1-13
Pierre Marie (1853–1940).

Figure 1-12
John Hughlings Jackson (1835–1911).

century. His style was direct, to say the least. One of his articles was so offensive to Déjerine that it provoked the latter to challenge Marie to a duel. His article questioning the empirical basis of the early claims concerning speech localization was entitled *"La troisiéme circonvolution frontale gauche ne joue aucun rôle spécial dans la fonction du langage"* ("The third frontal convolution plays no special role at all in the function of language").[44] Marie believed that there was just one basic form of aphasia, a posterior aphasia, which was a type of general intellectual loss not specific to language per se. He held that the speech problems of anterior aphasics were motoric in nature. When aphasia is viewed this way, a network of specialized centers is superfluous. A movement

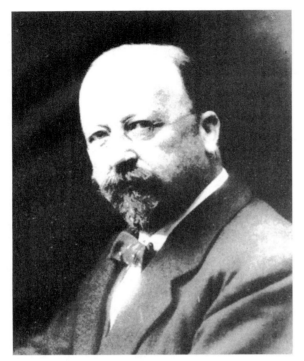

Figure 1-14
Henry Head (1861–1940).

architectonic maps, followed by many others, including those of Korbinian Brodmann,[58] whose cortical maps of the human brain have had the most widespread application. While these workers did not agree on the number and location of cortical areas (the Vogts counted over 200, Brodmann only 52[3]) it could not be contested that there were clear regional neuroanatomic differences.

The late nineteenth century also saw the beginnings of the modern study of memory and vision. Theodule Ribot introduced the distinction between anterograde and retrograde memory impairments and observed what is now known as "Ribot's law," that the most recently laid down memories were the most vulnerable to brain damage.[59–61] Ribot can also be credited with describing preserved learning in amnesia, thus anticipating the distinction between declarative and nondeclarative forms of memory that has been so intensively investigated in our own recent times. An ad-

ditional contribution to memory research in the latter nineteenth century was the description by Wernicke and Korsakoff (shown in Fig. 1-16) of the syndrome that bears their names, including Korsakoff's observations of what he called "pseudo-reminiscence," now known as confabulation.[70,71]

In 1881, Hermann Munk reported that when he ablated the occipital lobes of dogs, they seemed unable to recognize objects despite seeing well enough to navigate the visual environment.[72] Shortly thereafter, Lissauer presented one of the earliest clinical descriptions of visual recognition impairment in a human and suggested the distinction between apperceptive and associative impairment—a clinical dichotomy still in use today.[73] Freud would later introduce the term *agnosia* to describe these conditions.[74] In the decades that followed, the visuospatial functions of the right hemisphere finally attracted the attention of neu-

Figure 1-15
Kurt Goldstein (1878–1965).

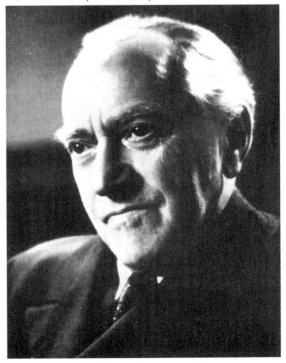

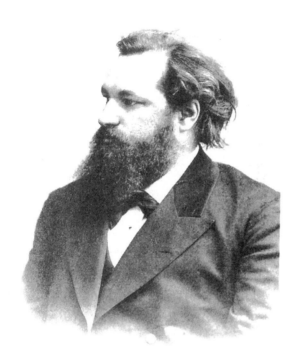

Figure 1-16
Sergei S. Korsakoff (1853–1900).

rologists and neuropsychologists.[67–69] The relatively delayed entry of this realm of functioning into the research arena is probably a result of the field's original focus on language and the left hemisphere, reflected in the nineteenth-century terminology of *major* and *minor hemisphere.*

THE RISE OF EXPERIMENTAL NEUROPSYCHOLOGY

Most of the advances described so far in this chapter were made by studying individual patients, or at most a small series of patients with similar disorders. In many instances, particularly before the middle of this century, patients' behavior was studied relatively naturalistically, without planned protocols or quantitative measurements. In the nineteen sixties and seventies, a different approach to the study of brain-behavior relations

took hold. Neurologists and neuropsychologists began to design experiments patterned on research methods in experimental psychology.

Typical research designs in experimental psychology involved groups of normal subjects given different experimental treatments (for example, different training or different stimulus materials), and the effects of the treatments were measured in standardized protocols and compared using statistical methods such as analysis of variance. In neuropsychology, the "treatments" were, as a rule, naturally occurring brain lesions. Groups of patients with different lesion sites or behavioral syndromes were tested with standard protocols, yielding quantitative measures of performance, and these performances were compared across patient groups and with non-brain-damaged control groups. Unlike the impairments studied previously in single-case designs, which were so striking that control subjects would generally have been superfluous, experimental neuropsychology often focused on group differences of a rather subtle nature, which required statistical analysis to substantiate.

The most common question addressed by these studies concerned localization of function. Often the localization sought was no more precise than left versus right hemisphere or one quadrant of the brain (which, in the days before computed tomography, often amounted to left versus right hemisphere with presence or absence of visual field defects and/or hemiplegia). Given the huge amount of research done during this period on language, memory, perception, attention, emotion, praxis, and so-called executive functions, it would be hopeless even to attempt a summary. For those interested in some examples of this approach, we cite here some classic papers from a variety of the active laboratories of the period, addressing the question "Is the right hemisphere specialized for spatial perception of properties such as location,[70–72] orientation,[73,74] and large-scale topography?[75,76]

The influential research program of the Montreal Neurological Institute also began during this period. In the wake of William Scoville's discovery that the bilateral medial temporal resection he performed on epileptic patient H. M. resulted in permanent and dense amnesia, Brenda Milner and her colleagues investigated this patient and groups of other operated epileptic patients. This enabled them to address questions of functional localization with the anatomic precision of known surgical lesions (e.g., see Refs. 77 and 78 for reviews of research from that period on frontal lobe function and temporal lobe function, respectively). At the same time, another surgical intervention for epilepsy, callosotomy, also spawned a productive and influential research program. Roger Sperry and his students and collaborators were able to address a wide variety of questions about hemispheric specialization by studying the isolated functioning of the human cerebral hemispheres.[79]

In addition to answering questions about localization, the experimental neuropsychology of the sixties and seventies also uncovered aspects of the functional organization of behavior. By examining patterns of association and dissociation among abilities over groups of subjects, researchers tried to determine which abilities depend on the same underlying functional systems and which are functionally independent. For example, the frequent association of aphasia and apraxia had been taken by some to support the notion that aphasia was not language-specific but was just one manifestation of a more pervasive loss of the ability to symbolize or represent ("asymbolia"). A classic group study by Goodglass and Kaplan[80] undermined this position by showing that severity of apraxia and aphasia were uncorrelated in a large sample of left-hemisphere-damaged subjects. A second example of the use of dissociations between groups of patients from this period is the demonstration of the functional distinction, by Newcombe and Russell, within vision between pattern recognition and spatial orientation.[81]

By the end of the seventies, experimental neuropsychology had matured to the point where many perceptual, cognitive, and motor abilities had been associated with particular brain regions, and certain features of the functional organization of these abilities had been delineated. Accord-ingly, it was at this time that first editions of some of the best-known neuropsychology texts appeared, such as those by Hécaen and Albert,[82] Heilman and Valenstein,[83] Kolb and Whishaw,[84] Springer and Deutsch,[85] and Walsh.[86]

Despite the tremendous progress of this period, experimental neuropsychology remained distinct from and relatively unknown within academic psychology. Particularly in the United States, but also to a large extent in Canada and Europe (the three largest contributors to the world's psychology literature), experimental neuropsychologists tended to work in medical centers rather than university psychology departments and to publish their work in journals separate from mainstream experimental psychology. An important turning point in the histories of both neuropsychology and the psychology of normal human function came when researchers in each area became aware of the other.

THE BIRTH OF COGNITIVE NEUROSCIENCE

Patient-based cognitive neuroscience was born when the theories and methods of cognitive psychology and neuropsychology were finally combined. Both fields had strong incentives to overcome their isolation. Let us begin by reviewing the state of cognitive psychology prior to the birth of cognitive neuroscience.

The central tenet of cognitive psychology is that cognition is information processing. Although the effects of damage to an information-processing mechanism might seem to be a good source of clues as to its normal operation, cognitive psychologists of the seventies were generally quite ignorant of contemporary neuropsychology.

The reason that most cognitive psychologists of the 1970s ignored neuropsychology stemmed from an overly narrow conception of information processing, based on the digital computer. A basic tenet of cognitive psychology was the computer analogy for the mind: the mind is to the brain as software is to hardware in a computer. Given that the same computer can run different programs and the same program can be run on different computers, this analogy suggests that hardware and software are independent and that the brain is therefore irrelevant to cognitive psychology. If you want to understand the nature of the program that is the human mind, studying neuropsychology is as pointless as trying to understand how a computer is programmed by looking at the circuit boards.

The problem with the computer analogy is that hardware and software are independent only for very special types of computational systems: those systems that have been engineered, through great effort and ingenuity, to make the hardware and software independent, enabling one computer to run many programs and enabling those programs to be portable to other computers. The brain was "designed" by very different pressures, and there is no reason to believe that, in general, information-processing functions and the physical substrate of those functions will be independent. In fact, as cognitive psychologists finally began to learn about neuropsychology, it became apparent that cognitive functions break down in characteristic and highly informative ways after brain damage. By the early 1980s, cognitive psychology and neuropsychology were finally in communication with one another. Since then, we have seen an explosion of meetings, books, and new journals devoted to so-called cognitive neuropsychology. Perhaps more important, existing cognitive psychology journals have begun to publish neuropsychological studies, and articles in existing neuropsychology and neurology journals frequently include discussions of the cognitive psychology literature.

Let us take a closer look at the scientific forces that drove this change in disciplinary boundaries. By 1980, both cognitive psychology and neuropsychology had reached states of development that were, if not exactly impasses, points of diminishing returns for the concepts and methods of their own isolated disciplines. In cognitive psychology, the problem concerned methodologic limitations. By varying stimuli and instructions

and measuring responses and response latencies, cognitive psychologists made inferences about the information processing that intervened between stimulus and responses. But such inferences were indirect, and in some cases they were incapable of distinguishing between rival theories. In 1978 the cognitive psychologist John Anderson published an influential paper[87] in which he called this the "identifiability" problem and took as his example the debate over whether mental images were more like perceptual representations or linguistic representations. He argued that the field's inability to resolve this issue, despite many years of research, was due to the impossibility of uniquely identifying internal cognitive processes from stimulus-response relations. He suggested that the direct study of brain function could, in principle, make a unique identification possible, but he indicated that such a solution probably lay in the distant future.

That distant future came to pass within the next 10 years, as cognitive psychologists working on a variety of different topics found that the study of neurologic patients provided a powerful new source of evidence for testing their theories. In the case of mental imagery, taken by Anderson to be emblematic of the identifiability problem, the finding that perceptual impairments after brain damage were frequently accompanied by parallel imagery impairments strongly favored the perceptual hypothesis.[88] The study of learning and memory within cognitive psychology was revolutionized by the influx of ideas and findings on preserved learning in amnesia, leading to the hypothesis of multiple memory systems.[89–91] In the study of attention, cognitive psychologists had for years focused on the issue of early versus late attentional selection without achieving a resolution, and here too neurologic disorders were crucial in moving the field forward. The phenomena of neglect provided dramatic evidence of selection from spatially formatted perceptual representations, and the variability in neglect's manifestations from case to case helped to establish the possibility of multiple loci for attentional selection as opposed to a single early or late locus. The idea of separate visual feature maps, supported by cases of acquired color, motion, and depth blindness, provided the inspiration for the most novel development in recent cognitive theories of attention—namely, feature integration theory.[92]

What did neuroscience gain from the rapprochement with cognitive psychology? The main benefits were theoretical rather than methodologic. Traditionally, neuropsychologists studied the localization and functional organization of *abilities,* such as speech, reading, memory, object recognition, and so forth. But few would doubt that each of these abilities depends upon an orchestrated set of *component cognitive processes,* and it seems far more likely that the underlying cognitive components, rather than the task-defined abilities, are what is implemented in localized neural tissue. The theories of cognitive psychology therefore allowed neuropsychologists to pose questions about the localization and functional organization of the components of the cognitive architecture, a level of theoretical analysis that was more likely to yield clear and generalizable findings.

Among patients with reading disorders, for example, some are impaired at reading nonwords (e.g., *plif*) while others are impaired at reading irregular words (e.g., *yacht*). Rather than attempt to localize nonword reading or irregular word reading per se and delineate them as independent abilities, neuropsychologists have been able to use a theory of reading developed in cognitive psychology to interpret these disorders in terms of damage to a whole-word recognition system and a grapheme-to-phoneme translation system, respectively.[93] This interpretation has the advantage of correctly predicting additional features of patient behavior, such as the tendency to misread nonwords as words of overall similar appearance when operating with only the whole-word system.

In recent years the neuroscience of every major cognitive system has adopted the theoretical framework of cognitive psychology in a general way, and in some cases specific theories have been incorporated. This is reflected in the content and organization of the present book. For the most intensively studied areas of behavioral neu-

rology and neuropsychology—namely, visual attention, memory, language, frontal lobe function, and Alzheimer's disease—integrated pairs of chapters review the clinical and anatomic aspects of the relevant disorders and their cognitive theoretical interpretations. Chapters on other topics will cover both the clinical and theoretical aspects together.

COMPLEMENTARY METHODS IN COGNITIVE NEUROSCIENCE: PATIENT STUDIES AND FUNCTIONAL IMAGING

Following its introduction in the 1970s, positron emission tomography (PET) was quickly embraced by researchers interested in brain-behavior relations. This technique provides images of regional glucose utilization, blood flow, oxygen consumption, or receptor density in the brains of live humans. Resting studies, in which subjects are scanned while resting passively, have provided a window on differences between normal and pathologic brain function in a number of neurologic and psychiatric conditions. With the use of radioactive ligands, abnormalities can be localized to specific neurotransmitter systems as well as specific anatomic regions. Activation studies, in which separate images are collected while normal subjects perform different tasks (typically one or more active tasks and one resting baseline) yielded new insights on the localization of cognitive processes. These localizations were not studied region by region, as necessitated by the lesion technique, but could be apprehended simultaneously in a whole intact brain.

Positron emission tomography was soon joined by other techniques for measuring regional brain activity, each of which has its own strengths and weaknesses. Single photon emission computed tomography (SPECT) was quickly adapted for some of the same applications as PET, providing a less expensive but also less quantifiable and spatially less accurate method for obtaining images of regional cerebral blood flow. With new developments in the measurement and analysis of electromagnetic signals, the relatively old techniques of electroencephalography (EEG) and event-related potentials (ERPs), as well as magnetoencephalography (MEG), joined the ranks of functional imaging techniques allowing some degree of anatomic localization of brain activity, with temporal resolution that is superior to the blood flow and metabolic techniques. Most recently, functional magnetic resonance imaging (fMRI) has provided a particularly attractive package of reasonably good anatomic and temporal resolution, using techniques that are noninvasive and can be implemented with equipment available for clinical purposes in many hospitals.

Much of the early work with functional neuroimaging could be considered a form of "calibration," in that researchers sought to confirm well-established principles of functional neuroanatomy using the new techniques—for example, demonstrating that visual stimulation activates visual cortex. As functional neuroimaging matured, researchers began to address new questions, to which the answers were not already known in advance. An important development in this second wave of research was the introduction of theories and methods from cognitive psychology, which specified the component cognitive processes involved in performing complex tasks and provided a means of isolating them experimentally. In neuroimaging studies of normal subjects, as with the purely behavioral studies of patients, the entities most likely to yield clear and consistent localizations are these component cognitive processes and not the tasks themselves. Starting in the mid-1980s, a collaboration between cognitive psychologist Michael Posner and neurologist Marcus Raichle at Washington University led to a series of pioneering studies in which the neural circuits underlying language, reading, and attention were studied by PET (see Ref. 94 for a review). Since then, researchers at Washington University and a growing number of other centers around the world have adapted neuroimaging techniques to all manner of topics in cognitive neuroscience.

To many psychologists and neuroscientists, cognitive neuroscience is equivalent to cognitive neuroimaging. At the very least, we hope this book shows this idea to be mistaken. Although

neuroimaging has had a huge and salutary effect on cognitive neuroscience, significantly expanding the range of questions that can be addressed, it has not replaced research with neurological patients. A full discussion of the complementary strengths and weaknesses of the two approaches could easily fill a chapter by itself, but a few of the most consequential differences can be summarized briefly here.

Lumping the different functional neuroimaging modalities together, they generally offer better spatial resolution than can be obtained in inferences from a few patients with focal brain lesions. Imaging also allows us to study normal brains, which lesion studies by definition do not. Furthermore, for some neurological conditions more than others there may be reason to suspect a degree of reorganization of remaining brain systems in response to damage. These are probably the greatest benefits of functional neuroimaging, although by no means the only ones.

The greatest weakness of neuroimaging is its inability to settle any issue concerning what might be called *mechanism*. An important goal of cognitive neuroscience is to identify the causal chain of neural events, or the mechanisms, underlying cognition. The data of functional neuroimaging are correlational: a certain area is activated when a certain cognitive process is occurring. Neuroimaging can never disentangle correlation from causation; in other words, it can never tell us which brain areas are causally involved in enabling a cognitive process. Activated regions could play a causal role or could be activated in an optional or even an epiphenomenal way. For this we must turn to studying the effects of brain damage, the "experiments of nature" that provide a direct test of the causal role of different brain areas by showing us how the system works in their absence. Given the complementary strengths of neuroimaging and patient studies, we predict that the most successful cognitive neuroscience research programs of the twenty-first century will be those that combine the two approaches.

REFERENCES

1. Pagel W: Medieval and Renaissance contributions to knowledge of the brain and its functions, in Poynter FNL (ed): *The Brain and Its Functions,* Oxford, England: Blackwell, 1958, pp. 95–114.
2. Clarke E. Dewhurst K: *An Illustrated History of Brain Function.* Berkeley, CA: University of California Press, 1972.
3. Finger S: *Origins of Neuroscience. A History of Explorations into Brain Function.* New York: Oxford University Press, 1994
4. Bakay L: *An Early History of Craniotomy.* Springfield, IL: Charles C Thomas, 1985.
5. Wozniak RH: *Mind and Body: René Descartes to William James.* National Library of Medicine, Bethesda, MD, and the American Psychological Association, Washington, DC, 1992.
6. Riese W: Descartes' ideas of brain function, in Poynter FNL (ed): *The Brain and Its Function.* Oxford, England: Blackwell, 1958, pp. 115–134.
7. Descartes R: *De homine figuris et latinitate donatus a Florentio Schuyl.* Leyden: Franciscum Moyardum and Petrum Leffen, 1662.
8. Descartes R: *Les passions de l'âme. Paris:* Henry Le Gras, 1649.
9. Clarke E, O'Malley CE: *The Human Brain and Spinal Cord.* Berkeley, CA: University California Press, 1968.
10. Willis T: *Cerebri anatome: Cui accessit nervorum descriptio et usus.* London: Martyn and Allestry, 1664.
11. Mazzolini RG: Schemes and models of the thinking machine. In Corsi P (ed): *The Enchanted Loom: Chapters in the History of Neuroscience.* New York: Oxford University Press, 1991, pp. 68–143.
12. Young RM: *Mind, Brain and Adaptation in the Nineteenth Century.* New York: Oxford University Press, 1990.
13. Stookey B: A note on the early history of cerebral localization. *Bull NY Acad Med* 30:559–578, 1954.
14. Ackerknecht EH: Contribution of Gall and the phrenologist to knowledge of brain function, in Poynter FNL (ed): *The Brain and Its Functions.* Oxford: Blackwell, 1958, pp. 149–153.
15. Pogliano C: Between form and function: A new science of man, in Corsi P (ed): *The Enchanted Loom: Chapters in the History of Neurosciences.* New York: Oxford University Press, 1991, pp. 144–203.
16. Brown JW, Chobor KL: Phrenological studies of aphasia before Broca: Broca's aphasia or Gall's aphasia? *Brain Lang* 43:475–486, 1992.
17. Flourens P: *Phrenology Examined* (Charles De Lucena Meigs, trans). Philadelphia: Hogan and Thompson, 1846.
18. Flourens P: *Recherches Expérimentales sur les Propriétés et les Fonctions du Système Nerveux dans les Animaux Vertèbras* (1824), 2d ed. Paris: Baillière, 1842.
19. Harrington A: Beyond phrenology: Localization theory in the modern era, in Corsi P (ed): *The Enchanted Loom. Chapters in the History of Neuroscience.* New York: Oxford University Press, 1991, pp. 207–239.
20. Bouillaud JB: *Traité clinique et physiologique de l'encephalite ou inflammation du cerveau.* Paris: Baillière, 1825.
21. Benton AL, Joynt RJ: Early descriptions of aphasia. *Arch Neurol* 3:205–221, 1960.
22. Benton AL, Joynt RJ: Three pioneers in the study of aphasia. *J His Med Sci* 18:381–383, 1963.
23. Joynt RJ, Benton AL: The memoir of Marc Dax on aphasia. *Neurology* 14:851–854, 1964.
24. Head H: *Aphasia and Kindred Disorders of Speech.* New York: Macmillan, 1926.
25. Stookey BL: Jean-Baptiste Bouillaud and Ernest Aubertin: Early studies on cerebral localization and the speech center. *JAMA* 184:1024–1029, 1963.
26. Critchley M: The Broca-Dax controversy, in Critchley M (ed): *The Divine Banquet of the Brain and Other Essays.* New York: Raven Press, 1979.
27. Joynt RJ: Centenary of patient "Tan": His contribution to the problem of aphasia. *Arch Intern Med* 108:953–956, 1961.
28. Broca P: Remarques sur le siège de la faculté du langage articulé: Suivies d'une observation d'aphemie. *Bull Soc Anat (Paris)* 6:330–357, 1861.
29. Broca P: Localisation des fonctions cérébrales: Sièe du langage articulé. *Bull Soc Anthropol (Paris)* 4:200–203, 1863.
30. Dax M: Lesions de la moitié gauche de l'encéphale coincident avec l'oublie des signes de la pensée. *Gaz hbd Méd Chir (Paris)* 2:259–262, 1865.
31. Dax G: Notes sur la même sujet. *Gaz hbd Méd Chir (Paris)* 2:262, 1865.
32. Broca P: Sur le siège de la faculté du langage articulé. *Bull Soc Anthropol* 6:337–393, 1865.
33. Berker EA, Berker AH, Smith A: Translation of Broca's 1865 report: Localization of speech in the third left frontal convolution. *Arch Neurol* 43:1065–1072, 1986.
34. Fritsch G, Hitzig E: On the electrical excitability of the cerebrum (1870), in von Bonin G (ed): *Some*

Papers on the Cerebral Cortex. Springfield, IL: Charles C Thomas, 1960, pp. 73–96.

35. Geschwind N: Wernicke's contribution to the study of aphasia. *Cortex* 3:449–463, 1967.

36. Wernicke C: *Der aphasische Symptomemkomplex: Eine psychologische Studie auf anatomischer Basis.* Breslau: Cohn und Weigert, 1874.

37. Lecours AR, Lhermitte F: From Franz Gall to Pierre Marie, in Lecours AR, Lhermitte F, Bryans B (eds): *Aphasiology.* London: Baillière Tindall, 1983.

38. Geschwind N: Carl Wernicke, the Breslau School and the history of aphasia, in Carterette EC (ed): *Brain Function:* Vol. III. *Speech, Language, and Communication.* Berkeley, CA: University of California Press, 1963, pp. 1–16.

39. Lichtheim L: On aphasia. *Brain* 7:433–484, 1885.

40. Liepmann H: Das Krankheitsbild der Apraxie ("motorische Asymbolie") auf Grund eines Falles von einseitiger Apraxie, *Monatschr Psychiatr Neurol* 8:15–44, 102–132, 182–197, 1900.

41. Liepmann H, Maas O: Fall von linksseitiger Agraphie und Apraxie bei rechtsseitiger Lähmung. *J Psychol Neurol* 10:214–227, 1907.

42. Déjerine J: Contribution à l'étude anatomopathologique et clinique des différentes variétés de cécité verbale. *CRH Séances Mem Soc Biol* 44:61–90, 1892.

43. Geschwind N: Disconnexion syndromes in animals and man. *Brain* 88:237–294, 585–644, 1965.

44. Brais B: The third left frontal convolution plays no role in language: Pierre Marie and the Paris debate on aphasia (1906–1908). *Neurology* 42:690–695, 1992.

45. Goldstein K: *The Organism.* New York: American Book, 1939.

46. Goldstein K: *Language and Language Disturbances.* New York: Grune & Stratton, 1948.

47. Lecours AR, Cronk C. Sébahoun-Balsamo M: From Pierre Marie to Norman Geschwind, in Lecours AR, Lhermitte F, Bryans B (eds): *Aphasiology.* London: Baillière Tindall, 1983.

48. Franz SI, Lashley KS: The retention of habits by the rat after destruction of the frontal portion of the cerebrum. *Psychobiology* 1:3–18, 1917.

49. Lashley KS, Franz SI: The effects of cerebral destruction upon habit-formation and retention in the albino rat. *Psychobiology* 1:71–139, 1917.

50. Lashley KS: *Brain Mechanisms and Intelligence: A Quantitative Study of Injuries to the Brain.* Chicago: University of Chicago Press, 1929.

51. Lashley KS: In search of the engram. *Symp Soc Exp Biol* 4:454–482, 1950.

52. Geschwind N: The paradoxical position of Kurt Goldstein in the history of aphasia. *Cortex* 1:214–224, 1964.

53. Harrington A: A feeling for the "whole": the holistic reaction in neurology from the fin de siècle to the interwar years, in Teich M. Porter R (eds): *Fin de Siècle and Its Legacy.* Cambridge, England: Cambridge University Press, 1990.

54. Vogt O, Vogt C: Zur anatomischen Gliederung des cortex cerebri. *J Psychol Neurol* 2:160–180, 1903.

55. Haymaker WE: Cecile and Oskar Vogt, on the occasion of her 75th and his 80th birthday. *Neurology* 1:179–204, 1951.

56. Campbell AW: Histological studies on cerebral localization. *Proc R Soc* 72:488–492, 1903.

57. Campbell AW: *Histological Studies on the Localization of Cerebral Function.* Cambridge, England: Cambridge University Press, 1905.

58. Brodmann K: *Vergleichende Lokalisationslehre der Grosshirnrinde in ihren Prinzipien dargestellt auf Grund des Zellenbaues.* Leipzig: Barth, 1909.

59. Levin HS, Peters BH, Hulkonen DA: Early concepts of anterograde and retrograde amnesia. *Cortex* 19:427–440, 1983.

60. Ribot T: *Diseases of Memory.* London: Kegan Paul, Trench, 1882.

61. Squire LR, Slater PC: Anterograde and retrograde memory impairment in chronic amnesia. *Neuropsychologia* 16:313–322, 1978.

62. Victor M, Adams RD, Collins GH: *The Wernicke-Korsakoff Syndrome and Related Neurologic Disorders due to Alcoholism and Malnutrition,* 2d ed. Philadelphia: Davis, 1989.

63. Victor M, Yakovlev PI: SS Korsakoff's psychic disorder in conjunction with peripheral neuritis: A translation of Korsakoff's original article with brief comments on the author and his contribution to clinical medicine. *Neurology* 5:394–406, 1955.

64. Munk H: Über die Functionen der Grosshirnrinde: Gesammelte Mitteilungen aus den Jahren. Berlin: Hirschwald, 1877–1880.

65. Lissauer H: Ein fall von seelenblindheit nebst einem Beitrage zur Theori derselben. *Arch Psychiatr Nervenkrankh* 21–222-270, 1980.

66. Freud S: Zur Auffassung der Aphasien. Leipzig and Vienna: Deuticke, 1891.

67. Paterson A, Zangwill OL: Disorders of visual space perception associated with lesions of the right cerebral hemisphere. *Brain* 40:122–179, 1944.

68. Hécaen H, Ajuriaguerra J, Massonet J: Les troubles visuoconstructives par lésion pariéto-occipitale droite. *Encéphale* 40:122–179, 1951.

69. Benton A: Neuropsychology: Past, present and future, in Boller F. Grafman J (eds): *Handbook of Neuropsychology.* New York: Elsevier, 1988, vol. 1, pp. 3–27.

70. Hannay HJ, Varney NR, Benton AL: Visual localization in patients with unilateral brain disease. *J Neurol Neurosurg Psychiatry* 39:307–313, 1976.

71. Ratcliff G, Davies-Jones GAB: Defective visual localization in focal brain wounds. *Brain* 95:46–60, 1972.

72. Warrington EK, Rabin P: Perceptual matching in patients with cerebral lesions. *Neuropsychologia* 8:475–487, 1970.

73. De Renzi E, Faglioni P, Scotti G: Judgement of spatial orientation in patients with focal brain damage. *J Neurol Neurosurg Psychiatry* 34:489–495, 1971.

74. Carmon A, Benton AL: Tactile perception of direction and number in patients with unilateral cerebral disease. *Neurology* 19:525–532, 1969.

75. Hécaen H, Tzortzis C, Masure MC: Troubles de l'orientation spatiale dans une épreuve de recherche d'itinéraire lors des lesions corticales unilaterales. *Perception* 1:325–330, 1972.

76. Semmes J, Weinstein S, Ghent L, Teuber HL: Correlates of impaired orientation in personal and extrapersonal space. *Brain* 86:747–772, 1963.

77. Milner B: Some effects of frontal lobectomy in man, in Warren JM, Akert K (eds): *The Frontal Granular Cortex and Behavior.* New York: McGraw-Hill, 1964.

78. Milner B: Memory and the medical temporal regions of the brain, in Pribram KH, Broadbent DE (eds): *Biological Bases of Memory.* New York: Academic Press, 1970.

79. Trevarthen C, Roger W: Sperry's lifework and our tribute, in Trevarthen C (ed): *Brain Circuits and Functions of the Mind: Essays in Honor of Roger W. Sperry.* Cambridge, England: Cambridge University Press, 1990.

80. Goodglass H, Kaplan E: Disturbance of gesture and patomime in aphasia. *Brain* 86:703–720, 1963.

81. Newcombe F, Russell W: Dissociated visual perceptual and spatial deficits in focal lesions of the right hemisphere. *J Neurol Neurosurg Psychiatry* 32:73–81, 1969.

82 Hécaen H, Albert ML: *Human Neuropsychology.* New York: Wiley, 1978.

83. Heilman KM, Valenstein E: *Clinical Neuropsychology.* New York: Oxford University Press, 1979.

84. Kolb B, Whishaw I: *Fundamentals of Human Neuropsychology.* New York: Freeman, 1980.

85. Springer SP, Deutsch G: *Left Brain/Right Brain.* San Francisco: Freeman, 1981.

86. Walsh KW: *Neuropsychology: A Clinical Approach.* New York: Churchill Livingstone, 1978.

87. Anderson JR: Arguments concerning representation for mental imagery. *Psychol Rev* 85:249–277, 1978.

88. Farah MJ: Is visual imagery really visual? Overlooked evidence from neuropsychology. *Psychol Rev* 95:307–317, 1988.

89. Schacter DL: Implicit memory: History and current status. *J Exp Psychol Learn Mem Cog* 13:501–518, 1987.

90. Squire L: *Memory and Brain.* New York: Oxford University Press, 1987.

91. Weiskrantz L: On issues and theories of the human amnesic syndrome, in Weinberger N, McGaugh JL, Lynch G (eds): *Memory Systems of the Brain.* New York: Guilford Press, 1985.

92. Treisman A: Features and objects: The fourteenth Bartlett lecture. *Q J Exp Psychol* 40A:201–237, 1988.

93. Coltheart M: Cognitive neuropsychology and the study of reading, in Marin IP, Marin OSM (eds): *Attention and Performance XI.* London: Erlbaum, 1985.

94. Posner MI, Raichle ME: *Images of Mind.* New York: Scientific American Library, 1994.

Chapter 2

THE LESION METHOD IN COGNITIVE NEUROSCIENCE

Hanna Damasio
Antonio R. Damasio

The lesion method aims at establishing a correlation between a circumscribed region of brain damage, a lesion and a pattern of alteration in some aspect of an experimentally controlled cognitive or behavioral performance. The brain-damaged region is conceptualized as part of a large-scale network of cortical and subcortical sites that operate in concert, by virtue of their interlocking connectivity, to produce a particular function. Given a theoretical framework for how such networks are constituted and carry out that particular function, a lesion is thus a *probe* to test a specific hypothesis. A lesion probe allows the investigator to decide whether damage to a component of the putative network, responsible for function X, alters the network behavior according to the predictions made for it. In other words, given a theory about the operations of a normal brain, lesions are a means to support or falsify the theory.

The subjects for the lesion method may be humans or animals. The lesions may have been produced by neurologic disease alone or incurred in the process of treating it (e.g., a surgical procedure). They may be small or large and may be studied in vivo or at postmortem. The indispensable requirements are that lesions be stable, well demarcated, and referable to a neuroanatomic unit. In this chapter we focus on human lesions, produced by neurologic disease or surgical ablation, and studied in vivo with modern neuroimaging techniques.

The lesion approach provided the first method in what was to become neuroscience. In the very least, it dates to Morgagni's demonstration of an association between unilateral brain disease and contralateral sensory and motor disabilities. Bouillaud's and Broca's finding of a correlation between speech and focal damage to the frontal lobe are reasonable signposts to mark the modern era of lesion studies.

In the latter decades of the nineteenth century, the lesion method led to pathbreaking discoveries. But although most of the findings have stood the test of time and gained wide acceptance, the theories that were associated with them did not. The pioneering neurologists conceived of the existence of brain centers capable of performing complex psychological functions with relative independence. What little interaction there was among those few and noncontiguous centers was achieved by unidirectional pathways. These concepts were subject to deserved criticism, the best known of which came from Sigmund Freud and Hughlings Jackson. As the theoretical account lost influence, the lesion method, which was closely interwoven with the theory, lost favor as a means of valid scientific inquiry.

The lesion method began to regain some prominence in the 1960s, perhaps as a reaction to the impasses of "equipotential" antilocalizationism and "black-box" behaviorism. The revival was spearheaded by Geschwind's reflections on the work of Wernicke, Lichtheim, Liepmann, and Déjerine and by the work of notable neuropsychologists, among whom were A. R. Luria, Henri Hécaen, Brenda Milner, Arthur Benton,

Hans-Lukas Teuber, and Oliver Zangwill. The full value of the lesion method, however, only began to be appreciated after the development of new neuroimaging technologies—computed tomography (CT), which had its inception in 1973, and magnetic resonance imaging (MRI), which emerged a decade later.

It has gradually become evident that the lesion method should be separated from the theoretical accounts historically connected with it. As with any other approach, this method has limitations and misapplications. Nonetheless, it is one entity, with its virtues and pitfalls, and the theoretical constructs that make use of it represent another. Nothing prevents practitioners of the lesion method from proposing the richest and most dynamic accounts of brain function.

In short, the classically discovered links between certain brain regions of the cerebral cortex and signs of neuropsychological dysfunction have been validated, remain a staple of clinical neurology, and allow for relatively accurate predictions of *localization of damage* from neurologic signs. That is, more often than not, the presence of certain neuropsychological defects indicates to the clinical expert that there is dysfunction in a specific brain area. These valid links, however, should not be taken to mean that the functions disturbed by the lesion were inscribed in the tissue that the lesion destroyed. The complex psychological functions, which usually constitute the target of neuropsychological studies in humans, are not localizable at that level.

The neural architectures revealed by neuroanatomy and neurophysiology and the cognitive architectures revealed by experimental neuropsychology suggest that single-center functions, single-purpose pathways, and unidirectional cascades of information process are unrealistic. Moreover, the residual performance that follows focal brain insults, and the ensuing patterns of recovery, suggest that knowledge must be widely distributed, at multiple neural levels, and complex psychological functions must emerge from the cooperation of multiple components of integrated networks.

Two key developments made human lesion studies rewarding again. First, lesion studies in nonhuman primates brought major advances to the understanding of the neural basis of vision and memory, as demonstrated, among others, by Mishkin and colleagues. Second, the advent of CT and MRI began to permit human lesion studies in vivo. It is apparent now that the lesion method is indispensable to cognitive neuroscience, especially when it comes to human studies. The *new* lesion method is not concerned with "localizing functions," nor is it a contest for "localizing lesions." It is a means to test, at systems level, hypotheses regarding *both* neural structure *and* cognitive processes. What investigators from Déjerine to Geschwind gleaned from single cases can now be replicated systematically in a suitable group of subjects. Hypotheses old and new, including some advanced by the pioneer neuropsychologists, can be tested experimentally.

Beyond their intrinsic value, the results from the new lesion method in humans provide a welcome complement to results from neuroanatomic and neurophysiologic experiments in animals. Lesion work in humans has revealed characteristics of neural systems that could not have been investigated in experimental animals. The example of linguistic processes is the most obvious. Lesion results have also been the source of hypotheses that were further investigated in animals and in humans. Ungerleider and Mishkin's study of ventral and dorsal visual pathways in nonhuman primates[1] was inspired by Newcombe's work in humans.[2] Conversely, Ungerleider and Mishkin's work was followed up in humans, and the inferotemporal system has now been anatomically and functionally fractionated.[3–5] Moreover, the lesion method offers the possibility of conducting in-depth experiments on some cognitive operations whose temporal characteristics are not suitable for other approaches (for instance, experiments requiring the monitoring of psychophysiologic variables).

We also see the lesion method as joining forces with two other approaches to the investigation of human brain function: electrophysiologic studies and functional imaging. The first includes the use of event-related potentials, the study of cognitive and behavioral changes induced by electrical stimulation of exposed cerebral cortex, and the direct recording of activity from cerebral cortex. The second involves the imaging of brain activity inferred from the differential emission of radio signals. It encompasses positron emission tomography (PET), single photon emission computed tomography (SPECT), and functional magnetic resonance imaging (fMRI). The combination of results from the lesion method with those from the other approaches will strengthen our conceptualization of the human brain and bring to light discrepancies that require new theorizing and experimentation. Many well-established facts from the lesion method remain the benchmark against which some results of the new dynamic methods must be measured. Moreover, the actual combination of procedures is likely to generate more powerful tools. This will become reality, for instance, with the performance of PET and fMRI studies in patients with focal lesions causing specific cognitive disorders.

The lesion method does have its limitations. Not every anatomic region of the human nervous system can be properly sampled by natural lesions, and the size of the lesions provides a natural limit to the structures the method can probe with confidence. And yet, in its modern incarnation, the approach provides data currently unavailable through other means.

Only a concerted set of approaches from the molecular to the systems levels, in both humans and experimental animals, can eventually provide answers to the questions currently posed in cognitive neuroscience. The lesion method is a key partner in systems-level studies.

THE MODERN PRACTICE OF THE LESION METHOD IN HUMANS

There are at least five prerequisites for the modern practice of the lesion method: first, the availability of fine-grained structural imaging of the living human brain; second, the availability of a reliable method for the anatomic study of lesion probes; third, access to a large pool of subjects with lesions in varied brain sites, so that hypotheses regarding the operation of different systems can be experimentally tested in comparable target subjects and in appropriate controls; fourth, the availability of reliable techniques for various cognitive measurements; and fifth, the guidance of testable hypotheses concerning the neural basis of specific cognitive processes at systems level. In the following pages, we discuss some of these requisites.

Neuroanatomy from Neuroimaging

For many years, we have conceptualized the systematic neuroimaging studies pursued in our laboratory as a means to practice *human neuroanatomy from imaging data,* i.e., a means for detection and description of a lesion and consideration of its placement in the context of the anatomic systems to which it belongs. This purpose, which requires detailed knowledge of human neuroanatomy, is distinguishable from the traditional role of neuroimaging in *clinical neurologic diagnosis,* i.e., the detection of structural alterations and the prediction of its possible neuropathologic basis. The original tool for these studies was the template technique,[6] but we have since developed a new technique for individualized lesion analysis based on the three-dimensional (3D) reconstruction of the human brain from high-resolution MRI.[7] This new technique is known as BRAINVOX. It permits us to identify reliably, in vivo, every major gyrus and sulcus of the human brain; to slice and reslice the human brain in whatever incidence is necessary for anatomic analysis; and to define and measure volumes or surfaces of interest in single cases and across groups. The technique dispenses with charting onto brain templates and permits instead a customized definition of each subject. We will comment on this technique first and complete this section with a review of the template technique.

BRAINVOX

BRAINVOX is a 3D volumetric imaging and analysis system. The software was originally developed to facilitate the 3D display and mapping of acquired human brain lesions using a volume-rendering approach, but it has grown to support a wide range of advanced multimodality neuroanatomic visualization and analysis techniques. Although BRAINVOX was designed for the analysis of high-resolution volumetric MRI, it can be used with CT and PET.

BRAINVOX consists of several interconnected software components: (1) a slice/contour–based tracing module, (2) a multivolume 3D rendering system, (3) a set of general-purpose volume-manipulation tools, (4) a basic volume–data-handling system, (5) a palette editor, and (6) a volumetric object-measurement system.

BRAINVOX allows for explicit definition of volumes bounded by tracings that can be separated from the full MRI volume. The software allows users to define many such volumes simultaneously, slice by slice, taking advantage of common borders, edge tracking, and flexible trace-editing tools. Volume and intersection volume statistics can be computed for all objects defined in this manner. Histograms of volumes and individual slices can be computed.

Lesion Analysis with BRAINVOX

Using the 3D reconstructed brain to determine which anatomic sectors of each hemisphere are damaged obviates the need to adjust the angle in which the MRI sections are obtained to the angle of available template systems. The accuracy of interpretation no longer depends on the "reading" of a template with the transferred lesion but rather on the direct reading from the identified landmarks in the unique brain in question.

The new technique permits a direct identification of gyri and sulci, comparable to what can be achieved at the autopsy table in a postmortem brain after the meninges have been removed. The technique permits the accurate marking of such structures in coronal axial or parasagittal slices, with the advantage that the extension of lesions into the depths of sulci can also be determined (Fig. 2-1).

Other advantages of the new technique are as follows. First, the identification of anatomic structures is based on each individual brain rather than on an idealized "average" brain. The standard landmarks of each area of interest can be localized in the brain of each individual subject rather than on a template. Although templates use anatomic constants, they cannot account for individual variation and thus introduce an error of measurement, albeit small in some cases. Second, because each area of interest has been customized for each subject, it is possible to determine with

---

Figure 2-1

Three-dimensional reconstruction (obtained from 124 contiguous thin coronal MRI slices) of the brain of a subject with an infarct in the left frontal lobe. Acutely, the subject had a nonfluent aphasia and mild paresis of the right face and arm. At the time of the MRI (1 year later), both language deficit and paresis had improved.

Several sulci were identified and color-coded on the 3D reconstructed brain: central sulcus (red), precentral sulcus (green), inferior frontal sulcus (yellow), superior frontal sulcus (brown), and sylvian fissure (magenta).

Inspection of the left lateral and top views of the brain shows that the area of infarct is centered on the precentral sulcus, which is clearly visible only in the top view. The most anterior sector of the precentral gyrus is damaged, as well as the posterior sector of the middle frontal and inferior frontal gyrus.

The brain volume was also resectioned in axial (ax), coronal (co), and parasagittal (ps) slices (as shown in the three rows of brain slices in the lower segment of the image). Whenever any of the slices intersected a color-coded sulcus, the color automatically appeared on the slice, thus permitting an accurate identification of sulci and of gyri. Resectioning allowed us to inspect the lesion in depth and show that it extended all the way to the insula, which is compromised in its most superior sector (best seen in slice ps-3).

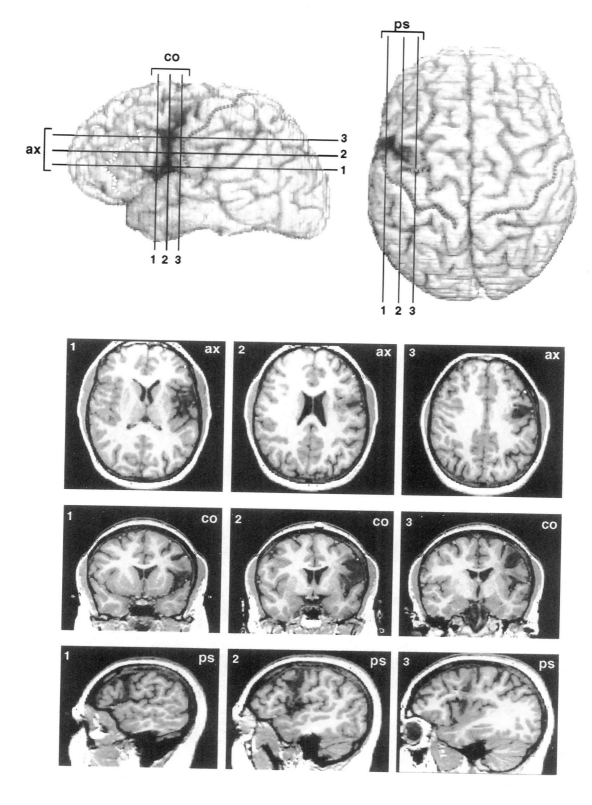

considerable rigor the proportion of a given area that has been destroyed by a lesion as well as the proportion of subjacent white matter that has been involved by the lesion (Fig. 2-2). Again, error is reduced.

This new technique requires a T_1-weighted MRI scan with contiguous thin slices (1.5 mm). For best results, the scan should be performed in the chronic stage. Regular MRI scans obtained for diagnostic purposes with thicker slices, interslice

Figure 2-2
Three-dimensional reconstruction of a human brain with a lesion in the left frontal lobe. The questions addressed here concerned the size of the lesion and the percentage of volume it occupied in the whole brain, in the left frontal lobe (LFL), and in some subdivisions of the frontal lobe: the pars triangularis (pars triang.) and the pars opercularis (pars operc.), the posterior half of the middle frontal gyrus (post. MFG), and the precentral gyrus in its inferior (inf. preCG) and middle thirds (mid. preCG). The limits of all of these regions of interest (ROI) were marked on the 3D reconstructed brain. On all coronal slices, the several ROIs are individually traced, as is the contour of the lesion. Six coronal slices are shown as an example. The different ROIs are color- and texture-coded. The automatically calculated absolute volumes and the percentage of damage in each of them are recorded on the top right-hand corner.

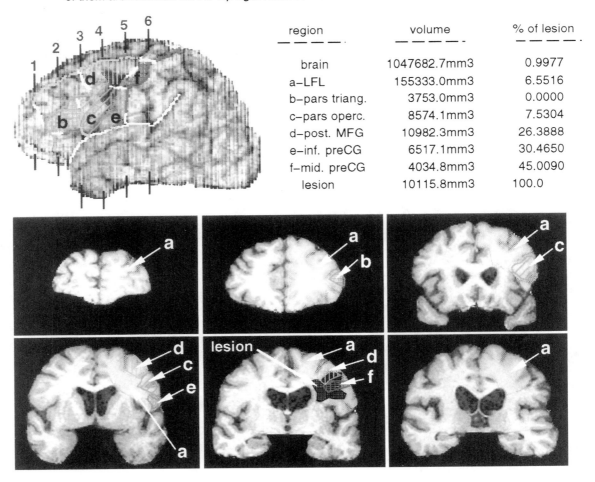

region	volume	% of lesion
brain	1047682.7mm3	0.9977
a–LFL	155333.0mm3	6.5516
b–pars triang.	3753.0mm3	0.0000
c–pars operc.	8574.1mm3	7.5304
d–post. MFG	10982.3mm3	26.3888
e–inf. preCG	6517.1mm3	30.4650
f–mid. preCG	4034.8mm3	45.0090
lesion	10115.8mm3	100.0

gaps, and other pulse specifications are not adequate for reconstruction. Furthermore, application of this elaborate procedure to acute lesions would be a waste of effort.

The Template Technique

Whenever MRI or CT scans are obtained with regular parameters (thick slices, and, in the case of MRI, interslice gaps), anatomic analyses must rely on the template technique.

The template technique relies on film transparencies of MRI or CT. For research purposes, it is advisable to have a technician collect all the films for a given case, mask the subject identification in all of them, and substitute a numerical entry code on the basis of which imaging data can be stored. This step ensures that the investigator performing the anatomic study is blind to the neurologic and neuropsychological data available for the same subject.

As with the previous technique, detailed knowledge of human neuroanatomy is indispensable. Needless to say, the investigator must be conversant with the imaging techniques themselves. The template technique relies on the availability of brain templates of the normal brain such as those published by us in 1989 and 1995. The key steps are as follows:

1. Determine the angle of incidence in which CT or MRI were obtained. This can be achieved on the basis of a pilot scan or by inspection of the lower axial slices in which the relative positions of structures in the three main cranial fossae can be observed.

2. On the basis of the above determination, select the set of templates that best fits the subject's films.

3. Chart the lesion on the templates at every level at which it occurs, using an X/Y plotting strategy.

4. Superimpose over the template an appropriate "in register" transparency that contains anatomic cells representing neural "areas of interest" in both gray and white matter structures. Each of those cells is limited by a linear boundary

and has a letter and number code on the basis of which it can be anatomically identified.

5. Assign the area of damage charted in the template to the cells that encompass the abnormal images.

6. Assign the estimation of the amount of involvement within target cells. We usually code this 0 when there is less than 25 percent involvement of the total, 1 if the involvement is between 25 and 75 percent; and 2 if more than 75 percent of the total area is damaged. This step can be achieved in two ways: (a) using a transparent square grid and counting the number of units involved by the lesion at each level, then calculating the percentage in relation to the total number of units encompassed by each area of interest (which is the sum of units occupied by the region at each template level); or (b) transferring the template system into computer software, tracing the lesion's limits as marked on the template with a digitizer, and then using automated determination of the percentage of area involved.

The number of cuts in the scan and in the correctly chosen set of templates may not coincide for two reasons: varied thickness of cuts and variations in individual brain size. Therefore, the investigator must search for the most appropriate scan/template matches, on a cut-by-cut basis, using all available anatomic constants—for example, ventricular system and prominent sulci. Fortunately, current MRI resolution provides such a wealth of landmarks that finding appropriate correspondences is no longer a daunting task. Correspondences are a necessary complement to the X/Y plotting approach. The results of X/Y plotting should be counterchecked by inspection of identifiable landmarks, since "blind" plotting may produce an inaccurate chart. This is why we do not advocate the use of fully automated lesion analysis with the template technique.

The major source of error in the template technique is the choice of the wrong template set. The key to the correct choice of templates is the inspection of *all* available brain cuts, especially the lower ones, which contain crucial landmarks for the determination of the incidence of a particular scan. In practical terms, it is necessary to compare the proportion of frontal lobe, temporal lobe, and posterior fossa structures shown in the scan with those seen in the various template sets and to select the best match. It is not possible to find the right match based on the inspection of high cuts alone, because in high-lying cuts, the cues from anatomic constraints such as the ventricular system or bony landmarks are lost.

Improved Template Technique

The availability of BRAINVOX and of 3D reconstructed normal brains has allowed us to improve the template technique. It is now possible to create "customized templates" for any set of CT or MRI slices. Instead of using published templates, a 3D reconstructed normal brain can be resliced so as to match the incidence of cut and the level of slices in the CT or MR images to be analyzed (Fig. 2-3). The key steps are as follows:

1. All major sulci are identified and color-coded in the 3D reconstructed normal brain.

2. The normal brain is resliced on the computer screen so as to match the slice orientation and thickness of the 2D images of the brain to be analyzed, creating an equal number of brain slices (the "customized template set"). The color codes generated in (1) are automatically transferred onto the single brain slices.

3. On each matched pair of normal/abnormal brain slices, the lesion is transferred in much the same manner as described for the basic template technique.

4. The result is a 3D transfer of the lesion, which can then be "read off" the normal 3D reconstructed brain.

Analysis of Groups of Subjects

Whenever a study involves a large number of subjects, it may be advantageous to create maps of lesion overlap. For this purpose we have developed a technique that permits the determination of the region of maximal overlap in terms of brain surface ("Map-2," a 2D map), or in volumetric terms ("Map-3," a 3D map). Each of these techniques entails the transfer of all individual lesions onto a normal reference brain.

For Map-2, the steps are as follows:

1. For each case, each view of the 3D brain showing the lesion is matched with the corresponding view of the normal reference brain, in terms of spatial coordinates.

2. The surface contour of the lesion is transferred from the subject's brain and fitted onto the normal reference brain, taking into account its relation to sulcal and gyral landmarks.

3. The lesions are then superimposed to form a surface map. A region of maximal lesion overlap is determined on the basis of the superimpositions and assigned a numerical weight based on the number of contributing lesions.

To obtain a Map-3, we transfer and fit the limits of all the target lesions onto the normal reference brain reconstructed in 3D (by transferring the contour of each lesion as seen in each slice into the corresponding slices of the reference brain in the way described above). The sum total of lesion contours for each case constitutes a 3D object. Given the collection of such objects, we then determine the intersection of their volumes in whatever plane we prefer. This allows us to determine overlap in both cortical "surface" and white matter "depth." We refer to the area of maximal overlap as the "center of volume."

Identifying Lesions with Computed Tomography and Magnetic Resonance Imaging

The identification of neuropathologic changes using CT depends on the detection, within a given brain region, of an x-ray absorption that departs from the norm. The presence of cerebral infarction, edema, or tumor at a specified anatomic location alters the standard x-ray absorption for that region and produces an abnormal image.

In the case of MRI, the identification of neuropathologic changes depends on the production of a locally different rate of hydrogen proton spinning, within the affected brain region, after the brain is exposed to a magnetic field. In other

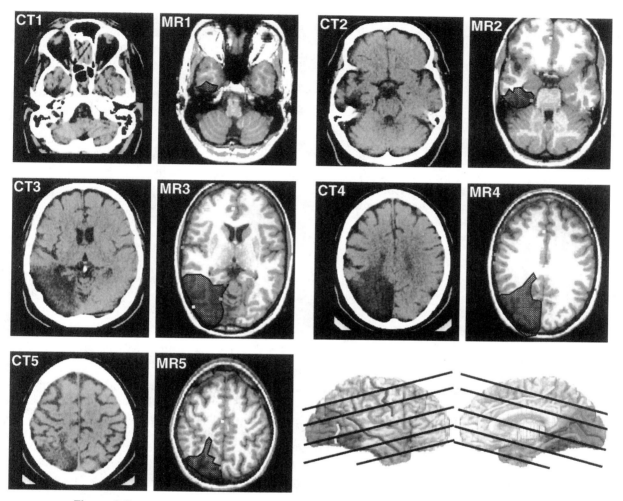

Figure 2-3

Demonstration of the improved template method. Brain CT (CT 1-5) of a subject who could not undergo an MRI study. A normal 3D reconstructed brain was resliced so as to match the orientation and level of the CT slices (MR 1-5). The lesion seen on the CT slices was transferred onto each matched MR slice, taking into account all identifiable sulci and gyri. Once the sulci were color-coded on the 3D reconstruction, the lesion could be read off each individual slice. The object defined by the transferred traces could be fused with the normal brain to visualize the lesion's surface extent (right lower corner).

words, after the brain is subjected to a magnetic field, with varied magnetic pulse sequence parameters, the presence of a pathologic brain region due to edema, infarction, or tumor will determine hydrogen proton spinning rates within the area that are different from what normally would be

expected for the given anatomic structure subjected to the same magnetic pulse sequence. Lesion-detection sensitivity with either method varies according to the specific procedure, the nature of the pathology, the stage at which the imaging measurement is made in relation to the onset of the pathologic process, and the quality of the equipment and proficiency of the technique.

The potential for false negatives or false positives is considerable, their magnitude depending on the factors listed above. For example, CT is often negative in the first 24 h following an infarct but is usually positive in the days after. However, in the second and third weeks after an infarct, because the infarcted tissue absorbs x-rays at the same rate as normal tissue, the CT may become negative again if not performed after the injection of a contrast-enhancing substance. Contrast seeps out of damaged vessels in the damaged region and increases the density of the area.

Neuroanatomic Resolution

The limits of resolution in the lesion method are set by the state of the technology. Current-generation CT and MRI scanners detect lesions as small as 1 mm on the plane of section. From the perspective of microstructure, these seemingly astounding resolutions are actually modest, since such small areas contain so many neurons and connections. Nonetheless, from the perspective of cytoarchitecture or of cortical regions defined neurophysiologically, this resolution is quite respectable. In short, current imaging technology visualizes neural structure at a level that permits the neuroanatomic definition of most lesions resulting from acquired neurologic disease or neurosurgical ablations.

Neither CT nor MRI can detect discrete cellular pathology except when a fairly large cortical region or subcortical nucleus is affected over a sizable surface or volume that turns out to be, in the aggregate, larger than the lower limit of resolution discussed above. This is why, in the early stages of degenerative dementia of either the Alzheimer or Pick types, when neuropsychological assessment already reveals marked cerebral dysfunction, CT and MRI studies may be so deceptively normal. At the same stage, however, dynamic neuroimaging using emission tomography procedures, of either the SPECT or PET types, may show changes in cerebral blood flow or metabolism.

Decreased radio signal in posterior temporal and temporoparietal regions is quite characteristic of Alzheimer's dementia.[8-11] This is probably the consequence of both local pathologic changes and local physiologic changes brought about by anterior temporal lesions.

In moderate to advanced stages of Alzheimer's disease, CT and MRI often show fairly widespread cerebral atrophy or ventricular enlargement. In addition, MRI studies may also show a reduction in the volume of medial temporal structures, the result of accumulated damage in entorhinal and perirhinal cortices, and subsequent degeneration in hippocampus.[12,13]

In Pick's disease, autopsy studies have shown repeatedly that the characteristic pathology is especially evident in the frontal and anterior temporal cortices,[14] and in moderate to advanced cases, anatomic analysis of CT or MRI of patients with progressive dementia does reveal severe atrophy localized to those regions.[15]

The Choice of Neuropathologic Specimens

The choice of pathologic specimen is a major technical consideration in the lesion method, given that the neuropathologic characteristics of infarctions, intraparenchymal hemorrhages, or varied types of tumor are entirely different.

Nonhemorrhagic infarctions provide the best specimens for neuroanatomic investigation and correlation with neuropsychological findings, because cerebral infarctions actually destroy brain parenchyma. The infarcted area is eventually replaced by scar tissue and by cerebrospinal fluid, and CT or MRI in the chronic state provide a clear demarcation of the infarct. In CT, the damage is depicted as an area of decreased density, seen as a darker area in the gray scale that accompanies the images. In MRI, infarctions show as a dark area in T_1-weighted images and a white bright signal region in T_2-weighted images.

Herpes simplex encephalitis provides comparable anatomic detail. In adults, the virus has an affinity for a limited set of brain structures, mostly within the limbic system, and it destroys those areas rather completely by a mechanism that includes vascular collapse. In the chronic state, both CT and MRI produce extremely accurate images of the involved territories.

In most other varieties of neuropathologic process, the precise anatomic definition of lesions is less accurate and the functional impact of the lesion itself is less well defined. For instance, earlier in their growth, *gliomas* infiltrate brain tissue by dislocating local populations of neurons but may not destroy them immediately. Moreover, the region of low or high density seen on the CT or MRI of such tumors corresponds not just to the tumor tissue but also to edema surrounding it and to brain tissue that may still be functionally competent. In other words, in such cases it may be impossible to decide that the brain parenchyma is destroyed or that the area is functionally inoperative, or, for that matter, that an area without apparent abnormality is free of tumor. For these reasons, we do not believe that patients with glial tumors are a first choice for the lesion method. This point is made clear in a study by Anderson and coworkers,[16] who compared the neuropsychological profile of patients with confirmed gliomas to that of patients with strokes in the same regions.

Where subjects with glial tumors pose problems for the lesion method, those in whom *meningiomas* have been excised and who have had a circumscribed ablation of brain tissue are actually ideal cases. The images from such cases are entirely appropriate to establish a link between the anatomic site of the ablation and the neuropsychological profile obtained *after* the ablation has taken place.

Patients who have had ablations for seizure treatment also afford a good opportunity for behavioral and anatomic studies. In those cases, MRI obtained with T_1-weighted images can help delineate the extent of brain tissue removal with extraordinary precision, although some caution is recommended in the interpretation of neuropsychological data obtained in such patients. Some patients who undergo surgical removal of brain tissue for the treatment of uncontrollable seizures may have developmental brain defects. Those whose seizures began early in life are likely to have had some degree of compensatory brain re-

organization before surgery. Frequent and longstanding seizural discharges may also produce changes elsewhere in the brain. The participation of such patients in lesion studies must be evaluated on an individual basis.

The inclusion in lesion method studies of subjects with *metastatic disease, intracerebral hemorrhages,* or *severe head injury* must also be decided on an individual basis, lest it contaminate otherwise valid results. For instance, data from patients with a single brain metastasis, removed surgically, and studied in the stable, postoperative state, concomitantly with a good-quality CT or MRI, are quite acceptable.

Intracerebral hemorrhages affect the brain by two different mechanisms. They destroy neural tissue, as nonhemorrhagic infarctions do, and they cause a space-occupying blood collection that displaces neurons, as tumors do. During the acute phase of a hemorrhage, neither CT nor MRI provides an accurate picture of the abnormality, because within the area of abnormal signal some neurons are truly destroyed, whereas others are simply displaced. The amount and location of tissue destruction can be estimated only after the resolution of the hematoma.

In conclusion, the specimen of choice for the purpose of establishing correlates between dysfunction and site of brain destruction are cases of nonhemorrhagic infarction and herpes encephalitis. Surgical ablations performed for the treatment of meningiomas also provide excellent material. Other material should be used on an individual basis, after careful assessment of the dynamics of lesion development.

Timing of Imaging

The timing of CT and MRI data collection is of the essence, especially in relation to subjects with stroke. Both CT and MRI may fail to show *any* abnormality when they are obtained immediately after the occurrence of a stroke. With modern-generation CT and MRI scanners, most images will be positive after 24 h. This is certainly not the case with older scanners, however. It is important to keep in mind that many CT (or even MRI) studies obtained less than 24 h after the onset of a stroke may be negative, especially when a patient with an acute stroke happens to have a CT or MRI that shows a well-demarcated area of low density with sharp margins. Such an image, early after stroke, should suggest a previous infarct, probably unrelated to the new set of symptoms.

Positive CT images obtained in the first week post onset usually show areas of abnormality that are far larger than the region of actual structural damage because of confounding phenomena—for example, edema. This commonly occurs and means that the results of observations and experiments conducted at later epochs should not be correlated with the anatomic analysis performed in the acute images.

When CT is obtained in the second or third week after a stroke's onset without intravenous infusion of a contrast-enhancing substance, the images are negative in a good number of cases. The image can change even after a previous CT obtained earlier showed a large area of decreased density. During this period, the damaged area can show the same density as the normal tissue. On the other hand, in contrast-enhanced CT images, those normal-looking areas will appear as areas of increased density (primarily due to seepage of contrast substance through the walls of newly formed vessels in the affected region). In the chronic stage, which we define as 3 months post onset and beyond, most CT studies of infarction are unequivocally positive. Even then, however, when strokes are small and located close to a major sulcus or to the wall of a ventricle, the chronic CT may mislead the observer, resembling images of focal "atrophy" with sulcal enlargement or images of ventricular dilatation. When no previous images are available for comparison with those obtained in the chronic stage, the correct interpretation and the establishment of an adequate behavioral/anatomic correlation may not be possible.

Similar problems befall MRI with images obtained with only one pulse sequence. T_1-weighted images obtained with an inversion recovery (IR) pulse sequence provide maximal anatomic detail. With this pulse sequence, however, infarctions appear as dark areas, in precisely the same range of grays used to depict the ventricular system or any region filled with cerebrospinal fluid, such as the cerebral sulci and fissures. When infarcts are small and close to one of these structures, they may not be readily distinguishable. Images obtained with different pulse sequences on MRI (proton density or T_2-weighted) show the damaged area as a region of intense bright signal, more easily distinguishable from the bright signals generated by white and even gray matter.

A meaningful relation between an anatomic image and a particular neuropsychological pattern require reasonable temporal closeness between the epochs at which the image and the neuropsychological data were obtained. Because, during the acute period, edema and brain distortion often occur, it is not easy to define precisely the location and amount of destroyed tissue. The pairing of such images with observations made in the chronic state may lead to error. Likewise for the inverse situation—that is, pairing the results of acute neuropsychological observations obtained in the acute state with the anatomy gleaned during the chronic stage. The most reliable anatomic and neuropsychological data are obviously those obtained in the chronic stage.

Other Considerations

A traditional limitation of the lesion method in humans has been the excessive reliance on single cases. Many of the important observations made in the past were uncontrolled and went unreplicated, the significance of the results being thus diminished. Notable exceptions—for instance, Milner's collection of epileptic patients with surgical ablations in temporal and frontal lobe, Newcombe's head injury project, or Gazzaniga's group of epileptics with split brain interventions—simply confirm the rule. In our laboratory, we have obviated this limitation by creating a continuously renewed population of patients with lesions in varied neural systems who would be willing to participate in neuropsychological experiments. The goal was to conduct multiple single-subject studies in target patients and in controls with an approach as rigorous as the one used in the traditional experimental setting and to make it possible to design and carry out experiments in which certain hypotheses regarding anatomy and function could be probed comprehensively, using many individual data sets.

It goes without saying that, given optimal neuroanatomic analysis, the lesion method will be only as successful as the quality of the cognitive tasks used in the experiments and the quality of the theoretical framework and hypotheses being tested. The rapidly evolving fields of cognitive science and experimental neuropsychology have provided investigators with many useful tasks applicable to most aspects of cognition and behavior likely to be studied with the lesion method. There are also many relevant theoretical developments concerning the conceptualization of both the cognitive and neural architectures in humans. The traditional divisions between behaviorist and cognitivist views seem to have been largely overcome by theoretical positions that combine the best of both (see, for examples, Refs. 17 to 19). The conceptualization of neural structures and of their operations, insofar as mental processes and behaviors are concerned, has also changed radically, as indicated at the beginning of this chapter. Neural signaling is seen as both massively parallel and massively sequential, and, no less importantly, massively recurrent. The prevalence of feedforward and feedback loops disposed along as well as across neural streams has been duly noted, and so has the convergent/divergent nature of those neuron streams. The dependence on timing mechanisms for the normal operations of these networks is well accepted.[20–24]

REFERENCES

1. Ungerleider LG, Mishkin M: Two cortical visual systems, in Ingle DJ, Mansfield RJW, Goodale MA (eds): *The Analysis of Visual Behavior.* Cambridge, MA: MIT Press, 1982.

2. Newcombe F, Russell WR: Dissociate visual, perceptual and spatial deficits in focal lesions of the right hemisphere. *J Neurol Neurosurg Psychiatry* 332:73–81, 1969.

3. Damasio A, Tranel D, Damasio H: Face agnosia and the neural substrates of memory. *Annu Rev Neurosci* 13:89–109, 1990.

4. Damasio AR, Damasio H, Tranel D, Brandt JP: Neural regionalization of knowledge access: Preliminary evidence. *Symposia on Quantitative Biology* 55:1039–1047, 1990.

5. Tranel D, Damasio H, Damasio AR, Brandt JP: Separate concepts are retrieved from separate neural systems: Neuroanatomical and neuropsychological double dissociations (abstr). *Soc Neurosci* 21:1497, 1995.

6. Damasio H, Damasio A: *Lesion Analysis in Neuropsychology.* New York, Oxford University Press, 1989; Japanese edition, Tokyo: Igaku-Shoin, 1992.

7. Damasio H: *Human Brain Anatomy in Computerized Images.* New York: Oxford University Press, 1995.

8. Chase TN, Foster NL, Fedio P, et al: Regional cortical dysfunction in Alzheimer's disease as determined by positron emission tomography. *Ann Neurol* 15(suppl):S170–S174, 1984.

9. Foster NL, Chase TN, Mansi L, et al: Cortical abnormalities in Alzheimer's disease. *Ann Neurol* 16:649–654, 1984.

10. Friedland RP, Budinger TF, Ganz E, et al: Regional cerebral metabolic alterations in dementia of the Alzheimer type: Positron emission tomography with (18F) Fluorodeaxyglucose. *J Comp Assist Tomogr* 7:590–598, 1983.

11. Rezai K, Damasio H, Graff-Radford N, et al: Regional cerebral blood flow abnormalities in Alzheimer's disease. *J Nucl Med* 26(5):105, 1985.

12. Hyman BT, Damasio AR, Van Hoesen GW, Barnes CL: Cell specific pathology isolates the hippocampal formation in Alzheimer's disease. *Science* 225:1168–1170, 1984.

13. Van Hoesen, Damasio A: Neural correlates of the cognitive impairment in Alzheimer's disease, in Plum F (ed): *The Handbook of Physiology.* Bethesda, MD: American Physiological Society, 1987, pp 871–898.

14. Escourelle R, Poirier J: *Manual of Basic Neuropathology.* Philadelphia: Saunders, 1978.

15. Graff-Radford NR, Damasio AR, Hyman BT, et al: Progressive aphasia in a patient with Pick's disease: A neuropsychological, radiologic and anatomic study. *Neurology* 40:620–626, 1990.

16. Anderson SW, Damasio H, Tranel D: The use of tumor and stroke patients in neuropsychological

research: A methodological critique. *J Clin Exp Neuropsychol* 10:32, 1988.

17. Kosslyn SM: *Image and Brain: The Resolution of the Imagery Debate.* Cambridge, MA: Bradford Books/MIT Press, 1994.

18. Damasio AR: *Descartes' Error: Emotion, Reason and the Human Brain.* New York: Grosset/Putnam, 1994.

19. Churchland PS, Sejnowski JF: *The Computational Brain: Models and Methods on the Frontiers of Computational Neuroscience.* Cambridge, MA: Bradford Books/MIT Press, 1992.

20. Damasio AR: The brain binds entities and events by multiregional activation from convergence zones. *Neural Comput* 1:123–132, 1989.

21. Damasio AR, Damasio H: Cortical systems for retrieval of concrete knowledge: The convergence zone framework, in Koch C (ed): *Large-Scale Neuronal Theories of the Brain.* Cambridge, MA: MIT Press, 1994, pp 61–74.

22. Crick F: *The Astonishing Hypothesis: The Scientific Search for the Soul.* New York: Scribner's, 1994.

23. Edelman G: *Neural Darwinism.* New York: Basic Books, 1987.

24. Rockland KS (ed): Special issue: Local cortical circuits. *Cerebral Cortex* 3:361–498, 1993.

Chapter 3

FUNCTIONAL IMAGING IN COGNITIVE NEUROSCIENCE

Marcus E. Raichle

Early discussions of the "mind-brain problem" treated the brain largely as a "black box." Then, in 1861, French surgeon and anthropologist Pierre Paul Broca described a clear relationship between a patient's difficulty speaking and an injury to a specific part of the patient's brain due to a stroke. Since this seminal observation, a vast body of scientific literature has accumulated implicating various parts of the human brain in specific aspects of human behavior, including language. The remarkable level of sophistication to which this work has risen is detailed in the preceding chapter by Drs. Antonio and Hanna Damasio.

The features of brain organization arising from the study of patients with brain injury nevertheless raise some questions of interpretation. The size and location of brain injury varies greatly from patient to patient, making a precise correlation between damage to a particular area of the brain and the function normally served by that area sometimes difficult to determine. Furthermore, each patient may be assumed to have some features of brain organization that are unique to him or her. Finally, it remains uncertain whether one can simply attribute a lost or disrupted function to a particular area of injury. Because of the interconnected nature of areas of the brain, injury in one area is likely to have effects on other areas that cannot necessarily be predicted from the location and size of the injury itself. Thus, as valuable as our insights concerning the organization of the human brain have been, from the study of patients with stroke and other types of brain in-

jury, it has remained an open question exactly how this information relates to the normal organization of the human brain.

Only recently have scientists interested in this question had the opportunity to explore it analytically—to peer inside the black box as it functions normally. This ability stems from the developments in imaging technology over the past 20 years, most notably positron emission tomography (PET) and magnetic resonance imaging (MRI). These techniques can now capture precisely localized physiologic changes in the normal human brain associated with behaviorally induced changes in neuronal activity.[1,2]

It is important to point out that the underlying assumptions of current brain-mapping studies with PET and functional MRI (fMRI) are not a modern version of phrenology. The phrenologists of the past century posited that single areas of the brain, often identified by bumps on the skull, uniquely represented specific thought processes and emotions. In contrast, modern thinking posits that single areas of the brain each contribute quite simple mental operations that form the elementary components of the observable behaviors. Observable behaviors and thought processes emerge through the cooperative interactions of many such areas. So, just as diverse instruments of a large orchestra are played in a coordinated fashion to produce a symphony, a group of diverse brain areas, each performing quite elementary and unique mental operations, work together in a coordinated fashion to produce human behavior. The prerequisite for such analyses is the conviction that complex behaviors can be broken down into sets of constituent mental operations.

HISTORY OF FUNCTIONAL BRAIN IMAGING

The modern era of medical imaging began in the early 1970s, when the world was introduced to a remarkable technique called x-ray computed tomography, now known as x-ray CT or just CT. South African physicist Allan M. Cormack and British engineer Sir Godfrey Hounsfield independently developed its principles. Hounsfield constructed the first CT instrument in England. Both investigators received the Nobel prize in 1979 for their contributions.

Computed tomography takes advantage of the fact that different tissues absorb varying amounts of x-ray energy. The denser the tissue, the more it absorbs. A highly focused beam of x-rays traversing the body will exit at a reduced energy level depending on the tissues and organs through which it passes. A beam of x-rays passed through the body at many different angles through a plane collects sufficient information to reconstruct a picture of that body section. It was crucial to the development of CT that clever computing and mathematical techniques emerged for processing the vast amount of information necessary to create the images themselves. Without the availability of sophisticated computers, the task would have been impossible to accomplish.

Computed tomography had two consequences. First, it changed the practice of medicine forever, because it was much superior to standard x-rays. For the first time, physicians could safely and effectively view living human tissue such as the brain with no discomfort or risk to the patient. Standard x-rays revealed only bone and some surrounding soft tissue. Second, CT immediately stimulated scientists and engineers to consider alternative ways of creating images of the body's interior using similar mathematical and computer strategies for image construction. These efforts went beyond the picture of human anatomy provided by CT to focus on function.

One of the first groups to be intrigued by the possibilities opened by CT consisted of experts in tissue autoradiography, a method used for many years in animal studies to investigate organ metabolism, biochemistry, and blood flow. In tissue autoradiography, a radioactively labeled compound is injected into a vein. After the compound has accumulated in the organ under investigation, the animal is sacrificed and the organ (e.g., the brain) removed for study. The organ is then carefully sectioned, and the individual slices are laid on a piece of film sensitive to radioactivity. Much as the film in a camera records a scene as it was originally viewed, this x-ray film records the distribution of radioactively labeled compound in each slice of tissue.

When the x-ray film is developed, scientists have a picture of the distribution of radioactivity within the organ and hence can deduce the organ's specific functions. The type of information is determined by the radioactive compound injected. A radioactively labeled form of glucose, for example, measures brain metabolism, because glucose is the primary source of energy for the cells of the brain. Central to functional brain imaging with PET is the measurement of brain blood flow, which is accomplished by the injection of radioactively labeled water.

Investigators adept at tissue autoradiography were fascinated when CT was introduced. They suddenly realized that if they could reconstruct the anatomy of an organ by passing an x-ray beam through it, as CT did, they could also safely reconstruct the distribution of a previously administered radioisotope. One had simply to measure the emission of radioactivity from the body section. This realization was the birth of autoradiography of living human subjects.

One crucial element in the evolution of human autoradiography was the choice of radioisotope. Workers in the field selected a class of radioisotopes that emit positrons, which resemble electrons except that they carry a positive charge. A positron produced within the tissue almost immediately combines with a nearby electron. The positron and electron annihilate one another in this interaction, emitting two high-energy gamma rays in the process. Since the gamma rays travel in nearly opposite directions, radiation detection devices arrayed in a circle around the organ of interest can detect the pairs of gamma rays and, with the aid of computers, locate their origin with remarkable precision. The crucial role of positrons in human autoradiography gave rise to the name positron emission tomography (PET).

More recently, another imaging technique has emerged and taken its place alongside PET in revealing the function of the human brain. This technique, MRI, derives from the potent laboratory technique known as nuclear magnetic resonance (NMR), which was designed to explore detailed chemical features of molecules. It garnered a Nobel prize for its developers, Felix Bloch of Stanford University and Edward Purcell of Harvard University, in 1972. The method depends on the fact that many atoms behave as little compass needles in the presence of a magnetic field. By skillfully manipulating the magnetic field, scientists can align the atoms. Applying radio-wave pulses to the sample under these conditions briefly perturbs the atoms from their aligned state in a precise manner. As a result, they emit detectable radio signals unique to the number and state of the particular atoms in the sample. Careful adjustments of the magnetic field and the radio-wave pulses yield particular information about the sample under study.

Nuclear magnetic resonance moved from the laboratory to the clinic when Paul C. Lauterbur of the University of Illinois found that NMR can form images by detecting protons. Protons are useful because they are abundant in the human body, being found primarily in water and fat. Using mathematical techniques again borrowed initially from x-ray CT but later modified extensively, images of the anatomy of organs of the living human body were produced that far surpassed in detail those produced by CT. Because the term *nuclear* made the procedure sound dangerous to some, NMR soon became known as magnetic resonance imaging. The current excitement over both PET and functional MRI (fMRI) for the imaging of normal brain function stems from the ability of these techniques to detect signals related to changes in neuronal activity through changes in local brain blood flow. Below, we turn briefly to the nature of these changes in blood flow and their relationship to changes in neuronal activity.

MEASURING BRAIN FUNCTION WITH IMAGING

Measurements of blood flow to local areas of the brain are at the heart of assessing brain function with either PET or fMRI.[2] The idea that blood flow is intimately related to brain function is a surprisingly old one. English physiologists Charles S. Roy and Charles S. Sherrington formally presented the idea in a publication in 1890 (for a detailed review of this history, see Refs. 2 and 3). They suggested that an "automatic mechanism" regulated the blood supply to the brain. The amount of blood depended on local variations in activity. Although subsequent experiments have amply confirmed the existence of such an automatic mechanism, no one is yet entirely certain about its exact nature. It obviously remains a challenging area for research.

Positron emission tomography measures blood flow in the human brain by adapting an autoradiographic technique for laboratory animals developed in the late 1940s by Seymour S. Kety of the National Institute of Mental Health and his colleagues (for a detailed review, see Ref. 3). Positron emission tomography relies on radioactively labeled water, specifically hydrogen combined with oxygen-15, a radioactive isotope of oxygen. The labeled water, which emits copious numbers of positrons as it decays, is administered into a vein in the arm. In less than a minute thereafter, the radioactivity accumulates in the brain, forming an image of blood flow.

Functional MRI measures a complex function of blood flow related to the fact that when blood flow increases during normal brain function, the amount of oxygen consumed by the brain does not.[3a] Under these circumstances, more oxygen is present locally in the tissue because the blood flow (i.e., supply) has increased but the demand for oxygen has not. Since the amount of oxygen in the tissue affects its magnetic properties, a fact first noted in 1935 by Linus Pauling,[4] fMRI can detect a change, which is often referred to as the "BOLD" or blood oxygen level-dependent effect.[5-7] An actual measurement of blood flow equivalent to that measured by PET with oxygen-15–labeled water has proven difficult with fMRI primarily because of the short "half-life" (i.e., the T_1 relaxation time) of the water protons in the fMRI experiment (i.e., the T_1 relaxation time of the water proton in brain tissue is approximately 1 s, whereas the half-life of oxygen-15–labeled water is 123 s, which is ideal for the measurement of blood flow in the human brain).

IMAGING STRATEGY

A distinct strategy for the functional mapping of neuronal activity has emerged during the past 15 years. Initially developed for PET, it has been extended, with modifications which will be discussed a bit further on, to fMRI.

This approach extends an idea first introduced to psychology in 1868 by Dutch physiologist Franciscus C. Donders. Donders proposed a general method to measure thought processes based on a simple logic. He subtracted the time needed to respond to a light (say, by pressing a key) from the time needed to respond to a particular color of light. He found that discriminating color required about 50 ms. In this way, Donders isolated and measured a mental process for the first time by subtracting a *control state* (i.e., responding to light) from a *task state* of interest (i.e., discriminating the color of the light).

The current functional imaging strategy is designed to accomplish a similar subtraction, but adding information about the areas of the brain that distinguish the task state from the control state. In particular, images of blood flow, or blood flow–related changes in the case of fMRI (i.e., the BOLD signal; see above), taken in a control state are subtracted from those obtained when the brain is engaged in the task. Scientists carefully choose the control state and the task state so as to isolate as well as possible a limited number of mental operations when subtracting the two states. Subtracting blood flow–dependent measurements made in the control state from those made in the task state should isolate those parts of the brain uniquely responsible for the performance of the task.

To obtain reliable data, scientists take the average of responses across many individual subjects (usually the case with PET) or of many experimental trials in the same person (usually the case with fMRI). Averaging enables researchers to detect changes in blood flow associated with mental activity that would otherwise easily be confused with spurious shifts resulting from statistical noise in the resulting images. The averaging of results across individuals has another important feature in that it gives us the opportunity to learn what features of brain organization we share. Knowledge of such common principles of brain organization is an essential basis for an understanding of the unique and universal capacity of humans for language, for example. The image subtraction and averaging strategy used for PET is illustrated in Fig. 3-1. A typical imaging paradigm used for fMRI is illustrated in Fig. 3-2.

The remainder of this review focuses on studies of language, largely from the author's own laboratory, for several reasons: (1) the work nicely illustrates the implementation of the strategies described above; (2) the work reflects substantial input from both cognitive scientists and neuroscientists; (3) results are promising in relation to cognitive theories of brain function, and (4) important lessons have been learned about how best to conduct functional imaging research and what conclusions to draw from the results of these studies. The following discussion is not intended as a review of functional imaging studies of language but, rather, as a review of functional brain imaging strategies as employed in laboratories throughout the world, using our studies of language for illustrative purposes only. For those interested in a more in-depth review of human cognition and functional brain imaging, a recently published book is recommended.[2]

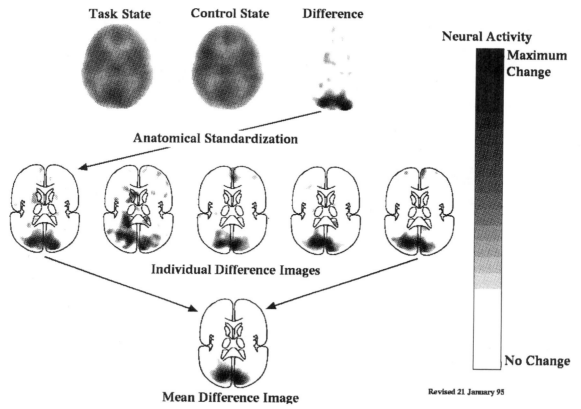

Figure 3-1

Image subtraction and image averaging are crucial steps in the development of PET images of brain function. In the top row are two PET blood-flow images in a normal human subject, one labeled Task State *and the other labeled* Control State. *These images represent horizontal slices throughout the center of the brain. In each image, the front of the brain is on top and the left side is to the reader's left. Areas that are darker have higher blood flow than those that are lighter. During the task state, the subject passively viewed a flashing annular checkerboard (i.e., a potent visual stimulus) while holding visual fixation on a small dot in the middle of the screen. During the control state, the subject simply maintained fixation. The difference in blood flow between the two states is shown in the difference image on the right. Once such a difference image is obtained, computer techniques are used to fit it to a standard brain so that comparisons can be made with other individuals (second row of difference images). From these individual difference images an averaged or mean difference image (bottom image) is made. Because the changes in blood flow are small, individual difference images tend to be somewhat variable due to the presence of statistical noise in the images and individual differences among the subjects. Therefore, averaging is necessary in order to determine the presence of significant changes that reflect changes common to a sample of all individuals. In such a process, noise is suppressed whereas consistent signals are enhanced. All of the remaining images in this chapter (with the exception of the fMRI images in Fig. 3-2) are mean difference images formed in the above manner.*

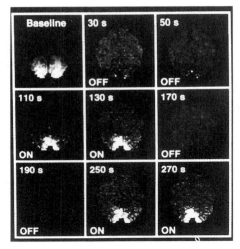

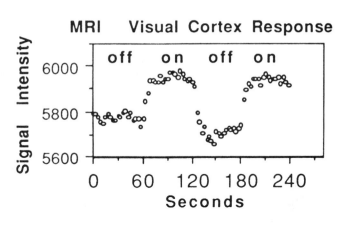

Figure 3-2

Data obtained by fMRI during visual stimulation in a single normal subject. The baseline image was acquired during darkness (upper left) *and was subtracted from the subsequent images obtained during darkness* (labeled OFF) *and during visual stimulation* (labeled ON). *A total of 80 images was obtained at the rate of one every 3.5 s. These images are oriented so that the front of the brain is on top and the visual cortices are on the bottom. Note the increase in signal intensity during visual stimulation. The graph on the right plots this signal intensity as a function of time and the presence or absence of a visual stimulus.* (From Kwong et al.,[7] with permission.)

STUDY OF LANGUAGE: AN EXAMPLE

The manner in which language skills are acquired and organized in the human brain has been the subject of intense investigation for more than a century. As recounted in Chap. 1, the Paris debate of 1861 spurred a number of investigators to examine the effects of focal brain lesions on the ability to speak, and, later, the ability to comprehend language. From these beginnings has emerged a concept of language organization in the human brain which, in broad outline, posits the following: information flows from visual and auditory reception areas to areas at the junction between the left temporal and parietal lobes for comprehension and then on to frontal areas for verbal response selection and speech production. As pointed out above, almost all of this information was gleaned from patients with brain damage. Could this organization represent the actual organization in the normal brain?

In the mid-1980s, the author and his colleagues Steven E. Petersen, Michael I. Posner, Peter T. Fox, and Mark A. Mintun began a series of experiments[8-11] designed to answer this question. We elected to begin our work with an analysis of the manner in which the normal human brain processes single words from perception to speaking. We designed our initial experiments in an hierarchical manner in which several levels of information processing of increasing complexity were employed. This design is in keeping with the experimental model discussed above. In these experiments, words were presented to the subjects either on a television monitor or through earphones. The presentation to follow focuses on those aspects of the study involving the *visual presentation* of words.

Opening the Eyes

Regardless of the task to be performed by our subjects, they were always asked to fix their gaze on a small fixation point in the middle of a television monitor. This was done to prevent the unwanted activation of brain areas concerned with saccadic eye movements from complicating our analysis. When one compares this simple act of opening one's eyes and fixing on a small dot in the middle of a television monitor with lying quietly with one's eyes closed (Fig. 3-3, top row), it is readily apparent that there is a significant increase in brain activity in the back of the brain in those areas known to respond to visual stimuli. It is important to realize that subsequent changes build upon this already present activity produced simply by opening the eyes and fixing the gaze.

Words as Passive Visual Stimuli

Putting common English nouns on the television monitor at the rate of one per second while subjects continued to fix their gaze on the fixation point produced a marked increase in the extent and complexity of brain activity in the visual areas of the brain, as shown in Fig. 3-3 (second row). The subjects were not instructed to process the words in any way, simply to fix their gaze on the fixation point. These results suggested that words had special properties as visual stimuli that had powerful effects on the visual system of the human brain. The question was what those properties might be. Clearly, further analysis of words as visual stimuli was needed.

In studying words as visual stimuli, we considered at least four properties as important contributors to the response we observed. First, words must be viewed as complex collections of *visual features*. They consist of varying numbers of units made up of connected lines with varying spatial orientations. Second these units of connected lines are not a random arrangement of lines but come from a unique set of 26 units representing the *letters* of the English alphabet. Third, the letters in words are not randomly distributed but are arranged in combinations of vowels and consonants according to the *rules* of the English language. These rules reflect the ways in which English letters can be put together to make words (orthography) and, to some extent, the ways in

which the letters are pronounced. Finally, words convey *meaning*.

It is reasonable to suppose that the responses we observed in the human visual system to the passive presentation of words represented a combination of responses to any or all of these features of words. We wished to begin the process of connecting, in the best possible way, active areas to specific features of words. To dissect the overall responses into their component parts, we needed to determine the component operations involved in reading a word. We believed at the outset that these operations related to visual features, letters and letter combinations, but not to the word meaning, which we did not expect to be processed in the visual system of the brain.

We devised four different visual stimuli,[10] shown in Table 3-1, that systematically varied the different features of the words. We then observed the effects of these different stimuli on the visual system of the brain as recorded by a PET scan. The four stimuli consisted of false fonts, consonant letter strings, pseudowords, and words; each represented one of the four suggested features of interest to us. The computer-generated false fonts incorporated all of the visual features of words but none of the other features. Consonant letter strings added the letter code but obviously could not be pronounced according to English rules of pronunciation. Pseudowords contained both consonants and vowels and could be pronounced because they had been arranged according to English rules of pronunciation. For most individuals, pseudowords do not convey meaning (an occasional individual will recognize a Hungarian word or the name of a neighbor inadvertently included among the pseudowords). Finally, words contain all of the aforementioned features plus meaning.

A group of normal individuals was instructed to observe the stimuli passively. By scanning the subjects as they were shown false fonts, consonant letter strings, pseudowords, or words, it was possible to distinguish among responses to the visual features, letters, orthographic regularity, and meaning. If the activation to words was attributable to the visual features of the stimulus and nothing else, then all stimuli should produce

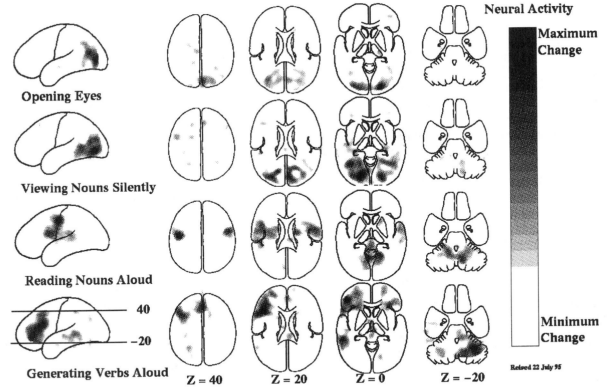

Opening Eyes

Viewing Nouns Silently

Reading Nouns Aloud

Generating Verbs Aloud

40

−20

Z = 40   Z = 20   Z = 0   Z = −20

Neural Activity

Maximum Change

Minimum Change

Revised 22 July 95

Figure 3-3

Four different task states are represented in these mean difference PET images from a group of normal subjects performing a hierarchically designed series of language tasks. Each row represents the mean difference between images of the designated task state and those of a control state. The images on the left represent projections of the changes as seen on the lateral surface of the brain with the front of the brain to the reader's left. The horizontal lines through the bottom left image denote the orientation of the horizontal slices throughout the same data as seen to the right of this first image. These horizontal images are oriented with the front of the brain on top and the left side to the reader's left. The markings Z = 40 and so on indicate millimeters above or below a horizontal plane through the brain at Z = 0. The row labeled Opening Eyes *indicates those areas of the brain with increased activity when subjects maintained fixation on a small dot of light in the middle of an otherwise blank television monitor, as compared with lying quietly with eyes closed. The row labeled* Viewing Nouns Silently *indicates those areas of the brain with increased activity when subjects passively viewed common English nouns as they appeared on the television monitor as compared to simply maintaining fixation on a small dot of light (row 1). The row labeled* Reading Nouns Aloud *indicates those areas of the brain with increased activity when subjects read aloud the nouns as they appeared on the screen. The control state was passively viewing the same nouns (row 2). Finally, the row labeled* Generating Verbs Aloud *indicates those areas of the brain with increased activity when subjects said aloud an appropriate verb for each noun as it appeared on the television monitor. The control state was reading the nouns aloud (row 3). Taken together, these difference images, arranged in a hierarchical fashion, are designed to demonstrate the spatially distributed nature of the processing going on in the normal human brain during a simple language task. By designing and presenting the experiment in this way, it is possible to take the first steps toward an understanding of the neural circuitry underlying various aspects of human language and the particular role played by individual areas within these circuits.*

Table 3-1

Example of the four types of visual stimuli

Words	Pseudowords	Letter strings	False fonts
ANT	GEEL	ѴSFFHT	ԶԱƎ
RAZOR	IOB	TBBL	ᒧԿᒧԱ
DUST	RELD	TSTFS	ԿDᒧԱ
FURNACE	BLERCE	JBTT	⊢ᒣᑒⴖ
MOTHER	CHELDINABE	STB	ԱԱᒧᒪᗷ
FARM	ALDOBER	FFPЩ	ԱⱵᑕᕼ

the same response. If the activation was attributable to the letters, then the activation should be produced only by letter strings, pseudowords, and words. If the activation was attributable to the orthographic regularity of words regardless of their meaning, then the results produced with words and pseudowords should be identical. Finally, if activation to words was attributable to the meaning of words, even during passive presentation, then words would produce a unique response. Thus, using the methods of cognitive science, we were able to break down the passive perception of words into a group of component mental operations and to set the stage for an imaging experiment designed to determine where in the brain these mental operations were implemented.

The results,[10] shown in Fig. 3-4, were of considerable interest. All four groups of stimuli produced responses in visual areas of the brain as compared with looking at a fixation point. The areas reacted to the complex visual features of the stimuli regardless of whether they consisted of groups of false fonts or letters. However, only pseudowords and words produced the dramatic responses originally observed with words alone. The heightened responses unique to words and pseudowords occurred along the inner surfaces of the left hemisphere of the brain, as shown in Fig. 3-4.

Two levels of analysis appear to be occurring in the visual system as we passively view words. At one level, the brain analyzes the visual features of the stimuli regardless of their relationships to letters and words. These visual features appear to be processed in multiple areas of the visual system on both sides of the brain. Responses to the false fonts that contain only meaningless features are particularly strong on the right side of the brain (not well illustrated in Fig. 3-4 because of the selection of slices).

At a second level, the brain analyzes the visual word form. It seems clear that visual stimuli incorporating the pronunciation rules of the English language uniquely activate a group of areas in the visual system of fluent readers of English. This coordinated response among a group of areas clustered in one part of the visual system must be acquired as we learn to read, and its existence is probably critical to the facility with which skilled readers handle words.

Reading Words Aloud

Following the hierarchical design of the original experiment, the subjects were next asked to read aloud the words (i.e., common English nouns) as they appeared on the television monitor in front of them. For most individuals fluent in their native language, this is an easy task to perform. One might easily envision that such a task could be performed effortlessly while, at the same time, another, unrelated task was being performed. The point is that such a task requires little of our conscious attention.

Not surprisingly for those knowledgeable about the location of the motor areas of the brain,

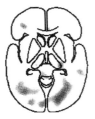 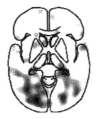 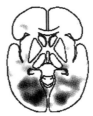

False Font   **Letter Strings**   **Pseudowords**   **Words**

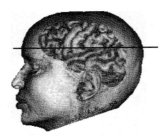

Figure 3-4
Four different task states are represented in these images: passive viewing of false fonts, letter strings, pseudowords, and words (see Table 3-1 for examples of each). In each instance, the control state was simply fixating on a small dot of light in the middle of an otherwise blank television monitor. The orientation of the slice of brain shown here is noted by the line through the figure at the bottom.

these areas were activated when individuals spoke the words they read on the television monitor. As shown in Fig. 3-3 (third row), these areas included the primary motor cortices in both cerebral hemisphere (Fig. 3-3, third row, Z = 40). In addition, other motor areas buried more deeply within the cerebral hemispheres (Fig. 3-3, third row, Z = 20) were also activated, including the cerebellum (Fig. 3-3, third row, Z = −20). At this point it should be noted that the act of speaking words, seen in its simplest form during reading aloud single words, did not produce activity in the classic areas of the left cerebral hemisphere known as Broca's and Wernicke's areas. This was probably one of the first surprises to emerge from the studies of language in normal people made with modern imaging techniques. The classic theories of language organization based on more than a century of research on patients with brain injury would have predicted clear-cut activity in these areas.

Although not mentioned above, listening to words does produce activity in posterior left temporal cortex at the temporoparietal junction in the region classically thought of as Wernicke's area. Furthermore, this area remains active when normal individuals repeat aloud the words they hear. However, it is important to the standard theory of

language organization that this area was not activated when the same individuals read aloud the words that were presented visually. Clearly, Wernicke's area as classically defined from studies of brain-injured patients is not active in an obligatory fashion when we speak. Critics of this new view are quick to point out that the new imaging techniques, such as PET and fMRI, might simply not have been sensitive enough to pick up a change in Wernicke's area when people read aloud. Were it not for the findings in the next stage of the experiment (generating verbs aloud for visually presented nouns) this would have been a difficult criticism to refute.

Generating Verbs Aloud

Generating a verb aloud for a noun presented visually (e.g., see *car*, say *drive*) may seem an unnecessarily complex next step in the hierarchical design of this experiment (linguists have been particularly critical!). After all, it involves a number of complex mental operations such as determining the meaning of the presented word (semantics) and the relation between the meaning of the word and the choice of an appropriate verb (syntax). Additionally, it is a very powerful episodic memory encoding task as well as a semantic retrieval task. Concerns about such issues obscure a most important difference between this task and reading or repeating words aloud. This difference lies in the requirement that the subjects devote considerable conscious attention to the task and, among other things, suppress the tendency to speak the word they see and to substitute an appropriate verb. Furthermore, this must be done rapidly, because in our experiments nouns were being presented at the rate of 40 to 60 per minute. It was very clear to us that subjects found this task difficult when they first attempted it. They often fell behind and occasionally skipped nouns.

The changes we observed in the brain (Fig. 3-3, bottom row) clearly indicated that this task of generating verbs for visually presented nouns placed a significant additional burden on the processing resources of the brain. In addition to areas previously activated, new areas within the left frontal (Fig. 3-3, bottom row, $Z = 40, 20$, and 0) and temporal (Fig. 3-3, bottom row, $Z = 0$) lobes were activated along with an area along the midline in front (Fig. 3-3, bottom row, $Z = 40$). Areas qualifying as Broca's and Wernicke's areas were clearly active, along with the surprising additional involvement of the right cerebellum (Fig. 3-3, bottom row, $Z = -20$). Recall that some of the cerebellum was active during reading aloud (Fig. 3-3, third row, $Z = -20$), but this additional activation in the right cerebellar hemisphere during verb generation represented a distinctly separate area. Whatever else might have been predicted about the neural substrate of this task, the right cerebellar hemisphere was not on anyone's mind prior to obtaining the results.

The fact that some areas of the motor system active during word reading (see Fig. 3-3, third row, $Z = 20$) were actually inactive during verb generation was an additional surprise. (Because of the nature of the color scale used in Fig. 3-3, where only positive differences between the task state and the control state can be shown, this inactivation cannot be illustrated. Suffice it to say that these areas, very active during reading aloud, were mysteriously inactive during verb generation.) This particular result (i.e., some areas being added while other areas were dropped) hinted at the possibility that the task of verb generation actually required *different* brain circuits rather than simply additional brain circuits for speech production. Our thinking in this regard was dramatically affected by an entirely serendipitous event.

While an additional group of subjects were being studied on the verb-generation task, a single subject was actually given practice on the task to ensure that he could do it with less difficulty and greater accuracy (never before had subjects practiced the verb-generation task prior to performing it in the PET scanner). Little did we suspect the effect this would have on our results. We immediately noticed that practice not only improved performance but also resulted in the failure to activate any of the areas seen in our previous study of verb-generation task (see Fig. 3-3, bottom row). In this individual, practice on the verb-generation task appeared to allow the brain to perform the task with the same circuits used for simple word reading aloud (for reference, see Fig. 3-3, row 3). If true, this was, indeed, a surprising finding. Therefore we set about studying the effect of practice on the brain circuits used for speech production.

Practice Effects

The first task was to examine in greater detail the actual effect of practice on the verb-generation task itself. What we learned[11] was that when normal subjects practiced generating verbs for the same list of 40 common English nouns, their reaction times became significantly shorter over a period of about 10 min. During this time, they were able to go through the same word list 10 times, each time being encouraged by the examiner to be as quick as possible in responding. Another remarkable feature of the learning process was the fact that as they became practiced, they became quite stereotyped in their responses. While each of the words on the list could be associated with several verbs, practice led to the repeated selection of just one verb. In a sense, an automated stimulus-response pattern of behavior had been established. If, after learning had occurred, a new word list was substituted, their behavior returned to the unpracticed state (i.e., significantly slower and unstereotyped). It should also be noted that regardless of the amount of practice or whether the subjects were speaking verbs or nouns, the actual time needed to say the word did not change. What did change was the time necessary to begin the response and the nature of the response (i.e., stereotyped versus not stereotyped). Armed with this more complete information concerning the behavioral effects of practice, we were in a position to evaluate the effect of practice on the brain circuits in a new imaging experiment.

In the new imaging experiment,[11] we studied normal subjects performing the verb-generation task to visually presented nouns, naively and after 10 min of practice. The control task was simply reading aloud the same words as they were presented on the television monitor. Consistent with our earlier experiments, the naive generation of verbs for visually presented nouns showed again the same brain areas involved, a reassuring finding, which supported our confidence in the imaging method. The changes with practice were dramatic. The areas in the frontal and temporal cortex in the left hemisphere and the right side of the cerebellum needed to accomplish the verb-generation task in the naive state (top row, Fig. 3-5) were completely replaced by areas deep within the brain hemispheres after a few minutes' practice (bottom row, Fig. 3-5). These latter areas were actually used as well for the far simpler task of reading nouns aloud. In addition, areas in left occipital cortex seen active during the passive visual presentation of words (see Fig. 3-3, second row, $Z = 0$) and unchanged during reading nouns aloud (see Fig. 3-3, third row, $Z = 0$) and naively generating verbs for visually presented nouns (see Fig. 3-3, fourth row, $Z = 0$) significantly increased their activity after practice on the verb-generation task (Fig. 3-6).

These results strongly support the hypothesis that we actually utilize different brain circuits when performing a task like verb generation for the first time than after practice when we have perfected or automated the task. Why should such an arrangement of brain circuitry be necessary? Why two circuits? Why not just do a better job of utilizing existing brain circuits as we learn? The

answer may not be simply that the brain needs two circuits, one for the nonconscious performance of highly automated tasks and the other for the performance of novel, nonautomated tasks. It may, instead, be related to our need to strike a balance between the efficiency conferred by automation of much of our behavior and the occasional need to modify our programmed behavior in accordance with unexpected contingencies in our environment. Only further research will allow us to clarify such issues. What is clear is that functional brain imaging adds a remarkable new dimension to our thinking about how language and other cognitive activities are implemented in the normal human brain.

Practical Implications

In our initial study of lexical processing,[8] we introduced the concept of hierarchical subtractions to modern functional imaging as a means of isolating the functional anatomy of specific mental operations (see Fig. 3-3). The logic of the subtraction analysis was that the passive presentation of nouns minus no presentation (i.e., fixation point only) would isolate areas involved in passive sensory processing (row 2, Fig. 3-3); reading aloud visually presented nouns minus the passive presentation of nouns would isolate areas involved in articulatory output and motor programming (row 3, Fig. 3-3); and the verb-generation task minus reading nouns aloud would isolate areas involved in high-level processes such as semantic analysis (row 4, Fig. 3-3).

In its simplest form, the type of hierarchical subtraction method used for the design of this study (see Fig. 3-3) involved accepting the assumption that processing done by previously added areas does not change with the addition or deletion of new areas (i.e., each area is functionally isolated). Also assumed in this approach is that the subject does not change strategies with the addition of another task, nor do the task combinations interact with each other.[12-14]

The limitations of the "additive" method were first discussed in terms of reaction-time studies of human performance.[12-14] For studies of this

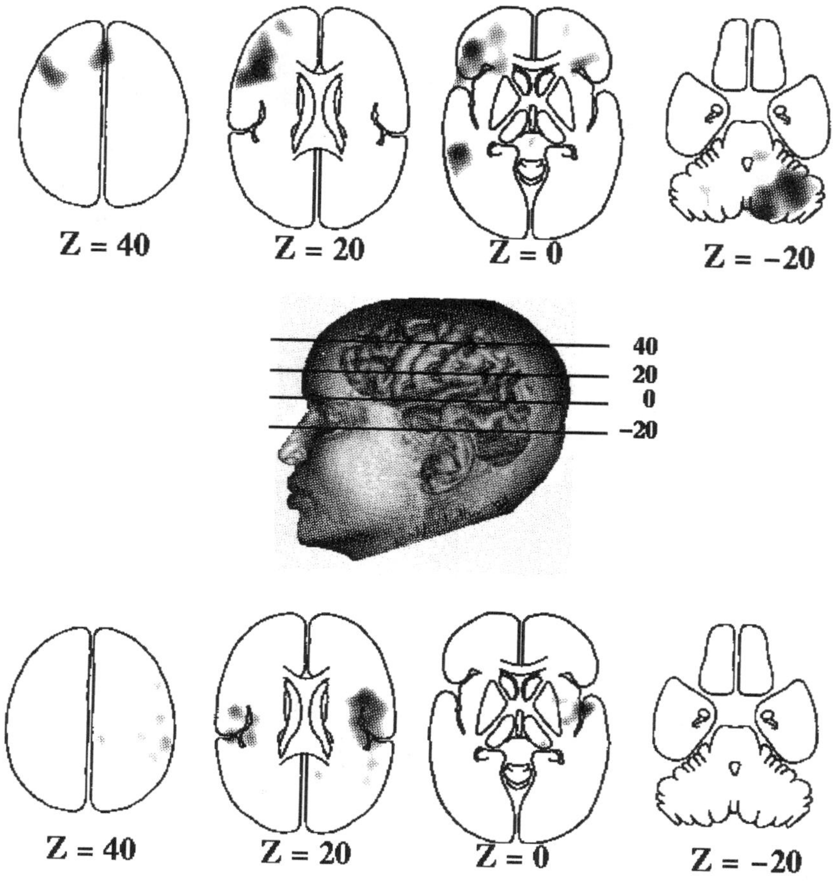

Figure 3-5
A single task state is represented in the images in this figure. In this task, subjects were asked to generate verbs aloud for visually presented common English nouns. The control state for these subtraction images was simply reading aloud the same visually presented nouns. The top row of images shows those areas of the brain used in the performance of this task when it is first undertaken. A brief period of practice markedly improves performance on this difficult task and dramatically alters the areas of the brain uniquely utilized for the task (bottom). Additional practice-induced changes are shown in Fig. 3-6.

type, the validity of the underlying assumptions cannot be directly tested and, as a result, controversy has occasionally arisen about their interpretation. For functional imaging studies, however, empirical testing is theoretically possible. The locations of areas added at different stages in a task hierarchy can be identified, and the magnitude of their activity at each level in the imaging sequence can be monitored. If a brain area is not functionally isolated, then the magnitude of its activity will be modulated by the addition of new tasks. In fact, our study of the effect of practice on the verb-generation task had its genesis in part because of the discovery that generation aloud of a verb appropriate to a visually presented noun (compared to reading the same noun aloud) modulated areas

activated by the reading aloud of the noun. Furthermore, these imaging results (see Figs. 3-5 and 3-6) clearly indicate that the actual areas supporting a task and their relationship with other areas can change dramatically as a result of practice. Such observations underscore the utility of combining the hierarchical subtraction method of psychology with modern functional imaging techniques such as PET and fMRI to further our understanding of the functional anatomy of the normal human brain. They should also impart a note of caution in placing neurobiological interpretations on behavioral data in the absence of direct information about how a process is actually implemented in the brain.

Because of the potential for rapid change in

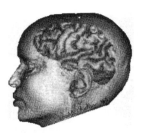
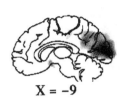

X = –9

Figure 3-6
The task state represented in Fig. 3-5 is again represented in this figure. In this task, subjects were asked to generate verbs aloud for visually presented common English nouns. The control state for these subtraction images was simply reading the same visually presented nouns aloud. The difference image to the right, which represents a sagittal slice of the brain 9 mm to the left of the midline, demonstrates the marked increase in blood flow in the medial occipital cortices occurring as the result of practice on the verb-generation task.

the use of brain circuitry resulting from the practice of an unfamiliar task, interpretation of repeated or time-intensive within-subject functional imaging measurements must be made with care. It would appear that 15 minutes of practice on an unfamiliar task such as the verb-generation task is sufficient to significantly alter the brain circuitry underlying the task. At what time these changes in brain circuitry actually occurred within this 15-min time period remains to be determined. That they may have occurred much earlier than 15 min remains a distinct possibility.

With regard to the actual imaging measurement duration and the effect of practice, the selection of an imaging measurement strategy will also be critical. In the study of the effect of practice on the verb-generation task, functional imaging was performed with PET and measurements of blood flow. The measurement of blood flow was selected because of its simplicity and also because of the short measurement time. The total measurement time for blood flow with PET is 40 s. This is to be contrasted with measurement of glucose metabolism, an equally good marker of neuronal activity,[3] which requires 30 to 45 min to complete.[15,16]

Clearly studies of the verb-generation task would have yielded very different results had such a lengthy measurement strategy been selected. The advent of fMRI with even more rapid measurements of functional change with the human brain than anything achievable with PET (see Fig. 3-2) portends an even more precise description of the events surrounding the shift in brain circuitry with practice.

THE TEMPORAL DIMENSION

While functional imaging studies with PET provide remarkable insights into the functional brain *anatomy* of neuronal circuits underlying various cognitive activities in the normal human brain, they do not provide any information on the temporal sequence of information processing within these circuits. Conceptually, one might think of a network of brain areas (see Fig. 3-3) as a group of individuals in the middle of a conference call. The temporal information sought would be equivalent to knowing who was speaking when and who was in charge. Such information is critical in understanding how specific brain areas are coordinated as a network to produce observable human behavior.

Viewing the temporally varying changes in brain activity revealed by fMRI (see Fig. 3-2) has raised the possibility that fMRI, with its speed of data acquisition approaching a few tens of milliseconds, might provide both the anatomy and the timing of information processing within functional brain circuits in the human brain. The stumbling block, however, is the speed of neuronal activity compared with the rate of change of the fMRI signal. Signals from one part of the brain can travel to another in as little as a few milliseconds. Unfortunately, changes in blood flow and blood oxygenation (which is dependent on changes in blood flow) often require several seconds to occur after the onset of a change in neuronal activity. In all likelihood, the only methods that respond quickly enough are the electrical recording techniques such as electroencephalography (EEG) and magnetoencephalography (MEG).

One might reasonably ask why these techniques have not been used to provide the types of maps now forthcoming from PET and fMRI. The limitations are spatial resolution and sensitivity. Even though great strides have been made, particularly with MEG, accurate localization of the source of brain activity remains difficult with electrical recording devices used in isolation. Furthermore, the resolution becomes poorer the deeper into the brain information is sought.

Neither PET nor fMRI suffers from this difficulty. They can both sample all parts of the brain with equal spatial resolution and sensitivity. Recently several successful attempts have been made to combine the spatial information from functional imaging studies with the temporal information from electrical studies.[17,18] One such attempt brought together investigators from our laboratory and the University of Oregon to study the temporal dynamics of the naive verb-generation task.[18] Event-related potentials (ERPs) were recorded during both verb generation and reading nouns aloud. Difference ERPs were then computed. From this study, it became clear that information processing unique to naive verb generation began in midline frontal cortices between 180 and 200 ms after the noun was presented. This was followed by a spread of activity laterally to the left prefrontal cortex between 220 and 240 ms. Only later did activity arise in the left posterior temporal cortex, peaking between 620 and 640 ms after stimulus onset (Fig. 3-7). These data, admittedly preliminary, provide important information about the role of specific areas of the brain in the information processing requirements underlying the verb-generation task. For example, the activation in posterior temporal cortex (see Fig. 3-3, fourth row, Z = 0, and Fig. 3-7) in the vicinity of the classic Wernicke's area is rather late to be involved in many rapid semantic tasks that produce reaction times much faster than 600 ms. The later Wernicke's area activation may relate more to the integration of word meanings to obtain the overall meaning of phrases, sentences, or other units more complex than words. Regardless of their fi-

nal interpretation, *combined data* of this type are likely to constrain our models of information processing in the human brain and certainly represent an important future direction in functional brain imaging.

RELATIONSHIP TO LESION STUDIES

Functional brain imaging studies in normal humans add a new dimension to the lesion-based studies of behavioral neurology and neuropsychology. Two examples will serve to illustrate this new relationship. In our studies of the processing of single words, which have been used primarily to illustrate the strategy and some of the new findings from functional brain imaging, a new role for the cerebellum was unexpectedly identified. The role of the cerebellum was expected when subjects read aloud words from a television monitor (see Fig. 3-3, third row, Z = −20), as would be the case for any overt motor activity. The presence of robust activity in the right cerebellar hemisphere during verb generation (see Fig. 3-3, fourth row, Z = −20) after subtraction of the activity associated with speaking a word (see Fig. 3-3, third row, Z = −20) was, indeed, a surprise. Although others had speculated about a role for the cerebellum in nonmotoric, cognitive activity,[19] direct evidence for this assertion in normal human subjects was lacking. The PET findings left little doubt about an important role, but the exact nature of the contribution of the cerebellum could not be determined from the imaging results in normals.

At this point we turned to the study of patients with lesions of the cerebellum.[20] Specifically, we wanted to know the performance of individuals who had lesions confined to the right cerebellar hemisphere. Such an individual was located and studied extensively over a period of 2 years.[20] Beginning with the task that produced the right cerebellar PET activation (see Fig. 3-3), we studied this 49-year-old right-handed male (RC1) with right cerebellar damage on a variety of tasks involving complex nonmotor processing. Whereas RC1's performance on standard tests of memory, intelligence, "frontal function," and language

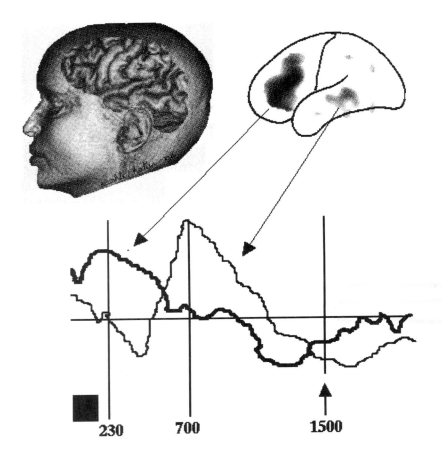

Figure 3-7
The PET difference image in this figure presents the increase in blood flow occurring in left frontal and temporal cortices during the naive performance of the verb-generation task (see Figs. 3-3 and 3-6 for additional information) along with selected event-related potential (ERP) difference (i.e., verb generation aloud minus reading nouns aloud) waveforms obtained for the same task. The arrows connect the PET blood-flow responses with difference ERP waveforms recorded at the nearest overlying electrode (heavy line = F7; light line = T5). The short horizontal bar below ERP waveforms indicates the visual presentation of the word and the vertical arrow indicates the response cue. Note that activity in frontal cortex precedes that in temporal cortex by over 400 ms. The numbers below the vertical lines represents times in milliseconds after presentation of the word. More complete descriptions of these ERP data are presented in Ref. 18.

skills was excellent, he had profound deficits in two areas: (1) practice-related learning and (2) detection of errors. Considered in relation to cerebellar contributions to motor tasks, the results suggested to us that some functions performed by the cerebellum may be generalized beyond a purely motor domain. Clearly this was an important advance in our understanding of human cerebellar function and its role in human cognition made possible by new knowledge from functional brain imaging of normals coupled with focused studies in patients with lesions.

Our experience with this patient, RC1, suggests to us a paradigm shift in which information about the organization of the normal human brain, obtained from modern functional imaging studies, uniquely guides the bedside evaluation of patients with specific lesions. RC1's very specific cognitive deficits were not apparent to him (remarkably, even during specific testing, he seemed almost completely unaware of his cognitive performance deficits). Likewise, his physicians were pleased to note that his classic cerebellar symptoms and signs of imbalance and incoordination had completely resolved. New knowledge of right cerebellar activation in normals and the specific class of tasks necessary to elicit this activation were critical to the evaluation of RC1 and future patients.

Experience with a second patient[21] reveals another aspect of the role played by functional imaging studies in the evaluation of patients with specific lesions. This patient (LF1) had a lesion of the left frontal cortex secondary to a stroke. Such lesions are known to produce speech-production impairments (nonfluent aphasia). These impairments vary from patient to patient and performance on certain speech-production tasks can be relatively preserved in some patients. It was, therefore, not entirely surprising to find that LF1 had a small island of preserved function. The task on which he performed entirely normally was word-stem completion. In this task, subjects are shown the first three letters of a word and asked to respond with the first word that comes to mind (e.g., see *str*, say *street*). Functional brain imaging in normals has shown that performance of this task activates a discrete area of left frontal cortex in Brodmann area 44.[22] This area had been completely destroyed in LF1.

A possible explanation for preservation of function under these circumstances is that areas outside left prefrontal cortex are used to compensate for the injured brain. We tested this hypothesis in LF1 by having him perform the word-stem completion task, which he was able to do normally despite the lesion in his left frontal cortex, while being scanned with PET. Remarkably, he activated an homologous region in the right frontal cortex. These findings are consistent with the hypothesis that preserved function can be the result of compensatory changes in the circuitry supporting the task performance. Building upon this experience, it should be possible to better understand the manner in which the human nervous system compensates for injury. Also, this experience should inject a note of caution in the behavioral interpretation of a lesion in the absence of a clear understanding of the function or functions performed by the lesioned area in the normal brain.

SUMMING UP

Modern functional brain imaging with PET and fMRI, complemented by ERPs, will play an important role in our understanding of the functional organization of the normal human brain. These new tools, guided by the principles of cognitive science, now permit us to dissect the basic mental operations underlying our behavior and to relate them to specific circuitry within the normal human brain. A glance back at Fig. 3-3 reveals that, as we undertake even relatively simple cognitive tasks, extensive areas of the brain are recruited to assist in the performance of these tasks. Although we can begin making statements about the roles of such groups of areas or circuits, it remains for further studies to determine the more basic mental operations to be assigned to the individual brain areas within a given circuit. The studies of words presented in this chapter give some indication of the manner in which such an analysis might proceed. This information—coupled with studies of patients with brain injury and guided anew by information from normals as well as more basic studies in laboratory animals using a variety of sophisticated techniques—bodes well for our future understanding of human brain function. Armed with such information, we will be in a much better position to appreciate the basis of human behavior.

REFERENCES

1. Posner MI, Petersen SE, Fox PT, Raichle ME: Localization of cognitive operations in the human brain. *Science* 240:1627–1631, 1988.
2. Posner MI, Raichle ME: *Images of Mind.* New York: Freeman, 1994.
3. Raichle ME: Circulatory and metabolic correlates of brain function in normal humans, in *Handbook of Physiology, The Nervous System. Higher Functions of the Brain.* Bethesda, MD: American Physiological Society, 1987, vol V, pp 643–674.
3a. Fox PT, Raichle ME, Minton MA, Deuce C: Nonoxidative glucose consumption during focal physiologic neural activity. *Science* 241:462–464, 1988.
4. Pauling L, Coryell CD: The magnetic properties

and structure of hemoglobin, oxyhemoglobin and carbonmonoxyhemoglobin. *Proc Natl Acad Sci USA* 22:210–216, 1936.

5. Ogawa S, Lee TM, Tank DW: Brain magnetic resonance imaging with contrast dependent on blood oxygenation. *Proc Natl Acad Sci USA* 87:9868–9872, 1990.

6. Ogawa S, Tank DW, Menon R, et al: Intrinsic signal changes accompanying sensory stimulation: Functional brain mapping with magnetic resonance imaging. *Proc Natl Acad Sci USA* 89:5951–5955, 1992.

7. Kwong KK, Belliveau JW, Chesler DA, et al: Dynamic magnetic resonance imaging of human brain activity during primary sensory stimulation. *Proc Natl Acad Sci USA* 89:5675–5679, 1992.

8. Petersen SE, Fox PT, Posner MI, et al: Positron emission tomographic studies of the cortical anatomy of single word processing. *Nature* 331:585–589, 1988.

9. Petersen SE, Fox PT, Posner MI, et al: Positron emission tomographic studies of the processing of single words. *J Cogn Neurosci* 1:153–170, 1989.

10. Petersen SE, Fox PT, Synder AZ, Raichle ME: Activation of extra striate and frontal cortical areas by visual words and word-like stimuli. *Science* 249:1041–1044, 1990.

11. Raichle ME, Fiez JA, Videen TO, et al: Practice-related changes in human brain functional anatomy during non-motor learning. *Cereb Cortex* 4:8–26, 1994.

12. Kulpe OO: The analysis of compound reactions, in Bradford-Tichener E (ed): *Outlines of Psychology.* New York: Macmillan, 1909, pp 410–422.

13. Donders FC: On the speed of mental processes (reprint). *Acta Psychol* 30:412–431, 1969.

14. Sternberg S: The discovery of processing stages: Extensions of Donders' method. *Acta Psychol* 30:276–315, 1969.

15. Sokoloff L, Reivich M, Kennedy C, et al: The [^{14}C]deoxyglucose method for the measurement of local cerebral glucose utilization: Theory, procedure and normal values in the conscious and anesthetized albino rat. *J Neurochem* 28:987–917, 1977.

16. Reivich M, Alavi A, Wolf A, et al: Glucose metabolic rate kinetic model parameters determination in humans: The lumped constants and rate constants for [^{18}F]fluorodeoxyglucose and [^{11}C]deoxyglucose. *J Cereb Blood Flow Metab* 5:179–192, 1985.

17. Heinze HJ, Mangun GR, Burchert W, et al: Combined spatial and temporal imaging of brain activity during visual selective attention in humans. *Nature* 372:543–546, 1994.

18. Snyder AZ, Abdullaev YG, Posner MI, Raichle ME: Scalp electrical potentials reflect regional cerebral blood flow responses during processing of written words. *Proc Natl Acad Sci USA* 92:1689–1693, 1995.

19. Leiner HC, Leiner AL, Dow RS: Does the cerebellum contribute to mental skills? *Behav Neurosci* 100:443–454, 1986.

20. Fiez JA, Petersen SE, Cheney MK, Raichle ME: Impaired non-motor learning and error detection associated with cerebellar damage. *Brain* 115:155–178, 1992.

21. Buckner RL, Corbetta M, Schatz J, et al: Preserved speech abilities and compensation following prefrontal damage. *Proc Natl Acad Sci USA,* 1996.

22. Buckner RL, Petersen SE, Ojemann JG, et al: Functional anatomical studies of explicit and implicit memory retrieval tasks. *J Neurosci* 15:12–29, 1995.

Chapter 4

COMPUTATIONAL MODELING IN COGNITIVE NEUROSCIENCE

Martha J. Farah

COGNITION AS COMPUTATION

If the insights of cognitive psychology had to be boiled down to a single statement, a good candidate would be "cognition is computation." Starting with the work of Allen Newell and Herbert Simon in the sixties,[1] psychologists have been able to explain a wide range of human behavior in terms of information encoded from the environment, information stored in memory, and mechanisms for combining these two sources of information to select appropriate actions.

Viewing cognition as computation freed the field of psychology from the constraints of Skinnerian behaviorism, in which all psychological explanation was confined to directly observable entities such as stimulus and response. According to behaviorism, to hypothesize about the internal mental states intervening between stimulus and response was unscientific, nonexplanatory, and downright mystical. The information processing of computers provided a concrete demonstration that the states intervening between stimulus and response could also be within the domain of objective science. Hypothesizing about the knowledge that caused a person to act one way rather than another is no more mystical than hypothesizing about the stored data in a computer that caused it to give one output rather than another. The computational view of the mind made it possible to have a *psychological* level of explanation —dealing with entities such as memory, knowledge, inference, and decision—that could be un- derstood as a function of perfectly nonmystical *physical* mechanisms.

There are many different ways that physical mechanisms can process information. The best known, and in many ways the most powerful, is the way computers work. Symbolically coded information is retrieved from a particular physical memory location, operated upon in a physically distinct central processing unit according to stored instructions, and then reentered into memory. Most of the early theories of cognitive psychology assumed this type of computational architecture. More recently, a very different computational architecture has been explored by computer scientists, psychologists, and neuroscientists, which has more in common with brains than with office computers. This is the parallel distributed processing (PDP) architecture. Because PDP is similar in many ways to neural information processing, PDP models have increasingly come to be used in neuropsychology.

Computation has played two roles in cognitive psychology and neuropsychology. In some cases theories are simply expressed in terms of the concepts of computation: the informational content and format of representations, the parallel or serial nature of searches, and the like. In other cases, researchers implement their theories as running computer simulations. With the advent of the PDP architecture, computer simulation is increasingly used. One reason for this is that the behavior of PDP systems is not always obvious or predictable by intuition alone.

PARALLEL DISTRIBUTED PROCESSING

Parallel distributed processing systems consist of a large number of highly interconnected neuronlike units. These units are connected to one another by weighted connections that determine how much activation from one unit flows to another. There is no central controller governing the behavior of the network. Rather, each part of the network functions locally and in parallel with the other parts, hence the first P in PDP. Representations consist of the pattern of activation distributed over a population of units, and long-term memory knowledge is encoded in the pattern of connection strengths distributed among a population of units, hence the D. Alternative terms for PDP include *connectionism* (not to be confused with the center-and-pathway approach of Wernicke and his followers, which has also been called connectionism), *brain-style computation,* and *artificial neural networks.* For more than the brief overview offered here, the reader is directed to Rumelhart and McClelland's classic two-volume book on PDP[2] or more recent books by Anderson[3] (for a technical introduction) or Bechtel and Abrahamsen[4] (for a conceptual and philosophical introduction).

There are many types of PDP networks with different computational properties. Among the features that determine network type are the activation rule, connectivity, and the learning rule. The activation rule governs how the activation values of units are updated given a certain input activation. Units' activations can be discrete or continuous, and activations may be increased in direct proportion to the sum of the inputs (a *linear activation function*) or as a nonlinear function of the inputs (generally a sigma-shaped function). The activation rule has a variety of consequences for network behavior, some of which are not immediately obvious. For example, as noted below, purely linear networks will not be able to learn certain kinds of associations.

A major distinguishing feature is connectivity, which can be unidirectional, in which case the network is called *feedforward,* or bidirectional, in which case it is called *interactive.* Feedforward networks may consist simply of a set of input units

and a set of output units. A pattern associator can be made from such a network if the weights between the first- and second-layer units are set so that each of a set of patterns of activation over the units in the first layer evokes an associated pattern over the units in the second layer. Some feedforward networks have an additional set of so-called *hidden units* interposed between the input and output units. With nonlinear systems, the additional set of units is useful in transforming the input patterns of activation to the desired output patterns; indeed, certain types of problems (such as associating input patterns 00 and 11 with one output and 01 and 10 with another, the "XOR" problem) can be solved only with hidden units. In *recurrent networks,* later layers loop back to earlier layers. In interactive networks, some or all connections are bidirectional. In recurrent and interactive networks, "downstream" units can influence "upstream" units; more than one processing step is therefore needed to arrive at their final activation state. These networks are said to "settle into" a stable state after the addition of an input pattern of activation.

Learning in neural networks consists of adjusting the weights between units so that, given a set of input activation patterns, in each case the network ends up in the desired activation state. For example, for a network to learn that a certain name goes with a certain face, the weights among units in the network are adjusted so that presentation of either the face pattern in the units representing faces or the name pattern in the units representing names causes the corresponding other pattern to become activated.

There is a wide variety of learning algorithms, and the choice depends in part on the type of network and the task to be learned. A learning rule proposed many decades ago by the neuroscientist Donald Hebb[5] forms the basis for many current learning algorithms. The gist of the *Hebb rule* is: Neurons that fire together wire together. In other words, when there is a positive correlation in the activity of two units, strengthen their connection so that future activation of one will be even more likely to activate the other. This form of the rule enables *unsupervised learning*—that is, learning without a teacher to direct what is learned. Networks that use unsupervised learning are called *self-organizing,* as they develop their own representations of regularities in their input—for example, developing edge representations from center-surround-like inputs[6] or semantic representations from patterns of word cooccurrence[7] (see Ref. 8 for additional information on self-organizing systems).

The Hebb rule can also be used to learn to associate patterns, but only if the input patterns are orthogonal, a rather stringent requirement. When the object is to learn to associate or complete patterns, then *supervised* learning is normally used. The *delta rule* is an example of a supervised learning rule that can be viewed as a variant of the Hebb rule. Both learning rules change weights proportionate with a comparison between activation values; in the case of supervised learning, the comparison is between desired activation value and actual activation value, an error measure. Networks with hidden units demand yet a further modification of the learning rule, as the weights to be changed do not directly link the input with the output units from which the error measure is derived. The *generalized delta rule,* or *backpropagation,* is often used in this case. With this rule, the error in the output units is propagated back to alter the weights of the (nonadjacent) input units.

Further discussion of learning rules is beyond the scope of this chapter, except to note that learning in PDP models is often not intended to simulate real learning. Rather, it is frequently used as a tool for setting the weights in a network so that the network can simulate some aspect of cognition in its mature end state. Backpropagation is sometimes criticized for being physiologically implausible. This may or may not be a valid criticism, depending on the goal of the simulation. For example, if one were interested in studying the effects of damage to the face-recognition system, one would need a model of face recognition that embodied a set of associations between facial appearance and other knowledge about people, on which one could inflict damage. As it is virtually impossible to "hand wire" networks of more than a few units, learning rules would be used to build in these associations. However, they would not be simulating in the way in which people learn face recognition. For this reason it might be less confusing to refer to learning algorithms for neural networks as weight-setting algorithms unless the learning process is explicitly being modeled.

How Realistic Are PDP Models?

Of course, there are cases when real human learning is the subject of the model, and then we are right to inquire whether or in what sense the model's learning is similar to human learning. More generally, it is important to consider whether PDP is a reasonable model for human brain function.

Parallel distributed processing models differ from real neural networks, including the human brain, in numerous ways: Even the biggest PDP networks are tiny compared to the brain; PDP models have just one kind of unit, compared to a variety of types of neurons; and just one kind of activation (which can act excitatorily or inhibitorily), rather than a multitude of different neurotransmitters; and so on. Yet these differences are not necessarily cause to reject the PDP approach. No model is identical in all respects to the system being modeled; models possess theory-relevant and theory-irrelevant attributes. Furthermore, science must often simplify nature in order to understand it. Parallel distributed processing models should be viewed as simplifications of the brain, possessing enough theory-relevant attributes of the brain to be informative on many questions but clearly leaving out or even contradicting many known aspects of brain function.

Among the theory-relevant aspects of PDP models are the use of distributed representations, the large number of inputs to and outputs from each unit, the modifiable connections between units, and the existence of both inhibitory and excitatory connections, summation rules, bounded activations, and thresholds. Parallel distributed processing models allow us to find out what aspects of behavior, normal and pathologic, can be explained by this set of theory-relevant attributes. Of course, some behavior may be explainable only with the incorporation of other features of neuroanatomy and neurophysiology not currently used in PDP models. This seems quite likely, and the discovery of such instances will be extremely informative with respect to the functional significance of these features of our biology. However, note that this problem does not apply to cases in which the current models perform well. In such cases, the only danger associated with nonrealism is that the model's success might depend on a theory-irrelevant simplification. For example, scale is generally treated as theory-irrelevant, but it is possible that certain mechanisms will work only for small networks or small amounts of knowledge. We must be on the lookout for such cases but also recognize that it is unlikely that the success of most models will happen to depend critically on their unrealistic features.

Spatial Analogies for Understanding the Behavior of PDP Networks

Spatial analogies are useful for visualizing certain aspects of network dynamics, including the way in which the network's patterns of activation change under the influence of an input and the way in which the ensemble of weights changes during learning. The activation state of the network at any point in time can be represented as a point in a high-dimensional space called *activation space.* The dimensions of this space represent the level of activation of each unit in the network, assuming a fixed set of weights. In addition to the dimensions representing the activation levels of the units, there is one additional dimension, representing the overall "fit" between the current activation pattern and the weights.

When units that are both active have a large positive weight between them, so that they reinforce each other's activation, this is an example of a good fit. If both units are active and the weight between them is negative (i.e., inhibitory), the fit will be poor. This measure of fit is called "energy," with low energy representing a better fit. The energy value associated with each pattern of activation defines a surface in activation space.

When an input pattern is presented to the network, the corresponding initial position in activation space is defined by the activation levels on the input units, along with resting-level values for the dimensions representing the other units in the network. The weights in the rest of the network will not fit well with uniform resting-level activation values over their portion of the network. Thus, the initial point in activation space will be in a region of high energy. As activation propagates through the network, the pattern of activation changes and the point representing this pattern moves along the energy surface in activation space. The movement will be generally downward, as the network lowers its energy, much as a ball rolls down a hill to lower its potential energy. To see why this would happen in terms of network dynamics rather than by analogy with rolling balls, consider the examples given earlier of high- and low-energy activation states. For example, active units connected by negative weights (a poor-fit, high-energy pattern) will tend to change their activations until one is active and the other is not (a good-fit, low-energy pattern).

The energy minima toward which the network tends are termed *attractors.* Attractors are useful in network computation not only for associating patterns and completing partial patterns but also for their ability to "clean up" a noisy input by transforming a pattern similar to a known pattern into that known pattern (i.e., a pattern just uphill from an attractor will roll down into the attractor).

The shape of the energy landscape is determined by the network's weights. In an untrained network, the landscape will be generally flat with random hills and valleys. When the network has learned a certain association, its weights will create an energy landscape in activation space in which the point corresponding to the input pattern and the attractor point corresponding to the complete associated pattern are connected by a smoothly and steeply sloping path that causes the one state to "roll" down into the other.

The weights that determine the attractor structure of activation space can themselves be used to define a space, and this space is useful for visualizing the process of learning. In *weight space,* each of the weights in a network corresponds to one dimension of a space, so that we can represent the sum total of the network's knowledge as a point in this high-dimensional space. If one additional dimension is now added to the space, representing the performance of the network at associating names and faces (an error measure of some sort), then there will be a surface defined by each combination of weights and their associated error measure. Learning consists of moving along this surface in weight space, changing weight values, until a sufficiently low point has been reached.

APPLICATIONS OF COMPUTATIONAL MODELING TO COGNITIVE NEUROSCIENCE

For most of the history of behavioral neurology and neuropsychology, the lesion method has been our primary source of insights into human brain organization. Yet the interpretation of lesion effects is not always as transparent as one would like. As early as the nineteenth century, authors such as John Hughlings-Jackson[9] cautioned that the brain is a distributed and highly interactive system, such that local damage to one part can unleash new modes of functioning in the remaining parts of the system. As a result, one cannot assume that a patient's behavior following brain damage is the direct result of a simple subtraction of one or more components of the mind, with those that remain functioning normally. More likely, it results from a combination of the subtraction of some components and changes in the functioning of other components that had previously been influenced by the missing components.

Parallel distributed processing provides a conceptual framework, and concrete tools, for reasoning about the effects of local lesions in distributed, interactive systems.[10] It has already proven helpful in understanding a number of different neuropsychological disorders. Each of the examples reviewed here constitutes a reinterpretation of a well-known disorder, with qualitatively different implications for the normal organization of the

brain and the functional locus of damage within that organization.

Deep Dyslexia: Interpreting Error Types

Patients with deep dyslexia (see Chap. 18) make two very different types of reading errors, which have been interpreted as indicating that two functionally distinct lesions are needed to account for these errors. Deep dyslexics make semantic errors, that is, errors that bear a semantic similarity to the correct word, such as reading *cat* as "dog." They also make visual errors—that is, errors that bear a visual (graphemic) similarity to the correct word, such as reading *cat* as "cot." The fact that both semantic and visual errors are common in deep dyslexia has been taken to imply that deep dyslexics have multiple lesions, with one affecting the visual system and another affecting semantic knowledge. However, a consideration of the effects of single lesions in a network with attractor states suggests that a single lesion is sufficient to account for these patients' errors. Furthermore, it suggests that mixtures of error types will be the rule rather than the exception when the system that has been damaged normally functions to transform the stimulus representation from one form that has one set of similarity relations (e.g., visual, in which *cot* and *cat* are similar) to another form with different similarity relations (e.g., semantic, in which *cot* and *bed* are similar).

Hinton and Shallice[11] trained the recurrent network shown in Fig. 4-1 to produce semantic representations of a set of words, given their printed orthography as input. The grapheme-to-"sememe" (their term for elements of semantic representation) mapping is carried out with the aid of hidden units, and the sememes are interconnected among themselves and connected to a final layer of semantic representation that connects, recurrently, back to the sememes. This pattern of connectivity in the semantic layers creates attractor states for the network. The input to the semantic layers need not be perfectly on target for the semantics of a particular word; as long as it is sufficiently similar to the correct semantics, which is an attractor state, it will be pulled in (i.e., as

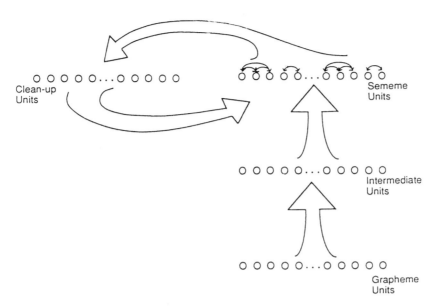

Figure 4-1
Hinton and Shallice's[11] PDP model of reading, in which visual graphemic representations are associated with semantic representations. Single lesions in this model produce a mixture of visual and semantic errors. (From Hinton and Shallice,[11] with permission.)

long as it falls in a region of activation space that slopes downward to the correct activation pattern, it will be transformed into that pattern). Damage to the network from the removal of units or connections distorts the shape of activation space. Figure 4-2 illustrates the normal attractor structure of a region of activation space containing *cot, cat,* and *bed* and the altered structure following damage to semantics. Whereas before damage, "cat" fell into the *cat* basin of attraction, after damage, the edges of the basins have shifted and "cat" falls into the *cot* basin of attraction. Thus, one need not hypothesize damage to visual representations to account for the visual errors in deep dyslexia.

Plaut and Shallice[12] have demonstrated the generality of Hinton and Shallice's account by replicating their simulation results with a variety of different networks, with different patterns of connectivity, and with different training procedures. As long as there are attractors that serve to transform input patterns whose similarity relations are based on visual appearance into semantic representations whose similarity relations are based on meaning, the landscape of the activation space will be organized by both visual and semantic similarity, and distortions of that landscape due

to network damage will result in both visual and semantic errors.

Neglect Dyslexia: Localizing the Functional Lesion

Patients with left visual neglect omit or misidentify letters on the left side of letter strings. When the letter string is a word, this pattern of performance is termed *neglect dyslexia* (see Chap. 18). Surprisingly, neglect dyslexics are more likely to report the initial letters of a word than of a nonword letter string, even when the initial letters of the word cannot simply be guessed on the basis of the end of the word.[13] This seems to imply that the breakdown in the processing of neglected stimuli comes at a late stage, after word recognition, for how else could lexical status (word versus nonword) affect performance?

The concept of attractors is helpful here, too, in localizing the functional lesion in neglect dyslexia at a stage prior to visual pattern recognition. Mozer and Behrmann[14] simulated neglect dyslexia by damaging the attentional mechanism in a computational model of printed word recognition so that attention is distributed asymmetri-

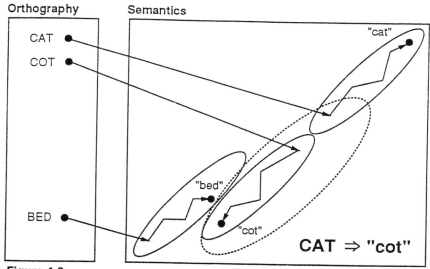

Figure 4-2

Part of the activation space of the Hinton and Shallice model, as represented by Plaut and Shallice,[12] showing attractors for three words. After damage to semantic units, the basins of attraction shift from those shown in solid lines to those shown in dotted lines, resulting in visual errors. (From Plaut and Shallice,[12] with permission.)

cally over letter strings. In their model, attention *precedes* word recognition. In fact, it gates the flow of information out of early visual feature maps. Neglect therefore results in full information from the right side of a letter string but only partial information from the left being transmitted to word representations.

According to this model, the errors that occur with nonword letter strings result from partial visual information about the letter features on the left side of the string, which is not sufficient to identify precisely which letters are present. In contrast, the same partial information about the initial letters of a word, with good-quality information about the remaining letters of a word, will result in an activation pattern that is similar to the activation pattern for that word. Because known words are attractors, the network will settle into the pattern of the word, complete with initial letters. In this way, it is possible to explain why neglect dyslexics read words better than nonwords without giving up the hypothesis that neglect is a disorder of visual perception, affecting stimulus processing prior to the word recognition stage.

Computational models make predictions that can be tested empirically. According to this model of neglect dyslexia, if the asymmetry of attention is too extreme, no information about the initial letters will get through to word representations and the resulting activation state will not fall within the basin of attraction for the word. Behrmann and colleagues tested this prediction with a patient who had severe neglect.[15] As predicted, he did not show better perception of the initial letters of words than of nonwords. Furthermore, when his attention was drawn to the left and the attentional asymmetry thereby was made less extreme, he then showed the usual difference between word and nonword letter strings. Conversely, a patient who normally showed this difference between words and nonwords was stopped from doing so by attentional manipulations that increased his attentional asymmetry.

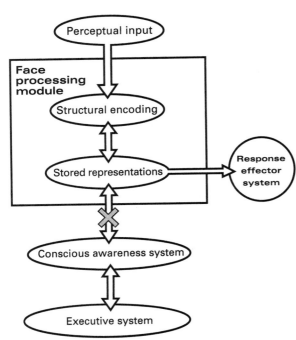

Figure 4-3
*A model proposed by De Haan, Bauer, and Greve[16]
to account for covert face recognition in prosopagnosia. There is a separate mechanism hypothesized
for conscious awareness, distinct from the mechanisms of face recognition, and covert recognition is
explained by a lesion at location 1, disconnecting
the two parts of the model. (From De Haan et al.,[16]
with permission.)*

Covert Face Recognition: Dissociation without Separate Systems

Prosopagnosia is an impairment of face recognition that can occur relatively independently of impairments in object recognition. A number of recent findings seem to suggest that the underlying
impairment, in at least some patients, is not in face
recognition per se but in awareness of recognition.
This would seem to imply that recognition and
awareness depend on dissociable and distinct
brain systems, as shown in Fig. 4-3.[16] My colleagues and I built a computer simulation that is
able to account for covert recognition in three
very different tasks.[17] The network is shown in
Fig. 4-4 and consists of face recognition units, semantic knowledge units, and name units (embod-
ying knowledge of people's facial appearance,
general information about them, and their names,
respectively). Hidden units were interposed between these layers to assist the network in learning to associate faces and names by way of semantic information. There is no part of the network
that is dedicated to awareness.

The first finding to be simulated was that
some prosopagnosics can learn to associate facial
photographs with names faster when the pairings
are true (e.g., Harrison Ford's face with Harrison

Figure 4-4
*A model proposed by Farah, Vecera, and O'Reilly[17]
to account for covert face recognition in prosopagnosia. The dissociation between overt and covert face
recognition emerges when the face-recognition system is damaged. (From Farah et al.,[17] with permission.)*

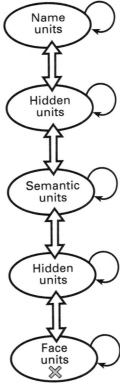

Ford's name) than when they are false (e.g., Harrison Ford's face with Michael Douglas's name).[18] This result was initially taken to imply that these patients were recognizing the faces normally and that the breakdown in processing lay downstream from vision, as shown in Fig. 4-3. However, when some of the face units were eliminated from our model, thus simulating a lesion in the visual system, the network also re-learned old face-name pairings faster than new ones. Why should this be? Recall that learning can be viewed as a process of moving through weight space. After damage, the network is in a high-error region of weight space for both old face-name pairings and new ones, and for this reason the network cannot overtly associate any faces with any names. However, that region of weight space is closer to a low-error region for the old pairings than for the new ones, because the residual weights (connecting intact units) have the correct values for the old pairings, and the learning process is therefore shorter.

A second finding, that previously familiar faces are perceived more quickly in the context of a same/different matching task, has also been interpreted as evidence for intact visual face pro-cessing.[18] However, after lesions to the face units in our model, the remaining face units settled into a stable state faster for previously familiar face patterns. This can be understood in terms of the distortion of the network's attractor structure after damage. The original structure was designed to take familiar face patterns as input and settle quickly to a stable state. After damage, these pat-terns will still find themselves on downward-sloping parts of the energy landscape more often than novel patterns, even if the energy minima into which they roll have changed.

Finally, in a task that requires classifying a printed name as belonging to an actor or a politi-cian, a face from the opposite occupational cate-gory shown in the background slows the responses of both normal subjects and a prosopagnosic, again implying that the face is recognized despite prosopagnosia.[18] In simulating this finding, face units were removed until the network's overt per-formance at classifying faces according to occupa-tion was as poor as the patient's. At this level of damage, wrong-category faces slowed perfor-mance in the name-classification task. This can be understood in terms of the distributed nature of representation in neural networks, which allows for partial representation of information when some but not all units representing a face have been eliminated. The partial information gener-ally raises the activation of the appropriate down-stream occupation units, thus biasing their responses to the printed names, but it is not gener-ally able to raise their activations above threshold to allow an explicit response to faces.

REFERENCES

1. Newell A, Simon HA: *Human Problem Solving.* Englewood Cliffs, NJ: Prentice Hall, 1972.
2. Rumelhart DE, McClelland JL: *Parallel Distributed Processing: Explorations in the Microstructure of Cognition.* Cambridge, MA: MIT Press, 1986.
3. Anderson JA: *An Introduction to Neural Networks.* Cambridge, MA: MIT Press, 1995.
4. Bechtel W, Abrahamsen A: *Connectionism and the Mind.* Cambridge, MA: Blackwell, 1991.
5. Hebb DO: *The Organization of Behavior.* New York: Wiley, 1949.
6. Linsker R: From basic network principles to neural architecture: Emergence of orientation-selective cells. *Proc Natl Acad Sci USA* 83:8390–8394, 1986.
7. Ritter H: Self-organizing maps for internal repre-sentations. *Psychol Res* 52:128–136, 1990.
8. Kohonen T: *Self-Organizing Maps.* New York: Springer-Verlag, 1995.
9. Jackson JH: On the anatomical and physiological localization of movements in the brain. *Lancet* 1:84–85, 162–164, 232–234, 1873.
10. Farah MJ: Neuropsychological inference with an in-teractive brain. *Behav Brain Sci* 17:90–104, 1994.
11. Hinton GE, Shallice T: Lesioning an attractor net-work: Investigations of acquired dyslexia. *Psychol Rev* 98:96–121, 1991.
12. Plaut DC, Shallice T: Deep dyslexia: A case study of connectionist neuropsychology. *Cog Neuropsy-chol* 10:377–500, 1993.
13. Sieroff E, Pollatsek A, Posner MI: Recognition of visual letter strings following injury to the posterior visual spatial attention system. *Cog Neuropsychol* 5:427–449, 1988.

14. Mozer MC, Behrmann M: On the interaction of selective attention and lexical knowledge: A connectionist account of neglect dyslexia. *J Cog Neurosci* 2:96–123, 1990.

15. Behrmann M, Moscovitch M, Black S, Mozer M: Perceptual and conceptual mechanisms in neglect dyslexia: Two contrasting case studies. *Brain* 113:1163–1183, 1990.

16. De Haan EHF, Bauer RM, Greve KW: Behavioral and physiological evidence for covert recognition in a prosopagnosic patient. *Cortex* 28:77–95, 1992.

17. Farah MJ, O'Reilly RC, Vecera SP: Dissociated overt and covert recognition as a emergent property of lesioned attractor networks. *Psychol Rev* 100:751–788, 1993.

18. De Haan EHF, Young AW, Newcombe F: Face recognition without awareness. *Cog Neuropsychol* 4:385–415, 1987.

Chapter 5

ANATOMIC PRINCIPLES IN COGNITIVE NEUROSCIENCE

M.-Marsel Mesulam

The student of human neuroanatomy faces many challenges. There is no universal agreement on terminology, no distinct boundaries that completely separate one region from another, and, in most instances, no one-to-one correspondence among lobar designations, traditional topographic landmarks, cytoarchitectonic boundaries, and behavioral specializations. One part of the brain can have more than one descriptive name and cytoarchitectonic (striate cortex), functional (primary visual cortex), and topographic (calcarine cortex) terms can be used interchangeably to designate the same area.

Cytoarchitectonic maps, especially that of Brodmann,[1] have introduced a useful and widely used approach to the parcellation of the cerebral hemispheres. Brodmann delineated individual architectonic areas on the basis of microscopic criteria. In contemporary usage, however, a statement such as "activation was seen in area 9" almost invariably means that the investigator estimated the area of activation to be in a part of the hemisphere analogous to the part that Brodmann designated area 9. This usage can lead to potential inaccuracies, since the topographic fit between the imaged brain slice and Brodmann's hand-drawn brain may not be exact and there may be interindividual differences in the distribution of cytoarchitectonic areas. Brodmann's map is also quite unclear about cytoarchitectonic designations for sulcal banks, which contain a very significant proportion of the cerebral cortex.

There is no immediate solution to these difficulties, but it is important to be aware of their existence. In this chapter, descriptive neuroanatomic designations are used whenever possible. For example, with regard to primary auditory cortex, the term *Heschl's gyrus,* which refers to an easily identifiable topographic landmark, is preferred to a cytoarchitectonic designation such as *area 41-42,* which is based on microscopic critera. When used, cytoarchitectonic designations follow the nomenclature of Brodmann. Since the anatomic information in this chapter is highly condensed, the reader may want to consult more comprehensive treatments of this subject by Brodmann (now available in English translation[1]), Duvernoy,[2] Nieuwenhuys and coworkers,[3] Pandya and Yeterian,[4] and Mesulam.[5]

Neurons of the central nervous system are engaged in three major operations: (1) reception and registration of sensory stimuli from outside and from within (input); (2) planning and execution of complex motor acts (output); and (3) intermediary processing interposed between input and output. Thought, language, memory, self-awareness and even many aspects of mood and affect constitute different manifestations of intermediary processing. The neural substrates for these intermediary processes are located principally within the limbic system and cortical association areas. From a behavioral point of view, therefore, the cerebral hemispheres can be divided into four major components: primary sensory cortex, primary motor cortex, association cortex, and limbic-paralimbic cortex (Table 5-1). It is the latter

Table 5-1

Types of cortical areas and their corresponding Brodmann numbers

Primary Sensory and Motor Cortex

Primary visual (area 17)

Primary auditory (areas 41, 42)

Primary somatosensory (areas 1, 2, 3 but mostly area 3b)

Primary motor (area 4 and caudal part of area 6)

Association Cortex

Unimodal visual (areas 18, 19, 20, 21, ? 37)

Unimodal auditory (area 22)

Unimodal somatosensory (area 5, rostral area 7)

Unimodal motor (rostral area 6, caudal area 8, area 44)

Heteromodal prefrontal (areas 9, 10, 11, 45, 46, 47, ? rostral area 8, rostral area 12, rostral area 32)

Heteromodal parietotemporal (areas 39, 40, caudal area 7, banks of superior temporal sulcus, ? area 36)

Limbic System (cortical components)

Corticoid formations (amygdala, substantia innominata, septal nuclei)

Allocortex (hippocampus, pyriform olfactory cortex)

Paralimbic cortex [insula (areas 14, 15), temporopolar cortex (area 38), caudal orbitofrontal cortex (caudal areas 11, 12, 13), cingulate complex (areas 23, 24, 33, 31, 26, 29) parolfactory region (area 25, caudal area 32), parahippocampal cortex (areas 28, 34, 35, 30)]

two components, those associated with intermediary processing, that are most relevant to behavioral neurology and neuropsychology and which will receive the most emphasis in this chapter.

CORTICAL TYPES

Regions of the cerebral cortex display a variety of architectures. The simplest type of cortex is located in the basal forebrain. Components of the basal forebrain such as the septal nuclei, the substantia innominata, and the amygdaloid complex are situated directly on the ventral and medial surface of the hemispheres and are thus considered part of the cortical mantle. These structures contain the simplest and most undifferentiated type of cortex. The organization of the constituent neurons is rudimentary and no consistent lamination or dendritic orientation can be discerned. These three components of the basal forebrain could be designated as having a "corticoid," or cortexlike, structure. Corticoid areas (especially the amygdala) have architectonic features that are in part cortical and in part nuclear.[5]

The next stage of cortical differentiation is known as allocortex. This type of cortex contains one or two principal bands of neurons arranged into moderately differentiated layers. The two allocortical formations of the brain are (1) the hippocampal formation, which also carries the designation of archicortex, and (2) the piriform or primary olfactory cortex, which is also known as paleocortex. Corticoid and allocortical formations collectively make up the limbic zone of cortex.

The next level of structural complexity is encountered in the paralimbic zone of the cerebral cortex (Fig. 5-1). These areas are intercalated between allocortex and isocortex so as to provide a gradual transition from one to the other. Allocortical cell layers often extend into the periallocortical component of paralimbic areas. Several gradual changes in the direction of increased complexity and differentiation occur from the allocortical toward the isocortical side of paralimbic regions. These changes include (1) progressively greater accumulation of small granular neurons in layer IV and then in layer II, (2) sublamination and columnization of layer III, (3) differentiation of layer V from layer VI and of layer VI from the underlying white matter, and (4) an increase of intracortical myelin, especially along the outer layer of Baillarger (layer IV).

There are five major paralimbic formations in the primate brain: (1) the caudal orbitofrontal cortex; (2) the insula; (3) the temporal pole; (4) the parahippocampal gyrus (includes the entorhinal, prorhinal, perirhinal, presubicular, and parasub-icular areas); and (5) the cingulate complex (includes the retrosplenial, cingulate, and parolfactory areas). These five paralimbic regions form

Figure 5-1

Distribution of functional zones in relation to Brodmann's map of the human brain. The boundaries are not intended to be precise. Much of this information is based on experimental evidence obtained from laboratory animals and must be confirmed in the human brain. Abbreviations: AA = auditory association cortex; AG = angular gyrus; A1 = primary auditory cortex; CG = cingulate cortex; F = fusiform gyrus; INS = insula; IPL = inferior parietal lobule; IT = inferior temporal gyrus; MA = motor association cortex; MPO = medial parietooccipital area; MT = middle temporal gyrus; M1 = primary motor area; OF = orbitofrontal region; PC = prefrontal cortex; PH = parahippocampal region; PO = parolfactory area; PS = peristriate cortex; RS = retrosplenial area; SA = somatosensory association cortex; SG = supramarginal gyrus; SPL = superior parietal lobule; ST = superior temporal gyrus; S1 = primary somatosensory area; TP = temporopolar cortex; VA = visual association cortex; V1 = primary visual cortex. (From Mesulam,[5] with permission.)

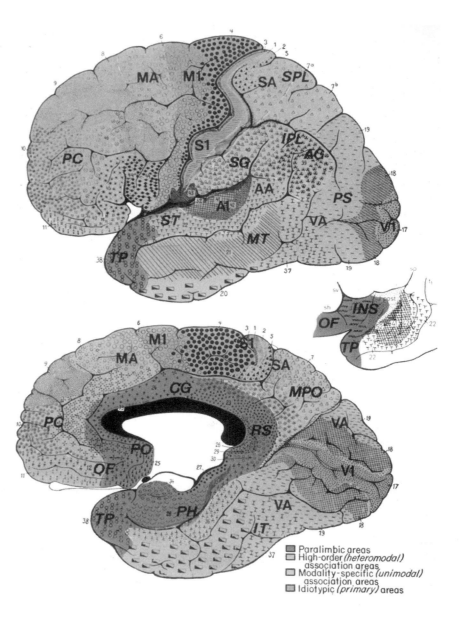

an uninterrupted girdle surrounding the medial and basal aspects of the cerebral hemispheres.[6]

The greatest extent of the cortical surface in the human brain consists of six-layered homotypical isocortex, also known as association cortex. Association isocortex can be subdivided into two major types: modality-specific (unimodal) isocortex and high-order (heteromodal) isocortex. Unimodal association isocortex is defined by three essential characteristics: (1) the constituent neurons are almost exclusively responsive to stimulation in only a single sensory modality; (2) the predominant cortical inputs are provided by the primary sensory cortex or by other unimodal regions in that same modality; (3) damage yields modality-specific deficits confined to tasks guided by cues in that modality.

The unimodal areas for the three major sensory modalities have been determined experimentally in the brain of the macaque monkey. Such experiments have shown that the superior temporal gyrus is the unimodal auditory association area, that the superior parietal lobule provides the somatosensory unimodal association area, and that the peristriate, midtemporal, and inferotemporal regions provide the unimodal association regions in the visual modality.[5]

The heteromodal component of isocortex is identified by the following characteristics: (1) neuronal responses are not confined to any single sensory modality, (2) the cortical inputs originate from unimodal areas in more than one modality and/or from other heteromodal areas, and (3) damage to this type of cortex leads to deficits that transcend any single modality. Some neurons in heteromodal association areas respond to stimulation in more than one modality, indicating the presence of direct multimodal convergence. More commonly, however, there is an admixture of neurons with different preferred modalities. Defined in this fashion, heteromodal cortex includes the types of regions that have been designated as high-order association cortex, polymodal cortex, multimodal cortex, polysensory areas, and supramodal cortex.[5]

There are essentially two and perhaps three major heteromodal fields in the brain of the monkey. One is in the prefrontal region, including the anterior orbitofrontal surface and the dorsolateral frontal convexity. The second heteromodal field includes the inferior parietal lobule and extends into the banks of the superior temporal sulcus and perhaps into parts of the midtemporal gyrus. There may be a third heteromodal region in the posterior part of the ventral temporal lobe.

There are some relatively subtle architectonic differences between unimodal and heteromodal areas. In general, the unimodal areas have a more differentiated organization, especially with respect to sublamination in layers III and V, columnarization in layer III, and more extensive granularization in layer IV and especially layer II. On these architectonic grounds, it would appear that heteromodal cortex is closer in structure to paralimbic cortex and that it provides a stage in the hierarchy of architectonic differentiation intercalated between paralimbic and unimodal areas.

The koniocortex of primary sensory areas and the macropyramidal cortex of the primary motor region constitute unique and highly specialized regions that can be designated as having an idiotypic architecture. There are two divergent opinions about these primary areas. One is to consider them as the most basic and elementary components of cortex; the other is to see these areas as the most advanced and highly differentiated components of the cortical mantle. I favor the latter point of view. The location of idiotypic regions is well known: the primary visual area covers the occipital pole and the banks of the calcarine fissure, the primary auditory cortex covers Heschl's gyrus on the supratemporal plane, the primary somatosensory cortex covers the postcentral gyrus, and the primary motor area is located in the precentral gyrus.

A GENERAL PLAN OF ORGANIZATION FOR PATTERNS OF BEHAVIORAL SPECIALIZATION AND NEURAL CONNECTIVITY IN CORTEX

The preceding discussion shows that the hemispheric surface can be subdivided into five zones (limbic, paralimbic, unimodal, heteromodal, and idiotypic) which collectively provide a spectrum of cytoarchitectonic differentiation ranging from the simplest to the most differentiated (Fig. 5-1).

All types of cortical areas, including association isocortex, receive direct hypothalamic projections.[7] For the great majority of cortical regions, this hypothalamic input is quite minor. The only exception is provided by the limbic structures. Thus, the septal nuclei, basal nucleus of the substantia innominata, amygdaloid complex, piriform cortex, and hippocampus stand out by the presence of substantial hypothalamic connections. Another major source of connections for limbic structures originates in the paralimbic zone. For example, the amygdala receives an extensive cortical input from the insula; the hippocampus from the entorhinal sector of the parahippocampal region; and the piriform cortex as well as the nucleus basalis from insular, temporopolar, and orbitofrontal paralimbic areas. Paralimbic areas have extensive monosynaptic connections with limbic and heteromodal areas; heteromodal areas with paralimbic and unimodal areas; unimodal areas with primary and heteromodal areas. Primary areas derive their major cortical connections from unimodal areas and major subcortical connections from the relevant thalamic relay nuclei.[5]

These patterns are relative rather than absolute. For example, the amygdala is also known to receive direct input from association isocortex, but this does not appear to be as substantial as the connections of this limbic structure with the hypothalamus and with paralimbic regions. In some cases, however, there are more rigid distinctions. The primary areas in the more advanced primates, for example, do not seem to receive any limbic or paralimbic cortical input. This may ensure that the initial processing of sensory information is not influenced by drive and mood. Perhaps this is why emotional state does not alter the shape of an object or the pitch of a sound. The adaptive value of this arrangement is evident. In other mammalian species such as the rat, however, this separation may be less complete, since direct connectivity between primary and paralimbic areas has been reported.[8]

Many cortical areas have connections with other constituents of the same functional zone.

These are extremely well developed within the limbic, paralimbic, and heteromodal zones. For example, of all the cortical neurons that directly projected to a subsector of prefrontal heteromodal cortex, 26 percent were located within unimodal areas, 13 percent in paralimbic regions, and 61 percent in other heteromodal cortex.[9] Furthermore, the insula as well as the cingulate cortex have interconnections with virtually each of the other paralimbic regions of the brain. Although unimodal regions may receive extensive input from other unimodal areas in the same modality, there is essentially no interconnectivity between areas belonging to different modalities. In a similar vein, except for the intimate interconnections between the primary somatosensory and motor areas, there are no neural projections among primary areas belonging to separate modalities. It appears, therefore, that there is a premium on channel width within the limbic, paralimbic, and heteromodal zones, whereas the emphasis is on fidelity within the unimodal and primary zones.

As noted above, the corticoid and allocortical areas, collectively designated as "limbic" structures, are the parts of the cerebral cortex that have the closest association with the hypothalamus. Through neural and also hormonal mechanisms, the hypothalamus is in a position to coordinate electrolyte balance, blood glucose levels, basal temperature, metabolic rate, autonomic tone, sexual phase, circadian oscillations, and even immunoregulation. The hypothalamus is essentially the head ganglion of the internal milieu and also a major coordinating structure for drives and instincts that promote the survival of the self and of the species. In keeping with these functions of the hypothalamus, areas in the limbic zone of the cerebral cortex assume an important role in the regulation of behaviors such as memory and learning, the modulation of drive, the emotional coloring of experience, and the higher control of hormonal balance and autonomic tone. These specializations of limbic structures are related to the maintenance of the internal milieu (homeostasis) as well as to the associated operations necessary for the preservation of the self and the species.[5]

At the other pole of the cytoarchitectonic

spectrum lie the most highly specialized primary sensory and motor areas. These are the parts of cortex that are most closely related to the extrapersonal space, since sensory input from the environment has its first cortical relay in primary koniocortical areas and motor cortex coordinates actions that lead to the manipulation of the extrapersonal world.

Intercalated between these two extremes, the zones of association and paralimbic cortex provide neural bridges that link the internal milieu to the extrapersonal environment. The heteromodal and unimodal areas are predominantly involved in perceptual elaboration and motor planning, whereas the paralimbic zone is involved predominantly in directing drive and emotion to the appropriate extrapersonal and intrapsychic targets. Collectively, the unimodal, heteromodal, and paralimbic areas enable the needs of the individual to be discharged according to relevant opportunities and limitations that exist in the environment.

Within the group of isocortical association areas, the unimodal association cortices provide the principal neuronal machinery for the modality-specific elaboration and encoding of sensory input. Unimodal areas can be divided into *upstream* and *downstream* components. Upstream components receive their major modality-specific information directly from the corresponding primary area, whereas the downstream areas receive their major modality-specific input from the corresponding upstream unimodal areas. In the visual modality, for example, the peristriate region (areas 18 and 19), constitutes an upstream unimodal association area, whereas inferotemporal cortex (areas 20 and 21) constitutes a downstream unimodal association area.

Heteromodal cortex receives convergent input from multiple unimodal areas, especially downstream unimodal areas, whereas paralimbic cortex acts as a relay between sensory association cortices and the limbic zone of the cerebral cortex.[4] Heteromodal and paralimbic formations support two major types of neural processing: (1) the associative linkage of unimodal sensory information into distributed templates that encode multimodal knowledge and (2) the integration of this information with drive and emotion. In contrast to the idiotypic and unimodal belts, which are characterized by relatively more "dedicated" and homogeneous neural mechanisms confined to single modalities of information processing, the heteromodal and paralimbic areas support a more "generalized" type of processing, with heterogeneous input-output relationships, so that no uniform behavioral specialization can be assigned to individual components of the paralimbic and heteromodal zones.

SUBCORTICAL STRUCTURES: STRIATUM AND THALAMUS

The striatum can be divided into three components: the caudate, the putamen, and the olfactory tubercle-nucleus accumbens complex. Each striatal component receives cortical input but none projects back to the cortex. The caudate and putamen, which are also collectively designated as the dorsal striatum, receive cortical input predominantly from association cortex and primary idiotypic areas. The dopaminergic input to these striatal components originates in the pars compacta of the substantia nigra. The cortical input to the olfactory tubercle-nucleus accumbens complex originates in limbic and paralimbic parts of the brain. The nucleus accumbens, for example, receives convergent input from the amygdala and the hippocampus. On the basis of this connectivity pattern, the nucleus accumbens-olfactory tubercle complex can be designated as the limbic striatum.[10] The dopaminergic innervation of the limbic striatum originates in the ventral tegmental area of Tsai, which is just medial to the substantia nigra, and dopamine turnover is higher in the limbic striatum than in the neostriatum.[11]

All parts of cortex project to the striatum. These corticostriatal projections obey a complex topographic arrangement. One feature of this arrangement is that the input from each cortical area forms multiple patches of axonal terminals within the striatum. Yeterian and Van Hoesen[12] made the interesting suggestion that terminal patches from separate cortical areas are more likely to show partial overlap if the relevant cortical areas are interconnected with each other. This implies that there may be some replication of corticocortical interaction patterns within the striatum.

The caudate may have a lesser role than the putamen in motor control. For example, motor cortex projects to the putamen but not to the caudate.[13] The head of the caudate receives most of its input from dorsolateral prefrontal cortex. It is therefore interesting to note that lesions in the head of the caudate yield deficits that are essentially identical to those that emerge upon ablating prefrontal cortex.[14] This raises the possibility that each striatal region may have behavioral specializations similar to those of the cortical area, from which it receives its major cortical input.

Lesions in the head of the caudate and in the putamen have been associated with aphasia and also with unilateral neglect. However, in almost all such cases the adjacent white matter is also involved, so that it is not possible to determine whether these deficits reflect damage to the striatum or to the adjacent fibers, which interconnect cortical areas related to language and attention. We have seen one ambidextrous patient with multi-infarct dementia who also had a substantial infarction in the head of the left caudate. This patient had no motor deficit, aphasia, or amnesia. His mental state deficits were characterized by a severe lack of judgment, insight, and planning. This patient raises the possibility that damage to the head of the caudate may give rise to mental changes similar to those seen in conjunction with prefrontal cortex lesions.[5]

The globus pallidus of the primate has four easily identifiable components: (1) the outer (lateral) segment, (2) the inner (medial) segment, (3) the ventral pallidum, and (4) the pars reticulata of the substantia nigra. The globus pallidus receives projections from the striatum and projects to the thalamus. The globus pallidus is thus an essential link in the striatopallidothalamocortical loops, which are thought to have important organizing roles in a number of complex behavioral domains.

There is essentially no disagreement about the crucial role of the globus pallidus in motor control. In humans, lesions of the globus pallidus are frequently associated with severe extrapyramidal disturbances. However, the relationship of the globus pallidus to movement may be quite complex and appears to involve substantial sensorimotor integration. For example, local cooling in the area of the globus pallidus in monkeys yields a severe and reversible breakdown of a learned flexion-extension movement, but only when the animal is blindfolded. In the presence of visual input, the deficit is no longer observed.[15]

The medial zone of the inner pallidal segment and also the ventral pallidum have close associations with limbic structures. For example, in contrast to the more dorsal parts of the pallidum, which receive their striatal input from the caudate and putamen, the ventral pallidum receives its major striatal projections from the nucleus accumbens. Furthermore, a substantial number of ventral pallidal neurons respond to amygdaloid stimulation.[16]

In the monkey, the core of the internal pallidal segment projects to the motor thalamus. However, a medial crescent of this pallidal segment projects predominantly to the lateral habenula, which is generally considered as a structure closely related to the limbic regions of the brain.[17] In keeping with this anatomic pattern, some types of pallidal lesions interfere with behaviors generally associated with limbic mechanisms. For example, MacLean[18] showed that damage to the medial globus pallidus of monkeys severely disrupts species-specific sexual display patterns. Thus, the ventral pallidum and the medial portion of the inner pallidal segment could be considered as having preferential limbic affiliations.

The pars reticulata of the substantia nigra is a caudal extension of the globus pallidus. There is evidence suggesting that this portion of the pallidal complex may participate in the programming of saccadic eye movements in response to actual or remembered targets.[19]

One function of the thalamus is to relay subcortical lemniscal inputs to cortical areas. Almost all thalamic nuclei have well-developed reciprocal connections with cortex. The one exception is the reticular nucleus, which receives subcortical and cortical input but does not project back to cortex.[20] There is very little interconnectivity among individual thalamic nuclei, so that there is very little interaction at the thalamic level among the different types of information that are being relayed to cortex. The one exception is provided by the reticular and intralaminar nuclei, which have extensive connections with other thalamic nuclei.

The large number of thalamic nuclei can be subdivided into several functional groups on the basis of their preferred cortical and subcortical projections.[5] The primary relay nuclei are the easiest to identify (Fig. 5-2). The caudal part of the ventroposterior lateral nucleus (VPL$_c$) and the principal division of the ventroposterior medial

nucleus (VPM) receive fibers from the medial lemniscus and quintothalamic tract and constitute the somatosensory relay nuclei of the thalamus. The lateral geniculate nucleus (LGN) and the part of the medial geniculate nucleus (MGN) that receives the brachium of the inferior colliculus are the primary relay nuclei for the visual and auditory modalities, respectively. Damage to the VPL$_c$ or to the LGN gives rise to hemihypesthesia and hemianopia, respectively. Since inputs from both ears reach the MGN in each hemisphere, unilateral damage to this thalamic nucleus does not lead to deafness in the contralateral ear. In fact, unilateral MGN lesions may be extremely difficult to detect clinically. The major thalamic input into primary motor cortex (M1) comes from the caudal ventrolateral nucleus (VL$_c$) and the oral ventroposterior lateral nucleus (VPL$_o$). The behavioral effects of lesions in these nuclei are poorly understood.

A second group of thalamic nuclei project predominantly to unimodal association areas (see Ref. 5 for a review of the evidence). In the rhesus monkey, the major thalamic projections to the somatosensory association cortex of the superior parietal lobule (area 5) come from the lateroposterior nucleus (LP) and perhaps also from the oral subdivision of the pulvinar nucleus (P$_o$). In the visual modality, the nuclei that provide the major projection to visual unimodal association areas include the inferior (P$_i$) and lateral (P$_l$) subdivisions of the pulvinar nucleus. In the auditory modality, the unimodal association region receives its major thalamic input from the anterior MGN and probably also from a ventral rim of the medial pulvinar. Thus, the MGN is the source of thalamic projections not only to A1 but also to the auditory association cortex. The motor association cortex receives its major thalamic input from the oral ventrolateral nucleus (VL$_o$) and from parts of the ventral anterior nucleus (VA).

A third group of thalamic nuclei have no specific modality affiliations and project predominantly to heteromodal and limbic cortex. The lateral part of the medial dorsal nucleus (MD) is the major thalamic nucleus for the prefrontal heteromodal fields, whereas the medial pulvinar nucleus (P$_m$) and parts of the adjacent lateral posterior nu-

Figure 5-2

Schematic diagram of the four major groups of thalamic nuclei. Abbreviations: AD = anterior dorsal; AM = anterior medial; AV = anterior ventral; LD = laterodorsal; LGN = lateral geniculate; LP = lateroposterior; MD = medialis dorsalis; MGN = medial geniculate; Pi = inferior pulvinar; Pl = lateral pulvinar; Pm = medial pulvinar; Po = oral pulvinar; VA = ventral anterior; VL = ventral lateral; VPL = ventroposterior lateral; VPM = ventroposterior medial. (From Mesulam,[5] with permission).

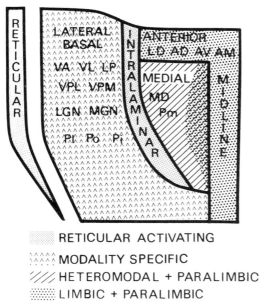

RETICULAR ACTIVATING

MODALITY SPECIFIC

HETEROMODAL + PARALIMBIC

LIMBIC + PARALIMBIC

cleus (LP) are the major nuclei for the heteromodal fields in the inferior parietal lobule and within the banks of the superior temporal sulcus.

The close interaction between cortical heteromodal and paralimbic zones is also reflected in the arrangement of thalamic connectivity patterns. Thus, the MD and P_m nuclei, which are the major nuclei for heteromodal cortical areas, also have extensive paralimbic connections. For example, the medial part of MD (including the magnocellular MD_{mc} component) is the major thalamic nucleus for the orbitofrontal paralimbic region, while the P_m has reciprocal projections with all components of the paralimbic belt and is probably the major nucleus for the temporopolar paralimbic area. The MD and P_m also have direct limbic connections. Thus, the medial and magnocellular parts of MD have connections with the amygdala, piriform cortex, and septal region. Furthermore, the P_m has also been shown to have reciprocal projections with the amygdaloid complex (see Ref. 5 for a review of the evidence).

Another group of dorsally and medially placed nuclei are collectively known as the nuclei of the "anterior tubercle." These nuclei include the anterior thalamic nucleus [including its dorsal (AD), ventral (AV), and medial (AM) components] and the laterodorsal nucleus (LD). They provide the major thalamic connections for the posterior cingulate cortex, the retrosplenial area, and some of the parahippocampal paralimbic areas. The anterior thalamic nucleus receives the mammillothalamic tract and is therefore an important component of the Papez circuit.

A number of nuclei that are situated close to the thalamic midline are collectively known as midline nuclei. These include the paratenial, paraventricular, subfascicular, central, and reuniens nuclei. These nuclei have extensive connections with paralimbic areas (e.g., temporal pole and anterior cingulate gyrus) and also with the hippocampal formation.

The effects of lesions in these nuclei are consistent with their patterns of cortical connectivity. For example, in the rhesus monkey, bilateral MD lesions reproduce deficits in spatial delayed alternation similar to those associated with prefrontal ablations.[21] On the other hand, more medial MD lesions, which also involve adjacent midline nuclei, lead to deficits in visual object recognition similar to those obtained after medial temporal ablations.[22] In some patients, even unilateral lesions in the more medial parts of the MD and in the anterior tubercle nuclei have been associated with severe amnestic conditions.[23] In Wernicke encephalopathy, involvement of the MD and P_m is thought to play a major role in the genesis of the amnestic state.[24] Lesions of the right pulvinar nucleus, including its medial component, have been described in conjunction with contralateral neglect for the left extrapersonal space.[25] Electrical stimulation of the left medial pulvinar has been reported to induce transient anomia.[26] These behavioral relations are consistent with the connections of the P_m with the parietotemporal parts of heteromodal cortex and with limbic-paralimbic structures.

A fourth group of thalamic nuclei are closely affiliated with the ascending reticular activating system. The reticular nucleus of the thalamus as well as the intralaminar nuclei (e.g., the limitans, paracentralis, centralis lateralis, centromedian, and parafascicularis) have strong associations with the ascending reticular activating pathways. In contrast to other thalamic nuclei, which have somewhat restricted projection zones, the intralaminar nuclei have more widespread connections and are also known as "diffuse projection nuclei."

THE ASCENDING RETICULAR ACTIVATING SYSTEM

The cerebral cortex has three sources of afferent neural projections: cortical, thalamic, and extrathalamic. The existence of corticocortical and thalamocortical projections had been established by classic neuroanatomic methodology. During the past 20 years, the advent of more powerful methods based on axonally transported tracers has helped to uncover a third set of subcortical but extrathalamic afferents with origins in the ventral tegmental area (dopaminergic), raphe nuclei (serotonergic), nucleus locus ceruleus (noradrenergic), hypothalamus (mostly histaminergic), and basal forebrain (cholinergic and GABAergic). These extrathalamic afferents exert a modulatory influence upon cortical activity and constitute important components of what is currently emerging as the modern concept of the ascending reticular activating system.[27]

Moruzzi and Magoun[28] had introduced the concept of a brainstem reticular activating system that acted to desynchronize the cortical electroencephalogram via a relay in the thalamus. Subsequent work revealed that a most important component in this system consists of a cholinergic reticulothalamic pathway that facilitates the activation of corticopetal relay neurons in the thalamus.[29–33] It is becoming quite clear that the original concept of the ascending reticular activating system (ARAS) needs to be expanded to include at least three interconnected sources of ascending projections, one in the brainstem, a second in the basal forebrain, and a third in the thalamus.

The brainstem contingent of the ascending activating pathways displays considerable complexity. In addition to ascending cholinergic projections from the laterodorsal tegmental and pedunculopontine nuclei, there are also dopaminergic projections from the substantia nigra–ventral tegmental area, serotonergic projections from the raphe nuclei, noradrenergic projections from the nucleus locus ceruleus, and excitatory amino acid projections from the rostral reticular formation.[27,34] The ascending monoaminergic projections are predominantly directed to the cerebral cortex (without a thalamic relay), whereas the ascending cholinergic and excitatory amino acid projections are directed predominantly to the thalamus. Although all thalamic nuclei receive cholinergic projections from the brainstem, the reticular and intralaminar nuclei are traditionally considered to have the most intimate relation to the ARAS.

The nucleus basalis of the substantia innominata provides the source of a very substantial cholinergic projection directed to the entire cerebral cortex and the amygdala. These projections have complex effects upon cortical neurons but generally tend to act as excitatory neuromodulators that increase the impact of behaviorally relevant sensory events upon cortical neurons.[35] The ascending corticopetal cholinergic projection originating from the nucleus basalis is a crucial telencephalic component of the ARAS.

The cerebral cortex is not only the target of ascending projections from the brainstem, basal forebrain, and thalamus but also the source of descending feedback projections to several components of the ARAS. Almost all parts of the cerebral cortex project to the reticular nucleus and therefore influence its inhibitory effect upon other thalamic nuclei.[20] The projection from the cerebral cortex to the reticular nucleus of the thalamus is mostly excitatory, whereas the projections to this thalamic nucleus from the brainstem cholinergic nuclei are inhibitory. The reticular nucleus is thus in a position to gate thalamocortical transmission in a way that reflects the integrated influence of the brainstem and cerebral cortex.

Although the basal forebrain projects to the entire cerebral cortex, it receives feedback projections from a very limited set of cortical areas, namely those that belong to the limbic and paralimbic zones of the cerebral cortex.[36] This asymmetry is a feature of all the other extrathalamic ascending pathways of the ARAS: they project widely to the cerebral cortex but receive very few reciprocal connections from the cerebral cortex.[37] These pathways of the ARAS collectively provide the physiologic matrix for modulating a wide range of cortical functions related to arousal and attention.

NEURAL NETWORKS

The anatomic substrate of individual cognitive domains takes the form of large-scale neurocognitive networks that contain interconnected cortical and subcortical nodes.[34] Each major node of such a network belongs to multiple intersecting networks. Consequently, the same cognitive domain may be disrupted after damage to several different regions of the brain, and damage confined to a single region may yield more than one type of cognitive deficit.

At least four large-scale neurocognitive networks can be identified in the human brain: the left hemisphere language network, the right hemisphere attentional network, the limbic system, and the frontal network.[34] The major cortical nodes of the language network are located in Broca's area (areas 44 and 45) and Wernicke's area (posterior part of area 22 and parts of areas 39 and 40) of the left hemisphere. These two nodes are interconnected with several perisylvian cortical areas and with specific regions of the thalamus and striatum. Damage to components of this network leads to distinct aphasic disturbances whose clinical features reflect the specializations of the primary lesion site. The three major cortical nodes of the attentional network are located in the frontal cortex, posterior parietal cortex, and cingulate gyrus of the right hemisphere. Damage to cortical or subcortical components of this network leads to the various manifestations of the spatial neglect syndrome. The limbic system includes the limbic and paralimbic cortical areas, limbic striatum, limbic nuclei of the thalamus, and hypothalamus. Damage to components of this network leads to deficits of retentive memory, emotion, motivation, and affiliative behaviors. The frontal network includes the heteromodal and paralimbic cortices of the frontal lobes, the head of the caudate nucleus, and the mediodorsal nucleus of the thalamus. Damage to components of this network leads to complex deficits of the attentional matrix, personality, and comportment.

Experimental investigation of interconnections between major cortical nodes of individual networks shows that pairs of such areas are interconnected not only with each other but also with an additional set of identical cortical areas.[38] This architecture of connectivity is compatible with parallel and distributed processing. In resolving a cognitive problem, a set of cortical areas interconnected in this fashion can execute an extremely rapid survey of a vast informational landscape until the entire system settles into a best fit with respect to the multiple goals and constraints engendered by the problem.[34] This computational architecture is quite compatible with cognitive tasks such as deciding which words best express a thought or how to reconstruct a specific complex

memory. There are no single "correct" solutions to such tasks but an entire family of possibilities, each leading to a different compromise within the relevant matrix of goals and constraints.

Anatomic experiments have shown that members of an interconnected pair of cortical areas in a network are likely to send interdigitating and partially overlapping projections to the striatum.[12] The striatum receives cortical input but does not project back to cortex and could act as an "efference synchronizer" for the set of cortical areas in a large-scale network.[34] Cortical areas have extensive corticocortical connections, so that each member of the association cortex is likely to belong to multiple intersecting networks. Thalamic subnuclei, however, have almost no interconnections among each other and may thus play an important role in setting coactivation boundaries for individual networks.[34] Cortical components, together with corresponding regions of the thalamus, striatum, and reticular pathways, make up large-scale distributed networks that provide the immediate anatomic substrates of individual cognitive domains.

Several computational models can be proposed for understanding how the central nervous system converts simple sensory input into knowledge and experience. One possibility is to postulate the existence of a hierarchical synaptic chain for the transfer of information from primary sensory areas first to upstream unimodal areas, then to downstream unimodal areas, and finally to multimodal areas where knowledge is encoded in convergent form. This convergent encoding model faces several serious objections.[39] An alternative selectively distributed processing model proposes that the most veridical building blocks of experience are encoded at the level of unimodal rather than heteromodal association cortex.[39,40] According to this model, heteromodal, paralimbic, and limbic areas of the cerebral cortex provide transmodal nodes for binding this modality-specific information into coherent but distributed (nonconvergent) multidimensional knowledge. Lesions that interrupt the flow of information within unimodal areas or from unimodal to transmodal areas result in disconnection syndromes such as pure alexia, pure word deafness, and pro-sopagnosia.[41]

Depending on their location, connectivity, and affiliations with specific large-scale networks, individual transmodal zones provide critical nodes for coordinating complex mental phenomena in the realms of memory encoding, retrieval, object recognition, language comprehension, and spatial awareness. The cerebral substrate for cognition is thus both distributed and regionally specialized but neither modular nor diffuse. This model, based predominantly on the anatomic organization of the cerebral cortex, lends itself to a variety of experimental approaches for probing the complex relationship between cerebral structure and cognitive phenomena.

REFERENCES

1. Brodmann K: *Localisation in the Cerebral Cortex.* London: Smith-Gordon, 1994.
2. Duvernoy H: *The Human Brain.* Vienna: Springer-Verlag, 1991.
3. Nieuwenhuys R, Voogd J, van Huijzen C: *The Human Central Nervous System.* Berlin: Springer-Verlag, 1988.
4. Pandya DN, Yeterian EH: Architecture and connections of cortical association areas, in Peters A, Jones EG (eds): *Cerebral Cortex.* New York: Plenum Press, 1985, vol 4, pp 3–61.
5. Mesulam M-M: Patterns in behavioral neuroanatomy: Association areas, the limbic system, and hemispheric specialization, in Mesulam M-M (ed): *Principles of Behavioral Neurology.* Philadelphia: Davis, 1985, pp 1–70.
6. Mesulam M-M, Mufson EJ: Insula of the old world monkey: I. Architectonics in the insulo-orbito-temporal component of the paralimbic brain. *J Comp Neurol* 212:1–22, 1982.
7. Mesulam M-M, Mufson EJ, Levey AI, Wainer BH: Cholinergic innervation of cortex by the basal forebrain: Cytochemistry and cortical connections of the septal area, diagonal band nuclei, nucleus basalis (substantia innominata), and hypothalamus in the rhesus monkey. *J Comp Neurol* 214:170–197, 1983.
8. Vogt BA, Miller MW: Cortical connections between rat cingulate cortex and visual motor and postsubicular cortices. *J Comp Neurol* 216:192–210, 1983.
9. Barbas H, Mesulam M-M: Organization of afferent input to subdivisions of area 8 in the rhesus monkey. *J Comp Neurol* 200:407–431, 1981.
10. Heimer L, Wilson RD: The subcortical projections of the allocortex: Similarities in the neural associations of the hippocampus, the piriform cortex and the neocortex, in Santini M (ed): *Golgi Centennial Symposium: Proceedings.* New York: Raven Press, 1975, pp 177–193.
11. Walsh FX, Thomas TJ, Langlais PJ, Bird ED: Dopamine and homovanillic acid concentrations in striatal and limbic regions of the human brain. *Ann Neurol* 12:52–55, 1982.
12. Yeterian EH, Van Hoesen GW: Cortico-striate projections in the rhesus monkey: The organization of certain cortico-caudate connections. *Brain Res* 139:43–63, 1978.
13. Künzle H: Bilateral projections from precentral motor cortex to the putamen and other parts of the basal ganglia: An autoradiographic study in *Macaca fascicularis. Brain Res* 88:195–209, 1975.
14. Iversen SD: Behavior after neostriatal lesions in animals, in Divac I, Oberg RGE (eds): *The Neostriatum.* Oxford: Pergamon Press, 1979.
15. Horel J, Meyer-Lohmann J, Brooks VB: Basal ganglia cooling disables learned arm movements of monkeys in the absence of visual guidance. *Science* 195:584–586, 1977.
16. Yim CY, Mogenson GJ: Response of ventral pallidal neurons to amygdala stimulation and its modulation by dopamine projections to nucleus accumbens. *J Neurophysiol* 50:148–161, 1983.
17. Parent A, de Bellefeuille L: Organization of efferent projections from the internal segment of the globus pallidus in primate as revealed by fluorescence retrograde labeling method. *Brain Res* 245:201–213, 1982.
18. MacLean PD: Effects of lesions of globus pallidus on species-specific display behavior of squirrel monkey. *Brain Res* 149:175–196, 1978.
19. Hikosaka O, Wurtz RH: Visual and oculomotor functions of monkey substantia nigra pars reticulata: III. Memory-contingent visual and saccade responses. *J Neurophysiol* 49:1268–1284, 1983.
20. Jones EG: Some aspects of the organization of the thalamic reticular complex. *J Comp Neurol* 162:285–308, 1975.
21. Isseroff A, Rosvold HE, Galkin TW, Goldman-Rakic PS: Spatial memory impairments following damage to the mediodorsal nucleus of the thalamus in rhesus monkeys. *Brain Res* 232:97–113, 1982.

22. Aggleton JP, Mishkin M: Visual recognition impairment following medial thalamic lesions in monkeys. *Neuropsychology* 21:189–197, 1983.

23. Michel D, Laurent B, Foyatier N, et al: Étude de la mémoire et du langage dans une observation tomodensitométrique d'infarctus thalamique paramedian gauche. *Rev Neurol (Paris)* 138:533–550, 1982.

24. Signoret J-L: Memory and amnesias, in Mesulam M-M (ed): *Principles of Behavioral Neurology.* Philadelphia: Davis, 1985, pp 169–192.

25. Cambier J, Elghozi D, Strube E: Lésion du thalamus droit avec syndrome de l'hémisphère mineur: Discussion du concept de négligence thalamique. *Rev Neurol (Paris)* 136:105–116, 1980.

26. Ojemann GA, Fedio P, VanBuren JM: Anomia from pulvinar and subcortical parietal stimulation. *Brain* 91:99–116, 1968.

27. Mesulam M-M: Cholinergic pathways and the ascending reticular activating system of the human brain. *Ann NY Acad Sci* 757:169–179, 1995.

28. Moruzzi G, Magoun HW: Brain stem reticular formation and activation of the EEG. *Electroencephalogr Clin Neurophysiol* 1:459–473, 1949.

29. Dingledine R, Kelly JS: The brainstem stimulation and acetylcholine-invoked inhibition of neurons in the feline nucleus reticularis thalami. *J Physiol* 271:135–154, 1977.

30. Hoover DB, Jacobowitz DM: Neurochemical and histochemical studies of the effect of a lesion of the nucleus cuneiformis on the cholinergic innervation of discrete areas of the rat brain. *Brain Res* 70:113–122, 1970.

31. Hoover DB, Baisden RH: Localization of putative cholinergic neurons innervating the anteroventral thalamus. *Brain Res Bull* 5:519–524, 1980.

32. McCance I, Phillis JW, Westerman RA: Acetylcholine-sensitivity of thalamic neurons: Its relationship to synaptic transmission. *Br J Pharmacol* 32:635–651, 1986.

33. Phillis JW, Tebecis AK, York DH: A study of cholinoceptive cells in the lateral geniculate nucleus. *J Physiol* 192:695–713, 1967.

34. Mesulam M-M: Large-scale neurocognitive networks and distributed processing for attention, language, and memory. *Ann Neurol* 28:597–613, 1990.

35. Mesulam M-M: Structure and function of cholinergic pathways in the cerebral cortex, limbic system, basal ganglia, and thalamus of the human brain, in Bloom FE, Kupfer DJ (eds): *Psychopharmacology: The Fourth Generation of Progress.* New York: Raven Press, 1994, pp 135–146.

36. Mesulam M-M, Mufson EJ: Neural inputs into the nucleus basalis of the substantia innominata (Ch4) in the rhesus monkey. *Brain* 107:253–274, 1984.

37. Mesulam M-M: Asymmetry of neural feedback in the organization of behavioral states. *Science* 237:537–538, 1987.

38. Morecraft RJ, Geula C, Mesulam M-M: Architecture of connectivity within a cingulo-fronto-parietal neurocognitive network for directed attention. *Arch Neurol* 50:279–284, 1993.

39. Mesulam M-M: Neurocognitive networks and selectively distributed processing. *Rev Neurol (Paris)* 150:564–569, 1994.

40. Seeck M, Schomer D, Mainwaring N, et al: Selectively distributed processing of visual object recognition in the temporal and frontal lobes of the human brain. *Ann Neurol* 37:538–545, 1995.

41. Geschwind N. Disconnection syndromes in animals and man. *Brain* 88:237–294, 1965.

Part II
PERCEPTION AND ATTENTION

Chapter 6

VISUAL OBJECT AGNOSIA

Martha J. Farah
Todd E. Feinberg

The term *visual object agnosia* refers to the impairment of object recognition in the presence of relatively intact elementary visual perception, memory, and general intellectual function. This chapter reviews the different subtypes of agnosia, their major clinical features and associated neuropathology, and their implications for cognitive neuroscience theories of visual object recognition.

The study of agnosia has a long history of controversy, with some authors doubting that the condition even exists. For example, Bay[1] suggested that the appearance of disproportionate difficulty with visual object recognition could invariably be explained by synergistic interactions between mild perceptual impairments on the one hand and mild general intellectual impairments on the other. The rarity of visual object agnosia has contributed to the slowness with which this issue has been resolved, but several decades of careful case studies have now shown, to most people's satisfaction, that agnosic patients may be no more impaired in their elementary visual capabilities and their general intellectual functioning than many patients who are not agnosic. Therefore, most current research on agnosia focuses on a new set of questions. Are there different types of visual object agnosia, corresponding to different underlying impairments? At what level of visual and/or mnestic processing do these impairments occur? What can agnosia tell us about normal object recognition? What brain regions are critically involved in visual object recognition?

APPERCEPTIVE AGNOSIA

Lissauer[2] reasoned that visual object recognition could be disrupted in two different ways: by impairing visual perception, in which case patients would be unable to recognize objects because they could not see them properly, and by impairing the process of associating a percept with its meaning, in which case patients would be unable to recognize objects because they could not use the percept to access their knowledge of the object. He termed the first kind of agnosia *apperceptive agnosia* and the second kind *associative agnosia*. This terminology is still used today to distinguish agnosic patients who have frank perceptual impairments from those who do not, although the implicit assumption that the latter have an impairment in "association" is now questioned.

Behavior and Anatomy

One might wonder whether apperceptive agnosics should be considered agnosics at all, given that the definition of agnosia cited at the beginning of this article excludes patients whose problems are caused by elementary visual impairments. The difference between apperceptive agnosics and patients who fall outside of the exclusionary criteria for agnosia is that the former have relatively good acuity, brightness discrimination, color vision, and other so-called elementary visual capabilities. Despite these capabilities, their perception of shape is markedly abnormal. For example, in the classic case of Benson and Greenberg,[3] pictures, letters, and even simple geometric shapes could not be recognized. Figure 6-1 shows the attempts of their patient to copy a column of simple shapes. Recognition of real objects may be somewhat better than recognition of geometric shapes, although this appears to be due to the availability of cues such as size and surface properties such as color, texture, and specularity rather than object shape. Facilitation of shape perception by motion of the stimulus has been noted in several cases of apperceptive agnosia. In most cases of apperceptive agnosia, the brain damage is diffuse, often caused by carbon monoxide poisoning. For a review of other cases of apperceptive visual agnosia, see Ref. 4.

Figure 6-1

The attempts of an apperceptive agnosic patient to copy simple shapes. (From Benson and Greenberg,[3] with permission.)

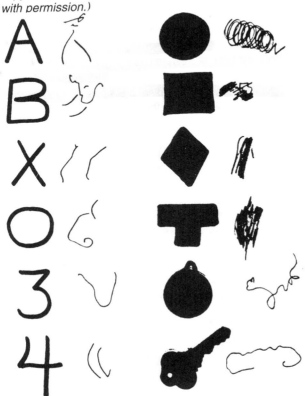

Interpretation of Apperceptive Agnosia

One way of interpreting apperceptive agnosia is in terms of a disorder of grouping processes that normally operate over the array of local features representing contour, color, depth, and so on.[4] Outside of their field defects, apperceptive agnosics have surprisingly good perception of local visual properties. They fail when they must extract more global structure from the image. Motion is helpful because it provides another cue to global structure in the form of correlated local motions. The perception of structure from motion may also have different neural substrates from static contour,[5] and may therefore be spared in apperceptive agnosia.

Relation to Other Disorders

Some authors have used the term *apperceptive agnosia* for other, quite different types of visual disorders, including two forms of simultanagnosia and an impairment in recognizing objects from unusual views or under unusual lighting conditions. *Simultanagnosia* is a term used to describe an impairment in perception of multielement or multipart visual displays. When shown a complex picture with multiple objects or people, simultanagnosics typically describe them in a piecemeal manner, sometimes omitting much of the material entirely and therefore failing to interpret the overall nature of the scene being depicted.

Dorsal simultanagnosia is a component of Balint's syndrome, in which an attentional limitation prevents perception of more than one object at a time.[4,6–8] Occasionally attention may be captured by just one part of an object, leading to misidentification of the object and the appearance of perception confined to relatively local image features. The similarity of dorsal simultanagnosia to apperceptive agnosia is limited, however. Once they can attend to an object, dorsal simultanagnosics recognize it quickly and accurately, and even their "local" errors encompass much more global shape information than is available to apperceptive agnosics. Their lesions are typically in the posterior parietal cortex bilaterally.

Despite some surface similarity to apperceptive agnosia and dorsal simultanagnosia, *ventral simultanagnosia* represents yet another disorder.[9] Ventral simultanagnosics can recognize whole objects, but are limited in how many objects can be recognized in a given period of time. Their descriptions of complex scenes are slow and piecemeal, but unlike apperceptive agnosics their recognition of single shapes is not obviously impaired. The impairment of ventral simultanagnosics is most apparent when reading, because the individual letters of words are recognized in an abnormally slow and generally serial manner (letter-by-letter reading, see Chap. 18). Unlike the case with dorsal simultanagnosics, their detection of multiple stimuli appears normal; the bottleneck is in recognition per se. Unlike apperceptive agnosics, they perceive individual shapes reasonably well. Their lesions are typically in the left inferior temporooccipital cortex.

Some patients have roughly normal perception and recognition of objects except when viewed from unusual perspectives or under unusual lighting. Their impairment has also been grouped with apperceptive agnosia by some, but for clarity's sake can also be called *perceptual categorization deficit* because they cannot categorize together the full range of images cast by an object under different viewing conditions. This disorder does not have great localizing value, although the lesions are generally in the right hemisphere and frequently include the inferior parietal lobe.[10]

ASSOCIATIVE AGNOSIA

Behavior and Anatomy

In associative agnosia, visual perception is much better than in apperceptive agnosia. Compare, for example, the copies made by the associative agnosics shown in Figs. 6-2 and 6-3 with the copies shown in Fig. 6-1. Nevertheless, object recognition is impaired. Associative agnosic patients may be able to recognize an object by its feel in their hand or from a spoken definition, demonstrating that they have intact general knowledge of the object in addition to being able to see it well enough to copy it, but they cannot recognize the same object

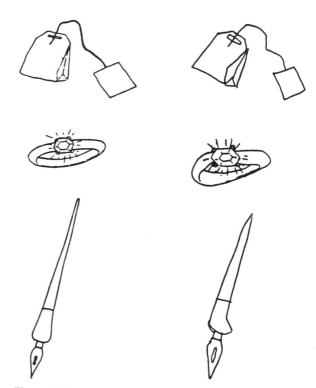

Figure 6-2

The copies of an associative agnosic patient with prosopagnosia and object agnosia. The patient did not recognize any of the original drawings. (From Farah et al.,[27] with permission.)

by sight alone. The impairment is not simply a naming deficit for visual stimuli; associative agnosics cannot indicate their recognition of objects by nonverbal means, as by pantomiming the use of an object or by grouping together dissimilar-looking objects from the same semantic category[11-16] (see Ref. 4 for a review of representative cases).

The scope of the recognition impairment varies from case to case of associative agnosia. Some patients encounter difficulty mainly with face recognition (see Chap. 7), while others demonstrate better face recognition than object recognition. Printed-word recognition is similarly impaired in some cases but not others. The selectivity of these impairments suggests that there is more than one

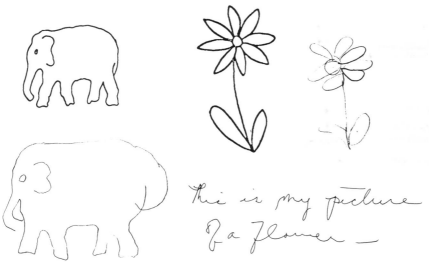

Figure 6-3
The copies of associative visual agnosic patients with alexia and object agnosia. The patients did not recognize the original drawings. Also shown is a sample of a patient's writing to dictation. After a delay, her own handwriting could not be read. (From Feinberg et al.,[16] with permission.)

system involved in visual recognition. According to one analysis,[17] there are two underlying forms of visual representation, one of which is required for face recognition, used for object recognition but not for word recognition, and the other of which is required for word recognition, used for object recognition and not required for face recognition. Indeed, if one regards associative agnosia as a single undifferentiated category, it is difficult to make any generalizations about the brain regions responsible for visual object recognition. Although the intrahemispheric location of damage is generally occipitotemporal, involving both gray and white matter, cases of associative agnosia have been reported following unilateral right-hemispheric lesions,[18] unilateral left-hemispheric lesions,[15,16,19,20] and bilateral lesions.[21–23] However, if one considers impairments in face and word recognition as markers for different underlying forms of visual recognition disorder, then a pattern emerges in the neuropathology. When face recognition alone is impaired or when face and object recognition are impaired but reading is spared, the lesions are generally either on the right or bilateral. De Renzi has proposed that the degree of right-hemispheric specialization for face recognition may normally cover a wide range, such that most cases of prosopagnosia become manifest

only after bilateral lesions, but in some cases a unilateral lesion will suffice (see Chap. 7). When reading alone is impaired or when reading and object recognition are impaired but face recognition is spared, the lesions are generally on the left. In a series of patients studied by us and additional cases of agnosia sparing face recognition culled from the literature, the maximum overlap in lesion locus was in the left inferior medial region involving parahippocampal, fusiform, and lingual gyri.[16] When recognition of faces, objects, and words is impaired, the lesions are generally bilateral.

Interpreting Associative Agnosia

Is associative agnosia a problem with perception, memory, or both? Associative agnosia has been explained in three different ways that suggest different answers to this question. The simplest way to explain agnosia is by a disconnection between visual representations and other brain centers responsible for language or memory. For example, Geschwind[24] proposed that associative agnosia is a visual-verbal disconnection. This hypothesis accounts well for agnosics' impaired naming of visual stimuli, but it cannot account for their inability to convey recognition nonverbally and may therefore be more suited to explaining *optic aphasia*, a form of anomia limited to impaired naming of visual stimuli (see Chap. 23). Associative agnosia has also been explained as a disconnection between visual representations and medial temporal memory centers.[23] However, this would account for a modality-specific impairment in new learning, not the inability to access old knowledge through vision.

The inadequacies of the disconnection accounts lead us to consider theories of associative agnosia in which some component of perception and/or memory has been damaged. Perhaps the most widely accepted account of associative agnosia is that stored visual memory representations have been damaged. According to this type of account, stimuli can be processed perceptually up to some end-state visual representation, which would normally be matched against stored visual representations. In associative agnosia, the stored representations are no longer available and recognition therefore fails. Note that an assumption of this account is that two identical tokens of the object representation normally exist, one derived from the stimulus and one stored in memory, and that these are compared in the same way as a database might be searched in a present-day computer. This account is not directly disconfirmed by any of the available evidence. However, there are some reasons to question it and to suspect that subtle impairments in perception may underlie associative agnosia.

Although the good copies and successful matching performance of associative agnosics might seem to exonerate perception, a closer look at the manner in which these tasks are accomplished suggests that perception is not normal in associative agnosia and suggests yet a third explanation of associative agnosia. Typically, these patients are described as copying drawings "slavishly"[25] and "line by line."[26] In matching tasks, they rely on slow, sequential feature-by-feature checking. It therefore may be premature to rule out faulty perception as the cause of associative agnosia. Recent studies of the visual capabilities of associative agnosic patients confirm that there are subtle visual perceptual impairments present in all cases studied.[4] If the possibility of impaired

recognition with intact perception is consistent with the use of a computational architecture in which separate perceptual and memory representations are compared, then the absence of such a case suggests that a different type of computational architecture may underlie object recognition. Parallel distributed processing (PDP) systems exemplify an alternative architecture in which the perceptual and memory representations cannot be dissociated (see Chap. 4; see also Ref. 4, Chap. 2, for a discussion of PDP models and agnosia). In a PDP system, the memory of the stimulus would consist of a pattern of connection strengths among a number of neuronlike units. The "perceptual" representation resulting from the presentation of a stimulus will depend upon the pattern of connection strengths among the units directly or indirectly activated by the stimulus. Thus, if memory is altered by damaging the network, perception will be altered as well. On this account, associative agnosia is not a result of an impairment to perception *or* to memory; rather, the two are in principle inseparable, and the impairment is better described as a loss of high-level visual perceptual representations that are shaped by, and embody the memory of, visual experience. It will thus be of great interest to see whether future studies of associative agnosics will ever document a case of impaired recognition with intact perception.

Relation to Other Disorders

As with apperceptive agnosia, a number of distinct disorders have been labeled associative agnosia by different authors. Visual modality–specific naming disorders exist and are usually termed *optic aphasia,* but they may on occasion be called *associative visual agnosia. Impairments of semantic memory* (see Chap. 23) will affect object-recognition ability (as well as entirely nonvisual abilities such as verbally defining spoken words) and perhaps for this reason have sometimes been called *associative visual agnosia.*

REFERENCES

1. Bay E: Disturbances of visual perception and their examination. *Brain* 76:515–530, 1952.

2. Lissauer H: Ein Fall von Seelenblindheit nebst einem Beitrage zur Theori derselben. *Arch Psychiatr Nervenkrankh* 21:222–270, 1890.

3. Benson R, Greenberg JP: Visual form agnosia. *Arch Neurol* 20:82–89, 1969.

4. Farah MJ: *Visual Agnosia: Disorders of Object Recognition and What They Tell Us about Normal Vision.* Cambridge, MA: MIT Press, 1990.

5. Marcar VL, Cowey A: The effect of removing superior temporal cortical motion areas in the macaque monkey: II. Motion discrimination using random dot displays. *Eur J Neurosci* 4:1228–1238, 1992.

6. Williams M: *Brain Damage and the Mind.* Baltimore: Penguin Books, 1970.

7. Girotti F, Milanese C, Casazza M, et al: Oculomotor disturbances in Balint's syndrome: Anatomoclinical findings and electrooculographic analysis in a case. *Cortex* 18:603–614, 1982.

8. Tyler A, Gelade G: A feature-integration theory of attention. *Cog Psychol* 12:97–136, 1980.

9. Kinsbourne M, Warrington EK: A disorder of simultaneous form perception. *Brain* 85:461–486, 1962.

10. Warrington EK: Agnosia: The impairment of object recognition, in Vinken PJ, Bruyn GW, Klawans HL (eds): *Handbook of Clinical Neurology.* Amsterdam: Elsevier, 1985.

11. Rubens AB, Benson DF: Associative visual agnosia. *Arch Neurol* 24:305–316, 1971.

12. Bauer RM, Rubens AB: Agnosia, in Heilman KM, Valenstein E (eds): *Clinical Neuropsychology,* 2d ed. New York: Oxford University Press, 1985.

13. Albert ML, Reches A, Silverberg R: Associative visual agnosia without alexia. *Neurology* 25:322–326, 1975.

14. Hécaen H, de Ajuriaguerra J: Agnosie visuelle pour les objets inanimes par lesion unilaterale gauche. *Rev Neurol* 94:222–233, 1956.

15. McCarthy RA, Warrington EK: Visual associative agnosia: A clinico-anatomical study of a single case. *Neurol Neurosurg Psychiatry* 48:1233–1240, 1986.

16. Feinberg TE, Schindler RJ, Ochoa E, et al: Associative visual agnosia and alexia without prosopagnosia. *Cortex* 30:395–412, 1994.

17. Farah MJ: Patterns of co-occurrence among the associative agnosias: Implications for visual object representation. *Cog Neuropsychol* 8:1–19, 1991.

18. Levine DN: Prosopagnosia and visual object agnosia: A behavioral study. *Neuropsychologia* 5:341–365, 1978.

19. Pilon B, Signoret JL, Lhermitte F: Agnosie visuelle associative rôle de l'hemisphere gauche dans la perception visuelle. *Rev Neurol* 137:831–842, 1981.

20. Feinberg TE, Heilman KM, Gonzalez-Rothi L: Multimodal agnosia after unilateral left hemisphere lesion. *Neurology* 36:864–867, 1986.

21. Alexander MP, Albert ML: The anatomical basis of visual agnosia, in Kertesz A (ed): *Localization in Neuropsychology.* New York: Academic Press, 1983.

22. Benson DF, Segarra J, Albert ML: Visual agnosia-prosopagnosia: A clinicopathologic correlation. *Arch Neurol* 30:307–310, 1973.

23. Albert ML, Soffer D, Silverberg R, Reches A: The anatomic basis of visual agnosia. *Neurology* 29:876–879, 1979.

24. Geschwind N: Disconnexion syndromes in animals and man: Part II. *Brain* 88:585–645, 1965.

25. Brown JW: *Aphasia, Apraxia and Agnosia: Clinical and Theoretical Aspects.* Springfield, IL: Charles C Thomas, 1972.

26. Ratcliff G, Newcombe F: Object recognition: Some deductions from the clinical evidence, in Ellis AW (ed): *Normality and Pathology in Cognitive Functions.* New York: Academic Press, 1982.

27. Farah MJ, Hammond K, Levine DN, et al: Visual and spatial mental imagery. *Cog Neuropsychol* 20:439–462, 1988.

Chapter 7

PROSOPAGNOSIA

Ennio De Renzi

Faces represent a class of stimuli that enjoy a special status in the study of visuoperceptual disorders and have been the subject of a number of investigations unparalleled by any other perceptual category. Historically, the main factors calling attention to them have been reports of patients who, following a brain lesion, manifest a deficit of recognition that is unique to familiar faces, or at least disproportionate with respect to other types of stimuli, and that is not accounted for by loss of knowledge about the biographic features of the unidentified people.

The earliest mention of the symptom was made by A. Quaglino,[1] an Italian ophthalmologist, who, in 1867, reported a patient suffering from left hemianopia, achromatopsia, and inability to recognize familiar faces—problems caused by a cerebrovascular accident. The patient's preserved ability to read words printed in very small type convinced the author that elementary visual deficits played no primary role in the patient's impairment. Although Quaglino recognized the cerebral origin of the disorder, the impact of his paper on the scientific community was practically nil. The symptom had to await Bodamer's report[2] in 1947 to be identified as a distinct form of agnosia, deserving a distinctive name (prosopagnosia, from the Greek word *prosopon,* meaning face).

Since the 1940s, more than a hundred case reports[3] have been published, and some patients have been extensively and repeatedly investigated. Yet it was not so much for its clinical frequency that prosopagnosia raised such a marked

interest as for the light it threw on the organization of the visual recognition system.

THE CLINICAL PICTURE

Patients are usually aware of their deficit and complain of it, although a few of them may be reluctant to speak about it because they feel ashamed of being unable to do such a simple thing as recognizing their closest relatives and friends, all the more as the organic nature of the symptom may go unrecognized. In two patients of mine, the ophthalmologist, to whom they had been referred by the family doctor, diagnosed a psychogenic disorder, baffled by their inability to recognize familiar faces in spite of normal acuity, campimetry, and visual object recognition.

Even upon superficial investigation, it is apparent that the failure to recognize people is restricted to the processing of facial features, and that these patients try to compensate for their handicap by relying on nonfacial cues, such as the subject's voice, gait, clothing, and so on. Sometimes they complain of seeing faces distorted or in a dim light, but they never fail to realize that they are looking at a face. With a few exceptions, they can discriminate its gender, race, and approximate age, although finer age estimation may be impaired.[4] Face recognition disorders do not extend to the identification of emotional expressions, which is preserved in the great majority of prosopagnosics, while it may be impaired in patients who do not have problems in recognizing familiar faces,[5] providing evidence that discrete neural structures subserve the two abilities (see later).

RECOGNITION OF FAMILIAR AND UNFAMILIAR FACES

Bodamer thought that the predominant deficit shown by his patients in recognizing faces justified the inference that these stimuli have a special status in the brain. This hypothesis found some support in subsequent studies, which showed that the processing of unknown faces differs from that of other categories of stimuli in being closely related to right hemispheric functioning. This is the kind of material most suitable for bringing out a right hemispheric advantage in recognizing laterally projected nonverbal stimuli. Interestingly, patients with right posterior lesions are more impaired than any other brain-damaged group in tasks requiring them to match to sample photographs of faces taken from different perspectives or in different conditions of illumination.[6-9] It was at first thought[7] that performance on unknown face matching tasks was strictly correlated with that on familiar face recognition and could represent a reliable index of the patient's skills in processing this unique category of stimuli. However, it was soon discovered that in brain-damaged patients, the correlation between familiar and unfamiliar face recognition is zero,[10] and that there are a few prosopagnosic patients who perform the unknown face tests correctly.[11,12] Morover, right brain–damaged patients who do very poorly on these tests yet have no difficulty in recognizing familiar faces. The conclusion drawn by Benton[13] was that there are two types of disorders related to face recognition—one concerning unknown faces, which is basically perceptual, and the other concerning familiar faces, which also entails an amnestic component.

LEVEL OF IMPAIRMENT IN PROSOPAGNOSIA

There have been several attempts to fractionate prosopagnosia according to the functional level at which face recognition is disrupted. A preliminary broad distinction, similar to that proposed by Lissauer[14] for object agnosia, is between apperceptive and associative (or amnestic) prosopagnosia.[15,16] However, this dichotomous classification can be further fractionated, based on the models recently proposed by cognitive psychologists to analyze how the flow of facial information is processed in normals. The most popular of them, elaborated by Bruce and Young,[17] envisages four stages that can be activated in a bottom-up or a top-down direction. The structural encoding stage represents the final product of perceptual analysis and yields a tridimensional, abstract representation of the stimulus, which is independent of the context and the viewpoint from which it is observed. If the face is known, the product of structural encoding is matched with its representation, stored in recognition units, and gives rise to a feeling of familiarity, though not yet permitting its identification. Recognition occurs when the firing of recognition units activates the identity nodes, a part of the semantic system that stores the information relevant to the identification of a person (when and where that person has been encountered, his or her profession, biography, and so on). Identity nodes can also be accessed from nonfacial inputs, such as the person's voice, way of walking, clothes, and so forth, and they have reciprocal connections with the people/name module. Its independence is shown by the dissociation between the ability to recognize a face and the failure to retrieve the corresponding name, occasionally exhibited by normals and, in a more massive way, by a few brain-damaged patients. In some cases the name is unavailable with any cue, verbal or visual (proper name anomia[18]); in others, the difficulty arises only on visual presentation of the face (prosopanomia[19]).

Damage at the level of structural encoding or at even earlier stages of perceptual processing is obviously implicated in cases where the inability to identify familiar faces appears in the context of a more general deficit of visual perception. Severe apperceptive agnosia[20-25] is always accompanied by prosopagnosia. More problematic is the assessment of the relevance of perceptual deficits to prosopagnosia, when the impairment outside the "face" category is apparent only for objects that are visually homogeneous or on tasks that are perceptually demanding, such as matching stimuli taken from different views, identifying incomplete or overlapping figures, discriminating patterns that differ for minimal features, and so on. When, in the sixties, it was found that right brain–damaged patients were impaired in matching photographs of unknown faces taken from different perspectives, the hypothesis was advanced that prosopagnosia represented the extreme end of a continuum of perceptual disorders, particularly evident for faces, because their physical similarity makes them hard to differentiate. However, as already mentioned, some prosopagnosics perform correctly these tests, possibly because their deficit is mainly amnestic. Also, the score on other tests of perception of facial features and facial configuration may not be predictive of familiar face recognition.[26] There have been attempts to ground the specificity of the patient's perceptual impairment on firmer evidence. Sergent and coworkers[27,28] proposed a sophisticated method to estimate the patient's ability to perform the configurational operations whereby facial features are processed in an interactive manner. De Renzi and coworkers[15] measured, in 100 normal subjects, the difference between the standardized scores of two-face perceptual tests and two-face memory tests and computed the internal and external tolerance limits of the difference in score distribution. These norms make it possible to identify prosopagnosics who are outliers either for an exceedingly poor performance on perceptual tests (apperceptive prosopagnosia), or for an exceedingly poor performance on memory tests (associative prosopagnosia). The question remains whether these measures also differentiate prosopagnosics from right brain–damaged patients who are not impaired in recognizing faces. McNeil and Warrington[26] have warned that scores on tests of facial features and facial configuration may not be predictive of familiar face recognition.

When the impairment of perceptual processing does not account for the inability to recognize familiar faces, a face-specific amnestic deficit must be considered. The identification of the stage at which the recognition process fails rests on performance on tests of familiarity (point to the one face in an array that is known; no recognition is required), of visual-verbal matching (point to the face named by the examiner), and of visual and verbal naming. Instead of the proper name, the knowledge of other semantic features (profession, nationality, and so on) can be required. Visual knowledge must be compared with knowledge elicited by the verbal presentation of information (name or some other qualifying feature) pointing to the same person. Prosopagnosics respond competently to verbal questions and can, therefore, be easily differentiated from patients who do not recognize familiar persons because they suffer from an amnesia specific for people[29–31] and are unable to retrieve information concerning them, no matter whether it is requested through the presentation of a face, name, or voice. The impairment may extend to knowledge about exemplars of other categories that have become famous in their individuality—for example, famous animals (Lassie), buildings (the Kremlin), or products that were much advertised in the past.[29]

Damage to identity nodes without involvement of recognition units should be manifest by the ability to perform familiarity tests, but there is just one case where a dissociation between sense of familiarity and recognition has been found.[32] All other patients fail on both types of tests. Further information on the level of impairment can be drawn from the study of nonconscious recognition.

NONCONSCIOUS FACE RECOGNITION

A fascinating phenomenon that has been pointed out in different neuropsychological domains, from blindsight to amnesia, neglect, and alexia, is the dissociation between what the patients overtly know about a stimulus and the implicit knowledge the patient manifests, through changes in behavior, in response to its presentation. The same holds in prosopagnosia, where patients who deny recognizing a face show a different pattern of physiologic or psychological responses depending on whether the face is familiar or unfamiliar. Among physiological procedures, positive findings have been reported with the galvanic skin reaction,[21,33] eye-movement scan paths,[34] and event-related potentials.[35] For instance, patient LF[21] was unable to choose which of five names successively spoken by the examiner corresponded to a famous face, but his skin conductance responses occurred more often and with a higher amplitude to true than to untrue names.

Paradigms based on psychological parameters have used learning and priming tasks, which have shown an advantage of familiar over unfamiliar faces. For instance, prosopagnosics learn to associate a familiar face with a name or a profession more successfully if the pairs are true than if they are untrue.[27,35–37] The effect, however, depended on the nature of the information provided or of the response required, since it vanished when only the first name instead of the full name of the person was given or when knowledge of specific instead of generic semantic information was required (e.g., not simply whether a face was that of a politician or a nonpolitician, but to what political party the person belonged).[38] Covert effects were also demonstrated by the interference exerted on a name-classification task (politicians versus nonpoliticians) by a distractor face, depending on whether it belonged to the same semantic category of the name[39] and by priming of name recognition by face primes.[36] In the one patient, who could be tested with physiologic as well psychological procedures, covert recognition was demonstrated on both.[40]

These findings provide evidence that some knowledge on faces that are not overtly recognized is still retained by some prosopagnosics and, if properly cued, can be activated. Note that unconscious recognition can also be shown when explicit decisions are requested, as in forced-choice tasks. Though the patients maintain that they are simply guessing, they respond faster in matching different views of familiar than of unfamiliar faces,[36] score above chance on a face-name matching test where the name or profession of a famous face must be chosen among alternatives,[26,27,32,37] and are able to pair two faces

of the same famous person across a 30-year age period much better than normal controls who are unfamiliar with that person.[27] Surprisingly, if the same forced-choice paradigm is used to assess familiarity, they score at chance.

An amazing finding, reported by Sergent and Poncet[27] and partially replicated[32,37] is the capacity shown by some prosopagnosic patients, if they are provided with partial information, to progressively attain a stage of transient recognition of faces they were initially unable to identify. When they were told that a set of nonrecognized faces belonged to the same professional category, they suddenly remembered it and then also succeeded in retrieving the associated names. Yet recognition was contingent on the spontaneous pop out of the category, since, no face could be named if the category was not retrieved or when the same exemplars that had been named were later presented intermingled with faces of other categories.

Implicit knowledge of familiar faces is not found in every prosopagnosic. Negative cases[21,28,41–43] are relevant to understanding the functional level of damage. The absence of covert recognition has been interpreted as evidence that recognition units are damaged, while its presence would indicate that they are intact but can only communicate with the identity nodes via an indirect route, which, though being able to alert the semantic system that the face is familiar, is inadequate to transmit the information needed for conscious recognition.[38,44]

Bauer[21] interpreted the overt-covert recognition dissociation in the light of the anatomic model,[45] which envisages two separate pathways for processing visual information—a ventral one linking the visual association cortex with the temporal limbic cortex and transmitting information about "what" the stimulus is and a dorsal one projecting to the superior temporal sulcus and then to the inferior parietal lobule and concerned with "where" the stimulus is. Lesion to the ventral occipitotemporal pathway would cause loss of conscious recognition but leave patent the dorsal occipitoparietal route, which, thanks to its reciprocal connections with the cingulate cortex, can mediate the emotional reaction to the nonrecognized face. The same interpretation was extended[46] to the manifestations of covert recognition, disclosed by psychological procedures, attributing to the dorsal system the unconscious processing of the information transmitted by the recognition units. This account, however, leaves unanswered the question of what the anatomic connections are that, in a forced-choice paradigm, make it possible to match a face with a name but not to make a familiarity judgment.

An alternative, simpler interpretation of the dissociation between overt and covert recognition is that a sensory percept reaches awareness only if the output from downstream centers attains a given threshold. Subthreshold information is not, however, lost and may be processed by unconscious mechanisms if we assume that they require a lower level of activation. Damage to the recognition units does not necessarily result in an all-or-none response. Depending on the degree of their impairment, they may either cease to fire (in which case covert recognition will also fail), or they may generate a reduced output that is inadequate to activate the identity nodes to the point of conscious recognition but is sufficient to raise their response above chance. In support of this contention, Farah and coworkers[47] built a computer simulation of face recognition that performed a variety of overt and covert tasks. When visual face perception was degraded by lesioning the model, overt recognition was eliminated, yet the model continued to show priming and interference from faces, facilitation in matching familiar faces, and savings in relearning face-name associations. The quality of covert recognition performance in prosopagnosic patients is also consistent with the hypothesis of a damaged, but not obliterated, face recognition system. The improvement patients show when confronted with familiar faces remains, in most cases, below the level found in normal subjects. Wallace and Farah[48] pointed out that normal subjects showed the same dissociation between overt recognition and savings in relearning, when overt recognition was hindered by delaying it over a 6-month period. Recognition units can also receive top-down information from names, and this may increase their activation.[37]

SPECIFICITY OF FACES

A question that has recurred ever since the earliest report of prosopagnosia is whether the deficit is confined to the category of faces or represents but one aspect of an impairment pervading other gnostic domains (although attention is unavoidably focused on the face recognition disorder because of its social implications). On this view, prosopagnosia would correspond to a mild visual agnosia.[49] Authors advocating the latter position have emphasized some features that would make faces particularly prone to disruption by brain damage. One is the great perceptual similarity of their external configuration and internal structure and the consequent need for a fine-grained discrimination system. The second is the high number—on the order of several hundred and even a few thousand—of unique exemplars of faces that must be stored in memory in order to ensure appropriate social relations. No comparison is possible with what happens with other categories of objects, where it is at most necessary that we recognize the individuality of those exemplars we own—it would be embarrassing to mistake one's own car in a parking lot or one's own overcoat on a coat tree—but we can use most objects interchangeably, without any need to retrieve the context in which we first met them and the network of associations that identifies them. This difference is reflected in the way object and face recognition is tested: the former is assessed by requiring the patient to name or provide semantic knowledge of the category to which the target belongs, the latter by requiring the recognition of that particular face.

From these considerations and from the finding that there are prosopagnosic patients who also show difficulty in recognizing the members of other categories (breeds of dogs, buildings, cars, articles of clothing) that, like faces, have great physical similarity, it has been argued[50,51] that the basic deficit of these patients concerns the identification of an exemplar within a class whose members have great perceptual similarity. If we extend the investigation to perceptual domains that share the same features, it will be apparent that the deficit is not specific for faces. For instance, some patients have been reported who were impaired in recognizing individual animals.[52,53]

However, there are data in the literature that contradict this assumption. Sergent and Signoret[54] had a patient who was particularly suitable to test it, since he was an expert on car makes and models, having made a hobby of collecting miniature cars. When he was presented with 210 photographs of cars, comprising 14 models from 15 makes, he was able to identify 172 of them correctly; and of the remaining 38, he correctly reported the company name for 31 and the model name for 22. Taking advantage of the fact that their patient was skillful in recognizing sheep faces, McNeil and Warrington[44] contrasted his ability to learn to associate sheep and human faces with arbitrary names and found that, differently from normal controls, he was poorer in learning faces than sheep. Farah and coworkers[55] tested the ability of a prosopagnosic to recognize faces and a variety of nonface objects, including a large set of similar-looking eyeglass frames, and found him to be disproportionately impaired with faces relative to normal subjects' performance. De Renzi[56] tested the hypothesis that if a prosopagnosic is asked to identify a specific object, "he will be just as incapable of evoking the history of a familiar object as he will be of evoking the history of a familiar face"[50] by asking his patient to recognize his own belongings when presented with other exemplars of the same class. The patient, who was a typical amnestic prosopagnosic, showed no difficulty in identifying his own electric razor, glasses, wallet, and necktie from among 6 to 10 exemplars of the same category and his own handwriting from among 9 samples of the same sentence written by other persons. The same behavior has been replicated in a second patient[15] and confirmed by Sergent and Signoret.[54] These authors, however, questioned the cogency of the finding, arguing that in these experiments recognition was contingent on the use of a forced-choice paradigm with a limited number of alternatives, a condition not comparable with that of unexpectedly encountering a familiar person and being unable to recognize him or her. In a forced-choice condition, the prosopagnosic patients did show correct recognition of the photograph of their own faces or of a close relative from among unknown faces when their names were provided. It must be emphasized, however, that when the same task was given using photographs of famous people as targets instead of those of close relatives, both patients failed. These results were not different from what De Renzi and coworkers[15,56] had reported in their patients when they were requested to point to the one face out of four that was familiar or to that whose name was given. Thus the aid provided by forced recognition was confined to a limited number of very familiar faces (no more than two faces were given to one patient and five to another) and may be related to unconscious rather than to conscious recognition, since, as already mentioned above, prosopagnosic patients score above chance on a forced-choice face-name matching test. It can be added that, were it true that a forced-choice paradigm is sufficient to show preserved knowledge in prosopagnosics, all experiments carried out to show covert recognition would be superfluous.

If faces have something special that deserves a separate organization in the brain, what is the psychological and the biological basis of their discrete treatment by the central nervous system? Farah and coworkers[57] have argued that face recognition differs from object recognition because the representation of the former is mainly based on overall structure, which is not parsed in the component parts, while that of the latter relies mostly on a preliminary decomposition into the local defining features. This hypothesis was borne out by a series of experiments that compared the contribution of part and whole representations to the perception of upright and inverted faces and the detrimental effect that masking parts or wholes exerts on the perception of upright and inverted faces, words, and houses. Thus, faces would lie at the end of a continuum, ranging from parts-based representations used for words to whole-based representations used for faces, with objects occupying an intermediate position and sharing either ability, depending on their structure. Farah[3,58] claimed that the different contribution that the holistic and analytic encoding of information make to these three classes of stimuli is borne out by the patterns of association with which the corresponding disorders appear. In its purest form, the disruption of the ability to decompose a stimulus into its parts results in alexia and that of encoding nondecomposed perceptual wholes in prosopagnosia. Object perception shares either encoding mechanism, depending on the features of the stimulus. It follows that there will never be a case of object agnosia without either alexia or prosopagnosia or a case of alexia associated with prosopagnosia in the absence of object agnosia. Support for this contention was found[3] in a review of the literature, but quite recently a case has been reported[59] that questions the former of the two assumptions. It remains, therefore, an open question whether the prevailing patterns of visual recognition impairment pointed out by the literature are indeed evidence of different encoding procedures depending on the nature of the stimulus or whether they reflect the degree of specialization that the left and right hemispheres have in processing and storing words, faces, and objects.

Face specificity also finds support in neurophysiologic data, which show the presence in the inferior temporal cortex and in the cortex of the superior temporal sulcus of cells that discharge selectively in response to the presentation of a face.[60,61] They may have different functional specification. Those in the inferior temporal cortex would be involved in the identification of single exemplars and would, therefore, be germane to the deficit in face recognition found in humans following damage to the same area. Those in the superior temporal sulcus would be sensitive to emotional expressions and to the direction of gaze,[62] a dimension that plays a paramount role in the social communication of monkeys. The superior temporal sulcus has strong connections with the amygdala, whose injury has been found in humans to cause a severe deficit in the comprehension of facial expressions and gaze directions.[63,64] The discrete anatomic organization of the abilities involved in face recognition and in the recognition of facial expressions is borne out by their dissociation produced by pathology. Most patients with prosopagnosia perform emotion-matching tasks

correctly, while the opposite pattern of impairment has been reported in nonprosopagnosic patients.[5] Two cases with selective impairment in naming and pointing to emotional expressions but integrity in understanding the meaning of facial affect have been reported following right temporal lobe damage;[65,66] this has been interpreted as being due to a category-specific bidirectional visuoverbal disconnection between intact visual semantic and verbal semantic representations for facial expressions. The locus of lesion of these patients (right middle temporal gyrus) tallies with the findings of a study[67] where neurons of the right middle temporal gyrus of epileptic patients showed a specific increase of their activity when the patients had to label facial expressions.

ANATOMIC CORRELATES OF PROSOPAGNOSIA

The ascendancy of the right over the left hemisphere in processing faces is beyond question, having been confirmed by many normal and clinical studies. What is a matter of debate is whether this asymmetry of function is so marked as to cause the inability to recognize familiar faces following a lesion confined to the right side or if bilateral damage is necessary to produce this result.

Bodamer[2] was cautious in drawing anatomic inferences from his cases, since they lacked autopsy, but he remarked that both showed evidence of bilateral lesions. Fifteen years later, a review of the available clinical cases[68] emphasized the presence in a substantial proportion of them of left visual field defects, a sign pointing to right brain damage. It was speculated that damage to this side played a crucial role in causing prosopagnosia. Although this paper was very influential in drawing attention to the possible specialization of the right hemisphere in face processing, its relevance to the anatomic basis of prosopagnosia was questioned by a subsequent review focusing on case reports with necroscopy documentation,[69] which pointed out that all of the patients had bilateral damage. New pathologic studies[70,71] corroborated this finding. Although Meadows[69] was cautious in drawing definite conclusions from his review of the literature—since there were also a few patients in whom surgery had shown a disease confined to the right hemisphere and in some bilateral cases the left lesion was located in areas having no relation to the processing of visual information—the view that bilateral damage is a necessary condition for the occurrence of prosopagnosia[50] gained overwhelming consensus. Yet the exceptions to the "bilaterality of damage" rule remarkably increased with the introduction of neuroimaging procedures, which made it possible to localize the lesion in a much greater number of patients. It must be stressed that while this source of information cannot compete with autopsy in terms of accuracy of localization, it has the great advantage of being available in practically every prosopagnosic, not only in those that come to autopsy (which may represent a biased sample) and that is available at the same time testing is carried out. A review of the pertinent literature published up to 1992[72] brought out 27 patients with evidence on computed tomography (CT) or magnetic resonance imaging (MRI)—complemented in 5 cases by positron emission tomography (PET)—of damage restricted to the right hemisphere, plus 3 cases with surgical documentation and 1 following right hemispherectomy. There is now also a case of prosopagnosia in which autopsy has shown an infarct in the territory of the right posterior cerebral artery.[73]

The pendulum is, therefore, shifting again toward the "unilaterality of lesion" thesis, to the effect that damage to the right brain may be sufficient to cause prosopagnosia. It is fair to recognize, however, that the exclusive specialization of this side of the brain for face recognition is far from attaining the same generality the left hemisphere has for language. For instance, in a consecutive series of 10 patients with an infarct of the right posterior cerebral artery, which supplies the occipitotemporal cortex involved in face recognition, none showed prosopagnosia,[72] while alexia was present in 13 consecutive patients out of 16 who had an infarct of the left posterior cerebral artery.[74] A likely inference suggested by these findings is that the degree of hemispheric asymmetry in face recognition is a dimension showing a wide range of functional variation in humans, such that only a minority of them have these skills preponderantly represented in the right brain.

The most frequent etiology of prosopagnosia is an infarct in the territory of the posterior cerebral artery, which encroaches upon the medial cortex of the occipital and temporal lobes and the inferior longitudinal fasciculus, running in the subjacent white matter. The role played in face recognition by these structures, in particular those of the right hemisphere, finds support in normal studies, showing that some physiologic parameters recorded from these areas are specifically activated by the presentation of familiar as opposed to unfamiliar faces. An enhancement of the late negative component (wave N500) of event-related cerebral potentials associated with familiar faces was recorded from the right occipital lead;[75] a different pattern of visual evoked potentials—recorded by depth electrodes inserted in the amygdala, hippocampus, and the superior and inferior temporal sulcus—is produced by the presentation of familiar and unfamiliar faces, and the difference is more marked on the right.[76] Two PET studies[77,78] agreed in showing a bilateral increase of cerebral blood flow in the striate and extrastriate cortex (lingual and fusiform gyri) when faces were processed as opposed to a resting condition, but they disagreed as to the side that was more activated when the face task involved memory. In one study,[78] changes were more marked in the right lingual, fusiform, and parahippocampal gyri; in the other[77] they were more marked in the left posterior hippocampus, and there was also a significant decrease of blood flow in the left superior temporal gyrus. Further studies are required to solve this contradiction.

CONGENITAL PROSOPAGNOSIA

Two cases with prosopagnosia dating back to early years of age and without evidence of an acquired cerebral disease have been reported.[41,79,80] Interestingly, both had a relative who complained of the same type of difficulty, which points to the genetic nature of the disorder. The first patient was reported by McConachie,[79] when she was 12 years old; she was tested again by De Haan and Campbell[41] 15 years later. Her disorder was prominent in face recognition, but extended to object recognition in only a minor degree, especially in discriminating items that belonged to a category made up of perceptually similar exemplars and in identifying figures seen from an unusual perspective. She was thought to fail at the stage where a fully specified code of a face must be constructed. Temple's[80] patient, on the contrary, was not impaired at the perceptual level and her deficit was specific for faces. It probably concerned the acquisition of stable stored representations. A third patient[43] with prosopagnosia dating back to childhood, when she incurred a meningoencephalitis, had difficulties similar to those of McConachie's[79] patient.

REFERENCES

1. Quaglino A: Empilegia sinistra con amaurosi- Guarigione- Perdita totale della percezione dei colori e della memoria della configurazione degli oggetti. Annotazione alla medesima di GB Borelli. *Giorn Oftalmol Ital* 10:106–117, 1867.
2. Bodamer J: Die Prosopagnosie. *Arch Psychiatr Nervenkrank* 179:6–53, 1947.
3. Farah M: Visual agnosia: Disorders of object recognition and what they tell us about normal vision. Cambridge, MA: MIT Press, 1990.
4. De Renzi, E, Bonacini MG, Faglioni P: Right posterior patients are poor at assessing the age of a face. *Neuropsychologia* 27:839–848, 1989.
5. Kurucz J, Feldmar G: Prosopo-affective agnosia as a symptom of cerebral organic disease. J Am Geriatric Soc 23:225–230, 1979.
6. Benton AL, Van Allen MW: Impairment in facial recognition in patients with cerebral disease. *Cortex* 4:314–358, 1968.
7. De Renzi E, Faglioni P, Spinnler H: The performance of patients with unilateral brain damage on face recognition tasks. *Cortex* 4:17–34, 1968.
8. De Renzi E, Spinnler H: Facial recognition in brain-damaged patients. *Neurology* 16:145–152, 1966.
9. Milner B: Visual recognition and recall after right temporal lobe excision in man. *Neuropsychologia* 6:191–209, 1968.
10. Warrington EK, James M: An experimental investigation of facial recognition in patients with unilateral cerebral lesions. *Cortex* 3:317–326, 1967.
11. Benton AL, Van Allen MW: Prosopagnosia and facial discrimination. *J Neurol Sci* 15:167–172, 1972.
12. Malone DR, Morris HH, Kay MC, Levin HS: Prosopagnosia: A double dissociation between the recognition of familiar and unfamiliar faces. *J Neurol Neurosurg Psychiatry* 45:820–822, 1982.
13. Benton AL: The neuropsychology of facial recognition. *Am Psychol* 35:176–186, 1980.
14. Lissauer H: Ein Fall von Seelenblindheit nebst einem Beiträge zur Theorie derselben. *Arch Psychiatr* 27:222–270, 1890.
15. De Renzi E, Faglioni P, Grossi D, Nichelli P: Apperceptive and associative forms of prosopagnosia. *Cortex* 27:213–221, 1991.
16. Hécaen H: The neuropsychology of face recognition, in Davies G, Ellis H, Shepherd J (ed): *Perceiving and Remembering Faces*. London: Academic Press, 1981, pp 39–54.
17. Bruce V, Young A: Understanding face recognition. *Brit J Psychol* 77:305–327, 1986.
18. Semenza C, Zettin M: Evidence from aphasia for the role of proper names as pure referring expressions. *Nature* 342:678–679, 1989.
19. Carney R, Temple CM: Prosopanomia? A possible category-specific anomia for faces. *Cogn Neuropsychol* 10:185–195, 1993.
20. Adler A: Course and outcome of visual agnosia. *J Nerv Ment Dis* 111:41–51, 1950.
21. Bauer RM: Autonomic recognition of names and faces in prosopagnosia: A neuropsychological application of the guilty knowledge test. *Neuropsychologia* 22:457–469, 1984.
22. Benson DF, Greenberg JP: Visual form agnosia: A specific defect in visual discrimination. *Arch Neurol* 20:82–89, 1969.
23. Campion J, Latto R: Apperceptive agnosia due to carbon monoxide poisoning: An interpretation based on critical band masking from disseminated lesions. *Behav Brain Res* 15:227–240, 1985.
24. De Renzi E, Lucchelli F: The fuzzy boundaries of apperceptive agnosia. *Cortex* 29:187–215, 1993.
25. Landis T, Graves R, Benson DF, Hebben N: Visual recognition through kinesthetic mediation. *Psychol Med* 12:515–531, 1982.
26. McNeil JE, Warrington EK: Prosopagnosia: A reclassification. *Q J Exp Psychol* 43A:267–287, 1991.
27. Sergent J, Poncet M: From covert to overt recogni-

tion of faces in a prosopagnosic patient. *Brain* 113:989–1004, 1990.

28. Sergent J, Villemure JG: Prosopagnosia in a right hemispherectomized patient. *Brain* 112:975–995, 1989.

29. Ellis AW, Young AW, Critchley EMR: Loss of memory for people following temporal lobe damage. *Brain* 112:1469–1483, 1989.

30. Evans JJ, Heggs AJ, Antoun N, Hodges JR: Progressive prosopagnosia associated with selective right temporal lobe atrophy: A new syndrome? *Brain* 118:1–13, 1995.

31. Kartsounis LD, Shallice T: Modality specific semantic knowledge loss for unique items. *Cortex.* In Press.

32. De Haan EHF, Young AW, Newcombe F: A dissociation between the sense of familiarity and access to semantic information concerning familiar people. *Eur J Cogn Psychol* 3:51–67, 1991.

33. Tranel D, Damasio AR: Knowledge without awareness: An autonomic index of facial recognition by prosopagnosics. *Science* 228:1453–1454, 1985.

34. Rizzo M, Hurtig R, Damasio AR: The role of scanpaths in facial recognition and learning. *Ann Neurol* 22:41–45, 1987.

35. Renault B, Signoret JL, Debruille B, et al: Brain potentials reveal covert facial recognition in prosopagnosia. *Neuropsychologia* 27:905–912, 1989.

35a. Bruyer R, Laterre C, Séron X, et al: A case of prosopagnosia with some preserved covert remembrance of familiar faces. *Brain Cogn* 2:257–284, 1983.

36. De Haan EHF, Young AW, Newcombe F: Face recognition without awareness. *Cogn Neuropsychol* 1:385–415, 1987.

37. Diamond BJ, Valentine T, Mayes AR, Sandel ME: Evidence of covert recognition in a prosopagnosic patient. *Cortex* 30:377–393, 1994.

38. Young AW, De Haan EHF: Boundaries of covert recognition in prosopagnosia. *Cogn Neuropsychol* 5:317–336, 1988.

39. De Haan EHF, Young AW, Newcombe F: Faces interfere with name classification in a prosopagnosic patient. *Cortex* 23:309–316, 1987.

40. De Haan EHF, Bauer RM, Greve KW: Behavorial and physiological evidence for covert recognition in a prosopagnosic patient. *Cortex* 28:27–95, 1992.

41. De Haan EHF, Campbell R: A fifteen year followup of a case of developmental prosopagnosia. *Cortex* 27:489–509, 1991.

42. Newcombe F, Young AW, De Haan EHF: Prosopagnosia and object agnosia without covert recognition. *Neuropsychologia* 27:179–191, 1989.

43. Young AW, Ellis HD: Childhood prosopagnosia. *Brain Cogn* 9:16–47, 1989.

44. McNeil JE, Warrington EK: Prosopagnosia: A face-specific disorder. *Q J Exp Psychol* 46A:1–10, 1993.

45. Mishkin M, Ungerleider LG, Macko KA: Object vision and spatial vision: Two cortical pathways. *Trends Neurosci* 6:414–417, 1983.

46. De Haan EHF, Young AW, Newcombe F: Covert and overt recognition in prosopagnosia. *Brain* 114:2575–2591, 1992.

47. Farah MJ, O'Reilly RC, Vecera SP: Dissociated overt and covert recognition as an emergent property of a lesioned neural network. *Psychol Rev* 100:571–588, 1993.

48. Wallace MA, Farah MJ: Savings in relearning face-name associations as evidence for "covert recognition" in prosopagnosia. *J Cogn Neurosci* 4:150–154, 1992.

49. Humphreys GW, Riddoch MJ: The fractionation of visual agnosia, in Humphreys GW, Riddoch MJ (eds): *Visual Object Processing: A Cognitive Neuropsychological Approach.* Hillsdale, NJ: Erlbaum, 1987.

50. Damasio AR, Damasio H, Van Hoesen GW: Prosopagnosia: Anatomical basis and behavioral mechanisms. *Neurology* 32:331–341, 1982.

51. Lhermitte F, Pillon B: La prosopagnosie: Rôle de l'hémisphère droit dans la perception visuelle. (A propos d'un cas consécutif à une lobectomie occipitale droite). *Rev Neurol* 131:791–812, 1975.

52. Assal G, Favre C, Anderes JP: Non-reconnaissance d'animaux familiers chez un paysan. *Rev Neurol* 140:580–584, 1984.

53. Bornstein B, Sroka, H, Munitz H: Prosopagnosia with animal face agnosia. *Cortex* 5:164–169, 1969.

54. Sergent J, Signoret JL: Varieties of functional deficits in prosopagnosia. *Cerebral Cortex* 2:375–388, 1992.

55. Farah MJ, Klein KL, Levinson K: Face recognition and within-category discrimination in prosopagnosia. *Neuropsychologia* 33:661–674, 1995.

56. De Renzi E: Current issues on prosopagnosia, in Ellis HD, Jeeves MA, Newcombe F, Young A (eds): *Aspects of Face Processing.* Dordrecht: Nijhoff, 1986, pp 243–252.

57. Tanaka JW, Farah MJ: Parts and wholes in face recognition. *Q J Exp Psychol* 46A:225–245, 1993.

58. Farah M: Patterns of co-occurrence among the associative agnosias: Implications for visual object representation. *Cogn Neuropsychol* 8:1–19, 1991.

59. Rumiani RI, Humphreys GW, Riddoch M: Pure visual agnosia without prosopagnosia or alexia: Evidence for hierarchical theories of visual recognition. *Visual Cognition* 1:181–226, 1994.

60. Desimone R: Face-selectivity cells in the temporal cortex of monkeys. *J Cogn Neurosci* 3:1–8, 1991.

61. Perret DI, Mistlin AJ, Chitty AJ: Visual neurons responsive to faces. *TINS* 10:358–364, 1987.

62. Perret DL, Hietanen JK, Oram MW, Benson PJ: Organization and functions of cells responsive to faces in the temporal cortex. *Phil Trans R Soc Lond B* 335:23–30, 1992.

63. Adolphs R, Tranel D, Damasio H, Damasio A: Impaired recognition of emotions in facial expressions following bilateral damage to the human amygdala. *Nature* 372:369–372, 1994.

64. Young AW, Aggleton JP, Hellawell DJ, et al: Face processing impairments after amygdalotomy. *Brain* 118:15–24, 1995.

65. Rapcsak SZ, Comer JF, Rubens AB: Anomia for facial expressions: Neuropsychological mechanisms and anatomical correlates. *Brain Lang* 45:233–252, 1993.

66. Rapcsak SZ, Kaszniak AW, Rubens AB: Anomia for facial expression: Evidence for a category specific visual-verbal disconnection syndrome. *Neuropsychologia* 27:1031–1041, 1989.

67. Ojemann JG, Ojemann GA, Lettich E: Neuronal activity related to faces and matching in human right nondominant temporal cortex. *Brain* 115:1–13, 1992.

68. Hécaen H, Angelergues R: Agnosia for faces (prosopagnosia). *Arch Neurol* 7:92–100, 1962.

69. Meadows JC: The anatomical basis of prosopagnosia. *J Neurol Neurosurg Psychiatry* 37:489–501, 1974.

70. Cohn R, Neumann MA, Wood DJ: Prosopagnosia: A clinicopathological study. *Ann Neurol* 1:177–182, 1977.

71. Nardelli E, Buonanno F, Coccia G, et al: Prosopagnosia: Report of four cases. *Eur Neurol* 21:289–297, 1982.

72. De Renzi E, Perani D, Carlesimo GA, et al: Prosopagnosia can be associated with damage confined to the right hemisphere: An MRI and PET study and a review of the literature. *Neuropsychologia* 32:893–902, 1994.

73. Landis T, Regard M, Blieste A, Kleihues P: Prosopagnosia and agnosia for noncanonical views: An autopsied case. *Brain* 111:1287–1297, 1988.

74. De Renzi E, Zambolin A, Crisi G: The pattern of neuropsychological impairment associated with left posterior cerebral artery infarcts. *Brain* 110:1099–1116, 1987.

75. Uhl F, Lang W, Spieth F, Deecke L: Negative cortical potentials when classifying familiar and unfamiliar faces. *Cortex* 26:157–161, 1990.

76. Seek M, Mainwaring N, Ives J, et al: Differential neural activity in the human temporal lobe evoked by faces of family members and friends. *Ann Neurol* 34:369–372, 1993.

77. Kapur N, Friston KJ, Young A, et al: Activation of human hippocampal formation during memory for faces: A PET study. *Cortex* 31:99–108, 1995.

78. Sergent J, Ohta S, MacDonald B: Functional neuroanatomy of face and object processing. *Brain* 115:15–36, 1992.

79. McConachie HR: Developmental prosopagnosia: A single case report. *Cortex* 12:76–82, 1976.

80. Temple CM: A case of developmental prosopagnosia, in Campbell R (ed): *Mental Lives: Case Studies in Cognition*. London, Blackwell, 1991.

Chapter 8

AUDITORY AGNOSIA AND AMUSIA

Russell M. Bauer
Tricia Zawacki

The term *auditory agnosia* refers to an impaired capacity to recognize sounds in the presence of otherwise adequate hearing as measured by standard audiometry. Historically, the term has been used broadly to refer to impaired capacity to recognize sounds in general and in a narrow sense to refer to a selective deficit in recognizing nonverbal sounds only. Terminological confusion abounds, with such terms as *cortical auditory disorder,*[1,2] *auditory agnosia,*[3,4] and *auditory agnosia and word deafness*[5] all being used to describe similar phenomena. In most cases, impairment in the recognition of both speech and nonspeech sounds is present to some degree. The relative severity of these impairments depends on lesion localization, on premorbid lateralization of linguistic and nonlinguistic skills in the individual patient, and on which hemisphere is first or more seriously damaged[6] (but see Ref. 7). Complicating the picture even further is the fact that many patients evolve from one disorder to another as recovery takes place.[8] In regard to generalized auditory agnosia, we prefer the theoretically neutral term *cortical auditory disorder,* and we first discuss this entity together with *cortical deafness.* We then discuss more "selective" deficits, including *pure word deafness* (a selective impairment in speech-sound recognition), *auditory sound agnosia* (selective impairment in recognizing nonspeech sounds), and *paralinguistic agnosias* (in which recognition of prosodic features of spoken language is impaired). Finally, we describe patients with *receptive (sensory) amusia,* loss of the ability to appreciate various characteristics of heard music. Table 8-1 lists the major clinical features of each syndrome.

CORTICAL DEAFNESS AND CORTICAL AUDITORY DISORDER

Patients with cortical deafness show profound impairments in processing auditory stimuli of any kind and often have electrophysiologic signs of primary impairment in auditory-perceptual acuity. The behavior of patients with cortical auditory disorders is similar, though auditory evoked responses are more often normal in this population. Both groups show a range of impairments in auditory perception, discrimination, and recognition that affect verbal and nonverbal material.[9,10] If present, aphasic signs are mild and do not prevent the patient from identifying visual or somesthetic stimuli. Difficulties in elementary auditory function, including temporal auditory analysis and localization of sounds in space, are common.

In our view, cortical auditory disorders and cortical deafness are related in much the same way as visual agnosia is related to cortical blindness. If so, then cortical auditory disorders can take apperceptive or associative[11] forms, though some degree of perceptual deficit is apparent in nearly all cases where the evaluation of auditory abilities has been sufficiently comprehensive. This statement is true even in cases where pure tone audiometry is relatively normal. Jerger and coworkers[12,13] reported impairments in auditory perception (ear

Table 8-1
Clinical features of various forms of auditory agnosia

	Cortical deafness	Cortical auditory disorder	Pure word deafness	Auditory sound agnosia	Sensory/ receptive amusia
Audiometric sensitivity	−	+/−	+	+	+
Speech comprehension	−	−	−	+	+
Speech repetition	−	−	−	+	+
Spontaneous speech	+	+[a]	+[a]	+	+
Reading comprehension	+	+	+	+	+
Written language	+	+	+	+	+
Recognition of familiar sounds	−	−	+	−	?
Musical perception	−	−	−[b]	−	+/−
Recognition of vocal prosody	−	−	+	?	−

Key: + = spared ability; − = impaired ability; ? = insufficient information in literature to generalize.
[a]May be some paraphasia.
[b]When tested (rarely), musical perception has been shown to be impaired in these patients.
Sources: Adapted from Buchman et al.[7] and Oppenheimer and Newcombe,[3] with permission.

suppression in dichotic listening, abnormal click fusion thresholds, and impaired discrimination of basic sound attributes) in patients with cortical auditory disorders. These sometimes evolve from a state of cortical deafness, making it difficult to distinguish between the two entities. Michel and colleagues[14] argued that the cortically deaf patient looks and feels deaf, whereas the patient with cortical auditory disorders insists that he or she is not deaf. This turns out to be a poor criterion, because the subjective experience of deafness in the former condition is typically so transient and patients in both groups are "deaf" when subjected to appropriate tests. Although it was once believed that bilateral cortical lesions involving primary auditory cortex resulted in total hearing loss, evidence from animal experiments,[15,16] cortical mapping of the auditory area,[17] and clinicopathologic studies in humans[18,19] indicate that complete destruction of primary auditory cortex does not lead to permanent loss of audiometric sensitivity. Thus, clinical, pathologic, and electrophysiologic data question the distinctive nature of cortical deafness[1,9,10]

and suggest that it is one of a spectrum of auditory impairments that runs from generalized disturbances in detecting and discriminating basic sound attributes to more complex and selective impairments in auditory recognition.

Cortical deafness is most often seen in bilateral cerebrovascular disease. The course is usually biphasic, with an initial deficit (often aphasia and hemiparesis) related to unilateral damage, followed by a second (contralateral) deficit associated with sudden transient total deafness.[12,13,20,21] A biphasic course is also typical of cortical auditory disorders. In cortical deafness, bilateral destruction of the auditory radiations or the primary auditory cortex (Heschl's gyrus) has been a constant finding.[20] The anatomic basis of cortical auditory disorders is more variable. Lesions can be quite extensive,[3] though the superior temporal gyrus and efferent connections of Heschl's gyrus are often involved. Two recent Japanese cases[22,23] suggest that cortical auditory disorders can result from bilateral lesions sparing the cortex entirely. Thus, the lesions in cortical auditory disorders seem to involve either intrinsic or disconnecting lesions of auditory association cortex, with relative sparing of Heschl's gyrus.

PURE WORD DEAFNESS (AUDITORY AGNOSIA FOR SPEECH, AUDITORY VERBAL AGNOSIA)

The patient with pure word deafness is unable to comprehend spoken language although he or she can read, write, and speak in a *relatively* normal manner.[7] Writing to dictation is typically impaired, though copying of written material is not. By definition, comprehension of nonverbal sounds is *relatively* spared, but nonverbal auditory recognition is impaired in the majority of cases in which it has been evaluated.[7] Thus, the syndrome is "pure" in that (1) the patient is *relatively* free of signs of posterior aphasia and (2) the impairment in speech sound recognition is disproportionately severe. The disorder was first described by Kussmaul.[24] Lichteim[25] later defined it as an isolated deficit and postulated a bilateral subcortical interruption of fibers from ascending auditory projections to the left "auditory word center." With few exceptions, pure word deafness has been associated with bilateral, symmetric corticosubcortical lesions of the anterior part of the superior temporal gyri with some sparing of Heschl's gyrus, particularly on the left. Some patients have subcortical lesions of the dominant temporal lobe only, presumably destroying the ipsilateral auditory radiation as well as callosal fibers from the contralateral auditory region.[26–28] It is generally agreed that the lesion profile results in a bilateral disconnection of Wernicke's area from auditory input.[29] The fact that it involves an unusually placed, circumscribed lesion explains the low incidence of pure word deafness. In the review performed by Buchman and colleagues,[7] the lesions in 30 of 37 reviewed cases were of cerebrovascular origin.

When first seen, the patient is often recovering from a Wernicke's aphasia, though occasionally pure word deafness may actually give way to a Wernicke's aphasia.[30–33] As the paraphasias and writing and reading disturbances disappear, the patient still does not comprehend spoken language but can communicate by writing. Deafness can be ruled out by normal audiometric pure-tone thresholds. At this point, the patient may experience auditory hallucinations or may exhibit transient euphoric[34] or paranoid[35] ideation. The inability to repeat poorly comprehended speech stimuli distinguishes pure word deafness from transcortical sensory aphasia; the absence of florid paraphasia and of reading and writing disturbance distinguishes it from Wernicke's aphasia. This having been said, it should be recognized that "aphasic" and "agnosic" symptoms may both be present, though different in degree, in the individual case.[7]

Many patients are responsive to speech input but complain of dramatic, sometimes aversive changes in their subjective experience of speech sounds.[8] The pure word deafness patient may complain that speech is muffled or sounds like a foreign language. Hemphill and Stengel's[36] patient stated that "voices come but no words." Klein and Harper's[31] patient described speech as "an undifferentiated continuous humming noise without any rhythm" and "like foreigners speaking in the distance." Albert and Bear's[30] patient said "words come too quickly" and, "they sound like a foreign language." The speech of these patients is often slightly louder than normal. Performance on speech perception tests is inconsistent and highly dependent upon context[37] and linguistic complexity.[38]

Many studies of pure word deafness have emphasized the role of auditory-perceptual processing in the genesis of the disorder.[1,8,12,30,38] Problems with temporal resolution[30] and phonemic discrimination[39–41] have also received attention. Auerbach and coworkers[38] suggest that the disorder may take two forms: (1) a prephonemic temporal auditory acuity disturbance associated with bilateral temporal lesions or (2) a disorder of phonemic discrimination attributable to left temporal lesions and closely linked to Wernicke's aphasia. Albert and Bear[30] suggest that the problem in pure word deafness is one of temporal resolution of auditory stimuli rather than specific phonetic impairment. Their patient demonstrated abnormally long click-fusion thresholds, and improved in auditory comprehension when speech was presented at slower rates. Saffran and colleagues,[41] on the other hand, showed that informing their patient of the nature of the topic under discussion significantly facilitated comprehension. Thus, the disorder appeared to arise at different levels in these two patients. This variability supports the contention of Buchman and coworkers[7] that pure word deafness describes a spectrum rather than an individual disorder.

On tests of phonemic discrimination, patients with bilateral lesions tend to show distinctive deficits for the feature of place of articulation.[38,39,42] Those with unilateral left hemispheric disease (LHD) show either impaired discrimination of voicing[41] or no distinctive pattern.[40] In dichotic listening, some patients show extreme suppression of right-ear perception,[30,41] suggesting the inaccessibility of the left hemispheric phonetic decoding areas (Wernicke's area) to auditory material that has already been acoustically processed by the right hemisphere. Several studies have reported brainstem and cortical auditory evoked responses in pure word deafness patients.[14] Brainstem auditory evoked potentials (BAEPs) are almost always normal, suggesting intact processing up to the level of the auditory radiations.[30,38,43] Results from studies of cortical auditory evoked potentials (AEPs) more variable, consistent with variable pathology.[38] For example, the patient of Jerger and colleagues[12] had no appreciable AEP, yet heard sounds. The patient of Auerbach and associates[38] showed normal P1, N1, and P2 responses to right-ear stimulation but had minimal response over either hemisphere to left-ear stimulation.

Although patients with pure word deafness are supposed to perform relatively well with environmental sounds, many show subnormal performances when such abilities are formally tested.[7] Similarly, the appreciation of music is often disturbed. Some patients may recognize foreign languages by their distinctive prosodic characteristics, and others can recognize *who* is speaking, suggesting preserved ability to comprehend para-

linguistic aspects of speech. Coslett and associates[44] described a word-deaf patient who showed a remarkable dissociation between the comprehension of neutral and affectively intoned sentences. He was asked to point to pictures of males and females depicting various emotional expressions. When instructions were given in a neutral voice, he performed poorly, but when instructions were given with affective intonations appropriate to the target face, he performed normally (at a level commensurate to his performance with written instructions). This patient had bilateral destruction of primary auditory cortex with some sparing of auditory association cortex, suggesting at least some direct contribution of the auditory radiations directly to association cortex without initial decoding in Heschl's gyrus.[44] These authors speculate that one reason why pure word deafness patients improve their auditory comprehension with lip reading is that face-to-face contact allows them to take advantage of visual cues (gesture and facial expression) that are processed by different brain systems. Another explanation is that lip reading provides visual information about place of articulation, a linguistic feature that is markedly impaired at least in the bilateral cases.[38] In either case, the preserved comprehension of paralinguistic aspects of speech in pure word deafness patients further reinforces the widely held belief that comprehension of speech and nonspeech sounds are dissociable abilities.

AUDITORY SOUND AGNOSIA (AUDITORY AGNOSIA FOR NONSPEECH SOUNDS)

Patients with auditory sound agnosia have selective difficulty recognizing and identifying nonverbal sounds. The disorder is rare, less common by far than pure word deafness, but its existence has raised interest because it suggests the same type of "domain-specificity" in the auditory system that has received much recent attention in the study of visual recognition disorders.[45–47] The lower incidence of auditory sound agnosia may be due in part to the fact that such patients are less likely to seek medical advice than are those with a disorder of speech comprehension and also because nonspecific auditory complaints may be discounted when pure tone audiometric and speech discrimination thresholds are normal. This is unfortunate, since normal audiometry does not rule out the possibility of primary auditory perceptual defects.[48,49]

Vignolo[9] argued that there may be two forms of auditory sound agnosia: (1) a perceptual-discriminative type associated mainly with right hemisphere damage and (2) an associative-semantic type associated with left hemisphere damage and linked with posterior aphasia. The former group makes predominantly acoustic (e.g., "man whistling" for birdsong) errors on picture-sound matching tasks, while the latter makes predominantly semantic (e.g., "train" for automobile engine) errors. This division follows the original classification of Kliest,[50] who distinguished between the ability to detect/perceive isolated sounds or noises and the inability to understand the meaning of sounds. In the verbal sphere, the analogous distinction (at least on the input side) is between pure word deafness (perceptual-discriminative) and transcortical sensory aphasia (semantic-associative). Relatively few cases of "pure" auditory sound agnosia have been reported.[51–55]

The patient of Spreen and colleagues[54] is a paradigm case. He was a 65-year-old right-handed male who complained of "nerves" and headache when seen 3 years after a left hemiparetic episode. Audiometric testing revealed moderate bilateral high-frequency loss and speech reception thresholds of 12 dB for both ears. The outstanding abnormality was the inability to recognize common sounds. There was neither aphasia nor any other agnosic deficit. Sound localization was normal, but scores on the pitch subtest of the Seashore Tests of Musical Talent were at chance level. The patient performed well on a matching-to-sample test, suggesting that his sound recognition disturbance could not be attributed to serious acoustic disturbance. He claimed no musical experience or talent and refused to cooperate with further testing of musical ability. Postmortem examination revealed a sharply demarcated old infarct of the

right hemisphere centering around the parietal lobe and involving the superior temporal and angular gyri as well as a large portion of the inferior parietal, inferior, and middle frontal gyri and the insula. Other cases with unilateral pathology were reported by Fujii and coworkers[52] (small posterior right temporal hemmorhagic lesion of the middle and superior temporal gyri), Neilsen and Sult[53] (right thalamus and parietal lobe), and Wortis and Pfeffer[55] (large lesion of the right temporoparietooccipital junction).

These data suggest that an inability to recognize environmental sounds can occur after unilateral right hemisphere damage. Such a defect is less commonly seen in the context of bilateral disease,[51] but these cases are less "pure" at least in the acute stage. The association of auditory sound agnosia with right hemisphere damage implies that acoustic processors within the right hemisphere are preferentially involved in dealing with nonlinguistic sounds. The left hemisphere is likely involved in providing linguistic labels for identified sounds, and in performing semantic-associative functions supporting sound recognition and identification.

"PARALINGUISTIC AGNOSIAS": AUDITORY AFFECTIVE AGNOSIA AND PHONAGNOSIA

The auditory speech signal conveys not only linguistic meaning but also—through variations in volume, timbre, pitch, and rhythm—information about the emotional state of the speaker. Recent clinical evidence suggests that comprehension of affective tone can be selectively impaired. Heilman and coworkers[56] showed that patients with hemispatial neglect from right temporoparietal lesions were impaired in the comprehension of affectively intoned speech (a deficit they called "auditory affective agnosia") but showed normal comprehension of linguistic speech content. Patients with left temporoparietal lesions and fluent aphasia showed normal comprehension of both linguistic and affective (paralinguistic) aspects of speech. Whether this defect is "agnosic" in nature remains to be seen, since auditory sensory/perceptual skills were not assessed. It is possible that auditory affective agnosia is a subtype of auditory sound agnosia (i.e., that it represents a category-specific auditory agnosia), but further studies are necessary before this can be asserted with any certainty.

Recent studies by Van Lancker and associates[57–59] have revealed another type of paralinguistic deficit after right hemisphere damage. In these studies, patients with unilateral right hemisphere damage showed deficits in discriminating and recognizing familiar voices, while patients with left hemisphere damage were impaired only on a task that required a discrimination between two famous voices. Although the exact nature of this distinction is elusive, it seems to parallel that between episodic (personally experienced) versus semantic (generally known) memory in amnesia research. Evidence from computed tomography (CT) suggested that right parietal damage resulted in voice-recognition impairment, while temporal lobe damage in either hemisphere led to deficits in voice discrimination. The authors refer to this deficit as "phonagnosia," but, like auditory affective agnosia, it remains to be seen whether it is truly agnosic in nature.

SENSORY (RECEPTIVE) AMUSIA

The subject of amusia has been reviewed in detail by Wertheim,[60] Critchley and Henson,[61] and Gates and Bradshaw.[62] *Sensory amusia* refers to an inability to appreciate various characteristics of heard music. Impairment of music perception occurs to some extent in all cases of auditory sound agnosia and in the majority of cases of aphasia[62] and pure word deafness, though its exact prevalence in such populations is unknown. Loss of musical perceptual ability is probably underreported because a specific musical disorder rarely interferes with everyday life.

Wertheim[60] believed that receptive amusia occurs more frequently with left hemisphere damage, while expressive musical disabilities are more apt to be associated with right hemisphere damage. More recent evidence suggests that music perception is a multicomponent process to which both hemispheres contribute in complex ways. Dichotic listening studies show that the right hemisphere plays a more important role than the left in the processing of musical and nonlinguistic sound patterns.[63,64] However, the left hemisphere appears to be important in the processing of sequential (temporally organized) material of any kind, including musical series. The dominant hemisphere may process heard music more analytically or with more attention to specific features of the music, such as temporal order or rhythm.[62,65] According to Gordon,[64] melody recognition becomes more dependent on sequential processing as time and rhythm factors become more important for distinguishing tone patterns (see Ref. 66). The multicomponential nature of music perception makes it difficult to define receptive amusia and to localize the deficit to a particular brain region. Further complicating the picture is the fact that pitch, harmony, timbre, intensity, and rhythm may be affected to different degrees and in various combinations in the individual patient.

Many clinical studies distinguish between "instant" perceptual processes governing judgments of pitch, harmony, timbre, and intensity (loudness) and more "sequential," time-dependent processes governing melody recognition and judgments of rhythm and duration. Tentative clinical support for this kind of distinction exists in a double dissociation between the perceptual processing of pitch and the processing of temporal sequences,[67] dissociations that also hold true for reading music and for singing. There is further evidence that aspects of musical denotation (the "real-world" events referred to by lyrics) and musical connotation (the formal expressive patterns indicated by pitch, timbre, and intensity) are selectively vulnerable to focal brain lesions.[68,69] Gordon and Bogen[70] reported that during the right hemispheric anesthesia by the WADA procedure, singing was impaired with disrupted pitch production but preserved rhythmic expression. Hallucinations of voices and musical sounds have been reported with electrical stimulation of the lateral and superior surfaces of the first temporal convolutions in either hemisphere with more frequent occurrence on the nondominant side.[71]

Peretz and colleagues[68] applied comprehensive nonverbal auditory testing to two patients with bilateral lesions of auditory cortex. In their patients, the perception of speech and environmental sounds was spared, but the perception of tunes, prosody, and voice was impaired. Based on these behavioral dissociations, they argue that music processing is distinct from the processing of speech or environmental sounds. Their data led them to argue for a task- and process-specific approach to the analysis of cases of auditory agnosia. They suggest that nominally "auditory" tasks should be broken down into their functional subcomponents and that more extensive component-based analysis of auditory processing deficits is warranted. For example, they distinguish between processes involved in the recognition of specific voices or musical instruments (which is timbre-dependent), and processes involved in recognition of tunes (which is pitch-dependent). The notion that nominally distinct classes of auditory material (e.g., melodies, prosody, and voice) share common processes may be critically important in developing a functional taxonomy of auditory recognition disorders in general and of amusia in particular.

This suggestion points out certain significant deficiencies in the evaluation of amusic patients. Although theories linking brain function to music perception have long been available,[60,72,73] such theories do not often contain sufficient process specificity to guide the clinical evaluation of amusic patients. Thus, for example, relatively little is known regarding which musical features will be most informative in constructing a neuropsychological model of music perception. Another obstacle to systematic study of acquired amusia is the variability of preillness musical abilities, interests, and experience (see Wertheim[60] for a system of classifying musical ability level). The cerebral organization of musical perception has been sug-

gested to be dependent upon on the degree of these preillness characteristics.[72]

SUMMARY

In this chapter, we have briefly reviewed major types of auditory recognition disorders. Although certain identifiable syndromes exist, our review suggests a bewildering array of clinical symptoms and assessment methods. A fundamental problem concerns the lack of a comprehensive theory of auditory cognition. Compared to vision, for example, we know relatively little about the cognitive architecture underlying auditory identification of voices or environmental sounds. This theoretical anarchy has led to terminologic confusion and has slowed development of a cognitive taxonomy of auditory disorders because it has been unsafe to assume that different authors are using such terms in the same way. Another problem is that relatively little agreement exists regarding necessary and sufficient methods of testing in patients with auditory recognition disturbances. Thus, for example, it is not uncommon for claims of a specific defect in one area of auditory processing to be made when, in fact, such specificity is a spurious result of incomplete testing. This problem has been noted by others,[9] and it is obvious that further theoretical development in the area of auditory recognition disturbances will depend on the ability of researchers to devise more comprehensive and theoretically driven assessments of auditory function.[68]

Despite these problems, some progress has been made in identifying potentially important dissociations within auditory recognition disturbances that may eventually reveal the underlying structure of higher auditory processes. Dissociations between verbal (pure word deafness) and nonverbal (auditory sound agnosia) deficits and between perceptual-discriminative and semantic-associative forms of recognition disturbance have been described. Recent findings of impairments in recognizing affective prosody, tunes, and voice are exciting because they raise the further possibility of "category-specificity"[47,74,75] (or process-specificity) in auditory recognition, as has been described for vision (see Chaps. 6 and 7).

It seems clear at this point that further divisions within the concept of auditory agnosia are necessary and that a more comprehensive, process-based approach to evaluating auditory function is required. If this approach is developed further, the important building blocks in the structure of auditory cognition will eventually become apparent through behavioral dissociations.[46] In our view, the clinical approach to a patient suspected of auditory agnosia should consist, at a minimum, of the following steps. First, extensive testing of nonauditory language functions and of general neuropsychological status should be conducted in order to rule out the contribution of aphasia or dementia to the auditory recognition deficit. Second, detailed testing of auditory-perceptual abilities should be conducted, including but not necessarily limited to pure tone audiometry, speech-detection thresholds, temporal auditory acuity (e.g., click fusion thresholds), auditory discrimination,[76] and sound-localization tasks. When possible, brainstem and cortical auditory evoked responses should be evaluated in order to ascertain the "level" at which the patient's deficit occurs. Third, a broad evaluation of auditory capacities should be conducted, including evaluation of the patient's ability to recognize speech, environmental sounds, and music. Performance in other areas not typically assessed in these patients (e.g., voice recognition, singing and related expressive behavior, and evaluation of the patient's ability to recognize linguistic and nonlinguistic prosody) should be assessed. In order to sharpen the hazy distinctions between auditory agnosia (identification and recognition disturbances) and auditory comprehension deficits associated with aphasia, it might also be fruitful to routinely subject aphasic groups to the same kind of comprehensive auditory testing instead of assuming that their impairment in speech comprehension is a straightforward consequence of linguistic impairment. The interested reader should consult Peretz and associates[68] for a useful and reasonably comprehensive instantiation of this kind of approach to the study of auditory agnosias.

REFERENCES

1. Kanshepolsky J, Kelley J, Waggener J: A cortical auditory disorder. *Neurology* 23:699–705, 1973.
2. Miceli G: The processing of speech sounds in a patient with cortical auditory disorder. *Neuropsychologia* 20:5–20, 1982.
3. Oppenheimer DR, Newcombe F: Clinical and anatomic findings in a case of auditory agnosia. *Arch Neurol* 35:712–719, 1978.
4. Rosati G, DeBastiani P, Paolino E, et al: Clinical and audiological findings in a case of auditory agnosia. *J Neurol* 227:21–27, 1982.
5. Goldstein MN, Brown M, Holander J: Auditory agnosia and word deafness: Analysis of a case with three-year follow up. *Brain Lang* 2:324–332, 1975.
6. Ulrich G: Interhemispheric functional relationships in auditory agnosia: An analysis of the preconditions and a conceptual model. *Brain Lang* 5:286–300, 1978.
7. Buchman AS, Garron DC, Trost-Cardamone JE, et al: Word deafness: One hundred years later. *J Neurol Neurosurg Psychiatry* 49:489–499, 1986.
8. Mendez MF, Geehan GR: Cortical auditory disorders: clinical and psychoacoustic features. *J Neurol Neurosurg Psychiat* 51:1–9, 1988.
9. Vignolo LA: Auditory agnosia: A review and report of recent evidence. In Benton AL (ed): *Contributions to Clinical Neuropsychology*. Chicago: Aldine, 1969.
10. Lhermitte F, Chain F, Escourolle R, et al: Etude des troubles per-ceptifs auditifs dans les lesions temporales bilaterales. *Rev Neurol* 128:329–351, 1971.
11. Teuber H-L: Alteration of perception and memory in man, in Weiskrantz L (ed): *Analysis of Behavioral Change*. New York: Harper & Row, 1968.
12. Jerger J, Weikers N, Sharbrough F, Jerger S: Bilateral lesions of the temporal lobe: A case study. *Acta Oto-Laryngologica,* 258(suppl):1–51, 1969.
13. Jerger J, Lovering L, Wertz M: Auditory disorder following bilateral temporal lobe insult: Report of a case. *J Speech Hearing Dis* 37:523–535, 1972.
14. Michel J, Peronnet F, Schott B: A case of cortical deafness: Clinical and electrophysiological data. *Brain Lang* 10:367–377, 1980.

15. Massopoust LC, Wolin LR: Changes in auditory frequency discrimination thresholds after temporal cortex ablation. *Exp Neurol* 19:245–251, 1967.

16. Dewson JH, Pribram KH, Lynch JC: Effects of ablation of temporal cortex upon speech sound discrimination in the monkey. *Exp Neurol* 24:279–291, 1969.

17. Celesia GG: Organization of auditory cortical areas in man. *Brain* 99:403–414, 1976.

18. Mahoudeau D, Lemoyne J, Dubrisay J, Caraes J: Sur un cas dagnosie auditive. *Rev Neurol* 95:57, 1956.

19. Wohlfart G, Lindgren A, Jernelius B: Clinical picture and morbid anatomy in a case of "pure word deafness." *J Nerv Ment Dis* 116:818–827, 1952.

20. Leicester J: Central deafness and subcortical motor aphasia. *Brain Lang* 10:224–242, 1980.

21. Earnest MP, Monroe PA, Yarnell PA: Cortical deafness: Demonstration of the pathologic anatomy by CT scan. *Neurology* 27:1172–1175, 1977.

22. Kazui S, Naritomi H, Sawada T, Inque N: Subcortical auditory agnosia. *Brain Lang* 38:476–487, 1990.

23. Motomura N, Yamadori A, Mori E, Tamaru F: Auditory agnosia: Analysis of a case with bilateral subcortical lesions. *Brain* 109:379–391, 1986.

24. Kussmaul A: Disturbances of speech, in von Ziemssien H (ed): *Cyclopedia of the Practice of Medicine.* New York: William Wood, 1877.

25. Lichteim L: On aphasia. *Brain* 7:433–484, 1885.

26. Kanter SL, Day AL, Heilman KM, Gonzalez-Rothi LJ: Pure word deafness: A possible explanation of transient-deterioration after extracranial-intracranial bypass grafting. *Neurosurgery* 18:186–189, 1986.

27. Liepmann H, Storch E: Der mikroskopische Gehirnbefund bei dem Fall Gorstelle. *Monatsschr Psychiatr Neurol* 11:115–120, 1902.

28. Schuster P, Taterka H: Beitrag zur Anatomie und Klinik der reinen Worttaubbeit. *Z Neurol Psychiatr* 105:494, 1926.

29. Geschwind N: Disconnexion syndromes in animals and man. *Brain* 88:237–294, 585–644, 1965.

30. Albert ML, Bear D: Time to understand: A case study of word deafness with reference to the role of time in auditory comprehension. *Brain* 97:373–384, 1974.

31. Klein R, Harper J: The problem of agnosia in the light of a case of pure word deafness. *J Mental Sci* 102:112–120, 1956.

32. Gazzaniga M, Glass AV, Sarno MT: Pure word deafness and hemispheric dynamics: A case history. *Cortex* 9:136–143, 1973.

33. Ziegler DK: Word deafness and Wernicke's aphasia: Report of cases and discussion of the syndrome. *Arch Neurol Psychiatry* 67:323–331, 1942.

34. Shoumaker RD, Ajax ET, Schenkenberg T: Pure word deafness (auditory verbal agnosia). *Dis Nerv Sys* 38:293–299, 1977.

35. Reinhold M: A case of auditory agnosia. *Brain* 73:203–223, 1950.

36. Hemphill RC, Stengel E: A study of pure word deafness. *J Neurol Psychiatry* 3:251–262, 1940.

37. Caplan LR: Variability of perceptual function: The sensory cortex as a categorizer and deducer. *Brain Lang* 6:1–13, 1978.

38. Auerbach SH, Allard T, Naeser M, et al: Pure word deafness: Analysis of a case with bilateral lesions and a defect at the prephonemic level. *Brain* 105:271–300, 1982.

39. Chocholle R, Chedru F, Bolte MC, et al: Etude psychoacoustique d'un cas de surdite corticale. *Neuropsychologia* 13:163–172, 1975.

40. Denes G, Semenza C: Auditory modality-specific anomia: Evidence from a case of pure word deafness. *Cortex* 11:401–411, 1975.

41. Saffran EB, Marin OSM, Yeni-Komshian GH: An analysis of speech perception in word deafness. *Brain Lang* 3:255–256, 1976.

42. Naeser M: The relationship between phoneme discrimination, phoneme/picture perception, and language comprehension in aphasia. Presented at the Twelfth Annual Meeting of the Academy of Aphasia, Warrenton, Virginia, October 1974.

43. Stockard JJ, Rossiter VS: Clinical and pathologic correlates of brainstem auditory response abnormalities. *Neurology* 27:316–325, 1977.

44. Coslett HB, Brashear HR, Heilman KM: Pure word deafness after bilateral primary auditory cortex infarcts. *Neurology* 34:347–352, 1984.

45. Bauer RM: Agnosia, in Heilman KM, Valenstein E (eds): *Clinical Neuropsychology,* 3d ed. New York: Oxford University Press, 1993, pp 215–278.

46. Farah MJ: *Visual Agnosia: Disorders of Object Vision and What They Tell Us about Normal Vision.* Cambridge, MA: MIT Press/Bradford, 1990.

47. Farah MJ, Hammond KM, Mehta Z, Ratcliff G: Category-specificity and modality-specificity in semantic memory. *Neuropsychologia* 27:193–200, 1989.

48. Buchtel HA, Stewart JD: Auditory agnosia: Apperceptive or associative disorder? *Brain Lang* 37:12–25, 1989.

49. Goldstein MN: Auditory agnosia for speech ("pure word deafness"): A historical review with current implications. *Brain Lang* 1:195–204, 1974.

50. Kliest K: Gehirnpathologische und Lokalisatorische Ergebnisse uber Horstorungen, Geruschtaubheiten und Amusien. *Monatsschr Psychiatr Neurol* 68:853–860, 1928.

51. Albert ML, Sparks R, von Stockert T, Sax D: A case study of auditory agnosia: Linguistic and nonlinguistic processing. *Cortex* 8:427–433, 1972.

52. Fujii T, Fukatsu R, Watabe S, et al: Auditory sound agnosia without aphasia following a right temporal lobe lesion. *Cortex* 26:263–268, 1990.

53. Nielsen JM, Sult CW Jr: Agnosia and the body scheme. *Bull LA Neurol Soc* 4:69–81, 1939.

54. Spreen O, Benton AL, Fincham R: Auditory agnosia without aphasia. *Arch Neurol* 13:84–92, 1965.

55. Wortis SB, Pfeffer AZ: Unilateral auditory-spatial agnosia. *J Nerv Ment Dis* 108:181–186, 1948.

56. Heilman KM, Scholes R, Watson RT: Auditory affective agnosia. Disturbed comprehension of affective speech. *J Neurol Neurosurg Psychiatry* 38:69–72, 1975.

57. Van Lancker DR, Kreiman J: Unfamiliar voice discrimination and familiar voice recognition are independent and unordered abilities. *Neuropsychologia* 25:829–834, 1988.

58. Van Lancker DR, Kreiman J, Cummings J: Voice perception deficits: Neuroanatomical correlates of phonagnosia. *J Clin Exp Neuropsychol* 11:665–674, 1989.

59. Van Lancker DR, Cummings JL, Kreiman J, Dobkin BH: Phonagnosia: A dissociation between familiar and unfamiliar voices. *Cortex* 24:195–209, 1988.

60. Wertheim N: The amusias, in Vinken PJ, Bruyn GW (eds): *Handbook of Clinical Neurology.* Amsterdam: North-Holland, 1969, vol 4.

61. Critchley MM, Henson RA: *Music and the Brain: Studies in the Neurology of Music.* Springfield, IL: Charles C Thomas, 1977.

62. Gates A, Bradshaw JL: The role of the cerebral hemispheres in music. *Brain Lang* 4:403–431, 1977.

63. Blumstein S, Cooper W: Hemispheric processing of intonation contours. *Cortex* 10:146–158, 1974.

64. Gordon HW: Auditory specialization of the right and left hemispheres, in Kinsbourne M, Smith WL (eds): *Hemispheric Disconnection and Cerebral Function.* Springfield, IL: Charles C Thomas, 1974.

65. Krashen SD: Mental abilities underlying linguistic and nonlinguistic functions. *Linguistics* 115:39–55, 1973.

66. Mavlov L: Amusia due to rhythm agnosia in a musician with left hemisphere damage: A nonauditory supramodal defect. *Cortex* 16:331–338, 1980.

67. Peretz I: Processing of local and global musical information by unilateral brain-damaged patients. *Brain* 113:1185–1205, 1990.

68. Peretz I, Kolinsky R, Tramo M, et al: Functional dissociations following bilateral lesions of auditory cortex. *Brain* 117:1283–1301, 1994.

69. Gardner H, Silverman H, Denes G, et al: Sensitivity to musical denotation and connotation in organic patients. *Cortex* 13:242–256, 1977.

70. Gordon HW, Bogen JE: Hemispheric lateralization of singing after intracarotid sodium amylobarbitone. *J Neurol Neuorsurg Psychiatry* 37:727–738, 1974.

71. Penfield W, Perot P: The brain's record of auditory and visual experience. *Brain* 86:595–696, 1963.

72. Bever TG, Chiarello RJ: Cerebral dominance in musicians and nonmusicians. *Science* 185:137–139, 1974.

73. Hecaen H: Clinical symptomotology in right and left hemispheric lesions, in Mountcastle VB (ed): *Interhemispheric Relations and Cerebral Dominance.* Baltimore: Johns Hopkins University Press, 1962.

74. Warrington EK, Shallice T: Category-specific semantic impairments. *Brain* 107:829–854, 1984.

75. Damasio AR: Category-related recognition defects as a clue to the neural substrates of knowledge. *Trends Neurosci* 13:95–98, 1990.

76. Chedru F, Bastard V, Efron R: Auditory micropattern discrimination in brain damaged subjects. *Neuropsychologia* 16:141–149, 1978.

Chapter 9

DISORDERS OF BODY PERCEPTION

Georg Goldenberg

LEVELS OF INFORMATION ABOUT ONE'S BODY

In this chapter we distinguish three levels at which information about one's body is perceived and represented, as outlined below.

A Body-Centered Reference System for Motor Actions

Information about the current configuration and position of one's body is a necessary prerequisite for the planning and execution of most movements aimed at external targets. Reaching with the hand for a visually presented object requires that the retinotopic coordinates of the perceived object be transformed into body-centered coordinates. This transformation has to take into account the current position of the eyes relative to the head and of the head relative to the trunk. In addition to the representation of the target in body-centered coordinates, the brain must also represent the initial arm configuration in order to plan the trajectory. Single-cell recordings in monkeys have provided evidence that cells in Brodmann's areas 7 and 5 in the posterior parietal lobe are informed about the current position and configuration of the eyes, head, body, and limbs and perform the computations necessary for transforming visually perceived locations into body-centered coordinates.[1-4]

Reaching for an object is a highly automatized task. One need not pay attention to the position and configuration of one's body in order to accurately reach for a seen object. Assessment of the body-centered reference frame and computation of the target's location in body-centered coordinates take place automatically and without necessitating conscious awareness of one's body.

Awareness of One's Own Body

One can, of course, pay attention to the position and configuration of one's own body. Vestibular, kinesthetic, tactile, and visual perceptions provide information about the actual position and configuration of one's body; but even without distinct afferences from these channels, one has a basic "feeling" of where one's body parts are. One can point to the tip of one's nose without a mirror even if the nose does not itch. This basic awareness of the limits and the spatial layout of one's own body has been conceptualized as a mental "body schema."[6]

General Knowledge about the Human Body

General knowledge about human body and body parts can be of different kinds.[6] On the one hand, there is lexical and semantic knowledge, which defines the names, categories, and functions of body parts. This knowledge specifies, for example, that the wrist and ankle are both articulations or that the mouth is for speaking and the ear for hearing. On the other hand, there is topographic knowledge about the spatial layout of body parts. This knowledge provides information about the positions of individual body parts, the proximity relations that exist between them, and the boundaries that define each body part. For example, it specifies that the nose is in the middle of the face and that its upper end is contiguous to the forehead with the line of the eyebrows marking the border between them.

One's own body is one instance of the general configuration of human bodies. Pointing on command to parts of one's own body therefore assesses both awareness of one's own body and general knowledge about the human body.

With this classification in mind, we will discuss the following neuropsychological symptoms: optic ataxia, body-part phantoms, unilateral neglect, autotopagnosia, finger agnosia, and impaired imitation of gestures in ideomotor apraxia.

OPTIC ATAXIA

Optic ataxia was originally described in association with apraxia of gaze and simultanagnosia but has since then been recognized as an independent symptom that can occur without the other elements of Balint syndrome.[8–11] Patients with optic ataxia cannot accurately reach for visually perceived external targets. They move a hand into the approximate vicinity of the target and then start searching movements with the hand widely opened. Optic ataxia can occur in association with a general disorder of visuospatial perception, but there are patients who can give accurate judgments about the location and orientation of the objects they are unable to find with the hand.[10] By contrast, such a patient can reach without hesitation or error to parts of his or her own body. Asked to touch the tip of the nose or a finger, they do so as fast and accurately as normal persons.

One interpretation of optic ataxia is that the basic disorder concerns the transformation of retinotopic locations into a body-centered reference frame necessary for movement planning. The patients can reach for parts of their own bodies accurately because they are a priori coded in body-centered coordinates. At the same time, successful pointing to body parts indicates that awareness of the patient's own body is preserved as well as general conceptual knowledge about the human body.

Anatomic data support this interpretation. Lesions in optic ataxia are centered around the intraparietal sulcus and regularly affect human area 5 in the adjacent superior parietal lobe.[9,10] This location coincides with the location of neurons that have been found to be responsible for transformations from retinotopic to body-centered coordinates in monkeys (see above).

BODY-PART PHANTOMS

The occurrence of phantom limbs has been among the first[5] and continues to be among the most impressive arguments for the contention that the brain houses a mental body schema which underlies and modifies the way we experience our own bodies. After an amputation, about 90 percent of adults experience a phantom of the lost limb.[12–14] Initially, the phantom may be experienced in exactly the same way as the true limb was experienced before amputation. Over time, the experience may become less natural. Particularly where there is an upper limb phantom, the representation of the proximal portion may become weaker and eventually vanish, leading to the strange sensation of a hand belonging to one's own body but being disconnected from it. Alternatively, a shrinking of the proximal portions may lead to "telescoping" and give rise to the belief that the phantom arm is shorter than the other arm or even that a phantom hand resides within the amputation stump.[13,15]

Phantom experiences are not restricted to limbs but have also been reported after the loss of eyes,[16] teeth, external genitalia, and the female breast.[14] Phantoms of the amputated breast occur in about 40 percent of women who undergo mastectomy.[17–21] In about one-third of them, the phantom is limited to the nipple.[18] This restriction of the phantom to the most distal portion of the body part resembles the overrepresentation of the hand and fingers in upper limb phantoms.

Phantoms occur not only after amputation but can be caused by nervous system lesions provided that they interrupt all afferents from the affected body part. This may be the case with lesions of the peripheral nerves, the plexus, and the spinal cord but also with subcortical cerebral lesions.[12,14,22] If the deafferented limb is still present and visible, the phantom may be experienced as an additional, supernumerary limb.[14,22]

The occurrence of sensations in phantoms has been discussed in relation to plastic changes in synaptic connectivity of neurons in the primary sensory cortex. It has been demonstrated that phantom limb sensations can be induced by stimulation of the amputation stump or, in the case of upper limb phantoms, the face, and that there is an exact and reproducible correspondence between the locations of the actual and referred sensations leading to a "remapping" of the phantom on either the stump or the face.[15,23–25] Particularly remapping from the face to the hand is a strong argument in favor of the view that the phantom sensation arises in the primary sensory cortex, as the portion of the postcentral sensory cortex devoted to the face is adjacent to that devoted to the fingers and the hand. Converging evidence for neuronal plasticity in the primary sensory cortex has come from magnetencephalographic investigations showing an enlargement of the primary sensory field of the face in patients with upper limb phantoms.[25] Recently, remapping of sensory stimulation has also been demonstrated in patients with breast phantoms.[26] Tactile sensations from the ipsilateral dorsal thorax, the shoulder, and the pinna were referred to the amputated breast, mainly to the nipple. According to Penfield's homunculus, the somatosensory representations of the stimulated regions could be adjacent to the former representation of the amputated breast.

It is important to emphasize that remapping of stimulations concerns phantom sensations and not the very existence of the phantom. The basic experience of the phantom's existence persists even if no stimulation is applied to corresponding zones of intact body. Consequently, the demonstration that the source of phantom sensations resides in the primary sensory cortex does not nec-essarily indicate that primary sensory cortex is the neural substrate of the phantom itself.

Further insight into the cerebral substrate of body-part phantoms is provided by observation of patients who have lost the basic experience of the phantom after cerebral lesions. There are a few patients on record in whom a cortical lesion of the posterior parietal lobes abolished a phantom limb on the opposite side of the body.[12,27,28] In one of them (case 2), the clinical evidence strongly suggests preservation of the primary sensory cortex.[28] It can be concluded that integrity of the posterior parietal lobes is necessary for phantom limbs and that integrity of the primary sensory cortex is not sufficient. As there are no observations of restricted postcentral regions in patients with phantom limbs, it cannot be said whether integrity of the posterior parietal lobes is sufficient or integrity of the primary sensory area necessary for phantom limbs.

Body part phantoms are the most direct manifestation of a mental body schema that continues to exist even if it has lost its correlate in the real body. One interesting question is whether this mental body schema is innate or acquired by experience. An argument for the native predetermination of the representation of one's own body is the occurrence of limb phantoms in persons with congenital absence of limbs or with amputations in early childhood.[12,13,29] However, the frequency of phantom limbs in persons who lost their limbs before the age of 6 appears to be only some 10 percent as compared to about 50 percent in persons amputated between 6 and 10 years and 90 percent in persons amputated later (Piorreck, cited in Ref. 13). This increase would suggest that the mental body schema is at least enhanced and made more durable by continuing experience of the intact body. The case for a significant shaping of the body schema by experience is even stronger for breast phantoms. Girls do not have phantoms of their "congenitally absent" future breasts. In adult women, the frequency of breast phantoms diminishes with advancing age at mastectomy.[17–21] This apparent weakening of the mental representation of the breast might reflect the age-related decline of the breasts' volume and tension. Thus, the breasts' mental representations change in accord with the biological changes of the breasts across the life cycle. It would appear highly improbable that the course of these alterations is innately preprogrammed in the neural substrate of the body schema.

NEGLECT OF ONE-HALF OF THE BODY

Patients with hemineglect may neglect not only one-half of external space but also one-half of their own body. When combing, washing, shaving, or dressing, they restrict grooming to the nonneglected half of the body. When asked to indicate with the normal hand the midline of the body, they deviate to the healthy side,[11,30] as if the nonneglected half of the body were thinner or completely absent. When asked to touch the neglected hand with the normal one, the reaching movement may end at the shoulder or even at the midline of the trunk.[31]

Only a few studies have looked for the possibility that personal neglect of one-half of the body dissociates from extrapersonal neglect of one-half of surrounding space. A group study found only 1 out of 97 right-brain-damaged patients in whom personal neglect was not associated with extrapersonal neglect, while the reverse dissociation was far more frequent. Another group study[32] included only right-brain-damaged patients who displayed evidence of neglect on conventional tests like star cancellation. As these tests assess neglect in extrapersonal space, there was a priori no possibility of finding a patient in whom personal neglect was not associated with extrapersonal neglect. However, the authors found that success on tasks sensitive to personal neglect correlated only weakly with success on tasks sensitive to extrapersonal neglect. The same group then published a single case study of a patient who, after a right parietal hemmorhage, displayed conspicuous neglect of the left half of his own body but no sign of neglect of extrapersonal space even in extensive testing.[33]

In view of the paucity of systematic observation, it would be premature to speculate as to the location of lesions responsible for personal as opposed to extrapersonal neglect. It is not even clear whether the preponderance of left-sided hemineglect applies to personal neglect, as the large studies that established this hemispheric asymmetry were all restricted to measures of extrapersonal neglect.

Body part phantoms and neglect of one-half of the body are both disorders that concern the awareness of the patient's own body. Kinematic analyses do reveal abnormalities of reaching to external targets in patients with left hemineglect.[11,34,35] The patients were selected for having neglect of extrapersonal space, and it is not clear whether they had personal neglect at all. In any case, the abnormalities are different from those shown by patients with optic ataxia. Movements toward targets in the neglected half of space are slowed down and the movement path may deviate toward the nonaffected side of space, but the patients ultimately reach visible targets accurately and without searching. Apparently they are able to translate retinotopic localization into body-centered coordinates.

General knowledge about the human body is preserved in patients with phantom limbs or personal hemineglect. They are able to point on command to body parts on a model and even on their own bodies provided that these parts are not amputated or, respectively, neglected.[33] There are, however, reports of impaired performance on visuoconstructional tasks involving the human body, like assembling a human figure from its parts or judging the laterality of rotated hands[33,36] in patients with personal hemineglect. As the affected patients had right brain damage, it is questionable whether these symptoms were due to a lack of topographic knowledge about the human body or an expression of general visuoconstructional difficulties.

AUTOTOPAGNOSIA

Taken literally, the term *autotopagnosia* would indicate an inability to recognize locations on one's own body, but it is generally understood as designating the inability to localize body parts on one's own body as well as on another person or on a model of the human body. The term *somatotopagnosia*[37] would be more appropriate but has not found wide acceptance.

Earlier case reports of autotopagnosia have been criticized as demonstrating nothing more than the effects of general mental deterioration or of aphasia on the task of pointing to body parts on verbal command,[38] but since then several carefully conducted single-case studies have established the independence of autotopagnosia from aphasia and dementia and have drawn a consistent clinical picture of "pure" autotopagnosia:[1,39-41] when asked to point to body parts on themselves, on another person, or on a model of the human body, the patients commit errors. The majority of these errors are "contiguity" errors, in which the patient points to a different body part in the vicinity of the designated one. Less frequent are "semantic" errors which confuse body parts of the same category—as, for example, the elbow and the knee. Errors occur not only when the body parts are designated by verbal command but also when they are shown on pictures or even when the examiner demonstrates correct pointing and the patient tries to imitate. Patients with pure autotopagnosia are able to name the body parts when they are pointed at by someone else or shown on pictures, and although they invariably have left-sided brain lesions (see below), several of them were not aphasic at all.[6,39,40,43] Some patients were asked to give verbal descriptions of body parts. They could describe the function and the individual visual appearance of body parts but got lost when asked to describe their location.[6,39,40] According to the classification proposed in the opening of this chapter, this pattern of deficits would correspond to a selective loss of knowledge about the spatial layout of the human body.

The selectivity of this spatial disturbance has been disputed. It has been found that single patients committed errors also when asked to point to single parts of other multi-part objects than the human body as, for example, a bicycle or a house,[40,43] and it has been concluded that they suffer from a general inability to "analyze a whole into its parts." However, since this proposal was published, additional reports have documented patients with autotopagnosia who could locate the parts of multipart objects other than the human body.[6,39,41]

There are patients with autotopagnosia in whom localizing of individual fingers was found to be preserved.[40,42] We discuss further differences between autotopagnosia and finger agnosia in the next section but want to stress now that the preserved ability to differentiate the individual fingers of the hand is a further argument against a general deficit of "analyzing a whole into its parts."

Reaching to external targets and hence the computation of body-centered coordinates is unimpaired in autotopagnosia. Awareness of one's own body is difficult to assess formally, as autotopagnosia itself affects reaching for body parts. There are, nonetheless, observations suggesting that awareness of the patient's own body is preserved in autotopagnosia. One patient could correctly point to body parts when asked where certain garments are worn.[41] Another patient could locate her body parts when small objects where fixed to them and she was asked to point either to the objects or, after they had been removed, to their remembered locations.[6] Apparently these patients could orient themselves on their own bodies. Autotopagnosia seems to result from the inability to link preserved spatial orientation on one's own body with general knowledge about the human body.

The lesions in cases of pure autotopagnosia are remarkably uniform. They always affect the posterior parietal lobe of the left hemisphere.[39-43] In a group study of patients with left- or right-sided brain damage, errors in pointing to body parts occurred only in left-brain-damaged patients.[44] In this unselected sample, there were no cases of pure autotopagnosia. The patients who committed errors in localizing body parts were all aphasic and had on average larger lesions than patients who performed without error.

FINGER AGNOSIA

Finger agnosia was originally been described as part of the "Gerstmann syndrome,"[45] which is a combination of finger agnosia with right-left confusion, acalculia, and agraphia. However, it has been demonstrated that these are unrelated symptoms, which may or may not happen to occur together.[46]

The value of verbal tasks of finger identification has been called into question because they may be more sensitive to language disorders than to defective orientation on the body.[38,44] However, a considerable number of brain-damaged patients fail on nonverbal tasks of finger localization, like pointing on a drawing of a hand to fingers touched on the patient's own hand.[38,44,47]

Finger agnosia has been considered as a minor form of autotopagnosia,[45] but whereas autotopagnosia as characterized by errors in pointing to proximal body parts has been observed exclusively in patients with left brain damage, finger agnosia occurs with approximately equal frequency in patients with left and right brain damage.[38,44,47,48] We have already mentioned that there are patients with autotopagnosia in whom identification of fingers is preserved. If they are compared with those right-brain-damaged patients who have difficulties with the localization of fingers but not with pointing to proximal body parts,[44] there emerges a double dissociation between autotopagnosia and finger agnosia.

Common neuropsychological wisdom would suggest that a task which is sensitive to both left- and right-hemispheric damage does not tap a single psychological function. Presumably, disturbances of finger localization have different reasons in left- and right-brain-damaged patients.

IDEOMOTOR APRAXIA

Ideomotor apraxia is a symptom of left brain damage, which is usually considered as a disorder of motor control.[49-52] (See Chap. 27.) In particular, defective imitation of gestures has been considered as testifying a deficit of motor execution. In the words of De Renzi, "Since the examiner provides the model and the patient has only to copy it, errors can only be due to a deficit of motor execution."[51] This argument seems to be particularly convincing if novel and meaningless gestures are

to be imitated. Whereas imitation of familiar and meaningful gestures could be mediated by preexisting knowledge of the gestures' spatial configuration, imitation of meaningless gestures appears to test a direct route from visual perception to motor execution.[53-55]

There is, however, an alternative interpretation of the task demands of imitation of meaningless gestures. It proposes that general topographic knowledge about the human body mediates the transition from visual perception to motor execution.[56-59] Application of this knowledge reduces the multiple visually perceived details of the demonstrated gesture to simple relationships between a limited number of significant body parts, which can easily be implemented in routine motor programs. As a further advantage, translating the gesture's visual appearance in terms of the human body produces an equivalence between demonstration and imitation that is independent of the particular angle of view under which the demonstration is perceived.

The idea that defective imitation of gestures is due to a lack of topographic knowledge about the human body likens it to autotopagnosia. The parallel between defective imitation of meaningless gestures and autotopagnosia was strengthened by a study by the author who examined imitation of three kinds of gestures: for imitation of hand postures, the patients were required to copy different positions of the hand relative to the head while the configuration of the fingers remained invariant; for imitation of finger postures, patients were asked to replicate different configurations of the fingers, and the position of the whole hand relative to the body was not considered for scoring; for imitation of combined gestures, both a defined position of the hand relative to the body and defined configuration of the fingers were required.[59] Regardless of whether imitations of hand positions and finger configurations were tested each on their own or together, they proved to show differential susceptibility to left and right brain damage. Whereas imitation of finger configurations was about equally impaired in left- and right-brain-damaged patients, defective imitation of hand positions occurred exclusively in left-brain-damaged patients, and whereas controls as well as right-brain-damaged patients committed fewer errors with hand positions than with finger configurations, the reverse was the case in left-brain-damaged patients. This dissociation between gestures requiring orientation relative to the proximal body and gestures requiring orientation within the hand closely resembles the above-mentioned dissociation between autotopagnosia and finger agnosia.

A lack of general knowledge about the human body should lead to errors regardless of whether gestures are to be replicated on another body or on oneself. Indeed, patients who display apraxia on imitation of hand positions commit more errors than either left-brain-damaged patients without apraxia or right-brain-damaged patients when trying to replicate the same positions on a manikin.[57]

REFERENCES

1. Mountcastle VB, Lynch JC, Georgopoulos A, et al: Posterior parietal association cortex of the monkey: Command functions for operations within extrapersonal space. *J Neurophysiol* 38:871–908, 1975.
2. Andersen RA: Visual and eye movement functions of the posterior parietal cortex. *Annu Rev Neurosci* 12:377–403, 1989.
3. Bizzi E, Mussa-Ivaldi FA: Motor control, in Boller F, Grafman J (eds): *Handbook of Neuropsychology.* New York: Elsevier, 1990, vol 2, pp 229–244.
4. Stein JF: The representation of egocentric space in the posterior parietal cortex. *Behav Brain Sci* 15: 691–700, 1992.
5. Pick A: Zur Pathologie des Bewußtseins vom eigenen Körper—Ein Beitrag aus der Kriegsmedizin. *Neurol Zentralbl* 34:257–265, 1915.
6. Sirigu A, Grafman J, Bressler K, Sunderland T: Multiple representations contribute to body knowledge processing. *Brain* 114:629–642, 1991.
7. Balint R: Seelenlaehmung des "Schauens," optische Ataxie, räumliche Störung der Aufmerksamkeit. *Monatsschr Psychiat Neurol* 25:51–81, 1909.
8. Rondot P, de Recondo J, Dumas JLR: Visuomotor ataxia. *Brain* 100:355–376, 1977.
9. Damasio AR, Benton AL: Impairment of hand movements under visual guidance. *Neurology* 29: 170–178, 1979.
10. Perenin MT, Vighetto A: Optic ataxia: A specific disruption in visuomotor mechanisms: I. Different aspects of the deficit in reaching for objects. *Brain* 111:643–674, 1988.
11. Jeannerod M: *The Neural and Behavioural Organization of Goal-Directed Movements.* Oxford, England: Clarendon Press, 1988.
12. Poeck K: Zur Psychophysiologie der Phantomerlebnisse. *Nervenarzt* 34:241–256, 1963.
13. Poeck K: Phantome nach Amputation und bei angeborenen Gliedmaßenmangel. *Dtsche med Wochensch* 46:2367–2374, 1969.
14. Frederiks JAM: Phantom limb and phantom limb pain, in Frederiks JAM (ed): *Handbook of Neurology:* New York: Elsevier, 1985, vol 1, pp 395–404.
15. Haber WE: Observations on phantom-limb phenomena. *Arch Neurol Psychiatry* 75:624–636, 1956.
16. Cohn R: Phantom vision. *Arch Neurol* 25:468–471, 1971.
17. Simmel ML: A study of phantoms after amputation of the breast. *Neuropsychologia* 4:331–350, 1966.
18. Jarvis JH: Post-mastectomy breast phantoms. *J Nerv Ment Dis* 144:266–272, 1967.
19. Jamison K, Wellisch DK, Katz RL, Pasnau RO: Phantom breast syndrome. *Arch Surg* 114:93–95, 1979.
20. Weinstein S, Vetter RJ, Sersen EA: Phantoms following breast amputation. *Neuropsychologia* 8: 185–197, 1970.
21. Kroner K, Krebs B, Skov J, Jorgensen HJ: Immediate and long-term phantom breast syndrome after mastectomy: Incidence, clinical characteristics and relationship to pre-mastectomy breast pain. *Pain* 36:327–334, 1989.
22. Halligan PW, Marshall JC, Wade DT: Three arms: A case study of supernumerary phantom limb after right hemisphere stroke. *J Neurol Neurosurg Psychiatry* 56:159–166, 1993.
23. Ramachandran VS: Behavioral and magnetoencephalographic correlates of plasticity in the adult human brain. *Proc Natl Acad Sci USA* 90: 10413–10420, 1993.
24. Ramachandran VS, Rogers-Ramachandran D, Stewart M: Perceptual correlates of massive cortical reorganization. *Science* 258:1159–1160, 1992.
25. Flor H, Elbert T, Knecht S, et al: Phantom-limb pain as a perceptual correlate of cortical reorganization following arm amputation. *Nature* 375:482–484, 1995.
26. Aglioti S, Cortese F, Franchini C: Rapid sensory remapping in the adult human brain as inferred from phantom breast sensation. *NeuroReport* 5:473–476, 1994.

27. Head H, Holmes G: Sensory disturbances from cerebral lesions. *Brain* 34:102–254, 1911.

28. Appenzeller O, Bicknell JM: Effects of nervous system lesions on phantom experience in amputees. *Neurology* 19:141–146, 1969.

29. Melczack R: Phantom limbs and the concept of a neuromatrix. *Trends Neurosci* 13:88–92, 1990.

30. Karnath HO: Subjective body orientation in neglect and the interactive contribution of neck muscle proprioception and vestibular stimulation. *Brain* 117:1001–1012, 1994.

31. Bisiach E, Perani D, Vallar G, Berti A: Unilateral neglect: Personal and extrapersonal. *Neuropsychologia* 24:759–767, 1986.

32. Zoccolotti P, Judica A: Functional evaluation of hemineglect by means of a semistructured scale: Personal and extrapersonal differentiation. *Neuropsychol Rehab* 1:33–44, 1991.

33. Guariglia C, Antonucci G: Personal and extrapersonal space: A case of neglect dissociation. *Neuropsychologia* 30:1001–1010, 1992.

34. Chieffi S, Gentilucci M, Allport A, et al: Study of selective reaching and grasping in a patient with unilateral parietal lesion. *Brain* 116:1119–1137, 1993.

35. Mattingley JB, Phillips JG, Bradshaw JL: Impairment of movement execution in unilateral neglect: A kinematic analysis of directional bradykinesia. *Neuropsychologia* 32:1111–1134, 1994.

36. Coslett HB: The role of the body image in neglect. *J Clin Exp Neuropsychol* 11:79, 1989.

37. Gerstmann J: Problems of imperception of disease and of impaired body territories with organic lesions: Relation to body scheme and its disorders. *Arch Neurol Psychiatry* 48:890–913, 1942.

38. Poeck K, Orgass B: An experimental investigation of finger agnosia. *Neurology* 19:801–807, 1969.

39. Ogden JA: Autotopagnosia: Occurrence in a patient without nominal aphasia and with an intact ability to point to parts of animals and objects. *Brain* 108:1009–1022, 1985.

40. De Renzi E, Scotti G: Autotopagnosia: Fiction or reality? *Arch Neurol* 23:221–227, 1970.

41. Semenza C: Impairment of localization of body parts following brain damage. *Cortex* 24:443–450, 1988.

42. Assal G, Butters J: Troubles du schéma corporel lors des atteintes hémisphériques gauches. *Schweiz Med Rundsch* 62:172–179, 1973.

43. Poncet M, Pellissier JF, Sebahoun M, Nasser CJ: A propos d'un cas d'autotopagnosie secondaire à une lésion pariéto-occipitale de l'hémisphère majeur. *Encephale* 61:1–14, 1971.

44. Sauguet J, Benton AL, Hecaen H: Disturbances of the body schema in relation to language impairment and hemispheric locus of lesion. *J Neurol Neurosurg Psychiatry* 34:496–501, 1971.

45. Gerstmann J: Zur Symptomatologie der Hirnläsionen im Übergangsgebiet der unteren Parietal- und mittleren Occipitalwindung. *Nervenarzt* 3:691–696, 1930.

46. Benton AL: The fiction of the "Gerstmann syndrome." *J Neurol Neurosurg Psychiatry* 24:176–181, 1961.

47. Gainotti G, Cianchetti C, Tiacci C: The influence of the hemispheric side of lesion on nonverbal tasks of finger localization. *Cortex* 8:364–381, 1972.

48. Kinsbourne M, Warrington EK: A study of finger agnosia. *Brain* 85:47–66, 1962.

49. Liepmann H: *Drei Aufsätze aus dem Apraxiegebiet.* Berlin: Karger, 1908.

50. Poeck K: The two types of motor apraxia. *Arch Ital Biol* 120:361–369, 1982.

51. De Renzi E: Apraxia, in Boller F, Grafman J (eds): *Handbook of Neuropsychology.* New York: Elsevier, 1990, vol 2, pp 245–263.

52. Heilman KM, Rothi LJG: Apraxia, in Heilman KM, Valenstein E (eds): *Clinical Neuropsychology.* New York: Oxford University Press, 1993, pp 141–164.

53. Barbieri C, de Renzi E: The executive and ideational components of apraxia. *Cortex* 24:535–544, 1988.

54. Rothi LJG, Ochipa C, Heilman KM: A cognitive neuropsychological model of limb praxis. *Cog Neuropsychol* 8:443–458, 1991.

55. Roy EA, Hall C: Limb apraxia: A process approach, in Proteau L, Elliott D (eds): *Vision and Motor Control* Amsterdam: Elsevier, 1992, pp 261–282.

56. Morlaas J: *Contribution à l'étude de l'apraxie.* Paris: Amédée Legrand, 1928.

57. Goldenberg G: Imitating gestures and manipulating a mannikin—The representation of the human body in ideomotor apraxia. *Neuropsychologia* 33:63–72, 1995.

58. Goldenberg G, Hermsdörfer J, Spatt J: Ideomotor apraxia and cerebral dominance for motor control. *Cog Brain Res.* In press.

59. Goldenberg G: Defective imitation of gestures in patients with left and right hemisphere lesions. *J Neurol Neurosurg Psychiatry.* In press.

Chapter 10

NEGLECT I: CLINICAL AND ANATOMIC ISSUES

Kenneth M. Heilman
Robert T. Watson
Edward Valenstein

Neglect is a failure to report, respond, or orient to stimuli that are presented contralateral to a brain lesion, when this failure is not due to elementary sensory or motor disorders.[1] Many subtypes of neglect have been described. A major distinction is between neglect of perceptual input, termed *sensory neglect* or *inattention*, and neglect affecting response outputs, termed *motor* or *intentional neglect*. Some further distinctions are outlined below.

Sensory neglect involves a selective deficit in awareness, which may apply to all stimuli on the affected side of space (*spatial neglect*) or be confined to stimuli impinging on the patient's body (*personal neglect*). It may even affect awareness of one side of internal mental images (*representational neglect*). The perceptual modalities affected by neglect may also vary: Subtypes of sensory neglect exist for the visual, auditory, and tactile modalities. The deficit in awareness is accompanied by an abnormal attentional bias. Attention is usually biased toward the ipsilesional side but in rare cases may be contralesional. Once attention is engaged on an ipsilesional stimulus, subjects may have difficulty disengaging their attention to move it to the contralesional side. If the lack of awareness and attentional bias are present only when there is a competing stimulus at a more ipsilateral location, the disorder is termed *extinction*. Many patients with neglect recover and become able to detect isolated contralesional stimuli but continue to manifest extinction.

Motor or *intentional neglect* involves a response failure that cannot be explained by weak-ness, sensory loss, or unawareness. There may be a failure to move a limb (*limb akinesia*), or the limb can be moved but only after a long delay and strong encouragement (*hypokinesia*). Patients with intentional neglect who can move may make movements of decreased amplitude (*hypometria*). They may also have an inability to maintain posture or movements (*impersistence*). Patients with motor neglect who can move their contralesional limb may fail to move this limb (or have a delay) when they are also required to move their ipsilateral limb (*motor extinction*). Limb akinesia, hypokinesia, hypometria, and motor impersistence can affect some or all parts of the body, including limbs, eyes, or head. The elements of intentional neglect discussed above can be *directional* (toward the contralesional hemispace) or *spatial* (within the contralesional hemispace). Patients with motor neglect may have intentional biases such that there is a propensity to move toward ipsilesional space. There may also be impaired ability to disengage from motor activities (*motor perseveration*).

TESTING FOR NEGLECT

In this brief review we cannot address all aspects of testing; therefore, for a complete discussion and list of references, the reader is referred to Heilman and coworkers.[1]

Inattention or Sensory Neglect

To test for inattention, the patient is presented with unilateral stimuli on either the ipsilesional or contralesional side in random order. If a patient fails to detect more stimuli on the contralesional side than the ipsilesional side, it would suggest that the patient is suffering from inattention. However, if the patient totally fails to detect any stimuli on the contralesional side, it is often difficult to tell whether or not the patient has inattention or a sensory loss. The auditory modality is the least difficult in which to dissociate inattention and sensory loss because sounds made on one side of the head project to both ears, and each ear projects to both the ipsilateral as well as the contralateral hemisphere. Therefore, if a patient is unaware of noises made on one side of his or her head, this unawareness cannot be explained by a sensory defect and suggests that the patient has inattention. In the visual modality, because unawareness may be hemispatial (body-centered) rather than retinotopic, having the patient deviate the eyes toward ipsilateral hemispace may allow him or her to become aware of stimuli projected to the contralesional portion of the retina. In regard to tactile neglect, one may have to use caloric stimulation of the ear to see if the patient can detect stimuli during such stimulation. One may also use psychophysiologic techniques such as evoked potentials or galvanic skin responses to see whether patients who are unaware of stimuli demonstrate autonomic signs of stimulus detection.[2]

Extinction

To test for extinction, one may randomly intermix the unilateral stimuli described above with bilateral simultaneous stimuli. The stimuli can be given in any modality (e.g., visual, auditory, tactile). When a subject has hemianopia, extinction may even occur within the ipsilesional visual field.

Intentional or Motor Neglect

Patients who have severe limb akinesia may appear to have a hemiparesis. An arm may hang off the bed or wheelchair. Sometimes, with strong encouragement by the examiner, it can be demonstrated that such a patient has normal strength. However, some patients will still not move, and

one may have to rely on brain imaging to learn whether the corticospinal tract is involved. In patients with motor neglect, the lesion should not involve the corticospinal system. Magnetic stimulation may also be helpful in demonstrating that the corticospinal tract is normal.[3] As we discussed, patients with hypokinesia are reluctant to move the affected arm or only move it after delay. However, once they have moved, their strength may be normal. To test for hypometria, the arm is passively moved or the patient is shown a line and asked to make a movement of the same length. Patients with hypometria will undershoot the target. To test for impersistence, the patient is asked to sustain a posture. Patients with impersistence cannot maintain postures. As mentioned, patients can be tested for forms of motor neglect by using the limbs, eyes, or even head. They can be tested in ipsilateral versus contralateral hemispace and in an ipsilesional versus contralesional direction.

Spatial Neglect

Four clinical tests are commonly used to assess for spatial neglect. In the line bisection task, the patient is given a long line and asked to indicate its midpoint (Fig. 10-1). Although horizontal lines are most commonly used (intersection of the coronal and axial planes), neglect has been reported in the vertical dimension (both up neglect and down neglect) and in the radial dimension (near neglect and far neglect).

In general, the longer the line, the greater the percentage of error. Placing the line in contralesional hemispace can also increase the severity of the error, as can putting cues on the ipsilesional side.

In performing the cancellation task, a sheet of paper that contains targets is placed before the patient and the patient is asked to mark out (cancel) all the targets (Fig. 10-2). Increasing the number of targets can increase the sensitivity of this test. Increasing the difficulty with which one discriminates targets from distractors can also increase the sensitivity of this task.

In testing drawing, the patient should be asked to draw spontaneously as well as to copy

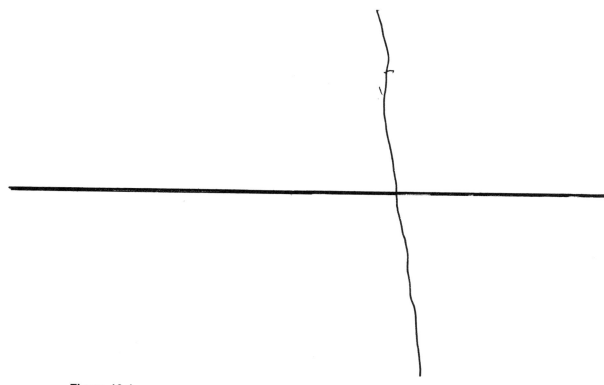

Figure 10-1

Line bisection task performed by a patient with a right hemisphere infarction and left hemispatial neglect. (From Dr. Todd E. Feinberg with permission.)

figures (Figs. 10-3 and 10-4). Copying asymmetrical nonsense figures may be more difficult than copying well-known symmetrical figures.

In testing for representational neglect, one should ask a subject to image a familar scene and then report what he or she sees. A patient with representational neglect will recall more objects from the ipsilesional than the contralesional part of the image.

At times it may be difficult to dissociate sensory attentional disorders from motor intentional disorders. In general, the best means of doing this is by performing cross-response tasks where the subject responds in one side of space to a stimulus presented on the opposite side. Video cameras, strings and pulley, or mirrors can be used in the performance of a cross response task.

To dissociate intentional from representa-

tional defects, one can use a fixed-aperture technique. To do this, an opaque sheet with a fixed window is placed over a sheet with targets so that only one target can be seen at a time, thereby reducing attentional demands. In one-half the trials, the subject moves the top sheet; in the other trials, the subject moves the target sheet. A failure to explore one portion of the target sheet in both conditions suggests a representational defect, and a failure to explore opposite sides of the target sheet in direct and indirect conditions suggests a motor intentional deficit.[4]

To dissociate neglect of one side of the environment from neglect of one side of the person, one can ask the patient to lie down on his or her side. This decouples the environmental left and right from the body's left and right. If the patient has a right hemispheric lesion, is lying on the right

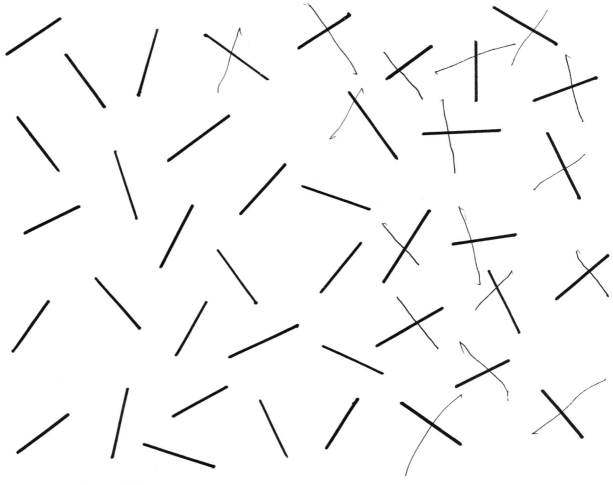

Figure 10-2
Cancellation task of same patient as in Fig. 10-1. (From Dr. Todd E. Feinberg with permission.)

side, and now fails to detect targets toward the ceiling, the neglect is body-centered. However, if the patient continues to neglect targets on his or her left side, the neglect is environmentally centered.[5,6]

PATHOPHYSIOLOGY

As the foregoing review suggests, neglect is not a homogeneous syndrome. The neglect syndrome

not only has many manifestations but also many levels of explanation. For a more complete discussion see Heilman and coworkers.[1] The heterogeneity of neglect is apparent on an anatomic level as well.

In humans, neglect is most often associated with lesions of the inferior parietal lobe (IPL), which includes Brodmann's areas 40 and 39. However, neglect has also been reported from dorsolateral frontal lesions, medial frontal lesions that include the cingulate gyrus, thalamic-mesencephalic

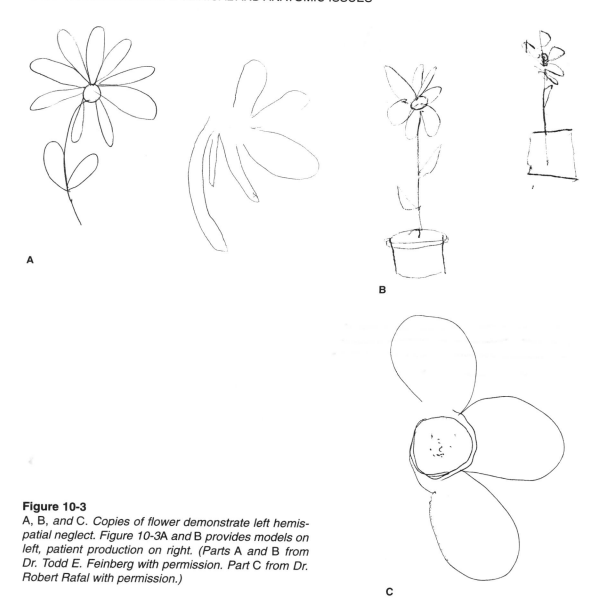

Figure 10-3
A, B, and C. Copies of flower demonstrate left hemispatial neglect. Figure 10-3A and B provides models on left, patient production on right. (Parts A and B from Dr. Todd E. Feinberg with permission. Part C from Dr. Robert Rafal with permission.)

lesions, basal ganglia, and white matter lesions. Because there is a limit on the anatomic, physiologic, and behavioral research that can be done in humans, much of what we know about the pathophysiology of the neglect syndrome comes from research on old-world monkeys. Monkeys also have an IPL; however, their IPL is Brodmann's area 7. In humans, the intraparietal sulcus separates the superior parietal area, Brodmann's area 7, from the inferior parietal lobule, Brodmann's areas 40 and 39. Some have thought that the IPL of monkeys is a homologue of the IPL in humans. Others, however, have thought that both banks of the superior temporal sulcus (STS) are the homologue of the inferior parietal lobule in humans. Recently, we[7] demonstrated that neglect in mon-

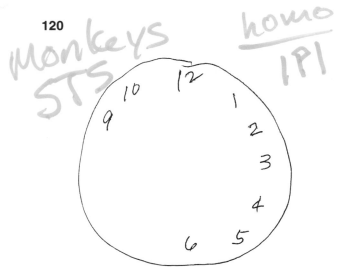

Monkeys STS   homo IPI (handwritten annotations)

Figure 10-4
Clock drawn by a patient with left hemispatial neglect.
(From Dr. Robert Rafal with permission.)

keys is associated with ablation of the STS region and not the IPL. These results suggest that, in regard to neglect, it is the monkeys' STS that is the homologue of the humans' IPL.

Anatomic studies of the STS of monkeys have provided some information as to why this area produces neglect when ablated. The STS is composed of multiple subareas and is one of the sites of multimodal sensory convergence. Visual, auditory, and somatosensory association cortices all project to portions of the STS. In addition, the STS has reciprocal connections to other multimodal convergence areas such as monkeys' IPL (Brodmann's area 7). Because ablation of area 7 in monkeys, a multimodal convergence area, was not associated with neglect, we do not believe that ablation of a sensory convergence area alone can account for the unawareness that is seen with neglect syndrome. Therefore, Watson and coworkers[7] have proposed a role for monkeys' STS or humans' IPL in awareness.

Mishkin and colleagues[8] suggested that the visual system, when presented with stimuli, performs dual parallel processes. Whereas the ventral division is important for determining the type of stimulus ("What is it?"), the dorsal system codes the spatial location of the stimulus ("Where is

it?"). In monkeys the "where" system is in part mediated by the posterior portion of Brodmann's area 7 or the monkey's IPL, and the "what" system is in part being mediated by the inferior visual association cortex found in the ventral temporal lobe. It has been long recognized that bilateral ventral temporal lesions in humans and monkeys induce visual object agnosia, a deficit in the "what" system. In contrast, biparietal lesions in monkeys induce deficits of visual spatial localization but not object discrimination. Watson and coworkers[7] posited that these "where" and "what" systems integrate in the banks of monkeys' STS or in the inferior parietal lobule of humans. According to Watson and colleagues,[7] lesions of monkeys' STS and humans' IPL induce unawareness or neglect not only because this is the area that receives polymodal sensory input but also because it is a convergence site of these perceptual-cognitive systems that deal with both the "what" and "where" aspects of environmental awareness. Both anatomic and electrophysiologic data substantiate the hypothesis that monkeys' STS is an area of convergence of these two systems (see Watson and coworkers).[7] Watson and colleagues[7] also proposed that similar areas important for spatial localization and object identification may also exist in the auditory and tactile systems and that these modalities may also converge in the STS.

Although there is anatomic and physiologic evidence that there is convergence from the Brodmann's area 7 "where" system and the ventral temporal lobes' "what" system, this cannot account for the observation that ablation of the STS induces unawareness. The STS receives input not only from these "what" and "where" systems but also from the cingulate gyrus and the dorsolateral frontal lobe. In earlier studies, we have demonstrated that lesions in both these areas are also able to induce neglect. The dorsolateral prefrontal region is important in the mediation of goal-directed behavior and may provide the STS with information that is not directly stimulus-dependent or related to immediate drives and biological needs but rather directed at long-term goals. The cingulate gyrus is part of the limbic system and may provide the STS with information about biological needs and drives. Because monkeys' STS or humans' IPL is supplied with "what" and "where" conative and motivational information, it may be able to make attentional computations.

Monkeys' STS has reciprocal connections with the ventral temporal "what" region and the parietal "where" region. Therefore, after the STS region (or the IPL in humans) performs an attentional computation, it may reciprocally influence the neurons in the ventral temporal lobe and Brodmann's area 7 regions.

Electrical stimulation of the STS is capable of activating the midbrain reticular formation more than stimulation of surrounding posterior regions. Therefore, the superior temporal sulcus appears to be important in the cortical control of arousal, and the supermodal synthesis that we discussed above may also lead to neuronal activation in the ventral temporal "what" and dorsal area 7 "where" systems. Therefore, if the STS in monkeys or the IPL in humans is dysfunctional, it not only fails to make attentional computations but also cannot arouse or activate directly or indirectly those areas that determine both location of objects and their identity. This failure of activation may prevent the monkey or human from being aware that there is a stimulus in the space opposite the STS or IPL (human) lesion.

Bisiach and Luzzati[9] have demonstrated that subjects with neglect may also have an inability to image those objects in scenes that would fall into contralesional hemispace. In addition, Heilman and coworkers[10] have demonstrated a hemispatial antegrade memory deficit associated with neglect. Therefore, lesions of the IPL in humans may be associated with the inability to activate old memory or form new memories of objects that are located in contralesional hemispace. In monkeys, the STS has strong reciprocal connections with the hippocampus. The hippocampus has also been posited to be important in retroactivation of sensory association areas,[11] and a partial (spatial) failure of retroactivation may account for the imagery-memory deficits.

In monkeys and humans, spatial neglect can often be distinguished from deafferentation by observing exploratory behaviors. Deafferented subjects fully explore their environment. However, patients with neglect often fail to fully explore the neglected portion of space. Theoretically, if we ablated both area 7 (the "where" system) and the ventral temporal cortex (the "what" system in monkeys), we suspect that these animals would continue to be able to explore their contralateral hemispace. The failure to explore contralesional space that we observed in animals with STS lesions and humans with IPL lesions may be related to the reciprocal connections that the STS has with the frontal arcuate gyrus region. The frontal arcuate gyrus region or frontal eye field is important for the initiation of purposeful saccades to important visual targets. The periarcuate region is important for the initiation of voluntary arm movements to important visual stimuli. It has been demonstrated that lesions of this region, as well as the basal ganglia and thalamus, which are all part of an intentional functional network, may induce motor intentional neglect. However exploratory defects may be also seen with posterior STS lesions in monkeys or IPL lesions in humans. In monkeys the frontal arcuate area and periarcuate regions have strong connections with both area 7 and the STS. Whereas the STS may be critical in activating both periarcuate and arcuate regions, area 7 may be important for providing these frontal regions with the spatial maps needed to make purposeful exploratory limb and eye movements. In addition to the dorsolateral frontal lobe, the motor intentional network also comprises the medial frontal lobes, including the cingulate gyrus, the basal ganglia, and the thalamic cortical loops as well as input from the STS or IPL. Whereas the attentional and intentional networks are highly interactive, they do not entirely overlap. Therefore one may, as we discussed, see neglect fractionate into motor intentional and sensory attentional components.

Although neglect can be in association with both right and left hemispheric lesions, neglect is in general more severe and frequent with right hemispheric lesions. These asymmetries appear to be related to asymmetrical representations of space and the body. For example, whereas the left hemisphere primarily attends to the right side, the right hemisphere attends to both sides.[12,13] Similarly, while the left hemisphere prepares for right-side action, the right prepares for both.[12]

TREATMENT AND MANAGEMENT OF NEGLECT

Because patients with neglect may be unaware of stimuli, they should avoid both driving and working with tools or machines that might cause injury to themselves or others. Their environment should be adjusted such that interactions with people and objects take place in the space that is ipsilateral to the damaged hemisphere.

Behavioral training paradigms have been used to teach patients with neglect to explore contralateral space. Although these procedures may be successful in the laboratory, they often fail to generalize to the environment. Similarly, prisms may be used to shift images from the contralateral to the ipsilateral side. Again, although this may improve performance on some tasks in the laboratory, these prisms do not seem to dramatically improve quality of life for patients with neglect.

Dynamic novel stimuli strongly summon attention in normal subjects. Butter and colleagues[14] used dynamic stimuli in the contralateral field of patients with neglect. Many patients showed a dramatic improvement following the treatment. However, because even hemianopic patients improved with dynamic stimuli, it is possible that these stimuli activate subcortical structures such as the colliculus. The colliculus receives more ipsilateral than contralateral input from the eyes. Lesions of the ipsilateral colliculus can reduce neglect (see Sprague[15]). Therefore, patching the ipsilateral eye may reduce the severity of neglect because it reduces ipsilateral collicular activation.[16] Irrigating the contralesional ear with cold water (caloric stimulation) may also dramatically improve neglect. Unfortunately, this improvement is only temporary. Last, pharmacologic therapy has been tried. If the dopaminergic system is unilaterally destroyed with toxins, animals may show neglect.[17] Corwin and associates[18] demonstrated that animals with neglect from frontal lesions improved with dopamine agonists. Fleet and colleagues[19] reported two patients who seemed to improve with dopamine agonist therapy. However, double-blind controlled studies with dopamine agonists must still be performed on subjects with neglect. These studies should also learn whether dopamine therapy helps intentional or attentional neglect or both.

REFERENCES

1. Heilman KM, Watson RT, Valenstein E: Neglect and related disorders, in Heilman KM, Valenstein E (eds): *Clinical Neuropsychology.* New York: Oxford University Press, 1993.
2. Valler G, Sandroni P, Rusconi ML, Barberi S: Hemianopia, hemianesthesia, and spatial neglect: A study with evoked potentials. *Neurology* 41: 1918–1922, 1991.
3. Triggs WJ, Gold M, Gerstle G, et al: Motor neglect associated with a discrete parietal lesion. *Neurology* 44:1164–1166, 1994.
4. Gold M, Shuren J, Heilman KM: Proximal intentional neglect: A case study. *J Neurol Neurosurg Psychiatry* 57:1395–1400, 1994.
5. Mennemeier MS, Wertman E, Heilman KM: Neglect of near peripersonal space: Evidence for multidirectional attentional systems in humans. *Brain* 115:37–50, 1992.
6. Ladavas E: Is the hemispatial deficit produced by right parietal damage associated with retinal or gravitational coordinates. *Brain* 110:167–180, 1987.
7. Watson RT, Valenstein E, Day A, Heilman KM: Posterior neocortical systems subserving awareness and neglect: Neglect after superior temporal sulcus but not area 7 lesions. *Arch Neurol* 51:1014–1021, 1994.
8. Mishkin M, Ungerleider LG, Macko KA: Object vision and spatial vision: Two cortical pathways. *Trends Neurosci* 6:414–417, 1983.
9. Bisiach E, Luzzati C: Unilateral neglect of representational space. *Cortex* 14:129–133, 1978.
10. Heilman KM, Watson RT, Schulman H: A unilateral memory deficit. *J Neurol Neurosurg Psychiatry* 37:790–793, 1974.
11. Damasio AR: Time locked multiregional retroactivation: A systems-level proposal for the neural sub-

strates of recall and recognition. *Cognition* 33:25–62, 1989.

12. Heilman KM, Van Den Abell T: Right hemisphere dominance for attention: The mechanisms underlying hemispheric asymmetries of inattention (neglect). *Neurology* 30:327–330, 1980.

13. Pardo JV, Fox PT, Raichle ME: Localization of a human system for sustained attention by positron emission tomography. *Nature* 349:61–64, 1991.

14. Butter CM, Kirsch NL, Reeves G: The effect of lateralized dynamic stimuli on unilateral neglect following right hemisphere lesions. *Restorative Neurol Neurosci* 2:39–46, 1990.

15. Sprague JM: Interaction of cortex and superior colliculus in mediation of visually guided behavior in the cat. *Science* 153:1544–1547, 1966.

16. Posner MI, Rafal RD: Cognitive theories of attention and rehabilitation of attentional deficits, in Mier MJ, Benton AL, Diller L (eds): *Neuropsychological Rehabilitation.* New York: Guilford, 1987.

17. Marshall JF: Somatosensory inattention after dopamine-depleting intracerebral 6-OHDA injections: Spontaneous recovery and pharmacological control. *Brain Res* 177:311–324, 1979.

18. Corwin JV, Kanter S, Watson RT, et al: Apomorphine has a therapeutic effect on neglect produced by unilateral dorsomedial prefrontal cortex lesions in rats. *Exp Neurol* 36:683–698, 1986.

19. Fleet WS, Valenstein E, Watson RT, Heilman KM: Dopamine agonist therapy for neglect in humans. *Neurology* 37:1765–1771, 1987.

Chapter 11

NEGLECT II: COGNITIVE NEUROPSYCHOLOGICAL ISSUES

Robert D. Rafal

This chapter reviews some of what has been learned about the cognitive neuropsychology of visual attention from the study of patients with neglect. The mutually supporting contributions of neurology and psychology have enriched both disciplines. Theories and methods for studying visual attention in normal people have contributed to our understanding of neglect; at the same time, a better understanding of neglect has helped illuminate some of the tougher theoretical issues in cognitive science.

DISENGAGING ATTENTION AND THE MECHANISM OF EXTINCTION

Does the phenomenon of extinction indicate that the parietal lobe is involved in controlling the orienting of attention? It had been argued[1,2] that an attentional explanation is not necessary to explain extinction. Instead, extinction could simply result from sensory competition. That is, although parietal lobe lesions do not produce hemianopia, they might nevertheless cause visual perceptions to be more weakly represented in the contralesional than in the ipsilesional field. Under conditions of sensory competition, the weakest sensory signal might not be perceived.

The most direct evidence for an attentional explanation of extinction was provided in an experiment in which it was shown that attending to the ipsilesional visual field could cause extinction, even under conditions where there was no com-

peting visual target to be reported in the ipsilesional field.[3] Patients with lesions of the parietal lobe were asked to respond, by pressing a key, to the appearance of a target in the visual field either ipsilateral or contralateral to the lesion. The target was preceded by a cue that could summon attention to target location (valid cue) or to the wrong location (invalid cue). As illustrated in Fig. 11-1, the cue was either a brightening of one of the possible target locations or an arrow in the center of the display instructing the subject where to expect the forthcoming target signal. The results showed that patients with parietal lesions, even those who did not have neglect or show clinical extinction on conventional examination, demonstrated an "extinction-like reaction-time pattern": slow detection of targets in the contralesional field when attention had been summoned to the ipsilesional field. Detection reaction time (RT) in the field opposite to the lesion (contralesional field) was not much slowed (and in some patients not slowed at all compared to the ipsilesional field) if a valid cue was given. Therefore, the patients were able to use the cue to move their attention to the contralesional field; when they did so, their performance for contralesional targets was relatively unimpaired. When, however, a cue summoned attention toward the ipsilesional field and the target subsequently occurred in the opposite, contralesional field (invalid cue), detection RT slowed dramatically. This extinction-like RT pattern occurred even after the cue disappeared. That is, the extinction effect occurred when atten-

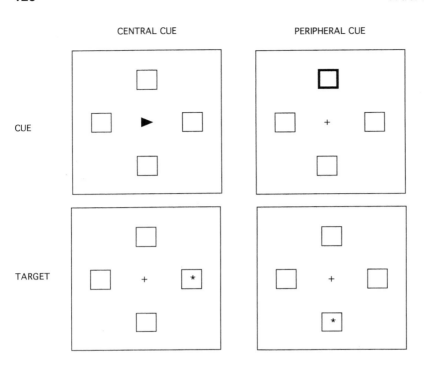

CENTRAL CUE

PERIPHERAL CUE

CUE

TARGET

Figure 11-1
The experimental displays used to assess the orienting of spatial attention in a detection reaction time task. The subject's task is to press a button as soon as the target, an asterisk, appears in any of four locations. Preceding the presentation of the target is a cue that directs attention to one particular location. The cue can be central, in the form of an arrow (top left panel), *or peripheral, as when one box brightens* (top right panel). *When the cue directs attention to the location of the target, it is said to be a valid cue* (bottom left panel); *when it directs attention to a different location from the target, it is said to be invalid* (bottom right panel).

tion was directed ipsilesionally, even though there was no competing target signal to detect there. So it was not sensory competition that caused the extinction-like RT performance, but a difficulty in disengaging attention from the ipsilesional field.

The disengaging of attention has been hypothesized to be one of a number of elementary operations underlying the orienting of spatial attention.[4] Support for this framework comes from a replication of the cued detection RT experiment comparing patients with lesions of the temporoparietal junction (TPJ) to patients with progressive supranuclear palsy (PSP) who have degeneration of the midbrain.[5] Figure 11-2 shows the results of this experiment. The effects of valid and invalid cues are measured by differences in RT between the affected visual hemifield and the more normal hemifield. For TPJ-lesioned patients, this is the difference between ipsilesional and contralesional fields; for patients with PSP, the difference is between vertical and horizontal attention shifts (because PSP affects vertical movements of the eyes

and of attention more than horizontal). Patients with TPJ lesions show the extinction-like RT pattern, with no impairment for valid cues and an impairment for invalid cues only when attention is engaged ipsilesionally. This can be interpreted as an impairment of the *disengage* operation. In contrast, patients with midbrain lesions show a deficit in orienting only with valid cues, reflecting a difficulty in moving attention to its target location. This can be interpreted as an impairment in the *move* operation.

EXTINCTION AND NEGLECT: DISENGAGING ATTENTION DURING VISUAL SEARCH AND EXPLORATION

The foregoing experiments, and a number of others, examined the effect of parietal lesions on detection of a luminance change in a relatively uncluttered field.[6–9] The results show that the extinction phenomenon is caused by a deficit in at-

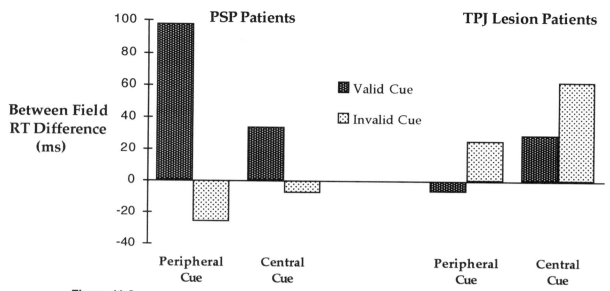

Figure 11-2

Covert orienting in patients with progressive supranuclear palsy and temperoparietal junction lesions. The results are depicted as the difference in detection RT between the more affected and the more normal visual fields. A greater difference in a given condition, thus, indicates a greater impairment in orienting in that condition. For the PSP patients (left) and the TPJ lesion patients (right) the between field detection RT differences are shown (in ms) for valid and invalid peripheral and central cues. The PSP patients are more impaired in the valid cue condition, especially with peripheral cues; whereas the TPJ lesion patients are more impaired in the invalid cue conditon, especially for central cues.

tention. Yet extinction is just one component of the neglect symptom complex. Other symptoms of neglect include defective exploratory behavior as revealed by tasks like line bisection, drawing, and cancellation. To understand how the deficit in disengaging attention can contribute to deficient exploration, we must examine attentional search in a cluttered field, where many objects are competing for attention. This is a more typical situation in the real world.

Eglin and coworkers[10] studied visual search in patients with neglect using a task developed by Treisman.[11] They varied the side of a predesignated conjunction target (one defined by a specific color and shape, requiring the conjunction of more than one feature to identify) among a variable number of distractors and measured the time to find the target. When distractors were present,

they could occur in either the ipsilesional or contralesional field. As long as no distractors appeared on the ipsilesional side of the display, no differences were found in locating a target on the neglected and intact sides. In other words, in displays that were limited to the ipsilesional side of a page, there were no objects to attract attention to the intact side and therefore nothing from which to disengage attention. Under these circumstances, the patients searched the display on the left as readily as they searched displays on the right. In contrast, for bilateral displays, in which distractors were present in both fields, search times increased as a function of the number of distractors or objects in the ipsilesional field. Each distractor on the intact side tripled the search time to locate the contralesional target. That is, the difficulty in disengaging attention from the ipsilesional field of distractors to move attention to the contralesional field depended on the number of items in the display.

Mark and colleagues[12] provide an elegantly simple demonstration that patients with neglect have difficulty in disengaging attention when ipsilesional items are present. They used a line cancellation task, a conventional bedside method for demonstrating and measuring neglect. The patient is shown a page filled with lines and asked to "cross them all out." Typically, a patient with left hemineglect fails to cross out many of the items on the left side of the page. Mark and coworkers[12] compared this conventional cancellation task with another condition in which they asked the patient to erase all the lines. As each line was erased and thus no longer present, the patient no longer had to disengage from it before moving on. Performance was strikingly better in this erasure task than in the conventional line cancellation task.

LOCAL PERCEPTUAL BIASES AFTER LESIONS OF THE RIGHT TEMPOROPARIETAL JUNCTION EXACERBATE VISUAL NEGLECT

Some patients with parietal lobe lesions may have extinction but not exhibit any of the exploratory deficits of neglect on drawing, copying, cancellation, or bisection tasks. In fact, extinction appears to be just as frequent after left as after right hemispheric lesions. However, other components of the syndrome, including deficits in exploration of contralesional space, are much more frequent after right hemispheric lesions, especially those that involve the right temporoparietal junction.[14] So while a deficit in disengaging attention may be a satisfactory explanation for extinction, it seems that other factors, perhaps specific to right hemispheric lesions, are at work in patients with the full-blown syndrome of neglect.

The observations of Eglin and coworkers[10] and Mark and colleagues,[12] discussed in the last section, show that the difficulty in disengaging attention is greater when attention is more actively

engaged. Factors that cause attention to become more actively engaged in the ipsilesional field will exacerbate the problem of disengaging attention and, hence, will exacerbate visual neglect. One effect of a lesion of the right temporoparietal junction (TPJ)—but not the left TPJ—is that it causes attention to become locked onto local perceptual details.[14] Figure 11-3[15] shows the copying of a patient with a large stroke of the right hemisphere and that of a patient with a large stroke involving the left hemisphere. The right hemispheric lesion causes almost complete exclusion of the global organization of the figure, while the left hemispheric lesion causes the exclusion of local detail.

The conjoint effects of the local bias with a difficulty in disengaging attention combine in producing some classic constructional signs of neglect in paper-and-pencil tasks. Consider, for example, a patient writing a number on to a clock face. She will be more successful if, as she is writing each number, she remains oriented to her task with reference to the whole clock. If her attention becomes excessively focused on the number she is writing and she loses sight of the whole clock, she will have more difficulty in disengaging from that number to fill in the rest of the numbers in the

Figure 11-3

Drawings of hierarchical stimuli by two patients. A. The figure which the patients were asked to copy is a hierarchical pattern in which the large letter at the global level is an M, constructed from small Z's at the local level. B. Global organization is lost in this drawing by a patient with a right hemispheric lesion. C. Only the global organization of the figure is preserved while the local details are lost in this copy by a patient with a left hemispheric lesion. (From Delis, et al.,[15] with permission.)

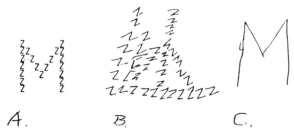

correct location on the clock face. As she writes a number on the clock face, her attention becomes stuck there, and the difficulty in disengaging attention causes the numbers drawn subsequently to be bunched up together next to it. On the other hand, if the clock face remains uncluttered with other numbers, patients with neglect are better able to remain oriented to the whole clock face. Di Pellegrino[16] showed that neglect patients can put a single number in the appropriate location on a clock face as long as they are given a separate sheet for each number.

Halligan and Marshall[17] have shown the importance of the local bias as a contributor to neglect and how the local bias and the deficit in disengaging attention interact to determine neglect behavior. They asked their patient to bisect a horizontal line. In one condition, they also presented a vertical line at the right end of the line that was to be bisected. Before asking the patient to bisect the horizontal line, they gave their patient a task that required attending to the full extent of the vertical line. This obliged the patient to expand the "attentional spotlight" from the point at the end of the horizontal line, and this improved subsequent bisection performance on the horizontal line. By helping to overcome the tendency of the patient to become hyperengaged in a small focus of attention at the end of the line to be bisected, they were able to mitigate the neglect. Perhaps this expansion of attention to a more global level explains why patients with neglect make less bisection error when bisecting a rectangle than when bisecting a line, and why the higher the vertical extent of the rectangle, the less the bisection error.[19]

ORIENTING BIAS AND HEMISPHERIC RIVALRY

One model of the neurobiological basis of spatial attention postulates that each hemisphere, when activated, mediates an orienting response in the contralateral direction.[19–21] According to this account, neglect results from a unilateral lesion because of a breakdown in the balance of hemispheric rivalry such that the nonlesioned hemisphere generates an unopposed orienting response to the side of the lesion. Experimental observations in patients with hemineglect provide some support for this view. Ladavas and colleagues[22] showed that, in patients with neglect, detection performance was best for the most ipsilesional targets, and detection of these ipsilesional targets was even better than for normal control subjects. These results suggest that patients with neglect hyperorient toward the ipsilesional field.

One variant of the hemispheric rivalry account emphasizes putative mutually inhibitory callosal connections between the hemispheres. According to this account, when one hemisphere is lesioned, homologous regions of the opposite hemisphere, which normally receive inhibitory projections from the damaged region, become disinhibited and hyperorient attention to the ipsilesional side. A recent study[23] has obtained some support for this hypothesis by examining the effects of transcranial magnetic stimulation (TMS) on thresholds for tactile perception detection in normal subjects. A suprathreshold (i.e., sufficiently strong to activate a twitch in the contralateral thumb when applied over motor cortex) TMS stimulus transiently inactivates subjacent cortex. This study examined whether the hemisphere opposite the TMS stimulus would show signs of disinhibition, manifested as a reduced threshold to detect a tactile stimulus in the thumb *ipsilateral* to the TMS lesion. Results supported the attentional disinhibition account by showing a reduced ipsilateral tactile threshold after parietal (3 or 5 cm posterior to motor cortex) TMS but not when TMS was applied at control locations over the motor cortex or 5 cm anterior to it.

Another mechanism that has been suggested for ipsilesional hyperorienting postulates a corticosubcortical interaction. According to this account, the unlesioned parietal lobe becomes disinhibited tonically increasing activity in the superior colliculus ipsilateral to it; whereas the colliculus on the side of the lesion loses some normally present tonic activation. As a result, parietal lesions also produce an imbalance in the activity of subcortical structures involved in orienting, such as the superior colliculus. The contralesional superior colliculus becomes disinhibited, and this results in exaggerated reflexive orienting to signals in the ipsilesional field.

Sprague's experiments in the cat confirmed that this kind of corticosubcortical interaction is important in regulating visually guided orienting behavior.[24] Cats were first rendered blind in one visual field by removing occipital and parietal cortex. It was then shown that vision in this field improved if the *opposite* superior colliculus were removed. A similar result is obtained if the inhibitory connections are severed between the contralesional substantia nigra pars reticulata and the ipsilesional colliculus.[25,26]

This "Sprague effect" is thought to work in the following way. Parietooccipital projections to the ipsilateral superior colliculus normally exert a tonic facilitation on it. After parietal lesions, the colliculus looses this tonic activation, and at the same time the opposite (contralesional) colliculus is in fact hyperactive due to increased activation from its parietal lobe, which, as we saw earlier, is disinhibited. The unilateral parietal lesion therefore also produces a subcortical imbalance between the two hemispheres. Moreover, this imbalance is sustained and aggravated by the mutually inhibitory connections between the two colliculi themselves. The more active contralesional superior colliculus is released from inhibition. The disinhibited contralesional colliculus produces disinhibited reflexive orienting to ipsilesional signals. Once attention is reflexively drawn to the ipsilesional field, the disengage deficit causes attention to get stuck there—resulting in neglect. If the contralesional superior colliculus is then removed (or the fibers of passage from the substantial nigra pars compacta to the opposite colliculus), the hyperorienting, and hence neglect, is ameliorated.

The Sprague effect demonstrates (at least in cats) that neglect is aggravated by disinhibition of subcortical visual pathways on the side opposite the cortical lesions and that prevention of visual input to this colliculus can alleviate neglect. Are there any practical applications of this phenomenon in rehabilitation? It is obviously not an option to surgically remove the contralesional superior colliculus in humans who have suffered parietal lobe strokes. It is possible, however, to decrease contralesional collicular activation and reflexive orienting by occluding the ipsilesional eye with a patch.[27] Indeed, patching the eye on the side of the lesion has been shown to help reduce symptoms of neglect.[28]

It seems likely that both cortical and subcortical imbalances contribute to the rightward bias of attention in patients with neglect. The subcortical imbalance is presumably more pronounced during the period of extensive diaschisis in the acute stage following the ictus. This imbalance is thought to produce not just a turning bias but also a shift in the spatial frame of reference such that the contralesional space is more weakly represented.[20,29] The effect of the rightward bias on spatial representation can be reduced transiently by production of a countervailing orienting bias through vestibular activation using a caloric stimulus. Vestibular activation can transiently alleviate not only visual[30,31] and somatosensory[32] neglect, but also the lack of awareness of the deficit (anosognosia).[33] A shift in spatial representation by vibration of neck muscles[34] or by optokinetic stimulation[35] can also decrease neglect.

PERCEPTUAL AND MOTOR NEGLECT

As reviewed in Chap. 10, the neural circuitry controlling spatial attention is a distributed network involving cortical and subcortical structures (see also Ref. 36). Within this network, there appear to be several specialized if interconnected circuits for regulating different kinds of behavior. Consider the different kinds of representations of space that would be needed for performing some common, simple tasks. A representation of space for generating an eye movement to a visual signal requires retinotopic coordinates. One for controlling reaching requires an egocentric representation of space—a scene-based representation in which location in the environment is coded and remains constant even if the eyes move. In monkeys, areas of parietal lobe have been identified in which retinotopically mapped information is gated by eye position.[37] For reaching, moreover, this representation must be integrated with a reference frame mapped relative to hand position.[38] This kind of representation of near peripersonal space may not, however, be adequate for throwing, which may require a separate representation of distant space.[39] The representations of space that might be adequate for reaching to a stationary object may not suffice to reach for an object that is moving. For this, one wants an object-based representation that updates the changing location of parts of the object relative to an egocentric reference frame. Finally, consider the problem of remembering the location of a cache of food relative to some geographic landmark or the problem of remembering the locations of cities on a map. For this one wants an allocentric reference frame in which the relative locations of objects are represented in a frame of reference totally independent of the viewpoint of the individual. For navigating while moving in the environment, this allocentric map must be continually updated and integrated with some enduring record of changes in body position with regard to this allocentric reference frame—for example, the "place" cells that have been identified in rat hippocampus.[40]

Given that there may be many such independent circuits that might be affected by some lesions and spared in others, it is not surprising that the manifestations of visual neglect may vary from patient to patient. In some, neglect may be more perceptual; in others, more motor. While this distinction may be better appreciated as a continuum rather than a dichotomy, the distinction between disorders of attention and intention has been a useful one.[41] Some patients with a more pure attentional disorder (typically those with more posterior lesions sparing frontal lobes) may have visual extinction and other perceptual deficits but no motor bias against turning contralesionally, moving the limbs contralateral to the lesion, or reaching into the contralesional field (directional hypokinesia).[42,43] Other patients who do not show extinction or other signs of perceptual neglect may, nevertheless, have a motor bias causing

neglect behavior in cancellation and construction tasks. Many patients with neglect have both perceptual and motor components affecting performance in these types of tasks. The relative contributions of these components may vary from patient to patient, depending on the size and location of the lesion in each patient and the task used to assess neglect.

Performance on many of the tests used clinically to diagnose neglect and measure its severity can be influenced by both motor and perceptual factors. Errors in line bisection or missed items in a cancellation task could be caused by perceptual neglect, motor neglect, or a combination of the two. Failure to cross out the leftmost items on a cancellation task, for example, could be due to failure to see the leftmost items or to a motor bias against moving toward the left.

Several ingenious studies have recently dissociated perceptual and motor components of neglect to measure their effects independently. Bisiach[44] first demonstrated this dissociation between perceptual and motor neglect by using a pulley device in a bisection task. Patients with neglect bisected lines under two conditions. In one, movement of the pencil toward the left (contralesional) direction required movement of the hand to the left. In this standard version of the task, a deficit in bisection could be due to perceptual neglect, motor neglect, or a combination of both. In the other version of the task, the pulley device required rightward movement of the hand to move the pencil to the left. Patients in whom neglect was exclusively due to a motor bias against moving the hand toward the left could be expected to improve their bisection performance in this version of the task. Some patients, those in whom neglect was dominantly perceptual, showed an equal amount of neglect in both versions of the task. Some patients showed some improvement in bisection with the pulley, and some, those in whom neglect was dominantly a motor bias, had no neglect under the pulley condition. These patients with more pure motor neglect tended to have more frontal lesions. Similar dissociations between perceptual and motor neglect have been also demonstrated using other devices, such as TV cameras[42] and mirrors[45] to separate out motor bias contributions to neglect. While there are clear tendencies for motor neglect to be more associated with more frontal lesions, the anatomic substrates relating to perceptual and motor neglect remain to be more precisely specified.[46]

Some simple bedside tests have recently been introduced to separate motor bias from perceptual neglect. Gold and colleagues[47] used a fixed-aperture technique in a cancellation task in which an opaque sheet with an aperture is placed over the page. The task can be done in one of two ways. In the standard task, the top sheet with the aperture is moved leftward by the patient during the cancellation task. In this task, both motor and perceptual neglect can influence performance. In the other condition, the bottom sheet is moved to the right by the patient in order to expose items on the left side of the page. In this version of the task, motor bias to the left cannot contribute to neglect performance, allowing for a purer assessment of perceptual contributions to neglect.

An elegant companion test to line bisection has been introduced[48] to determine whether motor neglect is contributing to bisection errors in an individual patient. Patients who manifest bisection errors are shown prebisected lines that may be bisected in the middle or to the left or right of midline. The patients are asked to point to the end of the line that is *closest* to the bisection mark. The critical condition is that in which the line is bisected in the middle. Patients in whom bisection error is due exclusively to a motor bias to the right would be expected to point to the right end of the line in this condition. In fact, several of the patients who were studied pointed to the left end of the line. This result indicates that, in these patients, their bisection errors were not due to a motor bias toward the right. These important observations suggest, in fact, that patients with perceptual neglect perceive the left side of the line as being shorter.

A more recent study has confirmed that neglect reduces perceived length. Milner and co-workers[49] showed patients with neglect two horizontal bars on a sheet of paper, one in each visual field, and asked them to judge which bar was

shorter. On the critical trial in which the bars were equal in length, the patients indicated the bars in the left field to be shorter. In a control test in which vertical bars were shown, no such asymmetry in length judgment was evident. These findings indicate that patients with perceptual neglect experience compression of the left side of space.

This result may seem to be contradicted by a recent study of oculomotor behavior in patients with visual neglect.[50] Patients with left hemineglect, when asked to look straight ahead in the dark, deviated their eyes to the right of objective midline. This observation is consistent with the rightward hyperorienting described earlier, when we considered the hemispheric rivalry account of neglect. However, these patients did not show any asymmetry of oculomotor exploration around their subjective midline. That is, although they deviated their eyes rightward of true midline, eye movements to the left of their subjective midline were as great as eye movements to the right of it. This result would seem to indicate that there is a shift in perceived center of the egocentric world but no compression of spatial representation to the left of this center. However, the study of Karnath and associates[50] measured eye movements in the dark, presumably in relation to far extrapersonal space. That of Milner and coworkers[49] examined attention in relation to objects being manipulated in near peripersonal space. In the next section, we will see that neglect can be greatly influenced by the frame of reference in which it is examined and that the operations of visual attention are contingent on the requirements made of it for perception and action.

WHAT IS NEGLECTED IN NEGLECT?

It is now clear that visual neglect is not simply blindness in one visual field or even a lack of attention restricted to one visual field. Although neglect is greater for objects to the left (for right hemineglect) of fixation, it does not have the sharp retinotopic boundaries of hemianopia. Rather, it seems to operate over a gradient.[22] Using the cueing task described earlier, it has been shown, for example, that an extinction-like RT deficit can occur for detecting the leftmost of two stimuli in the right visual field,[7] even though this event is in the "good" field (and is in fact closer to the fovea). In this sense neglect seems to operate as a directional bias independent of visual field. However, neglect does, also, differentially affect the two visual fields. Baynes and coworkers[6] showed that vertical shifts of attention from an invalid cue were slower in the contralesional than the ipsilesional visual field.

So while it is clear that neglect is a deficit in attending to visual information, we still need to consider what it is that is neglected. We have seen that several different representations of space are maintained in the brain. Neglect could result from a degradation of any of these representations or of the ability to attend to any of them. Thus, what is neglected in neglect may differ from patient to patient, depending on which representations of space are involved by the lesion; in any given patient, what is neglected may depend on the requirements of the task at hand.

Reference Frames of Visual Neglect

Extrapersonal space exists independent of the viewpoint of the observer. Even when we are lying down (or standing on our heads), "up" and "down" remain the same, determined by the gravitational field. Ladavas[51] first showed that when patients with neglect tilted their heads, neglect was manifest not in terms of visual field but in terms of "gravitational" coordinates.

However, Fig. 11-4 shows a striking demonstration, using a test devised by Lynn Robertson, that neglect is not always manifest in terms of simple environmental (gravitational) coordinates. The examiner tests for extinction by wiggling a finger on each of his hands. In one condition, the examiner's body and face are rotated to the left (that is, the reference frame is rotated counterclockwise). In this condition the patient detects the upper finger wiggle and extinguishes the lower; that is, there is extinction of the left side of the reference frame. In contrast, when the examiner's body and face are rotated to the right (that is the reference frame is rotated clockwise), the

patient now detects the lower finger wiggle and extinguishes the upper. That is, there is now extinction of the opposite spatial location, but this again is on the left side of the reference frame. In this case, then, neglect is not manifest with reference to gravitational coordinates but with reference to the principal axis of the attended object.

It seems that visual neglect does not simply affect a visual field mapped in retinotopic coordinates nor even simply one side of egocentric space. It can be manifest in object-based coordinates. To understand how neglect can operate in object-based coordinates for objects that are neglected—an apparent contradiction—we must first consider to what degree visual objects can be represented in the neglected field outside of the focus of attention.

Figure-Ground Segregation and Grouping in Visual Neglect

When we look at the two drawings on the left (*A*) and right (*B*) of Fig. 11-5,[52] we normally see bright-green objects on a dim red background (both because the green is brighter and because its area is smaller than that of the dim red). Driver and colleagues[53] showed a patient with left hemineglect figures like these; they asked him to remember the shape of the dividing line between red and green and to then match this line with the probe shapes (shown under the study shapes in Fig. 11-5). Notice that the boundary to be remembered is on the left side of the page in *A* and on the right in *B*; yet for *A*, the boundary to be remembered lies on the right side of the green object, while in *B* it lies on the left side of the green object. The patient's task did not require any judgment about either the perceived object (green) or its ground (red). His task was only to attend to the shape of the line bordering the two colored areas. Were neglect manifest strictly with respect to egocentric space, more errors would have been expected for *A* than for *B*. The results showed the exact opposite pattern. The patient was much more accurate in condition *A*, where the contour to be remembered was on the right side of the object but on the left side of the page,

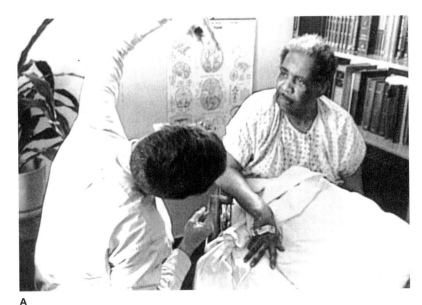

A

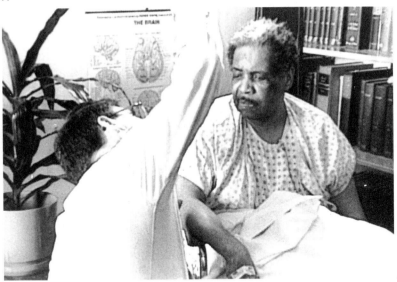

B

Figure 11-4
*Reference frames and ne-
glect. This patient detected a
single finger wiggling in his
contralesional field but did not
see it when a finger was also
wiggled simultaneously in the
ipsilesional* (right) *field (extinction). The test illustrated here
demonstrates the depen-
dence of extinction on the reference frame of the patient.
When the examiner rotates
clockwise* (A), *there is extinction of the lower stimulus,
which is still the left side of
the object, and the patient
looks up. When the examiner
rotates counterclockwise* (B),
*there is extinction of the up-
per stimulus, which is still the
left side of the object, and the
patient looks down. (From
Rafal,[75] with permission.)*

than in condition *B,* where the contour to be remembered was on the left side of the object but
on the right side of the page. Although the green
shape on the left side in *A* was in the neglected
field and while judgments about the object were
not relevant to the task at hand, the patient's attention was nevertheless summoned to it.

In this example, neglect operated with regard to the reference frame of the object. These
observations tell us two important things: (1) the
processes for segregating figure from ground can
operate preattentively in the neglected field and
(2) attention operates at a later stage on candidate
objects generated by these preattentive processes.

Figure 11-5

A patient with left hemispatial neglect was shown figures like those shown here and asked to report verbally whether the contour dividing red (hatched) *and bright-green* (white) *areas of a rectangle matched the probe line presented immediately below the rectangle following its offset. Normally the small bright-green region is seen as figure against the dim red background. Although not required to identify figure or ground, the patient showed more neglect for the left side of the figure* (B), *even though this figure was in the right visual field. (Adapted from Driver et al.,[53] with permission.)*

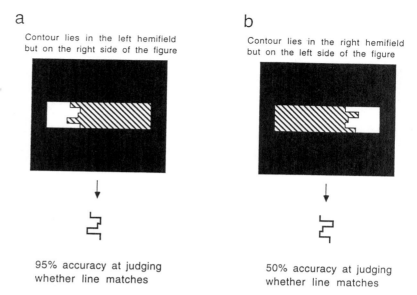

a

Contour lies in the left hemifield but on the right side of the figure

95% accuracy at judging whether line matches

b

Contour lies in the right hemifield but on the left side of the figure

50% accuracy at judging whether line matches

The object-based neglect of objects segregated from ground is nicely shown by the drawings of similar shapes shown in Fig. 11-6.[54]

Another preattentive process that is preserved in patients with unilateral neglect is the segregation of figure from ground based on symmetry. The effect of symmetry in preattentively generating candidate objects was first demonstrated by showing a patient with visual neglect pictures in which isoluminant red and green areas were alternated across a page. Either the red or the green areas on each page were symmetrical. The patient was asked to report simply whether the red or green areas appeared to be "in front." Normal individuals see symmetrical regions as being the figure and report them to be in front of the ground. Like any normal individual, the patient reported symmetrical regions to be in front, indicating that he had perceived the symmetrical objects as the figure. When he was asked to judge whether the shapes were symmetrical or not, he performed at chance. That is, even though his neglect prevented him from reporting whether or not shapes were symmetrical, he nevertheless

Figure 11-6

Object-based neglect is demonstrated by the copying performance of a patient with left hemispatial neglect. When asked to copy the black object, the patient did well, since the jagged contour is on the right side of the black object. When asked to copy the white object, the patient was unable to copy the jagged contour, since it is on the left side of the object being attended. (From Marshall and Halligan,[54] with permission.)

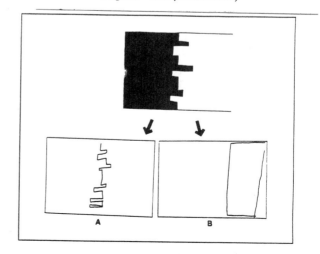

A   B

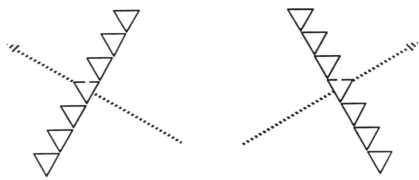

Figure 11-7

The figures used by Driver and coworkers[55] to study axis-based visual neglect. Three patients with left hemispatial neglect were asked to report whether or not the triangle in the center had a gap in it. Because of grouping of the triangles, triangles on the left were seen as pointing toward the northwest, so that the gap in the top of the central triangle is on the right side of its principal axis, whereas the triangles on the right are seen as pointing toward the northeast, so that the gap in the top of the central triangle is on the left side of its principal axis. All three patients had more neglect (missed seeing the gap) in the condition shown on the right than in the condition shown on the left. (From Driver et al.,[55] with permission.)

perceived symmetrical shapes as the objects in the visual scene.

Once candidate objects are preattentively segregated from background, they may then be grouped with other objects based on gestalt principals. Figure 11-7 shows a task used to test whether grouping is preserved in visual neglect.[55] The patient's task was simply to determine whether or not there was a gap in the top of the central triangle. The principal axis of the triangle (i.e., which way it appeared to point) was manipulated by the way in which the central triangle was grouped with the others. In the figure on the right, the alignment of the triangles (from southwest to northeast) causes them to appear to be pointing toward the northwest; the gap in the top of the central triangle is perceived to appear on the right side of its perceived principal axis. In the figure on the left, the alignment of the triangles (from southeast to northwest) causes them to appear to be pointing toward the northeast. The gap in the top of the central triangle is perceived to appear on the left side of its perceived principal axis. Results in three patients with left hemineglect showed that all missed more of the gaps in the

condition on the right, in which the gap was on the perceived left of the triangle. These results demonstrate that grouping is preserved in visual neglect and that attention operates in the reference frame of the group such that visual neglect is determined based on the principal axis of the group.

Object-Centered Neglect

The results of the experiment shown in Fig. 11-7[55] provide a more formal proof of the phenomenon shown in Fig. 11-4. After figure-ground segmentation occurs preattentively, candidate objects become represented to which attention may then be directed. Attention is allocated to the attended object aligned with its principal axis. Neglect is then manifest for parts of the object or other objects contralateral to the primary axis of the attended object. If, as shown in Fig. 11-4, the principal axis of the attended object moves or rotates, neglect moves or rotates with it.[56] Behrman and Tipper showed object-based neglect which actually moved to the ipsilesional side of the object after it rotated. Reaction time was measured to targets appearing in either the left (contralesional) or right (ipsilesional) side of a dumbbell. Patients were slower to respond to targets on the left. If the dumbbell rotated, however, such that the two sides of the dumbbell reversed field, RTs were prolonged for targets on the right.

Object-based neglect has also been inferred from the reading errors of neglect patients. In a striking demonstration of neglect dyslexia,[57] a patient with right hemineglect made more errors at the end of the word regardless of the orientation of the word on the page—that is, even when the word was upside down, such that the right end of the word was in the left visual field. Patients with neglect have also been shown to make more reading errors when they read pronounceable nonwords than when they read words.[58–60] This shows that word forms are preattentively processed and integrate the constituent letters into a single object. The study by Brunn and Farah[59] incorporated cancellation or line bisection tasks along with the reading task. Less neglect was found on these secondary tasks when the primary task required reading a word as opposed to a nonword. This finding suggests that word processing causes an automatic deployment of attention to encompass the word and, in patients with left neglect, this draws their attention to the left.

Not all attempts to identify object-based neglect have been successful; a contrast of the studies that demonstrated object-based neglect and those that did not is instructive. Farah and colleagues[61] asked patients to name colors surrounding pictures of common objects. When the pictures were rotated, the colors neglected did not rotate with the object; that is, neglect remained location-based rather than object-based. Behrman and Moscovitch[62] used the same paradigm and confirmed the lack of object-based neglect with object drawings. However, object-based neglect was manifest in the special case where the objects were asymmetrical letters. That is, object-based neglect was manifest when the object's identity was uniquely defined by its principal axis.

Spatial Representations and Neglect

Neglect can result not only in the failure to perceive or to respond to contralesional signals or objects but also to a lack of conscious access to the contralesional side of visual images stored in memory.[65] Bisiach and Luzzatti[64] asked patients with left hemineglect to imagine themselves in the Piazza del Duomo in Milan. In one condition, they asked the patients to imagine themselves at one end of the square, looking toward the cathedral dominating the other end of the square, and to describe what they would be able to see. In another condition, the patients were asked to imagine themselves standing on the cathedral steps facing the opposite way. In both circumstances, the patients reported fewer landmarks on the contralesional side of the mental image. (For non-Milanese clinicians, a baseball imagery task may be substituted. In one condition, the patient is asked to imagine herself as the catcher and to name the positions of all the players that she would be able to see. Then the patient is told to imagine being in center field and is asked the same question.)

These kinds of observations have engendered an account of neglect in which the parietal lobes are assumed to maintain a representation of space in viewer-centered coordinates, and that parietal lesions produce a degradation of the contralesional representation. In an elegant experimental test of this account, Bisiach and coworkers[65] had patients view cloudlike shapes that were passed slowly behind a slit (so that only part of the shape could be seen at any moment). The task required that a mental image be generated and maintained as the slit moved over the shape they were attempting to remember. The patients were shown two shapes that could be either the same or different, and they were asked to respond whether the shapes were the same or not. On the trials in which the shapes were different, they could be different on the patients' left or right side. The patients made more errors on this task when shapes were different from each other on the contralesional end than on the ipsilesional end.

We need to know more about the neuroanatomic and pathophysiologic basis for the deficit of spatial representation in neglect.[66] Some authors have considered spatial representation in terms of oculomotor coding,[67,68] while others have emphasized spatial working memory.[69] Recent reports show that perceptual neglect and neglect of internal imagery may be dissociated. Two patients with perceptual neglect and mainly parietal lesions did not evidence neglect in visual imagery,[70] whereas a patient with a frontal lesion causing neglect of imagined scenes did not have perceptual neglect.[71]

CONCLUDING REMARKS

In neglect, a constellation of symptoms is seen affecting both perception and exploratory behavior. Which symptoms (and with what severity) occur in any given patient depends upon the extent and location of the lesion, its chronicity, and the premorbid cognitive architecture of the individual. Across the rather heterogeneous population of patients with elements of the neglect syndrome, the pathophysiologic mechanisms underlying each of the component symptoms are diverse. We are just beginning to understand some of these: hyperreflexive orienting toward the ipsilesional side or to local elements in the visual scene; impaired ability to disengage attention; a deranged internal representation of space, which is not only shifted but contracts contralesionally; impaired voluntary orienting toward the contralesional field; a motor bias toward the ipsilesional side that causes defective contralesional exploratory behavior; deficient ability to generate contralesional voluntary saccades; and failure of contralesional stimuli to produce arousal. The manifestations of neglect in an individual patient may not simply represent the additive contributions of each of these mechanisms, depending on which are affected by the lesion, but rather an interaction between them.[72]

The study of neglect has advanced our understanding of preattentive vision and the functions of attention in object recognition and the control of goal-directed behavior. We have learned that the visual scene is parsed preattentively into candidate objects and that attention then operates on these objects to afford awareness and recognition of them and to guide subsequent action. We are developing a better understanding of the plight of these patients and of their perplexing behavior. These insights can be applied to fashioning more rational approaches to their rehabilitation.[73–75]

REFERENCES

1. Bender MB, Feldman M: The so-called "visual agnosias." *Brain* 95:173–186, 1972.
2. Bay E: Disturbances of visual perception and their examination. *Brain* 76:515–530, 1953.
3. Posner MI, Walker JA, Friedrich FJ, Rafal R: Effects of parietal injury on covert orienting of visual attention. *J Neurosci* 4:1863–1874, 1984.
4. Posner MI, Inhoff AW, Friedrich FJ, Cohen A: Isolating attentional systems: A cognitive-anatomical analysis. *Psychobiology* 15:107–121, 1987.
5. Rafal RD, Posner MI, Friedman JH, et al: Orienting of visual attention in progressive supranuclear palsy. *Brain* 111:267–280, 1988.
6. Baynes K, Holtzman HD, Volpe BT: Components of visual attention: Alterations in response pattern to visual stimuli following parietal lobe infarction. *Brain* 109:99–114, 1986.
7. Posner MI, Walker JA, Friedrich FJ, Rafal RD: How do the parietal lobes direct covert attention? *Neuropsychologia* 25:135–146, 1987.
8. Morrow LA, Ratcliff GCP: The disengagement of covert attention and the neglect syndrome. *Psychobiology* 16:261–269, 1988.
9. Egly R, Driver J, Rafal R: Shifting visual attention between objects and locations: Evidence from normal and parietal lesion subjects. *J Exp Psychol Gen* 123:127–161, 1994.
10. Eglin M, Robertson LC, Knight RT: Visual search performance in the neglect syndrome. *J Cogn Neurosci* 1:372–385, 1989.
11. Treisman A, Gelade G: A feature integration theory of attention. *Cogn Psychol* 12:97–136, 1980.
12. Mark VW, Kooistra CA, Heilman KM: Hemispatial neglect affected by non-neglected stimuli. *Neurology* 38:1207–1211, 1988.
13. Vallar G: The anatomical basis of spatial neglect in humans, in Robertson IH, Marshall JC (ed): *Unilateral Neglect: Clinical and Experimental Studies.* Hillsdale, NJ, Erlbaum, 1993, pp 27–62.
14. Robertson LC, Lamb MR, Knight RT: Effects of lesions of the temporal-parietal junction on perceptual and attentional processing in humans. *J Neurosci* 8:3757–3769, 1988.

15. Delis DC, Robertson LC, Efron R: Hemispheric specialization of memory for visual hierarchical stimuli. *Neuropsychologia* 24:205–214, 1986.

16. Di Pellegrino G: Clock-drawing in a case of left visu-spatial neglect: A deficit of disengagement. *Neuropsychologia* 33:353–358, 1995.

17. Halligan PW, Marshall JC: Right-sided cueing can ameliorate left neglect. *Neuropsychol Rehabil* 4:63–73, 1994.

18. Vallar G: Left spatial hemineglect: An unmanageable explosion of dissociations? No. *Neuropsychol Rehabil* 4:209–212, 1994.

19. Kinsbourne M: Mechanisms of neglect: Implications for rehabilitation. *Neuropsychol Rehabil* 4:151–153, 1994.

20. Kinsbourne M: Hemi-neglect and hemisphere rivalry, in Weinstein EA, Friedland RP (ed): *Advances in Neurology.* New York, Raven Press, l977, pp 41–49.

21. Kinsbourne M: Orientational bias model of unilateral neglect: Evidence from attentional gradients within hemispace, in Robertson IH, Marshall JC (ed): *Unilateral Neglect: Clinical and Experimental Studies.* Hillsdale, NJ, Erlbaum, 1993, pp 63–86.

22. Ladavas E, Del Pesce M, Provinciali L: Unilateral attention deficits and hemispheric asymmetries in the control of visual attention. *Neuropsychologia* 27:353–366, 1989.

23. Seyal M, Ro T, Rafal R: Perception of subthreshold cutaneous stimuli following transcranial magnetic stimulation of ipsilateral parietal cortex. *Ann Neurol* 38:264–267, 1995.

24. Sprague JM: Interaction of cortex and superior colliculus in mediation of peripherally summoned behavior in the cat. *Science* 153:1544–1547, 1966.

25. Wallace SF, Rosenquist AC, Sprague JM: Recovery from cortical blindness mediated by destruction of nontectotectal fibers in the commissure of the superior colliculus in the cat. *J Comp Neurol* 284:429–450, 1989.

26. Wallace SF, Rosenquist AC, Sprague JM: Ibotenic acid lesions of the lateral substantia nigra restore visual orientation behavior in the hemianopic cat. *J Comp Neurol* 296:222–252, 1990.

27. Posner MI, Rafal RD: Cognitive theories of attention and the rehabilitation of attentional deficits, in Meir RJ, Diller L, Benton AL (ed): *Neuropsychological Rehabilitation.* London, Churchill Livingstone, 1987.

28. Butter CM, Kirsch NL, Reeves G: The effect of lateralized dynamic stimuli on unilateral spatial neglect following right hemisphere lesions. *Restor Neurol Neurosci* 2:39–46, 1990.

29. Karnath H-O: Disturbed coordinate transformation in the neural representation of space as the crucial mechanism leading to neglect. *Neuropsychol Rehabil* 4:147–150, 1994.

30. Rubens AB: Caloric stimulation and unilateral visual neglect. *Neurology* 35:1019–1024, 1985.

31. Cappa SF, Sterzi R, Vallar G, Bisiach E: Remission of hemineglect and anosognosia after vestibular stimulation. *Neuropsychologia* 25:775–782, 1987.

32. Vallar G, Bottini G, Rusconi ML, Sterzi R: Exploring somatosensory hemineglect by vestibular stimulation. *Brain* 116:71–86, 1993.

33. Bisiach E, Rusconi ML, Vallar G: Remission of somatoparaphrenic delusion through vestibular stimulation. *Neuropsychologia* 29:1029–1031, 1991.

34. Karnath HO, Christ K, Hartje W: Decrease of contralateral neglect by neck muscle vibration and spatial orientation of trunk midline. *Brain* 116:383–396, 1993.

35. Pizzamiglio L, Frasca R, Guariglia C, et al: Effect of optokinetic stimulation in patients with visual neglect. *Cortex* 26:535–540, 1990.

36. Mesulam MM: A cortical network for directed attention and unilateral neglect. *Ann Neurol* 4:309–325, 1981.

37. Zisper D, Anderson R: A back-propagation programmed network that simulates response properties of a subset of posterior parietal neurons. *Nature* 331:679–684, 1988.

38. Graziano MSA, Yap GS, Gross CG: Coding of visual space by premotor neurons. *Science* 266:1054–1057, 1994.

39. Rizzolatti G, Camarda R: Neural circuits for spatial attention and unilateral neglect, in Jeannerod M (ed): *Neurophysiological and Neuropsychological Aspects of Spatial Neglect.* Amsterdam, North-Holland, 1987, pp 289–314. (Stelmach GE, Vroon PA, eds. *Advances in Psychology;* vol 45).

40. O'Keefe J: Hippocampus, theta, and spatial memory. *Curr Opin Neurobiol* 3:917–924, 1993.

41. Heilman KM, Valenstein E, Watson RT: The neglect syndrome, in Fredricks JAM (ed): *Clinical Neuropsychology.* New York, Elsevier 1985, pp 153–183.

42. Coslett HB, Bowers D, Fitzpatrick E, et al: Directional hypokinesia and hemispatial inattention in neglect. *Brain* 113:475–486, 1990.

43. Heilman KM, Bowers D, Coslett HB, et al: Directional hypokinesia: Prolonged reaction times for

leftward movements in patients with right hemisphere lesions and neglect. *Neurology* 35:855–859, 1985.

44. Bisiach E, Geminiani G, Berti A, Rusconi ML: Perceptual and premotor factors of unilateral neglect. *Neurology* 40:1278–1281, 1990.

45. Tegner R, Levander M: Through a looking glass: A new technique to demonstrate directional hypokinesia in unilateral neglect. *Brain* 113:1943–1951, 1991.

46. Mattingley JB, Bradshaw JG, Phillips JG: Impairments of movement initiation and execution in unilateral neglect: Directional hypokinesia and bradykinesia. *Brain* 115:1849–1874, 1992.

47. Heilman KM, Valenstein E, Watson RT: The what and how of neglect. *Neuropsychol Rehabil* 4:133–139, 1994.

48. Milner AD, Harvey M, Roberts RC, Forster SV: Line bisection errors in visual neglect: Misguided action or size distortion? *Neuropsychologia* 31:39–49, 1993.

49. Milner AD, Harvey M: Distortion of size perception in visuospatial neglect. *Curr Biol* 5:85–89, 1995.

50. Karnath H-O: Ocular space exploration in the dark and its relation to subjective and objective body orientation in neglect patients with parietal lesions. *Neuropsychologia* 33:371–378, 1995.

51. Ladavas E: Is the hemispatial deficit produced by right parietal damage associated with retinal or gravitational coordinates? *Brain* 110:167–180, 1987.

52. Baylis GC, Driver J: One-sided edge-assignment in vision: 1. Figure-ground segmentation and attention to objects. *Curr Dir Psychol Sci.* In press.

53. Driver J, Baylis G, Rafal R: Preserved figure-ground segmentation and symmetry perception in a patient with neglect. *Nature* 360:73–75, 1993.

54. Marshall JC, Halligan PW: Left in the dark: The neglect of theory. *Neuropsychol Rehabil* 4:161–167, 1994.

55. Driver J, Baylis GC, Goodrich SJ, Rafal RD: Axis-based neglect of visual shapes. *Neuropsychologia* 32:1353–1365, 1994.

56. Behrman M, Tipper SP: Object-based visual attention: Evidence from unilateral neglect, in Umilta C, Moscovitch M (ed): *Attention and Performance: XIV. Conscious and Nonconscious Processing and Cognitive Functioning.* Hillsdale, NJ, Erlbaum, 1994.

57. Hillis AE, Caramazza A: Deficit to stimulus-centered, letter shape representations in a case of "unilateral neglect." *Neuropsychologia* 29:1223–1240, 1991.

58. Friedrich FJ, Walker JA, Posner MI: Effects of parietal lesions on visual matching: Implications for reading errors. *Cogn Neuropsychol* 2:253–264, 1985.

59. Brunn JL, Farah MJ: The relationship between spatial attention and reading: Evidence from the neglect syndrome. *Cogn Neuropsychol* 8:59–75, 1991.

60. Sieroff E, Pollatsek A, Posner MI: Recognition of visual letter strings following injury to the posterior visual spatial attention system. *Cogn Neuropsychol* 5:427–449, 1988.

61. Farah MJ, Brunn JL, Wong AB, et al: Frames of reference for allocating attention to space: Evidence from the neglect syndrome. *Neuropsychologia* 28:335–347, 1990.

62. Behrman M, Moscovitch M: Object-centered neglect in patients with unilateral neglect: Effects of left-right coordinates of objects. *J Cogn Neurosci* 6:1–16, 1994.

63. Bisiach E: Mental representation in unilateral neglect and related disorders: The twentieth Bartlett Memorial Lecture. *Q J Exp Psychol* 46A:435–462, 1993.

64. Bisiach E, Luzzatti C: Unilateral neglect of representational space. *Cortex* 14:129–133, 1978.

65. Bisiach E, Luzzatti C, Perani D: Unilateral neglect, representational schema and consciousness. *Brain* 102:609–618, 1979.

66. Kinsella G, Olver J, Ng K, et al: Analysis of the syndrome of unilateral neglect. *Cortex* 29:135–140, 1993.

67. Duhamel JR, Colby CL, Goldberg ME: The updating of the representation of visual space in parietal cortex by intended eye movements. *Science* 255:90–92, 1992.

68. Gianotti G: The role of spontaneous eye movements in orienting attention and in unilateral neglect, in Robertson IH, Marshall JC (ed): *Unilateral Neglect: Clinical and Experimental Studies.* Hillsdale, NJ, Erlbaum, 1993, 107–122.

69. Funahashi S, Bruce CJ, Goldman RP: Dorsolateral prefrontal lesions and oculomotor delayed-response performance: Evidence for mnemonic "scotomas." *J Neurosci* 13:1479–1497, 1993.

70. Anderson B: Spared awareness for the left side of internal visual images in patients with left-sided extrapersonal neglect. *Neurology* 43:213–216, 1993.

71. Guariglia C, Padovani A, Pantano P, Pizzamiglio L:

Unilateral neglect restricted to visual imagery. *Nature* 364:235–237, 1993.

72. Humphreys GW, Riddoch MJ: Interactive attentional systems in unilateral visual neglect, in Robertson IH, Marshall JC (eds): *Unilateral Neglect: Clinical and Experimental Studies.* Hillsdale, NJ, Erlbaum, 1993, pp 139–168.

73. Robertson IH, Halligan PW, Marshall JC: Prospects for the rehabilitation of unilateral neglect, in Robertson IH, Marshall JC (eds): *Unilateral Neglect: Clinical and Experimental Studies.* Hillsdale, NJ, Erlbaum, 1993, pp 279–292.

74. Diller L, Riley E: The behavioural management of neglect, in Robertson IH, Marshall JC (eds): *Unilateral Neglect: Clinical and Experimental Studies.* Hillsdale, NJ, Erlbaum, 1993, pp 293–310.

75. Rafal RD: Neglect. *Curr Opin Neurobiol* 4:2312–2316, 1994.

Chapter 12

DISORDERS OF PERCEPTION AND AWARENESS

Martha J. Farah
Todd E. Feinberg

Perception and awareness of perception are normally inextricably related. Most people would say that one has not perceived an object if one is not consciously aware of it. Yet, recent findings in behavioral neurology and neuropsychology are forcing us to revise this notion of the relation between perception and conscious awareness. Brain-damaged patients may manifest considerable knowledge of stimuli or particular properties of stimuli of which they deny any conscious perceptual experience. Although these findings challenge the intuitive idea that part and parcel of perceiving something is being aware of it, they also offer us a unique opportunity for investigating the neural bases of consciousness. In this chapter we review six perceptual disorders in which perception and awareness are dissociated and relate these disorders to the three main schools of thought concerning the brain correlates of conscious awareness.

THE NEURAL CORRELATES OF CONSCIOUS AWARENESS: THREE TYPES OF PROPOSAL

A Localized System for Consciousness

The first and most straightforward account of the relation between consciousness and the brain is to conceive of particular brain systems as mediating conscious awareness. The great grandfather of this type of account is Descartes' theory of mind-body interaction through the pineal gland. The most direct and influential descendant of this tradition is the DICE (dissociated interactions and conscious experience) model of Schacter and coworkers shown in Fig. 12-1.[1] According to this account, there is some brain system or systems, the conscious awareness system (CAS), separate from the brain systems concerned with perception, cognition, and action, whose activity is necessary for conscious experience and only for conscious experience. In a variant of this view, a brain system could be necessary for conscious awareness and for other functions as well. For example, Gazzaniga[2] attributes many of the differences between what one would call conscious and unconscious behavior to the involvement of left-hemispheric interpretive mechanisms, closely related to speech.

Consciousness as a State of Integration

In contrast to the first type of proposal, the next two types explain the relations between conscious and unconscious information processing in terms of the dynamic states of brain systems rather than in terms of the enduring roles of particular brain systems themselves. According to Kinsbourne's "integrated field theory," conscious awareness is a brain state in which the various modality-specific perceptions, recollections, current actions, and action plans are mutually consistent.[3] Normally, the interactions among these disparate brain systems automatically bring the ensemble into an integrated state, continually updated to reflect the current information available in all parts of the

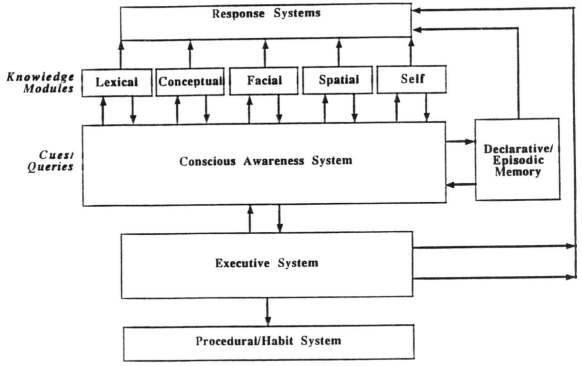

Figure 12-1
The DICE model (dissociated interactions and conscious experience) of Schacter and coworkers. (From Schacter et al.,[1] with permission.)

brain. Integration accounts have also been proposed by Crick and Koch[4] and by Damasio.[5] Crick and Koch limit themselves to the issue of visual awareness and equate the phenomenon of visual awareness with the binding together of the different, separately represented visual properties of a stimulus (e.g., color, shape, depth, motion) into a single integrated percept. They call upon the work of Singer and colleagues (e.g., Engel et al.[6]), who found synchronization of the oscillations of neuronal activity within visual cortex for different parts of the same representation of a stimulus and who suggested that this could be a mechanism for binding together the different parts of the representation. Crick and Koch suggest that synchronization across visual areas could enable both binding and conscious awareness of stimuli. Damasio[5] has proposed a similar identification of binding

with conscious awareness, which in his theory is accomplished via the "convergence zone" to which the separate representations all project.

Consciousness as a Property of Graded Representation

A third account emphasizes the graded nature of representation in neural networks and suggests that consciousness may be associated only with the higher-quality end of the continuum of degrees of representation. Experiments on subliminal perception in normal subjects dissociate perception and awareness by using very brief, masked stimulus presentations or by other experimental manipulations known to degrade the quality of the perceptual representation. According to this account, in both normal and in brain-damaged subjects there is a correlation between the quality of the perceptual representation and the likelihood of conscious awareness (e.g., Farah et al.[7]).

It is worth noting that these different types of explanation are not necessarily mutually exclusive. For example, the idea of a convergence zone fits the criteria for a particular brain area necessary for consciousness, as well as emphasizing integration of different brain areas.

DISSOCIATIONS BETWEEN PERCEPTION AND AWARENESS AFTER BRAIN DAMAGE

In a number of different disorders of perception, special tests have revealed surprisingly preserved visual processing in the absence of conscious awareness. What do these dissociations tell us about the neural correlates of visual awareness? Let us briefly review each dissociation with respect to the three proposals just outlined.

Blindsight

Representative Findings *Blindsight* refers to the preserved visual abilities of patients with damage to primary visual cortex for stimuli presented in regions of the visual field formerly represented by the damaged cortex. In the best-known case of blindsight, case DB, Weiskrantz and colleagues documented relatively preserved ability to point to stimulus locations, detect movement, discriminate the orientation of lines and gratings, and discriminate shapes such as X's and O's despite DB's denial that he was seeing the stimuli.[8] The pattern of preserved and impaired abilities has been found to vary considerably from case to case. Detection and localization of light and detection of motion are invariably preserved to some degree. In addition, many patients can discriminate orientation, shape, direction of movement, and flicker. Color vision mechanisms also appear to be preserved in some cases, as indicated by Stoerig and Cowey's[9] findings of normal-shaped spectral sensitivity functions. A good review of the blindsight literature can be found in Cowey and Stoerig.[10]

Proposed Mechanisms The mechanism of blindsight has been a controversial topic. Some researchers have argued that the phenomenon is mediated, directly or indirectly, by residual functioning of primary visual cortex. For example, Campion and coworkers[11] alleged that blindsight abilities are mediated by primary visual cortex, either indirectly, by light from the scotomatous region of the visual field reflecting off other surfaces into regions of the visual field represented by intact primary visual cortex, or directly, by residual functioning of lesioned areas of primary visual cortex. Fendrich and colleagues[12] have shown that small islands of preserved primary cortex can support certain visual discriminations in the absence of awareness. The explanation of blindsight as residual functioning of damaged primary visual cortex is consistent with the view that conscious awareness is correlated with the quality of a neural representation. However, this explanation meets several difficulties in accounting for the totality of the empirical data now available on blindsight. For example, it is difficult to see how scattered light would enable patient DB to perceive black figures on a bright background, nor how this account could explain the qualitative differences in his performance within his natural blind spot and his acquired blind region. Residual functioning of spared cortex is clearly not a possibility for subjects who show blindsight in one hemifield following hemidecortication, yet they, too, show a wide range of blindsight abilities.[13]

Other than spared primary visual cortex, what other neural systems might mediate the preserved abilities in blindsight? One possibility is the subcortical visual system, which consists of projections from the retina to the superior colliculus, and on to the pulvinar and cortical visual areas, as shown in Fig. 12-2. Evidence in favor of the subcortical mediation hypothesis includes the close functional similarities between the known specializations of the subcortical visual system and many of the preserved abilities in blindsight, such as detection and localization of onsets and moving stimuli, and the asymmetries observed between the nasal-temporal hemifields in some measures of blindsight, consistent with asymmetries in

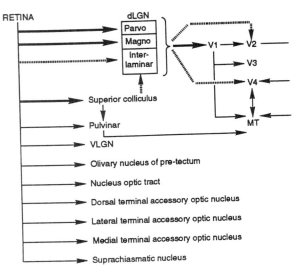

Figure 12-2
Cortical and subcortical visual pathways, including the two that may mediate blindsight: superior colliculus to pulvinar to extrastriate visual cortex, and lateral geniculate nucleus to extrastriate visual cortex.

retinal-collicular projections.[14] Thus according to this explanation, awareness is correlated with the activity of the cortical but not the subcortical visual system. This is consistent with the first of the proposals reviewed earlier, that some brain systems are endowed with conscious awareness and others are not.

Cowey and Stoerig have suggested that the cortical visual system, which projects from the retina to cortex by way of the lateral geniculate nucleus (LGN), may also contribute to blindsight.[15] They note that a population of cells in the LGN projects directly to extrastriate visual cortex and could therefore bring stimulus information into such areas as V4 and MT in the absence of primary visual cortex. According to this account, many of the same visual association areas are engaged in blindsight and in normal vision. What distinguishes normal vision and visual performance without awareness is that in the latter only a subset of the normal inputs arrive in extrastriate visual cortex. This type of mechanism fits most naturally with the third hypothesis, that represen-

tational quality is the critical factor for enabling conscious awareness.

Implicit Shape Perception in Apperceptive Visual Agnosia

Representative Findings   In apperceptive visual agnosia, patients are unable to name, copy, or match even the simplest shapes, such as squares or triangles, and cannot discriminate differently oriented line segments despite relatively preserved perception of brightness, color, motion, and acuity (see Chap. 6). Yet in at least one carefully studied case of apperceptive agnosia following carbon monoxide poisoning, good performance in a variety of visuomotor tasks implies the preservation of visual shape representations. Goodale and Milner[16] found that their patient DF reached toward a variety of objects with appropriate hand shapes for grasping. They went on to demonstrate that she could insert cards into slots of differing orientation while being unable to discriminate those orientations in purely perceptual tasks. A review of this work can be found in Milner and Goodale's recent book.[17]

Proposed Mechanism   Goodale and Milner[16] suggest that the dissociation between perception and awareness in their patient may result from an interruption in the flow of information from occipital to ventral visual areas needed for conscious object recognition. They hypothesize that the dorsal visual pathway, needed for spatial and visuomotor processing, normally operates without engendering conscious awareness, and that this pathway is relatively preserved in their patient. Thus, they endorse a variant of the first type of account, according to which conscious awareness accompanies the operation of some brain systems and not others.

Covert Recognition of Faces in Prosopagnosia

Representative Findings   Prosopagnosia is an impairment of face recognition following brain damage, which can occur relatively independently of impairments in object recognition and which is not caused by impairments in lower-level vision or memory (see Chap. 7). In some cases of prosopagnosia, there is a dramatic dissociation between the loss of face recognition ability as measured by standard tests of face recognition, as well as by patients' own introspections and the apparent preservation of face recognition when tested by certain indirect tests.[18]

For example, when prosopagnosics are required to learn to associate the facial photographs of famous people with the names of such people, some have been found to learn correct pairings faster than incorrect pairings.[19] Evidence of preserved recognition has also come from reaction time (RT) tasks in which the familiarity or identity of faces is found to influence processing time. In a visual identity match task with simultaneously presented pairs of faces, De Haan and colleagues[19] found that a prosopagnosic patient was faster at matching pairs of previously familiar faces than unfamiliar faces, as is true of normal subjects, even though he performed poorly at judging the familiarity of the faces. In so-called "priming" studies, photographs of faces have been found to influence the time needed to make decisions about printed names, such as those shown in Fig. 12-3.[19] For example, in deciding whether a name belonged to an actor or a politician, a prosopagnosic was found to be faster when an accompanying face also came from the same occupational category than when it came from another occupational category. Good reviews of research in this area may be found in Bruyer[20] and Young.[21]

Proposed Mechanisms The oldest and still predominant explanation of covert recognition is that the face-recognition system is intact in these patients but has been disconnected from other brain mechanisms necessary for conscious awareness (e.g., the model of De Haan and coworkers,[22] who base their account on the DICE model). Thus, the neural correlate of conscious awareness is taken to be activation of a particular brain system dedicated to conscious awareness.

Tranel and Damasio[23] also interpret covert

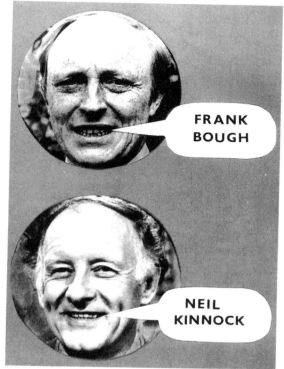

Figure 12-3
Examples of stimuli from the study of De Haan and colleagues. Subjects must classify the names as belonging to an actor or a politician. Their speed is influenced by the occupation of the faces. (From De Haan et al.,[19] with permission.)

recognition as the normal activation of visual face representations, disconnected from the convergence zones from whence representations in other areas of the brain can be activated. A similar idea is embodied in the computer simulation of Burton and colleagues.[24] These interpretations are most consistent with the second type of proposal discussed earlier in suggesting that conscious awareness requires the integration of representations across different brain areas; we cannot be consciously aware of an isolated, modality-specific representation.

It is also possible that covert recognition reflects the residual processing capabilities of a damaged but not obliterated visual face-recognition system. Farah and associates[7] trained a neural network to associate "face" patterns with "semantic" patterns and to associate these, in turn, with "name" patterns. As described in Chap. 4, we found that, at levels of damage to the face representations that led to poor or even chance performance in overt tasks, the network showed all of the behavioral covert recognition effects reviewed above: it relearned correct associations faster than novel ones, completed the visual analysis of familiar faces faster than unfamiliar, and showed priming and interference from the faces on judgments about names.

Unconscious Perception in Neglect and Extinction

Representative Findings Neglect is a disorder of spatial attention that generally follows posterior parietal damage and results in patients' failure to report or even orient to stimuli occurring on the side of space contralateral to the lesion (see Chaps. 10 and 11). Extinction is often viewed as a mild form of neglect, resulting in difficulty with contralateral stimuli only when an ipsilateral stimulus is presented at the same time. The behavior of patients with neglect and extinction suggests that they do not perceive neglected and extinguished stimuli. However, evidence is beginning to accumulate showing that, in at least some cases, considerable information about such stimuli is extracted by patients. As with covert recognition in prosopagnosia, this information is generally only detectable using indirect tests.

The first suggestion that patients with extinction may see more of the extinguished stimulus than is apparent from their conscious verbal report came from Volpe and coworkers.[25] They presented right-parietal-damaged extinction patients with pairs of visual stimuli, including drawings of common objects and three-letter words, one in each hemifield. On each trial, subjects were required to state whether the two stimuli shown were the same or different and to name the stimuli. Figure 12-4 shows the stimuli and results from a typical trial. Subjects did poorly at overtly identi-fying the stimuli on the left, sometimes remarking that they did not even see anything on the left, but they did well at same/different matching.

Berti and coworkers[26] used the paradigm of Volpe and associates to determine the level of processing to which extinguished stimuli were encoded. They included pairs of pictures that were physically different but depicted either the same object from a different view or different-looking exemplars of the same type of object, and they instructed their subject to say "same" if the two stimuli had the same name. The subject was able to do this, implying that extinguished stimuli are encoded to the level of meaning.

A recent study by McGlinchey-Berroth and colleagues[27] showed semantic priming by neglected pictures in a lexical decision task. On each trial of this experiment, subjects with left neglect viewed a picture in one hemifield, followed by a letter string in central vision to which they made a "word"/"nonword" response. When the picture was semantically related to the word, "word" responses were faster, and this was true even when the picture had been presented on the left side of the display. For a good review of these and other findings of unconscious perception after parietal damage, see Wallace.[28]

Proposed Mechanisms The earliest and most straightforward interpretation of these findings was offered by Volpe and colleagues,[25] who suggested that the stimulus processing was carried out normally and unconsciously in parietal-damaged patients but that the transfer of those representations to other parts of the system needed for conscious awareness was interrupted. This presupposes the first of the three kinds of relations between neural systems and consciousness—namely, the existence of particular localized systems needed for conscious awareness.

An alternative interpretation suggested by Kinsbourne[3] and Bisiach[29] is that the effects of parietal damage are to attenuate the influence of the percept on the rest of the system. This is consistent with the view that integration among neural systems is essential for awareness. However, insofar as the hypothesized failure of integration re-

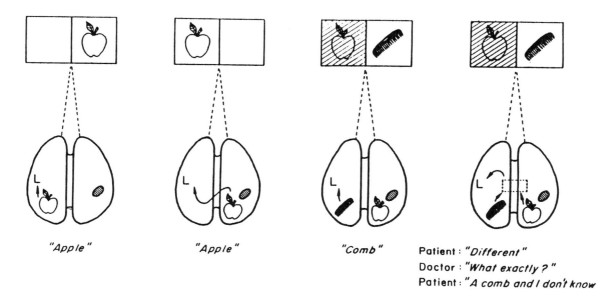

Figure 12-4
Typical trials from the experiment of Volpe and coworkers, showing extinction of the left stimulus with preserved same/different matching. (From Volpe et al.,[25] with permission.)

sults from the poor perception of neglected and extinguished stimuli, this interpretation is also consistent with the third type of proposal outlined earlier.

There is some support for the view that neglect and extinction impair perceptual processing and that the output of impaired perceptual processing can be used for perceptual same/different matching and partially activate appropriate semantic representations. Farah and coworkers[30] demonstrated that the dissociation described by Volpe and colleagues can be obtained with perceptual degradation with normal subjects and that it can be eliminated in patients when the perceptual demands of the same/different and naming tasks are matched. Also relevant is the simulation discussed in the previous section and Chap. 4 of semantic priming by faces after visual system damage. Although initially interpreted with respect to face perception and prosopagnosia, it nevertheless provides a generic demonstration that the output of impaired visual processing can evoke semantic information that will be detect-

able using indirect tests such as priming. Berti and associates[26] suggest that priming may underlie the matching performance of their patient, with the nonextinguished stimulus semantically priming the extinguished one.

Implicit Reading in Pure Alexia

Representative Findings Patients with pure alexia are impaired at reading, despite being able to write normally and understand spoken words. To the extent that they can read at all, they appear to do so in a "letter by letter" fashion, spelling the word to themselves before they can recognize it (see Chap. 18).

The first comprehensive investigation to suggest that pure alexics might understand more than they can report was carried out by Shallice and Saffran.[31] Their subject was able to discriminate words from nonword letter strings with relatively high accuracy with stimuli presented too quickly for him to reliably identify the words explicitly. Shallice and Saffran also demonstrated that their subject was able to make reasonably accurate semantic categorizations of briefly presented words, such as *animal* versus *nonanimal*. Coslett and Saffran[32] replicated and extended these findings with additional cases, showing that concrete words were understood better than abstract and that affixes were not processed (e.g., subjects would accept *elephanting* as a word). Perhaps their most striking finding is that their subjects performed the implicit reading tasks more accurately with extremely brief exposures of the words, such as 250 m, than with exposures of 2 s.

Proposed Mechanisms Although DICE has been applied to implicit reading (see Fig. 12-1), it fails to explain findings such as the concreteness effect, insensitivity to affixes, and improvement in performance with shorter presentations. A quality-of-representation account, whereby implicit reading is mediated by a degraded but not obliterated reading system, seems compatible with the first two findings, but it does not easily accommodate the third.

The most successful account at present attributes implicit reading to the right hemisphere, which is known to be deficient in knowledge of abstract words and morphology.[31,32] According to Coslett and Saffran, brief exposures may be necessary to foil the damaged but still dominant left hemisphere's letter-by-letter strategy. This interpretation implies that awareness of word recognition depends on the involvement of the left hemisphere and is thus an instance of the first type of explanation reviewed at the outset. It should be noted, however, that some implicit readers are aware of the information they glean from words (Shallice and Saffran;[31] personal observations). The core dissociation in implicit reading is between knowledge of certain word properties and knowledge of the specific word (e.g., knowing it is an animal but not knowing it is *camel*). It may be that only when tachistoscopic presentations are necessary to enable implicit reading does word knowledge dissociate from awareness, and this could be by the same mechanisms responsible for tachistoscopic subliminal perception in normal subjects.

Implicit Object Recognition in Associative Visual Agnosia

Representative Findings Associative visual agnosia is a disorder of visual object recognition not attributable to underlying primary perceptual or linguistic impairments (see Chap. 6). These patients perform adequately on figure copying tasks, thus distinguishing their disorder from apperceptive agnosia, and can name objects to verbal description, thus distinguishing their disorder from aphasia. They cannot demonstrate an object's use nonverbally through pantomime or other means, separating the disorder from optic aphasia.

In spite of their failures on tasks of explicit object recognition, residual object recognition abilities have been found in some of these patients. For instance, Taylor and Warrington[33] reported a patient with severe associative visual agnosia who was nonetheless able to place pictures in their proper orientation and sort pictures into basic categories. Similar abilities were reported in another associative visual agnosic by Jankowiak.[34]

We recently tested a patient with classic associative visual agnosia and alexia due to a dominant medial occipital infarction from a left posterior cerebral occlusion.[35,36] In spite of a severe defect in object naming, describing use, and pantomiming to visually presented objects, she showed a surprising ability to make semantic matches on forced-choice matching tasks with both pictures and words. Figure 12-5 shows an example of the picture-matching task. In an effort to assess the nature of the residual knowledge, we developed two tests of her metaknowledge on these tasks. On every trial, prior to responding, we assessed her "judgment of knowledge" by asking "Do you know what this picture is?" and, after she responded, we assessed her "judgment of accuracy" by asking "Are you sure or are you guessing?" We found three results of interest—first, overall accuracy varied directly with the number of choices, that is the more choices the worse her performance; second, while judgment of knowledge was poor overall, judgment of accuracy varied with performance accuracy. Under conditions of high accuracy (two-choice tasks) and low accu-

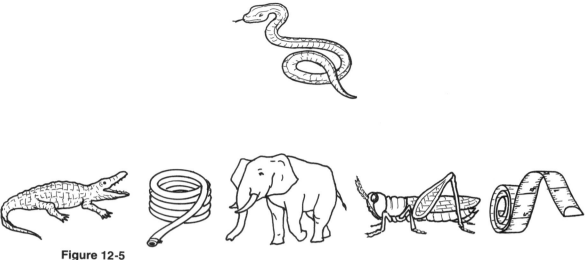

Figure 12-5
Example of five choice picture-to-picture matching tasks. Patient is asked which one is most like or goes with the target. Choices at bottom include two visual and two semantic foils.

racy (unlimited choice), the patient showed significant insight into her knowledge with better than chance judgment of accuracy on both tasks. When her accuracy was intermediate (five-choice tasks), her judgment of accuracy was poor. She thus showed her maximum level of insight when she had very much or very little knowledge. Finally, on the subset of trials in which she claimed no knowledge of the objects' identity during judgment-of-knowledge assessment, though the patient showed better than chance response accuracy, she still showed significant insight on judgment of accuracy, stating she was "sure" of her responses on almost 80 percent of trials where she was accurate, compared to only 25 percent of trials where her responses were inaccurate.

Proposed Mechanisms The findings that our patient's level of awareness was associated with her recognition performance is inconsistent with the view that the systems required for conscious awareness of recognition are disconnected from the recognition systems themselves. This fact coupled with the finding that performance accu-

racy varied with the number of choices is most consistent with the hypothesis of degraded knowledge. Additionally, while her residual reading abilities were consistent with those subserved by the right hemisphere,[31,32] there was no asymmetry in the accuracy of the patient's performance between the two hands. Our findings overall were most consistent with a degraded object-recognition system, whether left, right, or bilaterally represented, which is nonetheless accessible to either hemisphere.

GENERAL CONCLUSIONS

Heterogeneity at the Level of Phenomena

There are differences in the ways in which awareness is described by patients and operationalized by experimenters in these disorders. Blindsight patients may profess to be guessing on the basis of no subjective awareness or may respond with some confidence on the basis of a subjective experience that is nevertheless nonvisual—for example, sensing movement. In contrast, prosopagnosic subjects typically report absolutely no sense of familiarity when they view a face and have low confidence in their identifications, and apperceptive agnosics guess at shapes with low confidence. Similarly, in neglect and extinction subjects profess no awareness of the stimulus properties assessed in the matching or priming tasks on which they evince perception. Anecdotal evidence suggests that at times they even lack awareness that there was a stimulus. In implicit reading, awareness is not invariably dissociated from reading performance, although subjects who read implicitly under tachistoscopic conditions report being unaware of the information gleaned. Although implicit object recognition appears to occur without awareness, in at least one patient there was a systematic relation between her feeling of confidence in her "guesses" and their accuracy. In sum, the five disorders constitute a somewhat heterogeneous group from the point of view of awareness.

Heterogeneity at the Level of Mechanism

The five disorders also appear to be heterogeneous from the point of view of mechanism. For example, in blindsight, there are two types of mechanism that are currently under consideration, without any intended mutual exclusivity: subcortical mediation and extrastriate cortical mediation. As already discussed, there are consistent with the ideas that certain localized brain systems must be engaged and that a certain minimal quality of representation must be available for conscious awareness to take place. In apperceptive agnosia, preserved shape processing within the visual-motor system is also consistent with the idea that conscious awareness accompanies the functioning of certain localized brain systems and not others, although the empirical support for this interpretation is currently weak because of the diffuse nature of the one subject's brain damage.

The mechanisms responsible for the dissociations observed in covert recognition in prosopagnosia and unconscious perception in neglect and

extinction are not well established, and more evidence is needed to distinguish among the possible candidates. However, both syndromes currently seem explainable in terms of the quality of the representations available in each. In prosopagnosia, the poor quality of the representations is presumably due to a loss of stored perceptual knowledge of faces, whereas in neglect and extinction it is due to a more dynamic processing failure of the attention system.

Although the issue of mechanism is also far from settled in the case of implicit reading, the right-hemisphere hypothesis seems most promising at present. This is consistent with the view that certain localized brain systems are needed for normal aware perception. Recall, however, that some implicit readers appear to be aware of the information they perceive; therefore this syndrome may not be as relevant to understanding the neural correlates of conscious awareness as the other four.

General Implications for the Neural Correlates of Awareness

It should be clear that the five syndromes reviewed here are unlikely to share a common explanation. Although there is a family resemblance among them, closer inspection reveals that the kinds of perceptual abilities and the nature of subjective experience are not uniform. We may therefore need to consider the possibility that the relation between conscious awareness and neural systems is itself not explicable by just one of the types of account discussed earlier. For example, on the basis of the present review, it seems plausible that conscious awareness requires certain cortical perceptual regions to be engaged, and that, within these regions, a certain quality of representation is also necessary (thus denying consciousness to both the normal-quality functioning of the superior colliculus and to the impaired functioning of cortical face representations). Furthermore, it is possible that the importance of representational quality derives from the reduced ability of low-quality representations to influence the ambient state of integration across brain areas.

The foregoing conclusion about the neural correlates of awareness is both tentative and rather unconstrained, in that it leaves room for at least some versions of all three types of proposal outlined earlier. However, there is one type of proposal we can reject with reasonable confidence on the basis of the findings reviewed here: proposals that feature some component whose dedicated function is to enable awareness. Among all of the disorders, there is none for which visual perception has been convincingly demonstrated to be normal or near normal. This, in turn, deprives theories featuring a "consciousness awareness system" or "convergence zones" of their basic motivation, which is to explain a straightforward dissociation between perception and awareness of perception. On the basis of the evidence currently available, it seems unlikely that there are any brain systems needed for conscious awareness of perception that do not also play a role in perception per se.

REFERENCES

1. Schacter DL, McAndrews MP, Moscovitch M: Access to consciousness: Dissociations between implicit and explicit knowledge in neuropsychological syndromes, in Weiskrantz L (ed): *Thought without Language.* Oxford, England: Oxford University Press, 1988.
2. Gazzaniga MS: Brain modularity: Towards a philosophy of conscious experience, in Marcel AJ, Bisiach E (eds): *Consciousness in Contemporary Science.* Oxford, England: Clarendon Press, 1988.
3. Kinsbourne M: Integrated field theory of consiousness, in Marcel AJ, Bisiach E (eds): *Consciousness in Contemporary Science.* Oxford, England: Clarendon Press, 1988.
4. Crick F, Koch C: Function of the thalamic reticular complex: The searchlight hypothesis. *Semin Neurosci* 2:263–275, 1990.
5. Damasio AR: Synchronous activation in multiple cortical regions: A mechanism for recall. *Semin Neurosci* 2:287–296, 1990.
6. Engel AK, Konig P, Kreiter A, et al: Temporal coding in the visual cortex: New vistas on integration in the visual system. *Trends Neurosci* 15:218–226, 1992.
7. Farah MJ, O'Reilly RC, Vecera SP: Dissociated overt and covert recognition as on emergent property of lesioned attractor networks. *Psychol Rev* 100:571–588, 1993.
8. Weiskrantz L: *Blindsight: A Case Study and Implications.* Oxford, England: Oxford University Press, 1986.
9. Stoerig P, Cowey A: Wavelength sensitivity in blindsight. *Nature* 342:916–918, 1990.
10. Cowey A, Stoerig P: The neurobiology of blindsight. *Trends Neurosci* 14:140–145, 1991.
11. Campion J, Latto R, Smith YM: Is blindsight an effect of scattered light, spared cortex, and near-threshold vision? *Behav Brain Sci* 3:423–447, 1983.
12. Fendrich R, Wessinger CM, Gazzaniga MS: Residual vision on a scotoma: Implications for blindsight. *Science* 258:1489–1491, 1992.
13. Perenin MT: Visual function within the hemianopic field following early cerebral hemidecortication in man: II. Pattern discrimination. *Neuropsychologia* 16:696–708, 1978.
14. Rafal R, Smith J, Krantz J, et al: Extrageniculate vision in hemianopic humans: Saccade inhibition by signals in the blind field. *Science* 250:118–121, 1990.
15. Cowey A, Stoerig P: Projection patterns of surviving neurons in the dorsal lateral geniculate nucleus following discrete lesions of striate cortex: Implications for residual vision. *Exp Brain Res* 75:631–638, 1989.
16. Goodale MA, Milner DA: Separate visual pathways for perception and action. *Trends Neurosci* 15:20–25, 1992.
17. Milner AD, Goodale MA: *The Visual Brain in Action.* New York: Oxford University Press, 1995.
18. Bauer RM: Autonomic recognition of names and faces in prosopagnosia: A neuropsychological application of the guilty knowledge test. *Neuropsychologia* 22:457–469, 1984.
19. De Haan EHF, Young AW, Newcombe F: Face recognition without awareness. *Cog Neuropsychol* 4:385–415, 1987.
20. Bruyer R: Covert recognition of faces in prosopagnosia: A review. *Brain Cog* 15:223–235, 1992.
21. Young A: Covert face recognition, in Farah MJ, Ratcliff G (eds): *The Neuropsychology of High-Level Vision: Collected Tutorial Essays.* Hillsdale, NJ: Erlbaum, 1994.
22. De Haan EHF, Bauer RM, Greve KW: Behavioral and physiological evidence for covert recognition in a prosopagnosic patient. *Cortex* 28:77–95, 1992.
23. Tranel D, Damasio A: Knowledge without awareness: An autonomic index of facial recognition by prosopagnosics. *Science* 228:1453–1454, 1985.

24. Burton AM, Young AW, Bruce V, et al: Understanding covert recognition. *Cognition* 31:129–166, 1991.

25. Volpe BT, LeDoux JE, Gazzaniga MS: Information processing of visual stimuli in an "extinguished" field. *Nature* 22:724, 1979.

26. Berti A, Allport A, Driver J, et al: Levels of processing for visual stimuli in an "extinguished" field. *Neuropsychologia* 30:403–415, 1992.

27. McGlinchey-Berroth R, Milberg WP, Verfaellie M, et al: Semantic processing in the neglected visual field: Evidence from a lexical decision task. *Cog Neuropsychol* 10:79–108, 1993.

28. Wallace MA: Unconscious perception in neglect and extinction, in Farah MJ, Ratcliff G (eds): *The Neuropsychology of High-Level Vision: Collected Tutorial Essays.* Hillsdale, NJ: Erlbaum, 1994.

29. Bisiach E: Understanding Consciousness: Clues from unilateral neglect and related disorders, in Milner AD, Rugg MD (ed): *The Neuropsychology of Consciousness.* San Diego, CA: Academic Press, 1992.

30. Farah MJ, Monheit MA, Wallace MA: Unconscious perception of "extinguished" visual stimuli: Reassessing the evidence. *Neuropsychologia* 29: 949–958, 1991.

31. Shallice T, Saffran E: Lexical processing in the absence of explicit word identification: Evidence from a letter-by-letter reader. *J Cog Neuropsychol* 3:429–458, 1086.

32. Coslett HB, Saffran EM: Evidence for preserved reading in "pure alexia." *Brain* 112:327–359, 1989.

33. Taylor A, Warrington EK: Visual agnosia: A single case report. *Cortex* 7:152–161, 1971.

34. Jankowiak J, Kinsbourne M, Shalev RS, Bachman DL: Preserved visual imagery and categorization in a case of associative visual agnosia. *J Cogn Neurosci* 4:119–131, 1992.

35. Feinberg TE, Schindler RJ, Ochoa E, et al: Associative visual agnosia and alexia without prosopagnosia. *Cortex* 30:395–411, 1994.

36. Feinberg TE, Dyckes-Berke D, Miner CR, Roane DM: Knowledge, implicit knowledge and metaknowledge in visual agnosia and pure alexia. *Brain* 118:789–800, 1995.

Chapter 13

MISIDENTIFICATION SYNDROMES

Todd E. Feinberg
David M. Roane

Misidentification syndromes, sometimes referred to as delusional misidentification syndromes, describe conditions in which a patient incorrectly identifies and reduplicates persons, places, objects, or events. The most commonly reported form of misidentification for persons is known as *Capgras syndrome.* The syndrome was first reported in 1923 by Capgras and Reboul-Lachaux[1] who described a 53-year-old woman with a chronic paranoid psychosis who became convinced that multiple persons, including members of her family, had been replaced by imposters. She also asserted that there were several duplicates of herself. Since that time, hundreds of cases of Capgras syndrome have been reported. The essence of the disorder lies in the delusional belief that a person or persons, generally close to the patient, have been replaced by "doubles" or imposters.[2]

A related type of misidentification is the *Frégoli syndrome.*[3] First reported in 1927, the syndrome is named after the famous Italian actor Leopoldo Frégoli, who was extremely adept at impersonation. This condition involves the belief that a person who is well known to the patient is really impersonating, and hence taking on the appearance of, a stranger in the patient's environment. Several authors have commented on the relationship between Capgras and Frégoli syndromes.[4-6] Christodoulou[6] suggested that Capgras syndrome is characterized by a "hypoidentification" of a person known by the patient who is felt to be an imposter, while Frégoli syndrome was the manifestation of a "hyperidentification" in which a known person could be seen in the guise of others. The syndrome of *intermetamorphosis,* described by Courbon and Tusques,[7] is a related condition in which persons known to the patient

are believed to have exchanged identities with each other. In the delusion of subjective doubles,[8] the patients believe they themselves have been replaced. Other varieties of delusional misidentification syndromes exist, and different varieties may co-occur in any given patient.

The delusional misidentification syndromes are related to the syndrome of reduplicative paramnesia. For instance, Alexander and colleagues[9] described a case of Capgras syndrome following a head injury that resulted in a large right frontal subdural hematoma. The patient stated that his wife and five children had been replaced by a nearly identical family, and he persisted in his conviction even when challenged by his examiners. Alexander and associates suggested a similarity between their case and *reduplicative paramnesia,* a syndrome originally described by Pick[10] in 1903. Pick's patient was a 67-year-old woman who confabulated the existence of two clinics, both headed by Professor Pick. While Capgras syndrome had traditionally been considered a psychiatric condition, reduplicative paramnesia had generally been felt to be a neurologic disorder, since it was usually seen in the setting of brain disorders and was often associated with confusion and memory loss. It differed as well from Capgras syndrome in that it typically involved misidentification of places rather than persons. However, the distinction between the two conditions is not entirely clear. Cases of reduplication reported by Weinstein[11] in the setting of brain disease involved duplication of persons, events, body parts, and even the self. Furthermore, Weinstein's cases of reduplication were frequently associated with other psychiatric symptoms including other delusions, hallucinations, and mood changes. It has therefore become customary to group delusional misidentification and reduplicative paramnesia together.

The Capgras delusion is most commonly associated with psychiatric illness and is often accompanied by derealization and depersonalization[12,13] and by other paranoid symptomatology.[14,15] Literature reviews of patients with the Capgras delusion have demonstrated the diagnostic heterogeneity of this condition.[14,16,17] Schizophrenia, mood disorders, and organic conditions, including Alzheimer disease,[18] have all been associated with Capgras syndrome.

Misidentification and reduplication in general have been associated with a wide variety of medical and neurologic conditions.[19,20] In a large literature review of cases of reduplication, Signer[19] found cases due to drug intoxication or withdrawal, infectious and inflammatory disease, and endocrine disorders. Neurologic conditions included seizures, cerebral infarction, and head injury. Diffuse brain syndromes including delirium, dementia, and mental retardation accounted for over 40 percent of patients with diagnosable organic conditions. Electroconvulsive therapy has also been implicated in cases of misidentification.[21,22]

NEUROANATOMIC CORRELATES

In a report of 29 personally examined patients with misidentification for person, Joseph[23] found that 16 patients with abnormal computed tomography (CT) scans had bilateral cortical atrophy, including bifrontal atrophy (88 percent), bitemporal atrophy (73 percent), and biparietal atrophy (60 percent). Weinstein and Burnham suggested that bilateral and diffuse brain involvement with right-hemispheric predominance were the most common neurologic findings.[24] Along these lines, Feinberg and Shapiro[25] reviewed the anatomic correlates on a selected series of case reports of patients with misidentification-reduplication. They found that bilateral cortical involvement occurred frequently (62 percent of Capgras patients and 41 percent of reduplication cases). In considering those cases where cerebral dysfunction was unilateral, they found that right-hemispheric pre-

dominance in reduplication was highly significant (52 percent right versus 7 percent left), with a statistical trend for more frequent right-hemispheric damage in the smaller number of Capgras cases (32 percent right versus 7 percent left). Förstl and coworkers[20] grouped together a wide range of misidentification cases and found that 19 of 20 patients with focal lesions on brain CT scans showed right-sided abnormalities. In a subsequent study, Förstl and colleagues[26] focused on patients with dementia of the Alzheimer's type and found that patients with misidentification had significantly greater atrophy in the right frontal lobe than did demented controls. Based on three cases of head trauma, Benson and associates[27] suggested that reduplicative paramnesia occurred in the setting of bifrontal impairment in concert with damage to the posterior portion of the right hemisphere. Hakim and coworkers,[28] in a prospective study of 50 patients with alcoholism, found that 3 of 4 reduplicators had acute right-hemispheric lesions. They presumed all patients to have chronic bifrontal damage on the basis of their chronic alcohol use and neuropsychological test results. Finally, Fleminger and Burns[29] compared right- versus left-hemispheric asymmetries in CT scans of patients with misidentification. In one selected group, asymmetry was found, with greater right-hemispheric damage in the occipitoparietal area. In the analysis of a second group of patients, greater right-hemispheric damage could be detected in frontal, temporal, and parietal lobes.

At present, while some evidence suggests that a right-hemispheric lesion (particularly right frontal impairment[30]) can be both necessary and sufficient to produce misidentification, the bulk of cases support the argument that a right-hemispheric lesion is much more likely to be associated with misidentification in the context of bifrontal or diffuse cortical disturbance. This finding may reflect the greater tendency in these patients to demonstrate confabulation in general.

REPRESENTATIVE THEORIES

It has been suggested that delusional misidentification is a symptom, rather than a distinct syndrome, associated with various psychiatric and neurologic diagnoses.[31] Nonetheless, several explanations have attempted to account for a broad range of misidentification phenomena. Anatomic disconnection has been offered as a mechanism by several authors. Joseph[23] theorized that misidentification could result from hemispheric disconnection of cortical areas responsible for orientation. This could result in each hemisphere's maintaining an independent "image" of person, place, and time, which might lead to reduplication of entities in the environment. However, Ellis and colleagues[32] showed that patients with Capgras syndrome could judge face stimuli more rapidly with bilateral than with unilateral presentation, a finding that they suggested was inconsistent with the hemispheric disconnection hypothesis. Staton and coworkers[33] suggested that reduplication could be a failure to integrate previously stored memories and new information resulting from disconnection of the right hippocampus. Alexander and associates[9] considered that a disconnection of the right temporal and limbic area from the frontal lobes could alter the patients' familiarity for people and places and prevent them from utilizing available information appropriately.

The mechanisms proposed by Staton and associates[33] and Alexander and colleagues[9] attribute misidentification particularly to the loss of functions subsumed by the right hemisphere. Several investigators have emphasized other nondominant hemispheric functions, such as disorders of visuospatial orientation,[28,30] problem solving,[30] and the ability to determine the exact identity and uniqueness of stimuli[34] in the origin of delusional misidentification syndromes and reduplication. A recent study by Ellis and coworkers[32] confirmed that three Capgras patients lacked the normal right-hemispheric superiority for visual processing of faces.

A final disconnectionist account, formulated by Ellis and Young,[35] is based on the suggestion that there are two anatomically independent pathways for facial recognition: a "ventral route" subserving explicit recognition and a "dorsal route" responsible for recognition of the emotional significance of faces but not sufficient to allow for conscious identification.[36] While Capgras syndrome has been linked with prosopagnosia,[37-39] Ellis and Young[35] argue that the two are dissociable because they result from separate lesions. The ventral route disconnection causes prosopagnosia while the dorsal route interruption yields Capgras syndrome.

While the above theories emphasize anatomic disconnection, psychiatric factors have often been cited as etiologically significant for the development of Capgras syndrome. For instance, according to Enoch and Trethowan,[31] ambivalence is the "psychodynamic aspect" of Capgras syndrome. Simultaneous conflicting affects toward a significant object exist, and, through the mechanisms of projection and splitting, the actual object is misidentified and devalued while the normal attachment to the "original" is maintained.

Another point of view emphasizes the *interaction* of neurologic and psychiatric factors in DMS. Early important work emphasizing the link between neurologic and psychiatric factors in DMS can be found in the writings of Jacques Vié[4,40-42] who noted that the diverse DMS (*méconnaissance systématique*) such as Capgras and Frégoli syndromes were related to the neurologic syndromes of anosognosia of Babinski (unawareness of hemiplegia) and asomatognosia[43] (denial of ownership of limb). Vié pointed out that in all these conditions, systematic and selective misidentifications occurred that could not be explained solely on the basis of factors such as generalized confusion.

The position of Weinstein and Kahn,[11,24,44] because of its emphasis on psychological denial, is usually taken to represent a psychological theory. In actuality these authors also suggested that DMS occurred through an interaction of neurologic and psychiatric factors. They suggested that misidentification and reduplication were facilitated by brain alteration and that they represented a denial, representation of, or solution to the patient's problems. More recent analysis by other investigators has also suggested an interaction between neurologic and psychiatric factors.[45,46]

An additional link between neurologic and psychiatric causation of delusional misidentification syndromes is provided by the fact that dissociative symptoms occur in delusional misidentification syndromes associated with both neurologic and psychiatric disorders.[24] Capgras, in the original report,[1] emphasized the importance of the *sentiment d'étrangeté* in the production of the syndrome in his chronic paranoid patient. Many authors have provided additional support for the association of depersonalization/derealization with delusional misidentification syndromes (see Christodoulou[5,6,12]). Christodoulou has suggested that depersonalization/derealization symptoms, under certain circumstances (paranoia, cerebral dysfunction, charged emotional circumstances), may evolve into delusional misidentification syndromes. Weinstein and coworkers have noted that patients with retrograde amnesia after head injury may also display elements of depersonalization and derealization.[24,47] Feelings of altered familiarity also occur during psychomotor seizures and with temporal lobe stimulation (see Feinberg and Shapiro[25] for review).

A PROPOSED FRAMEWORK FOR DELUSIONAL MISIDENTIFICATION SYNDROMES

As noted by prior authors, we agree that DMS can be viewed as being especially related to, and perhaps a special instance of, dissociative disorders, and we regard the origin of these symptoms as a perturbation, as opposed to a loss, of personal relatedness. We suggest that DMS cleaves along the dimension of personal relatedness into three basic groups based upon the pattern of relatedness between the object (person, event, or experience) and the self. The various subtypes of DMS and reduplication can thus be characterized as showing a pattern of decreased (withdrawal) or increased (insertion of) personal relatedness (or both) between the self and the misidentified object or event.

Our basic dichotomization into patterns of withdrawal or insertion of personal relatedness corresponds in part to several previously suggested dichotomies (Table 13-1) and is consistent with the viewpoint that Capgras may be similar to jamais vu phenomena[25,48–51] and that Frégoli[49] and environmental reduplication[25,49–52] are similar to déjà vu phenomena. Our model (Table 13-1), however, differs in two fundamental ways from previously proposed models (see, for example, de Pauw[51]). First of all, as to the basic means of distinguishing Capgras from Frégoli, these syndromes have previously been categorized on the basis of physical versus psychological substitution or hypoidentification versus hyperidentification. In contrast we view the distinguishing feature to be alteration of personal relatedness or significance. Those syndromes exemplified by decreased relatedness may be said to represent a disavowal, estrangement, or alienation from persons, objects, or events, while those with increased relatedness are manifestations of an overrelatedness with elements in the environment.

We prefer the concept of an alteration in relatedness as opposed to an alteration in familiarity because many stimuli that the patient misidentifies, such as hospitals and aneurysms, are not particularly "familiar" in any sense of the word. Rather they are significant and actually do pertain to the self though the patient rejects them in spite of this.

Secondly, we argue that our approach is particularly useful in explaining instances where Capgras- and Frégoli-type misidentifications co-occur within a single misidentification (Table 13-2, col-

Table 13-1

Prior formulations of basic dichotomization of Capgras and Frégoli syndrome

Author		
Vié[4]	Illusion of negative doubles (Capgras)	Illusion of positive doubles (Frégoli)
Christodoulou[6]	Delusional hypoidentification	Delusional hyperidentification
Christoldoulou[5]	Physically identical, psychologically different	Physically different, psychologically identical
de Pauw[49–51]	Hypoidentification, denial of familiarity, jamais vu (Capgras)	Hyperidentification, affirmation of familiarity, déjà vu (environmental reduplication)
Feinberg and Shapiro[25]	Pathological unfamiliarity, jamais vu, substitute familiar for unfamiliar (Capgras)	Pathological familiarity, déjà vu, substitute unfamiliar for familiar (environmental reduplication)

Table 13-2
Proposed model of common DMS

Examples of misidentified entities	Mechanism supporting misidentification/reduplication and clinical examples		
	Withdrawal of personal relatedness	Insertion of personal relatedness	Combined withdrawal/insertion of personal relatedness
Persons	Misidentifies wife as "impostor" (Capgras–jamais vu)	Misidentifies stranger as son (Frégoli– déjà vu)	Misidentifies personal physician as a friend from home[44,53] (Capgras/Frégoli–jamais vu/déjà vu)
Hemiplegic arm[40,43,44,53] (asomatognosia)	Denies ownership of arm[50,51]		Misidentifies own arm as belonging to close friend[43,44,53]
Hospital[11,24,44,53,54] (environmental reduplication)	Calls the hospital a "branch" or "annex" of actual hospital[44]	Mislocates actual hospital closer to patient's own neighborhood[44,49–51]	Misidentifies hospital as "annex" of actual hospital and locates it closer to patient's own neighborhood[44]
Traumatic events[11,24,53,54] (temporal reduplication) i.e., car accident	Denies accident occurred to patient (jamais vécu)	Claims similar accident happened previously to patient (déjà vécu)	Minimizes own accident but claims reduplicated brother "Martin" killed in (fictitious) car accident[54]
Illness[11,24,44,53]	Denial of illness	Had similar illness previously	Patient denies illness but claims reduplicated child Bill called "Willie" had same illness as patient[44]
			Patient with aneurysm minimizes it and claims her relatives have aneurysms

umn 4). This occurs, for instance, in asomatognosia where the patient simultaneously denies ownership of the arm[43,44,53] (withdrawal of personal relatedness) while identifying the arm as belonging to a friend or relative (insertion of personal relatedness). In a similar fashion, when a patient with environmental reduplication claims he is located in a hospital "annex" in his own neighborhood, he is *both* denying the actual identity of his current location as well as inserting an element of personal relatedness.

The same pattern of withdrawal and insertion of relatedness occurs in reduplication of illness in the context of anosognosia. Thus a patient of Weinstein did not recognize her own illness, but claimed she had two children, Bill (real) and "Willie" (fictitious), and that "Willie" had an illness similar to hers.[44,53] We saw a patient who minimized the problems posed by her own aneurysm but claimed that several of her relatives had aneurysms. Finally, with regard to misidentification of a traumatic event, Baddeley and Wilson[54] described the patient RJ who denied that he was seriously injured in a car accident, yet simultaneously claimed to have two brothers named Martin: a Martin who actually existed and a fictitious "Martin" who was killed in a car accident. In these cases we hypothesize that the neurologic impairment facilitates the derealization/depersonalization (dissociation) of an actual person, place, or event, which is then replaced by some other personally significant relationship. Motivational factors appear important in determining both the withdrawal and insertion of significance.

CONCLUDING REMARKS

If a perturbation in personal relatedness to oneself or one's environment is an essential ingredient in delusional misidentification syndromes, one may ask whether this distortion is primarily a result of a neurologic lesion, a psychiatric mechanism linked with motivational variables, or both. Many theories emphasizing a neurologic etiology for Capgras syndrome[9,33,46] assert a limbic disconnection of current perceptions from past experience. This causes a reduced feeling of familiarity with environmental stimuli and a confabulation of "doubleness" to explain the disparity between current and past experience. These theories do not account for the selectivity of many cases of Capgras, their delusional nature, the lack of gross neuropathologic lesions in most cases, the occurrence of misidentification of relatively unfamiliar persons in many cases, the occurrence of misidentifications of the hyperfamiliar type, and the role of motivation. For instance, in regard to the last of these, it has been pointed out that in environmental reduplication, while abnormal spatial perception, poor visual memory, and other neuropsychological defects are evident, these patients often show, in addition, a pronounced desire to return home.[55]

Other theories describe the psychoanalytic viewpoint that derealization/depersonalization is the result of psychological defense mechanisms. As noted by Nemiah,[56] "From the earliest period of the development of psychoanalytic concepts, the experience of estrangement that is central to depersonalization phenomena has been viewed as a psychological defense." In this scenario, derealization/depersonalization occurs as a defense against irreconcilable affects or unacceptable and conflicting motivations. The ambivalence produces the delusion of "doubleness" through mechanisms such as "splitting."[31,57] While these theories can account for selectivity, delusional nature and the possibility of hypo- and hyperfamiliar misidentifications, they do not account for delusional misidentification syndromes occurring in the context of neurologic disease.

A mediating point of view is that the neurologic lesion, and certain neurologic lesions in particular, cause a distortion of normal sensation, memory, and awareness. The response to this distortion, particularly when it involves personally significant objects or events, creates the circumstances which, in the susceptible individual, results in derealization/depersonalization. It is upon this substrate that motivational variables may become evident.

REFERENCES

1. Capgras J, Reboul-Lachaux J: L'illusion des "sosies" dans un délire systématisé. *Bull Soc Clin Med Ment* 11:6–16, 1923.
2. Christodoulou GN: The delusional misidentification syndromes. *Br J Psychiatry* 14:65–69, 1991.
3. Courbon P, Fail G: Syndrome "d'illusion de Frégoli" et schizophrenie. *Ann Med Psychol* 85:289–290, 1927.
4. Vié J: Un trouble de l'identification des personnes: L'illusion des sosies. *Ann Med Psychol* 88:214–237, 1930.
5. Christodoulou GN: Delusional hyper-identifications of the Frégoli type. *Acta Psychiatry Scand* 54:305–314, 1976.
6. Christodoulou GN: The syndrome of Capgras: *Br J Psychiatry* 130:556–564, 1977.
7. Courbon P, Tusques J: L'illusion d'intermetamorphose et de charme. *Ann Med Psychol* 90:401–406, 1932.
8. Christodoulou GN: Syndrome of subjective doubles. *Am J Psychiatry* 135:249–251, 1978.
9. Alexander MP, Stuss DT, Benson DF: Capgras syndrome: A reduplicative phenomenon. *Neurology* 29:334–339, 1979.
10. Pick A: Clinical studies. *Brain* 26:242–267, 1903.
11. Weinstein EA, Kahn RL, Sugarman LA: Phenomenon of reduplication. *AMA Arch Neurol Psychiatry* 67:808–814, 1952.
12. Christodoulou GN: Role of depersonalization-derealization phenomena in the delusional misidentification syndromes, in Christodoulou GN (ed): *The Delusional Misidentification Syndromes.* Basel: Karger, 1986.
13. Spier SA: Capgras' syndrome and the delusions of misidentification. *Psychiatr Am* 22:279–285, 1992.
14. Kimura S: Review of 106 cases with the syndrome of Capgras. *Bibl Psychiatry* 164:121–130, 1986.
15. Todd J, Dewhurst K, Wallis G: The syndrome of Capgras. *Br J Psychiatry* 139:319–327, 1981.
16. Merrin EL, Silberfarb PM: The Capgras phenomenon. *Arch Gen Psychiatry* 33:965, 1970.
17. Signer SF: Capgras' syndrome: The delusion of substitution. *Clin Psychiatry* 48:147–150, 1987.
18. Mendez MF, Martin RJ, Symth KA, Whitehouse PJ: Disturbances of person identification Alzheimer's disease: A retrospective study. *J Nerv Ment Dis* 180:94, 1992.
19. Signer SF: Psychosis in neurologic disease: Capgras symptom and delusions of reduplication in neurologic disorders. *Neuropsychiatr Neuropsychol Behav Neurol* 5:138–143, 1992.
20. Förstl H, Almeida OP, Owen A, et al: Psychiatric, neurological and medical aspects of misidentification syndromes: A review of 260 cases. *Psychol Med* 21:905–950, 1991.
21. Weinstein EA, Linn L, Kahn RL: Psychosis during electroshock therapy: Its relation to the theory of shock therapy. *Am J Psychiatry* 109:22–26, 1952.
22. Hay GG: Electroconvulsive therapy as a contributor to the production of delusional misidentification. *Br J Psychiatry* 148:667–669, 1986.
23. Joseph AB: Focal central nervous system abnormalities in patients with misidentification syndromes, in Christodoulou GN (ed): *The Delusional Misidentification Syndromes.* Basel: Karger, 1986, p 68.
24. Weinstein EA, Burnham DL: Reduplication and the syndrome of Capgras. *Psychiatry* 54:78, 1991.
25. Feinberg TE, Shapiro RM: Misidentification-redu-

plication and the right hemisphere. *Neuropsychiatr Neuropsychol Behav Neurol* 2:39–48, 1989.

26. Förstl H, Burns A, Jacoby R, Levy R: Neuroanatomical correlates of clinical misidentification and misperception in senile dementia of the Alzheimer type. *Clin Psychiatry* 52:268, 1991.

27. Benson DF, Gardner H, Meadows JC: Reduplicative paramnesia. *Neurology* 26:147–151, 1978.

28. Hakim H, Verma NP, Greiffenstein MF: Pathogenesis of reduplicative paramnesia. *Neurol Neurosurg Psychiatry* 51:839–841, 1988.

29. Fleminger S, Burns A: The delusional misidentification syndromes in patients with and without evidence of organic cerebral disorder: A structured review of case reports. *Biol Psychiatry* 33:22–32, 1993.

30. Kapur N, Turner A, King C: Reduplicative paramnesia: Possible anatomical and neuropsychological mechanisms. *Neurol Neurosurg Psychiatry* 51:579–581, 1988.

31. Enoch MD, Trethowan WH: *Uncommon Psychiatric Syndromes.* Bristol: John Wright, 1979.

32. Ellis HD, de Pauw KW, Christodoulou GN, et al: Responses to facial and non-facial stimuli presented tachistoscopically in either or both visual fields by patients with the Capgras delusion and paranoid schizophrenics. *Neurol Neurosurg Psychiatry* 56:215–219, 1993.

33. Staton RD, Brumback RA, Wilson H: Reduplicative paramnesia: A disconnection syndrome of memory. *Cortex* 18:23–36, 1982.

34. Cutting J: Delusional misidentification and the role of the right hemisphere in the appreciation of identity. *Br J Psychiatry* 159:70–74, 1991.

35. Ellis HD, Young AW: Accounting for delusional misidentifications. *Br J Psychiatry* 147:239–248, 1900.

36. Bauer RM: The cognitive psychophysiology of prosopagnosia, in Ellis H, Felves M, Newcombe F, et al (eds): *Aspects of Face Processing.* Dordrecht: Nijhoff, 1986.

37. Shraberg D, Weitzel WD: Prosopagnosia and the Capgras syndrome. *Clin Psychiatry* 40:313–316, 1979.

38. Bidault E, Luaute JP, Tzavaras A: Prosopagnosia and the delusional misidentification syndromes. *Bibl Psychiatry* 164:80–91, 1986.

39. Lewis SW: Brain imaging in a case of Capgras' syndrome. *Br J Psychiatry* 150:117–120, 1987.

40. Vié J: Les méconnaissances systématiques. *Ann Med Psychol* (*Paris*) 102:410–455, 1944.

41. Vié J: Le substratum morbide et les stades évolutifs des méconnaissances systématiques. *Ann Med Psychol* (*Paris*) 102:410–455, 1944.

42. Vié J: Étude psychopathologique des méconnaissances systématiques. *Ann Med Psychol* (*Paris*) 102:1–15, 1944.

43. Feinberg TE, Haber LD, Leeds NE: Verbal asomatognosia. *Neurology* 40:1391–1394, 1990.

44. Weinstein EA, Kahn RL: *Denial of Illness: Symbolic and Physiological Aspects.* Springfield, IL: Charles C Thomas, 1955.

45. Gordon MacCallum WA: The interplay of organic and psychological factors in the delusional misidentification syndrome. *Bibl Psychiatry* 164:92–98, 1986.

46. Fleminger S: Delusional misidentification: An exemplary symptom illustrating an interaction between organic brain disease and psychological processes. 27:161–167, 1994.

47. Weinstein EA, Marvin SL, Keller NJA: Amnesia as a language pattern. *Arch Gen Psychiatry* 6:269–270, 1962.

48. Todd J, Dewhurst K, Wallis G: The syndrome of Capgras. *Br J Psychiatry* 139:319–327, 1981.

49. de Pauw KW, Szulecka TK, Poltock TL: Frégoli syndrome after cerebral infarction. *J Nerv Ment Dis* 175:433–438, 1987.

50. de Pauw KW: Delusional misidentification syndromes, in Bizon Z, Szyszkowski W (eds): *Proceedings of the 35th Congress Polish Psychiatrists.* Warsaw: Polish Psychiatric Association, 1989.

51. de Pauw KW: Delusional misidentification: A plea for an agreed terminology and classification. *Psychopathology* 27:123–129, 1994.

52. Sno HN, Linszen DH, DeJonghe F: Déjà vu experiences and reduplicative paramnesia. *Br J Psychiatry* 161:565–568, 1992.

53. Weinstein EA: Patterns of reduplication in organic brain disease, in Vinken PJ, Bruyn GW (eds): *Handbook of Clinical Neurology.* Amsterdam: North Holland Publishing Co., 1969.

54. Baddeley AD, Wilson B: Amnesia autobiographical memory and confabulation, in Rubin DC (ed): *Autobiographical Memory.* Cambridge: Cambridge University Press, 1986.

55. Ruff RL, Volpe BT: Environmental reduplication associated with right frontal and parietal lobe injury. *Neurol Neurosurg Psychiatry* 44:382–386, 1981.

56. Nemiah J: Dissociative disorders, in Kaplan HI, Sadock BJ (eds): *Comprehensive Textbook of Psychiatry.* Baltimore: Williams & Wilkins, 1989, vol 5.

57. Benson RJ: Capgras' syndrome. *Am J Psychiatry* 140:969–978, 1983.

Part III
LANGUAGE

Chapter 14

APHASIA I: CLINICAL AND ANATOMIC ISSUES

Michael P. Alexander

The clinical study of aphasia began in 1861 with the observations of Paul Broca.[1] Within 40 or 50 years, all of the basic clinical phenomena reviewed here had been described and many of the major flashpoints of clinical and theoretical disagreement had been identified. In the past 20 years, fresh interest has come to clinical aphasia research from two directions: modern neuroimaging and cognitive neurosciences. Together, they have additionally provided tools to carry out aphasia-related language experiments in normals. Furthermore, old questions such as cerebral laterality, the influence of handedness, the effects of gender and bilingualism on aphasia, and the mechanisms of recovery have been reexplored. Much of this chapter—which reviews the basic clinical features of aphasia—could have been written 20, 50, or even 100 years ago. In 1995, it is possible to consider this material with greater appreciation of the variability found in the basic syndromes, of their anatomic complexities, of the natural history of recovery, and (although here only briefly) of the cognitive and linguistic deficits that fundamentally underlie the classic syndromes. The chapters on neuroimaging and on cognitive analysis of aphasia should be read along with this chapter.

CLINICAL SYNDROMES

The description of syndromes of aphasia arose out of much the same motivation as the identification of other clinical neurologic syndromes: the need

to identify clinically useful associations between specific clusters of signs and the likely anatomy of the lesion producing them. The most clinically transparent signs of aphasia have generally been taken to be independent signs of brain damage. Thus, syndromes have been constructed out of reduced language output as well as impaired comprehension, repetition, and naming. Disorders of written language have been divided into additional syndromes only as reading and writing have been impaired beyond spoken language impairments. Using three independent signs will generate eight syndromes, assuming naming to be impaired in all aphasics.

Although these syndromes have reasonable clinical validity, there are numerous limitations to this type of syndrome construction. First, the syndromes depend on a sign being normal or not, much as a hemiparesis is present or absent; but the complexity of impairments in comprehension and language production are less amenable to simple dichotomous judgments. Thus, distinctions come to depend on the statistical properties and structural assumptions of the test. Second, there is no certainty that signs all have the same pathophysiologic mechanism in all patients. For comprehension at the sentence level, in particular, there may be several independent pathways to impairment.[2] Third, the syndromes are not stable even when the anatomy is. A patient with a temporoparietal stroke may have an initial Wernicke's aphasia, but, over weeks, language improves to reach the clinical diagnosis of conduction aphasia.[3] Does one conclude that the behavioral-anatomic correlations are with Wernicke's or conduction aphasia? Can one be certain that there are two distinct syndromes if they blur into each other? Should one conclude that only the early-phase correlations hold, that all correlations have built in corollaries about recovery, or that both are true? Fourth, most syndromes are polytypic—that is, they are defined by several criteria.[4] What do we conclude if only some of the criteria are met? Would this be a less severe syndrome? A subsyndrome? A different syndrome altogether?

Despite these limitations, the classic syndromes do have utility. They serve as a type of shorthand for clinical communications. If told that a patient has transcortical motor aphasia 2 weeks after a stroke, one would know approximately what to expect of language examinations, what the range of possible brain lesions would be, what the prognosis should be, and what some reasonable treatments might be. If inclined, one would even know what interesting cognitive neuroscience issues the patient might illuminate.

Broca's Aphasia

In Broca's aphasia, language output is nonfluent—that is, it is reduced in phrase length and grammatical complexity. This reduction can range from no recognizable output or repeated meaningless utterances to short, truncated phrases using only the most meaning-laden words (substantives). There is usually considerable hesitation and delay in production. Speech quality is impaired. Articulation is poor (dysarthria). Melodic line is disrupted (dysprosody), partly due to dysarthria but often more than just secondary to it. Volume is usually reduced at first (hypophonia). With time, speech takes on hyperkinetic (dystonic and spastic) qualities. Language comprehension is adequate although rarely normal. Response to word-recognition tasks, simple commands, and routine conversation is generally good. Response to multistep commands and complex syntactical requests is generally poor. Repetition is poor, although often better than speech. Relational words (functors—articles, conjunctions, modifiers, etc.)

may be produced in repetition, but they are exceedingly uncommon in spontaneous speech. Written language parallels spoken, although some patients, while never regaining useful speech, develop writing that is telegraphic. Oral reading is usually agrammatic; so-called deep dyslexia (see Chap. 18) may emerge with this.[5] Naming is usually poor, but it may be surprisingly good in chronic patients. All types of errors can occur, although semantic errors are most typical for substantive words.[6] Objects are frequently named better than are actions.[7]

Broca's aphasia is commonly accompanied by right hemiparesis, buccofacial apraxia, and ideomotor apraxia of the left arm (or both arms in the nonparetic case). Right-sided sensory loss and right visual field impairments (extinction and/or lower-quadrant deficit) are less frequent. Depression, frequently major, develops in approximately 40 percent of patients with Broca's aphasia.[8]

Many patients have fractional syndromes of Broca's aphasia. Because all of these fractional disorders are still taxonomically closer to Broca's aphasia than to any of the other seven classic diagnoses, many aphasia systems will classify them all as Broca's aphasia.[9] In analyzing reports of Broca's aphasia, it is crucial to understand the taxonomic rules of the report's assessment tool. If all fractional cases are considered Broca's aphasia, the clinicoanatomic correlations will seem imprecise. This is an example of the difficulty inherent in building syndromes with polytypic qualities. Analysis of the clinicoanatomic relationships within these fractional cases may be much more informative than lumping them all together on the basis of some overlap with the full syndrome.

Chronic Broca's Aphasia

This syndrome, as described above, often emerges out of global aphasia.[10] Damage can vary in extent; there does not seem to be a necessary and sufficient lesion profile. The most common pattern is extensive dorsolateral frontal, opercular, rolandic, and anterolateral parietal cortical damage plus lateral striatal and extensive paraventric-

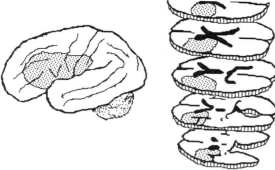

Figure 14-1
Typical lesion associated with severe chronic Broca's aphasia.

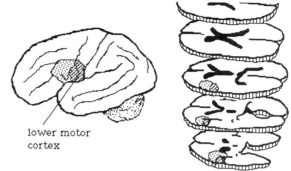

lower motor
cortex

Figure 14-2
Lesion distributions of incomplete forms of Broca's aphasia. The entire lesion would produce "acute" Broca's aphasia. The anterior component involved alone (stippled area) would typically evolve toward transcortical motor aphasia. The posterior component involved alone would typically evolve toward aphemia. In either case, the residual aphasia would be mild.

ular white matter damage (Fig. 14-1).[11] Particularly critical to chronic Broca's aphasia is the subcortical extension of the lesion.[12] Long-lasting mutism can be seen after anterior deep lesions, undercutting supplementary motor area and cingulate-caudate projections.[13] Deep anterior periventricular white matter lesions disrupt dorsolateral frontal-caudate systems involved in ready access to complex output procedures.[14] They may also disrupt ascending anterior thalamic-frontal projections. Anterior supraventricular deep white matter lesions disrupt callosal frontal projections. Large periventricular and subcortical white matter lesions can disrupt all of the long parietotemporal to frontal projection pathways. All the distant corticocortical systems will be disrupted. A combination of these systems' disruptions seems to be the structural basis of persistent Broca's aphasia even with subcortical lesions only.

Acute Broca's Aphasia

Infarctions or trauma that produce acute Broca's aphasia often involve the frontal operculum, lower motor cortex, lateral striatum, and subcortical white matter (Fig. 14-2).[9,15] These patients recover over weeks to months, with variable mixtures of initiation delay, syntactic simplification, paraphasias, speech impairment, and usually with impaired repetition.

"Broca's Area" Lesion

Damage to the frontal operculum (areas 44 and 46) produces an acute aphasic disorder roughly compatible with Broca's aphasia (Fig. 14-2), but there is quite rapid improvement usually to transcortical motor aphasia or even just mild anomic aphasia.[9,15] Damage to the dorsolateral frontal cortex (areas 44, 46, 6, and 9) produces classic transcortical motor aphasia[13] (discussed in detail below). Damage to the subcortical frontal white matter or even to the dorsolateral caudate nuclei may produce the same deficit.[14] These observations suggest the existence of a "frontal-caudate" regional network required for construction of complex output procedures of language—syntax and narrative discourse at a minimum. Damage to this system is part of classic Broca's aphasia.

Lower Motor Cortex Lesion

Damage to the lower 50 percent of the prerolandic gyrus can acutely produce a deficit pattern roughly compatible with mild Broca's aphasia, but there is rapid recovery to a much more limited disorder of speech—predominantly of articulation and prosody—sometimes called aphemia (Fig. 14-2).[16] Damage to the subcortical outflow of lower motor cortex can produce the same speech deficit, suggesting the existence of a local (rolandic) network for articulation and some aspects of prosody that project to the brainstem. This, too, is part of classic Broca's aphasia.

A rare variant of this restricted damage to motor systems of speech production is the foreign-accent syndrome.[17] A small number of cases have been described, usually emerging out of mild Broca's aphasia. In these patients, the predominant deficit is in speech prosody, but the quality of the prosodic deficit sounds to the listener like a foreign accent, not pathologic prosody. The reported lesions have all been in some component of the motor system for speech, either lower motor cortex[16] or putamen or deep connections between lower motor cortex and basal ganglia.[18,19] The precise speech impairment has not been consistent, and the foreign accent syndrome probably represents a heterogeneous group with partial damage to the motor speech apparatus.

For all of these variants and fractional syndromes of Broca's aphasia, some improvement can be expected. The severe cases that often emerge from global aphasia typically have better recovery of comprehension than of speech; this recovery that may continue over a very long time.[3,20] Minimal recovery of spoken or written output from essentially none to classic telegraphic output is usually accompanied by lesion extent throughout the deep frontal white matter from the middle periventricular region to the region anterior and superior to the frontal horn.[12] The outcome of the milder cases is partly determined by lesion size,[9] but for these smaller lesions, precise lesion site seems to best account for evolution into the various fractional systems.[10,15,16] In both severe and milder cases, some patients may recover by reorganizing cerebral functions to allow some right-brain control of speech. Evidence for this comes from patients with serial frontal lesions[21] and from temporary inactivation of the right brain (Wada test) after left-brain stroke has produced severe nonfluent aphasia.[22]

Wernicke's Aphasia

In this disorder, language output is fluent—that is, normal in mean phrase length, generally sentence-length, and using all grammatical elements available in the language. Content may be extremely paraphasic[6] or empty. Paraphasic speech conforms to the general rules of the language but contains substitutions at the phonemic level (phonemic paraphasias such as "smoon" for spoon), the word level (semantic paraphasias such as "cup" for spoon), or entirely novel but phonologically legal words (neologisms such as "snopel"). Empty speech may consist of either vague circumlocutions or single words (thing, one, unit, it, going, etc.). Lengthy, complex, phonologically rich output with varied neologisms is jargonaphasia. Although statements may be of sentence length, grammar may become quite imprecise, usually because of semantic ambiguity; this is paragrammatism.[23] Speech is normal. Language comprehension is poor at the levels of word recognition, simple commands, and simple conversation. Repetition is very poor. Written language is comparable to spoken. Naming is very poor. Errors are paraphasias, circumlocutions, and nonresponses.

Apraxia to command is common, but when the patient is given a model to imitate, performance can be extremely variable, from persistently severe apraxia to normal performance.[24] Deficits in the right visual field are common. In the acute phase, patients may be anosognosic; but with awareness of deficits, agitation and suspiciousness may emerge.

Fractional syndromes of Wernicke's aphasia are less common but can occur. Some patients have relatively better auditory comprehension (and usually repetition); others have relatively better reading comprehension. Severe limb apraxia (both ideomotor, even with imitation of gestures, and ideational) is sometimes seen.

The minimal lesion producing Wernicke's aphasia is damage to the superior temporal gyrus back to the end of the sylvian fissure (Fig. 14-3).[11] If damage includes additional adjacent structures, either the deep temporal white matter or the supramarginal gyrus or both, problems will be more

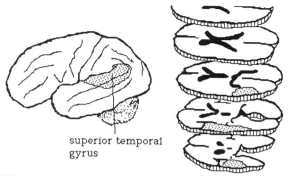

superior temporal
gyrus

Figure 14-3

Typical lesion producing Wernicke's aphasia. Persistence and severity would depend on lesion extent (see text).

persistent.[25–27] If damage includes middle and interior temporal gyri, initial deficits will be more severe, anomia will be more persistent, and reading comprehension will be poor even if auditory comprehension improves. Patients with lesions restricted to the superior temporal gyrus may have predominantly auditory comprehension difficulties with relatively little anomia and much less reading impairment. The differential effects of lesion placement in the posterior temporal lobe certainly reflect variable damage to converging regional networks for several language processing systems. The auditory language system may be more specifically temporal, thus the relatively greater impairment of auditory comprehension. Visual language processing surely emerges out of the more posterior temporooccipitoparietal association cortex.[28] Cross-modal lexical and semantic knowledge emerges out of a broad range of regions in the posterior association cortex, but available evidence highlights the inferior temporal and middle temporal/angular gyrus transition as the particularly key regions for word retrieval.[29]

Severe and persistent Wernicke's aphasia seems to require damage to all of these regions or to their deep functional connections. The mechanisms of recovery are not completely known. As noted above, the brain regions involved in lexical-semantic function are broadly distributed in posterior association cortex. Size of lesion in these re-

gions, extent of involvement of the superior temporal gyrus,[25,27] and extent of coincident damage to supramarginal and angular gyri[26] have all been implicated as factors in recovery of comprehension. Studies with positron emission tomography (PET) have demonstrated a variety of effects related to recovery. Heiss and colleagues, studying subacute recovery in a mixed group of aphasic syndromes, demonstrated that recovery of comprehension was proportional to recovery of resting blood flow in the surviving left hemisphere, particularly the temporoparietal junction.[30] Weiller and coworkers demonstrated that recovery in Wernicke's aphasia is closely related to a shift in PET activation to semantic tasks from left temporal in normals to right temporal in Wernicke's aphasics who recover.[31] The precise meaning of these related studies is not known, but they all converge on the importance of posterior association cortex, either left or, if it is too damaged, right for recovery of comprehension.

Pure word deafness is sometimes considered a separate syndrome reflecting exclusive impairment to the auditory language processing system.[32] Most patients are only relatively "pure," emerging out of Wernicke's aphasia with relatively better recovery of reading comprehension for anatomically specific reasons proposed above. Some patients have had only small left temporal lesions;[32] others have had bilateral temporal lesions.[33] Depending upon the relative size and location of the bilateral lesions, these patients may be effectively deaf[37] (cortical deafness: bilateral Heschl gyrus lesions) or have agnosia for the meaning of all sounds (machinery, animals, musical instruments, etc.) even though they hear them (auditory environmental agnosia: large right lesion, whatever the left lesion[34]). Also, depending on specific lesion sites, language output can be variably abnormal, although to be "pure," it should be normal. In this case, the implication is that underlying knowledge of word phonology is preserved because spontaneous production is normal. Depending on lesion site, "relatively pure" cases may have considerable phonemic paraphasia or anomia.

The mechanism of pure word deafness is presumably damage to a system that converts the acoustic signal into a phonologically meaningful stimulus.[33] This is necessary but not sufficient for comprehension; for example, normals can repeat sentences in languages phonologically similar to their native one without understanding anything. There must still be merger of the processed acoustic signal with a semantic system. In some patients with Wernicke's aphasia, the phonological process seems very impaired; in others, the mapping to semantics and in yet others both are impaired.

Conduction Aphasia

In conduction aphasia, language output is fluent. Content is paraphasic, usually predominantly phonemic.[6] There may be frequent hesitations and attempts to correct ongoing phonemic errors (so-called *conduit d'approche*). Speech is normal. Language comprehension is good except for auditory span. Repetition is poor, not always worse than spontaneous output but dominated by phonemic paraphasias on substantive words, particularly phonologically complex target words ("happy hippopotamus") or words embedded in phonologically complex sentences ("Dogs chase but rarely catch clever cats"). Written language is extremely variable in this syndrome. Writing is rarely better than speech, but it can be much more impaired. Oral reading is usually comparable to speech but can be better or worse. Reading comprehension is usually comparable to auditory but can be worse. Patients with the agraphia with alexia syndrome usually have conduction aphasia. Naming is also extremely variable, from extremely poor to nearly normal. Errors are paraphasias (phonemic especially).

Limb ideomotor apraxia is common initially but clears in most patients.[24] Right-sided sensory loss or visual field impairment (extinction and/or lower quadrant deficit) are common.

Most patients with conduction aphasia have prominently reduced auditory verbal short-term memory (STM), tested as digit-span, word-span, or sentence-length effect in repetition. There is, however, little specificity of the STM problem, as many patients with perisylvian aphasias have a similar problem. The STM deficit also has little

relevance to the language production problem, as similar output occurs in spontaneous output, oral reading and naming, as well as repetition. There is converging evidence that the inferior parietal lobule, particularly the supramarginal gyrus, is critical for all aspects of phonologic processing. Thus, lesions there have been blamed for pure STM deficits,[35] phonologic agraphia,[36,37] and phonologic alexia, all of which commonly emerge from conduction aphasia.

The necessary and sufficient lesion to produce conduction aphasia is damage to supramarginal gyrus[38] (Fig. 14-4). The classic correlation was with the arcuate fasciculus, putatively connecting temporal lobe to frontal lobe.[39] Lesions in subcortical parietal white matter disrupt this fasciculus and may represent the classic correlation.[40] Lesions in white matter deep to sensory cortex or in the subinsular extreme capsule as well as supramarginal cortex lesions may also produce conduction aphasia.[41] These observations suggest that temporoparietal short association pathways (i.e., a regional network) may support the phonologic output structure of speech. This network is required for phonologic accuracy in spontaneous output, repetition, oral reading, and naming. If disturbed phonologic structure of output is the hallmark of conduction aphasia, this would be the criterion structural basis.

Some patients have very extensive parietal

Figure 14-4
Typical lesion producing conduction aphasia. Smaller lesions within this region may also produce similar aphasia (see text).

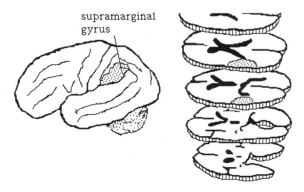

supramarginal gyrus

lesions with more severe anomia, agraphia, and limb ideomotor apraxia. Partial involvement of the superior temporal gyrus can produce initial Wernicke's aphasia that evolves into conduction aphasia with *very* paraphasic output and severe anomia. Again, the overlap of syndromes should be evident. Patients whose perisylvian arterial architecture just happens to catch the superior temporal lobe in a predominantly parietal stroke will have elements of pure word deafness (decreased auditory comprehension) with conduction aphasia (phonemic paraphasias, anomia, and agraphia). That combination would be indistinguishable from Wernicke's aphasia; in fact, it probably *is* Wernicke's aphasia except that recovery of comprehension would be "surprisingly" good.

Most patients with acute conduction aphasia have good recovery over a few weeks, although residual writing impairments, mild anomia, and occasional phonemic errors can be observed.[3] For the more severe cases with marked anomia and very paraphasic output, recovery is less complete. The combination of significant phonologic and semantic deficits despite good comprehension can be very long-lasting. Over time, patients become less neologistic and more empty and circumlocutory, even if the basic deficits do not improve.[42]

Global Aphasia

In many ways global aphasia is the easiest syndrome to define. By definition, patients have significant impairments in all aspects of language. Language output is severely limited—there is no more than "yes," "no," and a recurring stereotypic utterance ("da, da," "no way, no way," etc.). In some global aphasics (and Broca aphasics) the recurring utterance may be repeated rapidly in a richly inflected manner that suggests fluent output if only it could be comprehended.[43] This is not jargonaphasia; it has none of the phonological richness or preservation of grammatical infrastructure of jargonaphasia. The mechanism of this richly inflected stereotype is unknown, and it has no known prognostic significance.

Comprehension is very impaired. The Boston Diagnostic Aphasia Examination (BDAE)

definition allows comprehension up to the 30th percentile for an aphasic population.[44] This is compatible with considerable single-word comprehension. The language comprehension tasks most likely to be preserved in global aphasia are pointing to a named location on a map,[45] pointing to personally highly familiar names from multiple choice or acknowledging them when they are presented auditorily, and a small subset of commands ("take off your glasses," "close your eyes," "stand up").[24] Some global aphasics can do those tasks but little else. There is no repetition, naming, or writing.

Buccofacial and limb apraxia, to command and imitation, are nearly universal.[24] Right hemiplegia, hemisensory loss, and visual field impairments are all common but not invariable.

The most typical lesion involves or substantially undercuts the entire perisylvian region.[11] At least, this would require a combination of the Broca's and Wernicke's aphasia lesions, but much clinical variability is seen. Some patients with Broca's aphasia lesions present as global aphasics without evident temporal lesions.[46,47] Conversely, some patients with very extensive posterior lesions that extend into subrolandic white matter present with global aphasia without *any* definite frontal or even anterior periventricular lesion.[9] The mechanism of severe comprehension loss without a temporal lesion in a substantial fraction of global aphasics, is not known. The same effect is not seen without coincident frontal lesions—that is, even enormous cortical and subcortical parietal lesions alone do not cause such deficits in comprehension. The coincident frontal lesion may produce additional cognitive problems—such as inattention, underactivation, unconcern, poor problem solving (particularly relevant when the Token Test is the defining tool of comprehension), or perseveration—that interact with more modest phonologic/semantic deficits to produce more profound functional comprehension deficits. Alexander and associates have suggested that a sufficiently great lesion of the deep temporal white matter might undercut connections to the temporal lobe.[48] Naeser and colleagues found these deep temporal lesions to be associated with poor comprehension in many global aphasics.[25] There was good recovery of comprehension in cases with deep temporal lesions but intact temporal cortex. Heisse and co-workers have demonstrated a very high correlation between reduced temporoparietal blood flow in resting PET and poor comprehension, whatever the anatomic limits of the infarction.[30] Vignolo and associates[46] and De Renzi and colleagues,[47] who have provided the most meticulous description of global aphasia without temporal lesions, have not found that temporal white matter lesions easily account for the deficits in comprehension.

Some patients with global aphasia have no hemiparesis. As a group, they are likely to have only a large frontal lesion or separate frontal and temporal lesions.[49] The purely frontal lesions are again presumably causing a quasicomprehension deficit due to inattention, activation, perseveration, and so on. These patients are also likely to have a better prognosis, but absence of hemiparesis is not a guarantee of a good outcome, as the absence of hemiparesis only means that a small portion of paraventricular white matter has been spared.[50]

When caused by infarction, global aphasia has a poor prognosis. Smaller lesions (some without hemiparesis) will improve quickly. After infarction, patients still meeting taxonomic criteria for global aphasia at 1 month postonset have a very low probability of improving substantially.[3] Large hemorrhages may be associated with more late recovery, but by 2 months without improvement, the prognosis remains grim. Many patients show gradually improving comprehension over weeks and months and eventually reach taxonomic criteria for severe Broca's aphasia.

Transcortical Motor Aphasia

In this syndrome, language output is commonly viewed as nonfluent because there is substantial initiation block, reduction in average phrase length, and simplification of grammatical form.[13] Many patients with transcortical motor aphasia (TCMA) are initially mute and may remain mute or nearly so for days or weeks. Note that, if they are mute, repetition is obviously absent and, by strict taxonomic criteria, such patients would initially be called Broca's aphasics. Frank agrammatism is uncommon; responses are simply terse and delayed. Echolalia in various forms is frequently observed. Completely uninhibited echolalia is unusual, but fragmentary echoing, particularly of commands, may be observed. Incorporation echolalia is more common. The patient incorporates a portion of a question into the initial portion of his response. Speech quality is normal in the classic case. Repetition is, by definition, normal or at least vastly superior to spontaneous output. Recitation of even very complex overlearned material (e.g., the Lord's Prayer) may be flawless. Language comprehension is supposed to be normal, but, as observed above, the large frontal lesions most often associated with TCMA may produce substantial impairment of comprehension. Writing is usually similar to spoken output, but patients rarely write to dictation as well as they repeat. Reading comprehension parallels auditory. Oral reading may be quite normal if initial prompts are provided. Naming is quite variable; errors are nonresponses, semantic paraphasias, or perseverations.[6]

Transcortical motor aphasia may have any range of associated motor deficits, depending upon lesion site. The classic case has no motor deficit. Hemiparesis accompanies many cases of subcortical TCMA.[14] Inverted hemiparesis (leg worse than arm) and a contralateral grasp reflex accompany medial frontal TCMA.[13] Sensory loss and visual field deficits are not usually seen except in subcortical cases. Buccofacial apraxia may be seen, but limb ideomotor apraxia is less common.[24]

The classic patient has a large dorsolateral frontal lesion, typically extending into the deep frontal white matter (Fig. 14-5).[13] Identical cases have been reported with just a white matter lesion abutting the frontal horn of the lateral ventricle.[48] Very similar cases involve the capsulostriatal region, particularly the dorsolateral caudate and adjacent paraventricular white matter (Fig. 14-6).[14] The similarity of the aphasia associated with these disparate lesions is paralleled by the nearly identical reduction in blood flow seen on resting PET or single proton emission computed tomography (SPECT) in dorsolateral frontal cortex, whatever

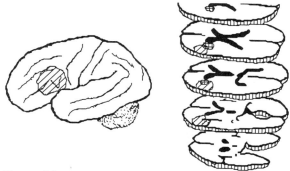

Figure 14-5

Typical lesions producing transcortical motor aphasia. Note overlap with Broca's area lesions (Fig. 14-2).

the lesion site.[51,52,57] The more posteriorly the lesion extends along the paraventricular white matter, the likelier the presence of dysarthria (see discussion of aphemia, above) and hemiparesis. Damage to the medial frontal lobe, particularly the supplementary motor area, produces TCMA-like disturbance.[53] Mutism may be more prolonged. When patients begin to speak, they rarely show any frankly aphasic qualities. They simply do not speak much.

Analysis of cortical and subcortical cases

Figure 14-6

Large lenticulostriate lesion, which is often associated with transcortical motor aphasia, frequently accompanied by speech disturbance and hemiparesis. Smaller lesion (cross-hatched area) may produce mild transcortical motor aphasia without motor deficits.

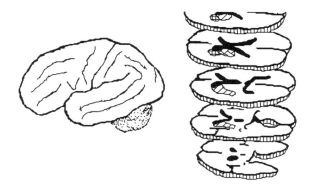

with TCMA suggests that one fundamental deficit is in generative language tasks.[14,54] The patients seem to have very limited capacity to generate complex syntax. They may reuse the syntax in a question they are asked (incorporation echolalia). They may produce short responses, even short sentences, quite well. When asked an open-ended question, however, they do not have timely access to the range of syntax needed to answer.[54,55] Bedside generative tasks—word-list generation, storytelling, or producing sentences using provided main verbs—will be impaired out of proportion to other language tasks. Patients with large dorsolateral frontal lesions may have little or no aphasia on standard tests but still be unable to tell a story or recite a narrative in normal fashion.

A second fundamental deficit in TCMA is reduction in activation to speak (or to write). Analysis of lesion site effects, particularly the profound mutism that occurs with medial frontal damage, suggests that reduced activation is due to loss of ascending dopaminergic pathways. The medial frontal regions are primary targets of the nonnigral dopaminergic system.[56] Bilateral damage to this system anywhere from the upper midbrain to the frontal cortex results in akinetic mutism,[57] evolving into less flagrant forms often called abulia.[58] Transcortical motor aphasia may represent a subsyndrome of akinetic mutism with more rapid clearing of mutism and less global akinesia because the lesion is only unilateral. The improvement in fluency and speech rate after administration of direct dopamine agonists supports this proposition.[59,60] Improvement with bromocriptine is almost uniquely seen in TCMA.

Transcortical Sensory Aphasia

In transcortical sensory aphasia (TCSA), language output is fluent. Content is very empty, with semantic paraphasia predominating. All patients make abundant use of one-word circumlocutions and nonspecific filler words, such as *one, things, does,* etc. Phonemic paraphasias and neologistic jargon are less common, so that output is more accurately described as extended English jargon. Content is also often perseverative. Speech quality is normal. Repetition is, by definition, normal. Language comprehension is impaired. In particular, single-word comprehension may be quite poor. When accompanied by accurate repetition of the test words and even their incorporation in sentences, ("A watch? I should know that. Is one of these a watch?"), the behavior has been called alienation of word meaning.[61] There may be category-specific comprehension impairments with particularly good performance at following commanded actions and very poor performance at pointing to named targets. Many patients will accept incorrect names or quibble over accuracy. ("You could call it a watch, but I don't think it is one.") Naming is poor, and again some category-specificity may be observed. Some patients are worse at naming animals, insects, and other animate objects than tools and other inanimate objects.[62] There is no important discrepancy between naming performance to different sensory modalities. Many patients respond quickly to phonemic cues but will then reject or be uncertain about the correct response. This behavior has been called a two-way naming impairment.[63] Written output may be similar to spoken, but patients usually do not write extensively and are very perseverative. Reading aloud and reading comprehension are both abnormal. In many patients reading comprehension is even worse than auditory comprehension.

Transcortical sensory aphasia has been described after lesions in middle and inferior temporal gyri (Fig. 14-7).[61] The temporal lesion may produce a right visual field defect if white matter extent reaches the geniculocalcarine pathways. Many cases of TCSA have unexpected lesion sites involving the entire perisylvian cortex, a lesion much likelier to produce global aphasia.[64] The mechanism for this is unknown, although some variant on bilateral language representation is usually recruited. Some cases with temporal lesions may also involve the inferior temporooccipital region—for instance, after posterior cerebral artery infarction. These patients will certainly have very impaired reading.[28] Many have associative agnosia.[65] Not only can they not name an object or point to a named object but they cannot

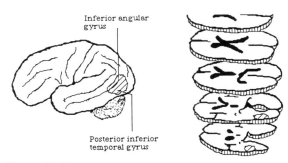

Figure 14-7
Typical lesion producing transcortical sensory aphasia. Lesions more medial and inferior, usually posterior cerebral artery infarctions, may produce similar aphasia (see text).

indicate its use or sort it into a correct functional category (i.e., put a pencil with chalk rather than with a knife). Thus, the deficit is not restricted to *lexical* semantic knowledge but involves actual semantic knowledge. This may be modality-specific, with visually presented tasks more impaired,[65] or it may affect all modalities equally.[66]

Transcortical sensory aphasia is almost monotypic in that it is fundamentally a disorder of semantic processing. Nevertheless, different aspects of semantic knowledge and access to semantic knowledge may be impaired in different cases. The inability of patients with TCSA to associate a name with an object is the result of a semantic disorder at the interface between language and semantic memory. When semantic memory is more globally affected, patients are unable to demonstrate recognition of objects by nonverbal means as well (see Chap. 23). This is most commonly seen in degenerative diseases with a predilection for temporal cortex, such as Alzheimer Disease, Pick Disease, and so-called Semantic Dementia.[29,62,67–69]

Anomic Aphasia

Anomic aphasia is a much less homogeneous grouping than any of the other classic syndromes. By definition, language is fluent, comprehension good, and repetition good. The only deficit in spoken language is in word retrieval. Paraphasias are infrequent. Word-finding problems usually produce filler words[6] or circumlocutions. Other impairments vary with lesion site.

Anomic aphasia is the residual state of many aphasic disorders after time for improvement.[21] As a primary diagnosis, anomic aphasia usually accompanies lesions in the same regions as TCMA or TCSA.[10,11]

As noted, most patients with TCMA are or at least become basically fluent but with terse, unelaborated utterances. When it is accompanied by word-finding deficits, this condition would qualify as anomic aphasia. Anomic aphasia is also the mildest form of TCSA, representing a deficit only in lexical retrieval from semantic stores. Thus, when anomic aphasia is caused by a dorsolateral frontal lesion, there are no accompanying neurologic signs. When it is caused by a deep frontal-striatal lesion, there may be dysarthria, hemiparesis, and buccofacial apraxia, depending upon lesion extent. When it is caused by a posterior association cortex lesion, there may be a visual field deficit and alexia, depending upon lesion extent. When anomic aphasia is the residual of partly recovered conduction or Broca's aphasia, the accompanying signs are as expected for those disorders.

Mixed Transcortical Aphasia

In mixed transcortical aphasia (MTA), language output is nonfluent. Comprehension is impaired. Naming is poor. Repetition is preserved. Echolalia and fragmentary sentence starters ("I don't . . . ," "Not with the . . .") are common. Speech quality is normal. Writing and reading are similarly reduced.

In the patient whose case report defined this syndrome, MTA was due to bilateral hypoxic neuronal loss in the arterial border zones,[70] but ischemic damage in the left border zones could presumably cause the same disorder. The implication is that MTA requires a combination of the lesions of TCMA and TCSA, with perisylvian structures allowing repetition preserved. Most cases are actually due to large frontal lesions in the region of

TCMA lesions. The comprehension defect is probably due to a mixture of frontal impairments, exactly as described for restricted frontal lesions and global aphasia. Comprehension improves, and patients evolve toward TCMA. Associated lesions are as described for TCMA.

Large anterior thalamic lesions also produce MTA.[71–73] Most cases have involved the anterior, ventrolateral, and dorsomedian nuclei at a minimum.[71,72] Damage to those three nuclei effectively deprives the frontal lobe of thalamic input and modulation. Patients are often mute initially. When they speak, the reduction in narrative and terseness of structure are similar to those of TCMA. The impairment in comprehension may be due to the speculative "frontal" mechanisms. The associated signs depend upon lesion extent out of the thalamus. Recovery of language is usually good.

CROSSED APHASIA AND APHASIA IN LEFT-HANDERS

The foregoing review is valid for most right-handers with lesions of the left hemisphere. For the 10 percent of the population that is left-handed and for the approximately 2 to 5 percent of the right-handed population that becomes aphasic after a right-brain lesion (crossed aphasia), some modifications of the clinical rules are required. For left-handers, the phenomenology of aphasia is complicated by the very issue of left-handedness. More than right-handers, all left-handers are not created equal; they vary greatly in degree and nature of hemispheric specialization for language. For both populations the phenomenology is further complicated by irregularities in lateral dominance for other typically lateralized functions, such as praxis and some aspects of visuospatial function. Only a brief summary of these issues is possible here.

Crossed Aphasia

The incidence of crossed aphasia has been reported as anywhere from 1 to 13 percent.[74–76] The stroke population[74] is least contaminated by possible bilateral lesions, but in all populations methodological limitations (defining handedness and aphasia testing strategies) leave the actual incidence uncertain. A reasonable estimate is 2 to 5 percent.

Patients with crossed aphasia fall into two broad categories. About 70 percent have a standard aphasia syndrome associated with, at least approximately, the lesion site expected in the left hemisphere.[77] All types of aphasia profiles can occur with the expected lesions (albeit in the right hemisphere). The other 30 percent have striking anomalies in the aphasia-lesion relationship.[77] In this group, unexpectedly mild aphasia syndromes occur despite large lesions that would typically cause a more severe aphasia. Conduction aphasia or phonologic agraphia have been seen despite large perisylvian lesions.[77,78] In other patients with large perisylvian lesions, transcortical sensory aphasia or anomic aphasia has been described.[64,87] Alexander and Annett have suggested that these anomalous cases point to possible discrepant lateralizations of phonologic and semantic functions.[79] Patients with crossed aphasia may have a better capacity for recovery.

Lateralization of praxis and visuospatial functions in crossed aphasia has not been as definitely addressed as the language functions. Castro-Caldos and coworkers claim that these functions show anomalous lateralization less frequently than language, asserting that praxis remains in the left hemisphere contralateral to the preferred right hand and that visuospatial functions remain in the right hemisphere.[74] Others have disputed this, arguing from case reports that all functions show a high rate of anomalous lateralization.[80] Alexander and coworkers have reviewed the case reports of anomalous visuospatial lateralization to the left hemisphere in right-handers.[81] They have proposed that there is a subset of right-handers who have chance lateralization of all functions. These authors, among others, have even proposed that a genetic basis for the inheritance of handedness and laterality of cognitive functions such as the right shift theory of Annett[77,79] can

account for the rates of all anomalies. The biological basis of crossed aphasia, however, remains unknown.

Aphasia in Left-Handers

Left-handers make up 10 percent of the population, but they are a much more heterogeneous group than right-handers. If a strict criterion for left-handedness is used, most of the left-handed population becomes relabeled as being mixed-handed.[76] Thus, some authorities simply refer to non-right-handers. The rate of cerebral lateralization of left-handers depends to some extent on the criteria used to define the group. Large studies of left-handed aphasics have been reasonably consistent, however, in finding that about 70 percent have left-brain lesions and 30 percent have right-brain lesions.[82] Hécaen has computed that approximately 15 percent probably would be aphasic after a lesion of either hemisphere; that is, they have bilateral language representation. Whether aphasic after left or right brain lesions, the proportion of cases with anomalous aphasia-lesion relationships is higher than in right-handers.[83] It has been claimed that left-handers have better recovery than right-handers,[82] but, as with crossed aphasia, this question is muddied by the higher proportion of mild aphasics.[83] It is also unclear if better recovery means bilateral language capacity so all functions have higher potential for recovery or divergent lateralization of functions so that some are left uninvolved by any lateralized lesion.[75,79,84] Both factors are probably operative, but in different patients.

Lateralization of praxis and visuospatial function shows anomalies at a rate similar to those of crossed aphasia. Every possible arrangement of impaired and preserved functions has been reported after left or right lesions.[94] Since the biological basis of neither handedness nor the lateralization of cognitive functions has been established, it remains an open question how these anomalies occur in left-handers as well as right-handers.

EFFECT OF ETIOLOGY

Infarctions

Almost all of the foregoing is based on the literature accumulated from strokes. Infarcts have numerous advantages for clinicoanatomic correlations. They are sudden in onset, and there is therefore no accommodation and compensation prior to clinical presentation. Boundaries between damaged and nondamaged brain are fairly precise, so correlations are clearer. Nevertheless, the vascular system cannot provide every topographic variation of brain injury; therefore much of what has come to us as classic syndromes could easily be partially artifactual correlations produced by the limited independence of lesions sites from infarctions.

There are some aphasic syndromes that are commonly believed to be caused by emboli because the distribution of infarction seems most plausibly to be in the territory of a branch of the middle cerebral artery. The fractional Broca's aphasias, conduction aphasia, and Wernicke's aphasia all seem likely to have an embolic basis when due to infarction. Global aphasia and Broca's aphasia require more extensive damage in the territory of the middle cerebral artery. There is, however, no basis for presuming an infarction mechanism simply on the basis of these aphasia types.

Hemorrhages

All of the rules established for infarctions apply for hemorrhages if the hemorrhage happens to be in the same brain topography as an infarction pattern. Patients with hemorrhages may be much more impaired initially because of physiologic deficits not primarily related to aphasia—mass effects, intraventricular blood, and so on. Hemorrhages are not constrained by vascular patterns, so entirely novel arrangements of lesions can be seen. This may be exemplified most clearly with lesions of the lenticulostriate region. Infarctions tend to be partially or completely limited to the middle cerebral artery perforators, but hemorrhages can dissect out of that limited region. Much

of the variability reported after lenticulostriate lesions[85] may be due to idiosyncratic extensions of hemorrhages.[86]

Trauma

Focal contusions can occur anywhere, depending upon the direction of the blow, skull fragments, and so forth. When the contusion is in a perisylvian region, the resulting aphasia will usually follow the rules established by infarctions. Conduction and Wernicke's aphasias may be seen with predominantly superficial lesions and so may be quite typical. Cortical contusions rarely cause injury deep enough to damage all of the required deep structures (see above) and thus to produce nonfluent aphasia. There is a strong tendency for traumatic contusions to arise from basal structures due to inertial effects. Focal contusions of the inferior temporal lobe will cause anomic aphasia. If the lesions are large and extend into lateral temporal lobe or hemorrhage dissects up into the deep temporal white matter, patients may present with Wernicke's aphasia or TCSA. Trauma can also cause large epidural or subdural hematomas that do not directly affect language zones. They cause cerebral herniation with entrapment of the posterior cerebral artery, causing occipitotemporal infarctions with alexia and anomia. This herniation-caused infarction can be superimposed on direct temporal contusion, resulting in a very severe fluent aphasia.

Tumors

The lesson for aphasia is no different than that for any cognitive function. In general, large tumors produce relatively much less cognitive impairment than an infarction of the same size would produce, but tumors produce symptoms qualitatively appropriate for the region involved. Tumors tend to infiltrate and gradually disrupt function, allowing substantial compensation as the disorder progresses. The conformity with patterns established by infarctions will be correlated largely with the malignancy and speed of growth of the tumor.

Herpes Simplex Encephalitis

Although rare, herpes simplex encephalitis (HSE) has a predilection for the medial temporal lobes, basal-medial frontal lobes, and insular cortices. Survivors of HSE frequently have severe amnesia.[62,87] Patients with extensive left-sided HSE lesions, including the inferotemporal lobe, commonly show category-specific semantic deficits.[62,87]

Dementia

The most common dementing illnesses—DAT and multi-infarct dementia (MID)—both cause language impairments. Dementia of the Alzheimer type typically presents with memory and language disturbances.[68] The language problem begins as anomia and is often misidentified by families as memory impairment. With time, the language disorder evolves toward TCSA, and the patients' semantic memory erodes.[88] The structure of this erosion is fairly predictable. Highly typical semantic associations survive longer than the semantic associations and attributes of low typicality.[88] For instance, the patients may still recognize the words and concepts behind "cat," but not the words and then even the concepts of "leopard," "fang," or "litter." It has been proposed that this slow erosion of semantic knowledge—first words and then concepts—is the fundamental cognitive deficit of DAT.[89] Its presumed pathologic basis is the loss of neurons in posterior association cortex.

If one of the infarcts is in the language zone, MID may cause aphasia directly. The more typical pathology of MID is, however, numerous small infarcts in subcortical regions. These lesions may produce a variety of motor speech impairments such as articulatory problems, hypophonia, dysprosody, and rate disturbances. A recognizable aphasic syndrome does not occur, but patients may show cognitive deficits similar to those seen with frontal lobe lesions, including disturbances in all aspects of generative language: reduced word-list generation, terse or unelaborate utterances, and poor narrative ability. It has been suggested that a single small infarct in the genu of the left internal capsule is sufficient to disconnect frontal-thalamic circuitry and produce these deficits.[90]

A rarer form of degenerative dementia, primary progressive aphasia, is virtually restricted to language deficits.[91] The most common form is progressive loss of semantics and has therefore also been called semantic dementia[92] (see Chap. 23). The presentation is usually similar to the language impairments of DAT—anomia initially progressing to TCSA and finally to loss of semantic concepts and knowledge. Unlike DAT, other cognitive functions remain intact in these cases. Pathology is restricted to the anterior inferior temporal lobes, and the histopathology is usually Pick disease.[69,92,93] Nonfluent forms of primary progressive aphasia have also been described;[94] however, the pathology has not always been established.

REFERENCES

1. Broca P: Perte de la parole. Ramollissement chronique et destruction partielle du lobe antérieur gauche du cerveau. *Bull Soc Anthropol* 2:235, 1861.
2. Goodglass H: *Understanding Aphasia.* San Diego, CA: Academic Press, 1983, pp 247–250.
3. Kertesz A, McCabe P: Recovery patterns and prognosis in aphasia. *Brain* 100:1–18, 1977.
4. Caramazza A: The logic of neuropsychological research and the problem of patient classification in aphasia. *Brain Lang* 21:9–20, 1984.
5. Marshall JC, Newcombe F: Patterns of paralexia. *J Psycholing Res* 2:175–199, 1973.
6. Ardila A, Rosselli M: Language deviations in aphasia: A frequency analysis. *Brain Lang* 44:165–180, 1993.
7. Kohn SE: Verb finding in aphasia. *Cortex* 25:57–69, 1989.
8. Robinson RG, Kubos KL, Starr LB, et al: Mood disorders in stroke patients: Importance of location of lesion. *Brain* 107:81–93, 1984.
9. Mazzocchi F, Vignolo LA: Localisation of lesions in aphasia: Clinical-CT scan correlations in stroke patients. *Cortex* 15:627–654, 1979.
10. Mohr JP, Pessin MS, Finkelstein S, et al: Broca's aphasia: Pathologic and clinical. *Neurology* 28:311–324, 1978.

11. Naeser MA, Hayward RW: Lesion location in aphasia with cranial computed tomography and the Boston Diagnostic Aphasia Exam. *Neurology* 28:545–551, 1978.

12. Naeser MA, Palumbo CL, Helm-Estabrooks N, et al: Severe nonfluency in aphasia: Role of the medial subcallosal fasciculus and other white matter pathways in recovery of spontaneous speech. *Brain* 112:1–38, 1989.

13. Freedman M, Alexander MP, Naeser MA: Anatomic basis of transcortical motor aphasia. *Neurology* 34:409–417, 1984.

14. Mega MS, Alexander MP: Subcortical aphasia: The core profile of capsulostriatal infarction. *Neurology* 44:1824–1829, 1994.

15. Alexander MP, Naeser MA, Palumbo C: Broca's area aphasia. *Neurology* 40:353–362, 1990.

16. Schiff HB, Alexander MP, Naeser MA, Galaburda AM: Aphemia: Clinical-anatomic correlations. *Arch Neurol* 40:720–727, 1983.

17. Monrad-Krohn GH: Dysprosody or altered "melody of language." *Brain* 70:405–415, 1947.

18. Blumstein SE, Alexander MP, Ryalls JH: The nature of the foreign accent syndrome: A case study. *Brain Lang* 31:215–244, 1987.

19. Graff-Radford NR, Cooper WE, Colsher PL, Damasio AR: An unlearned foreign "accent" in a patient with aphasia. *Brain Lang* 28:86–94, 1986.

20. Prin RS, Snow E, Wagenaar E: Recovery from aphasia: Spontaneous speech versus language comprehension. *Brain Lang* 6:192–211, 1978.

21. Basso A, Gardelli M, Grassi MP, Mariotti M: The role of the right hemisphere in recovery from aphasia: Two case studies. *Cortex* 25:555–556, 1989.

22. Kinsbourne M: The minor hemisphere as a source of aphasic speech. *Trans Am Neurol Assoc* 96:141–145, 1971.

23. Goodglass H: *Understanding Aphasia.* San Diego, CA: Academic Press, 1983, pp 107–109.

24. Alexander MP, Baker E, Naeser MA, et al: Neuropsychological and neuroanatomical dimensions of ideomotor apraxia. *Brain* 118:87–107, 1992.

25. Naeser MA, Helm-Estabrooks N, Haas G, et al: Relationship between lesion extent in Wernicke's area on computed tomographic scan and predicting recovery of comprehension in Wernicke's aphasia. *Arch Neurol* 44:73–82, 1987.

26. Kertesz A, Lau WK, Polk M: The structural determinants of recovery in Wernicke's aphasia. *Brain Lang* 44:153–164, 1993.

27. Selnes OA, Knopman DS, Niccum N, et al: Computed tomographic scan correlates of auditory comprehension deficits in aphasia: A prospective recovery study. *Ann Neurol* 13:558–566, 1983.

28. Henderson VW, Friedman RB, Teng EL, Weiner JM: Left hemisphere pathways in reading: Inference from pure alexia without hemianopia. *Neurology* 35:962–968, 1985.

29. Damasio A: Synchronous activation in multiple cortical regions: A mechanism for recall. *Semin Neurosci* 2:287–296, 1990.

30. Heiss W, Kessler J, Karbe H, et al: Cerebral glucose metabolism as a predictor of recovery from aphasia in ischemic stroke. *Arch Neurol* 50:958–964, 1993.

31. Weiller C, Isensee C, Rijintjes M, et al: Recovery from Wernicke's aphasia: A positron emission tomography study. *Ann Neurol* 37:723–732, 1995.

32. Takahashi N, Kawamura M, Shinotou H, et al: Pure word deafness due to left hemisphere damage. *Cortex* 28:295–303, 1992.

33. Auerbach SH, Allard T, Naeser MA, et al: Pure word deafness: Analysis of a case with bilateral lesions and a defect at the prephonemic level. *Brain* 105:271–300, 1982.

34. Fujii T, Fukatsu R, Watabe S, et al: Auditory sound agnosia without aphasia following a right temporal lobe lesion. *Cortex* 26:263–268, 1990.

35. Paulesu E, Frith CD, Frackowiack RSJ: The neural correlates of the verbal component of working memory. *Nature* 362:342–345, 1993.

36. Roeltgen DP, Sevush S, Heilman KM: Phonological agraphia: Writing by the lexical semantic route. *Neurology* 33:755–765, 1983.

37. Alexander MP, Friedman RB, Loverso F, Fischer RF: Lesion localization in phonological agraphia. *Brain Lang* 43:83–95, 1992.

38. Palumbo CL, Alexander MP, Naeser MA: CT scan lesion sites associated with conduction aphasia in Se K (ed): *Conduction Aphasia.* Hillsdale NJ: Erlbaum, 1992, pp 51–75.

39. Benson DF, Sheremata WA, Bouchard R, et al: Conduction aphasia: A clinicopathological study. *Arch Neurol* 28:339–346, 1973.

40. Mendez MF, Benson DF: Atypical conduction aphasia: A disconnection syndrome. *Arch Neurol* 42:886–891, 1985.

41. Damasio H, Damasio AR: The anatomical basis of conduction aphasia. *Brain* 103:337–350, 1980.

42. Kertesz A, Benson DF: Neologistic jargon: A clinicopathological study. *Cortex* 6:362–386, 1970.

43. Poeck K, de Bleser R, von Keyserlingk DG: Neurolinguistic status and localization of lesions in

aphasic patients with exclusively consonant vowel recurring utterances. *Brain* 107:199–217, 1984.

44. Goodglass H, Kaplan E: *The Assessment of Aphasia and Related Disorders.* Philadelphia: Lea & Febiger, 1983, p 97.

45. Wapner W, Gardner H: A note on patterns of comprehension and recovery in global aphasia. *J Speech Hearing Res* 29:765–771, 1979.

46. Vignolo LA, Boccardi E, Caverni L: Unexpected CT-scan finding in global aphasia. *Cortex* 22:55–69, 1986.

47. DeRenzi E, Colombo A, Scarpa M: The aphasic isolate. *Brain* 114:1719–1730, 1991.

48. Alexander MP, Naeser MA, Palumbo CL: Correlations of subcortical CT lesion sites and aphasia profiles. *Brain* 110:961–991, 1987.

49. Tranel D, Biller J, Damasio H, et al: Global aphasia without hemiparesis. *Arch Neurol* 44:304–308, 1987.

50. Legatt AD, Rubin AJ, Kaplan LR, et al: Global aphasia without hemiparesis. *Neurology* 37:201–205, 1987.

51. Alexander MP: Speech and language deficits after subcortical lesions of the left hemisphere: a clinical, CT, and PET study, in Vallar G, Cappa SF, Wallesch C-W (eds): *Neuropsychological Disorders Associated with Subcortical Lesions.* Oxford, England: Oxford Science Publications, 1991, pp 454–477.

52. Démonet JF, Puel M: "Subcortical" aphasia: Some proposed pathophysiological mechanisms and their rCBF correlates revealed by *SPECT. J Neuroling* 6:319–344, 1991.

53. Rubens AB: Transcortical motor aphasia. *Studies Neuroling* 1:293–306, 1976.

54. Luria AR, Tsvetkova LS: Towards the mechanism of "dynamic aphasia." *Acta Neurol Psychiatr Belg* 67:1045–1067, 1967.

55. Costello A de L, Warrington EK: Dynamic aphasia. *Cortex* 25:103–114, 1989.

56. Lindvall O, Bjorklund A, Moore RY, Stenevi U: Mesencephalic dopamine neurons projecting to neocortex. *Brain Res* 81:325–331, 1974.

57. Alexander MP: Disturbances in language initiation: Mutism and its lesser forms, in Joseph AR, Young RR (eds): *Movement Disorders in Neurology and Psychiatry.* Boston: Blackwell, 1992, pp 389–396.

58. Fisher CM: Abulia minor vs. agitated behavior. *Clin Neurosurg* 31:9–31, 1985.

59. Albert ML, Bachman DL, Morgan A, Helm-Estabrooks N: Pharmacotherapy for aphasia. *Neurology* 38:877–879, 1988.

60. Saba L, Leiguarda R, Starkstein SE: An open-label trial of bromcriptine in nonfluent aphasia. *Neurology* 42:1637–1638, 1992.

61. Alexander MP, Hiltbronner B, Fischer R: The distributed anatomy of transcortical sensory aphasia. *Arch Neurol* 46:885–892, 1989.

62. Warrington EK, Shallice T: Category-specific semantic impairment. *Brain* 107:829–854, 1984.

63. Benson DF: Neurologic correlates of anomia, in Whitaker H, Whitaker HA (eds): *Studies in Neurolinguistics.* New York: Academic Press, 1979, pp 293–328.

64. Berthier ML, Starkstein SE, Leiguarda R, et al: Transcortical aphasia. *Brain* 114:1409–1427, 1991.

65. Feinberg TE, Dyckes-Berke D, Miner CR, Roane DM: Knowledge, implicit knowledge and metaknowledge in visual agnosia and pure alexia. *Brain* 118:789–800, 1995.

66. Feinberg TE, Rothi LJG, Heilman KM: Multimodal agnosia after unilateral left hemisphere lesion. *Neurology* 36:864–867, 1986.

67. Riddoch MJ, Humphreys GW, Coltheart M, Funnell E: Semantic systems or system? Neuropsychological evidence re-examined. *Cogn Neuropsychol* 5:3–25, 1988.

68. Price BH, Gurvit H, Weintraub S, et al: Neuropsychological patterns and language deficits in 20 consecutive cases of autopsy-confirmed Alzheimer's disease. *Arch Neurol* 50:931–937, 1993.

69. Graff-Radford NR, Damasio AR, Hyman BT, et al: Progressive aphasia in a patient with Pick's disease. *Neurology* 40:620–626, 1990.

70. Geschwind N, Quadfasel FA, Segarra JM: Isolation of the speech area. *Neuropsychologia* 6:327–340, 1968.

71. McFarling D, Rothi LJ, Heilman KM: Transcortical aphasia from ischemic infarcts of the thalamus. *J Neurol Neurosurg Psychiatry* 45:107–112, 1982.

72. Graff-Radford NR, Damasio H, Yamada T, et al: Nonhemorrhagic thalamic infarction. *Brain* 108:485–516, 1985.

73. Cappa SF, Vignolo L: "Transcortical" features of aphasia following left thalamic hemorrhage. *Cortex* 19:227–241, 1979.

74. Castro-Caldas A, Confraria A, Poppe P: Nonverbal disturbances in crossed aphasia. *Aphasiology* 1:403–413, 1987.

75. Bryden MP, Hécaen H, DeAgostini M: Patterns of cerebral organization. *Brain Lang* 20:249–262, 1983.

76. Annett M: *Left, Right, Hand and Brain: The Right Shift Theory.* Hillsdale, NJ: Erlbaum, 1985.

77. Alexander MP, Fischette MR, Fischer RS: Crossed aphasia can be mirror image or anomalous. *Brain* 112:953–973, 1989.

78. Basso A, Capitani E, Laiacona M, Zanobio ME: Crossed aphasia: One or more syndromes? *Cortex* 1:25–45, 1985.

79. Alexander MP, Annett M: Crossed aphasia and related anomalies of cerebral organization: Case reports and a genetic hypothesis. *Brain Lang.* In press.

80. Trojano L, Balbi P, Russo G, Elefante R: Patterns of recovery in verbal and nonverbal function in a case of crossed aphasia. *Brain Lang* 46:637–661, 1994.

81. Fischer RS, Alexander MP, Gabriel C, et al: Reversed lateralization of cognitive functions in right handers. *Brain* 114:245–261, 1991.

82. Hécaen H, DeAgostini M, Monzon-Montes A: Cerebral organization in lefthanders. *Brain Lang* 12:261–284, 1981.

83. Basso A, Farabola M, Grassi MP, et al: Aphasia in left-handers. *Brain Lang* 38:233–252, 1990.

84. Naeser MA, Borod JC: Aphasia in lefthanders. *Neurology* 36:471–488, 1986.

85. Puel M, Démonet JF, Cardebat I, et al: Aphasies sous-corticales: Étude neurolinguistigue avec scanner x de 25 cas. *Rev Neurol* 140:695–710, 1984.

86. D'Esposito M, Alexander MP: Subcortical aphasia: Distinct profiles following left putaminal hemorrhages. *Neurology* 45:33–37, 1995.

87. DeRenzi E, Lucchelli F: Are semantic systems separately represented in the brain? The case of living category impairment. *Cortex* 30:3–25, 1994.

88. Smith S, Faust M, Beeman M, et al: A property level analysis of lexical semantic representation in Alzheimer's disease. *Brain Lang* 49:263–279, 1995.

89. Hodges JR, Salmon DP, Butters N: Semantic memory impairment in Alzheimer's disease: Failure of access or degraded knowledge? *Neuropsychologia* 30:301–314, 1992.

90. Tatemichi TK, Desmond DW, Prohovnik I, et al: Confusion and memory loss from capsular genu infarction: A thalamocortical disconnection syndrome? *Neurology* 42:1966–1979, 1992.

91. Weintraub S, Rubin NP, Mesulam MM: Primary progressive aphasia: Longitudinal course, neuropsychological profile and language features. *Arch Neurol* 47:1329–1335, 1990.

92. Hodges JR, Patterson K, Oxbury S, Funnell E: Semantic dementia. *Brain* 115:1783–1806, 1992.

93. Kertesz A, Hudson L, MacKenzie IRA, Munoz DG: The pathology and nosology of primary progressive aphasia. *Neurology* 44:2065–2072, 1994.

94. Mesulam MM: Slowly progressive aphasia without generalized dementia. *Ann Neurol* 11:592–598, 1982.

Chapter 15

APHASIA II: COGNITIVE ISSUES

Eleanor M. Saffran

As is evident from the preceding chapter, much was known about aphasia prior to the emergence of cognitive neuropsychology in the 1970s. Symptoms had been described, diagnostic and treatment protocols developed, anatomic correlates established, and models proposed that interpreted aphasic phenomena within an anatomic theory based on aphasic data (see Ref. 1 for a review). The cognitive neuropsychological approach represents a shift from clinical and anatomic concerns to an emphasis on functional architecture. One assumption that underlies this approach is that language breakdown patterns reflect the natural divisions of the language system and hence that the disorders reveal its componential structure. This school of neuropsychological research is closely tied to developments in cognitive psychology and psycholinguistics. Normative models guide the investigation of pathologic phenomena, which, in turn, provide fertile ground for testing and extending theories of language function.

The concern with functional architecture has implications not only for the types of questions that are addressed by aphasia research but also for methodology. Earlier investigators had relied extensively on the classic aphasia syndrome categories (e.g., Broca's aphasia, Wernicke's aphasia) as the basis for identifying and grouping subjects. While useful as behavioral descriptors and pointers to lesion site, the syndrome designations allow a considerable amount of variability.[2,3] Moreover, these fairly gross breakdown patterns did not map very neatly onto the models of nor-

mal language processing that psycholinguists were developing. The investigative focus therefore moved from what might be regarded as "typical" aphasic manifestations*—for example, the combination of receptive and expressive symptoms that define Wernicke's aphasia—to deficits that were (1) of a more circumscribed nature and (2) had some clear relationship to models of language processing.† An early statement of the assumptions underlying the approach was provided by Marin and colleagues:[4]

> . . . the behavior of the patient with organic brain disease largely reflects capacities which existed in the premorbid state. We should therefore be able to make some inferences about the organization of normal language function from patterns of functional preservation and impairment: if process X is intact where process Y is severely compromised or absent, and especially if the converse is found in other patients, there is reason to believe

---

*Although any experienced clinician would agree that many patients are not easily assigned to the classic syndrome categories.

†This is not to imply that the cognitive neuropsychology approach is without clinical relevance. The assumption is that analyses of disorders in terms of loci of disruption within processing models should provide the basis for developing treatment programs tailored to the underlying disturbance (e.g., Chap. 12 in Ref. 105).

that X and Y reflect different underlying mechanisms in the normal state. At the very least, the resulting matrix of intact and impaired functions should yield a taxonomy of functional subsystems. It may not tell us how these subsystems interact—but it should identify and describe what distinct capacities are available (e.g., it might, to take a hypothetical instance, describe a semantic process that is distinct from a syntactic process). The method is, of course, limited by the functional topology of the brain. Because functions may overlap in their anatomical substrates, we cannot state with assurance that every functional system which could *be observed* will *be observed. But* positive *evidence that functions are organized independently should be significant for a theory of the language process [pp. 869–870].*

It follows from this emphasis on dissociations that, for investigative purposes, greater value is placed on the purity of the impairment than on its frequency of occurrence in the aphasic population. Since circumscribed deficits are relatively rare, studies of single patients are not only admissible but, in the view of some investigators (e.g., Ref. 5), constitute the only valid source of neuropsychological data for the purpose of testing models of cognitive function (see Chap. 10 in Ref. 6 for discussion). Many cognitive neuropsychologists do not subscribe to this position, and group studies that involve sets of patients identified as having a particular cognitive impairment (e.g., "asyntactic" comprehension; see below) are not uncommon. Moreover, although the case study approach clearly departs from the random sampling from a population that is standard for behavioral research, the data are nevertheless cumulative. Delineation of an impairment in a single case report often leads to the identification of other patients with similar impairments and ultimately to compilations of data from a number of cases whose deficits appear quite similar (e.g., Refs. 7 and 8).

The cognitive neuropsychological approach is clearly well suited to the investigation of cognitive systems with modular architectures, that is, systems with components that are discrete and isolable, both functionally and anatomically (cf. Ref. 9). In a system so constituted, the effects of damage to a single component should be quite local; other components should continue to function much as they did before the damage was incurred (see Ref. 6 for discussion). According to this view, the behavioral deficit should directly reflect the nature of the underlying impairment; Caramazza[1] refers to this as the "transparency" assumption. We will return to this point again at the end of the chapter, after reviewing the major contributions of cognitive neuropsychology to the study of aphasia.

COMPONENTS OF LANGUAGE PROCESSING

Most psycholinguists would agree that a model of language processing should include the components identified in Fig. 15-1. The model distinguishes among three types of information—semantic, syntactic, and phonologic; it does not, however, specify the extent to which these forms of information are processed independently, a matter that is still much debated (see, for example, Refs. 10 to 12). The model includes procedures for recognizing and producing spoken words and for recovering and generating syntactic structures; the extent to which components are shared by the comprehension and production streams is another open question (e.g., Refs. 13 and 14). Language breakdown patterns are germane to both of these issues.

Assuming that the model is correct and that the processes and components identified in Fig. 15-1 can be disrupted independently, it should be possible to find patients with deficits that reflect breakdown at particular loci in the model. We will examine evidence for such disorders in the sections that follow.

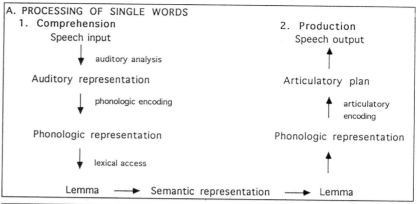

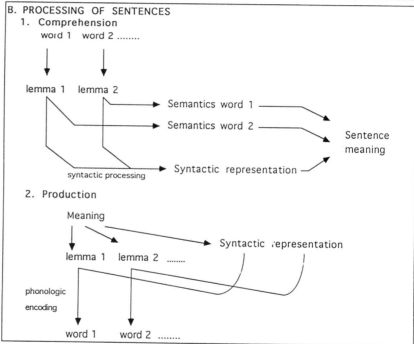

Figure 15-1

Stages in language processing. A. *Processing of single words. The lemma refers to a processing level at which the word is specified with respect to meaning and grammatical class but not encoded phonologically.* B. *Processing of sentences.*

DISORDERS OF LANGUAGE PROCESSING

Processing of Single Words: Comprehension

Impairments in the comprehension of spoken words are common in aphasia, and it is evident from Fig. 15-1 that there are a number of ways in which comprehension might fail: faulty phonologic processing prior to lexical access; loss of or impaired access to the phonologic forms of words; and/or loss of or impaired access to word meanings. Disorders of the first type can be ruled out by tests of phoneme perception and the second by lexical decision tasks in which the patient is asked to determine whether a string of phonemes is or is not a word. If a semantic deficit is present, it should be manifest not only on tests of auditory word comprehension but on written word comprehension and production tasks as well. This follows from the widely held assumption that comprehension and production, in both oral and written modalities, rely on a common conceptual base (cf. Ref. 14).

Phonologic Processing The task for the perceiver of spoken language is to recover meaningful units (words) from the complex and variable sound patterns produced by the human vocal tract. Phonemes, such as *d*, *ow,* and *t*, which are the basic building blocks of words, consist of several distinct frequency bands (formants) that may differ in their relative onset times as well as undergo transient shifts in frequency. These acoustic properties can vary depending on the context in which the phoneme occurs; compare the *d* sound in "ride" with the *d* sound in "rider." A further complication is that the boundaries between words are not systematically marked by gaps in the acoustic stimulus, as they are in written text. Thus the processing of speech input is a complicated matter, which, it has been argued, requires specialized mechanisms that are distinct from those used to process other types of acoustic stimuli (e.g., Ref. 15).

The fact that the processing of speech sounds can be selectively disrupted by brain damage supports this view. Disorders that meet this description are labeled "pure word deafness." They are the product of small lesions, usually embolic in nature, that affect the superior temporal lobe on the left, or, in other cases, bilaterally. In its pure form, the disorder is relatively rare. In most cases the lesion is more extensive, resulting in the set of symptoms associated with Wernicke's aphasia, which may include features of word deafness (e.g., Ref. 16).

The hallmark of pure word deafness is that the patient has great difficulty comprehending and repeating what he or she hears but can read and speak virtually normally. The audiometric exam is essentially normal, and nonspeech sounds are interpreted without difficulty. Some patients have shown suppression of right-ear input under dichotic listening conditions, suggesting that auditory input is being processed in the right hemisphere[17,18] (but see Ref. 19). Auditory comprehension improves significantly when lipreading is allowed (e.g., Ref. 19), speech is slowed down (e.g., Ref. 17), and/or contextual constraints are provided. For example, Saffran and coworkers[18] described a patient whose ability to repeat words was better with semantically constrained than random word lists. These observations suggest that the auditory information available for word identification is in some way inadequate or degraded. Studies in which speech perception has been carefully examined have demonstrated deficits in the discrimination and identification of phonemes (e.g., Refs. 18 to 20). Vowels, made up of steady-state formants, tend to be better preserved than consonants, in which there are transient frequency shifts (e.g., Ref. 20). The processing of nonspeech sounds has not been examined as systematically. Although word-deaf patients are generally able to identify environmental stimuli such as the sounds of animals and musical instruments, they have seldom been called upon to make fine-grained judgments outside the speech domain, involving, for example, the temporal and waveform parameters that are manipulated in speech perception tasks. In the few studies that have included such investigations, deficits in the resolution of repetitive click stimuli have been identified.[17,19,21] This finding points to an impairment in auditory processes that are essential to phoneme perception but are not necessarily specific to speech. Auerbach and co-workers[19] have suggested that there may, in fact, be two forms of word deafness, one reflecting impairment of prephonetic auditory processing and the other specific to phonetic operations. This proposal requires further investigation.

Lexical Processing Lexical access entails matching of the acoustic input to an entry in lexical memory that represents the word's phonologic form. Loss or degradation of lexical phonology is a possible cause of comprehension failure. Deciding whether a speech sound is a word or not (auditory lexical decision) should be impaired under these conditions, but it should still be possible to repeat words, treating them as one would normally treat nonwords. Lexical decision and comprehension of written words should be preserved. Deficits in word comprehension, with relatively preserved repetition, have been described under the label "word-meaning deafness."[22–24] These patients are reported to have no comparable difficulty with written words and may resort to writing down spoken words in order to understand them. However, data on lexical decision have not been provided, and evidence for the critical phenomenon—failure to comprehend spoken words that can be understood in written form—is limited to a small number of examples.

The model outlined in Fig. 15-1 also suggests the possibility of preserved access to phonologic form with failure of access to word meaning. Franklin and associates[25] have recently reported a case that meets this description, at least for abstract words. This patient performed well on phonologic processing and auditory lexical decision tasks but was impaired in the auditory—but not written—comprehension of abstract words. He also had difficulty repeating abstract words as well as nonwords. Word meaning was clearly a significant factor in his repetition performance, as further indicated by a tendency to produce semantic errors in repeating single words. This pattern of repetition performance is termed "deep dysphasia" (for case reports, see Refs. 26 to 28). As will be seen below, this is but one of several disorders in which particular types of words are disproportionately affected.

Semantic Processing Deficits that involve the loss of word meaning are frequently reported, although often in the context of other impairments (e.g., as in Wernicke's aphasia). Relatively pure cases have been described under the label "transcortical sensory aphasia," a disorder in which repetition is spared relative to comprehension and spontaneous production (e.g., Refs. 29 and 30). Semantic disturbances are also found in cases of herpes encephalitis (e.g., Refs. 31 and 32) and, in progressive form ("semantic dementia"), in association with degenerative brain disease (e.g., 33 and 34); these disorders involve damage to middle and inferior temporal lobe structures that lie out-

side the perisylvian zone usually associated with language function (see Chap. 23).

In some cases, the deficit is remarkably selective, affecting some categories of words more than others. The pattern that has been most frequently reported is a disproportionate loss of knowledge of biological kinds, such as animals, fruits, and vegetables; knowledge of artifacts, such as tools and furniture, is at least relatively preserved (see Ref. 35 for review). The semantic deficit is manifest on naming tasks as well as on a variety of measures of word comprehension. This "category-specific" disorder has most often been described in cases of herpes encephalitis but has also been found in one case of semantic dementia (e.g., Ref. 36). There have been attempts to account for this pattern in terms of confounding factors such as the greater visual complexity and lesser familiarity of animals relative to objects such as tools (e.g., Refs. 37 and 38), but the category differences have been shown to persist even when these factors are well controlled (e.g., Ref. 39). Moreover, the opposite pattern—better performance on living things—has been demonstrated in patients with frontoparietal lesions (see Ref. 35 for review). One possible account of this double dissociation is that biological kinds and artifacts depend in different degrees on different types of semantic information (e.g., Refs. 31 and 40). For example, animals are distinguished largely on the basis of perceptual characteristics such as shape and color (compare *lion* and *tiger,* for example), while artifacts are defined primarily by their function (namely, the diverse objects that qualify as radios).

These considerations are compatible with the view that semantic memory is distributed across subsystems specialized for different types of knowledge (but see Ref. 41). Figure 15-2, from Allport,[42] illustrates such a model: the shape of a telephone is stored in one subsystem, its sound in another, its function (not shown) in still another. Although represented in different subsystems, the properties of an object are linked in memory by virtue of the fact that they consistently occur together. When some features of an object (e.g., its shape) are accessed, properties that reside in

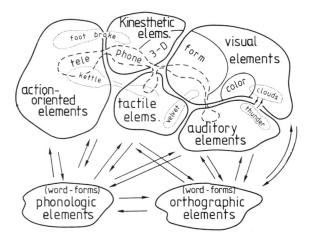

Figure 15-2
Schematic of a distributed model of conceptual representation. (From Allport,[42] with permission.)

other subsystems (e.g., function) are automatically activated, instantiating the distributed activation pattern that corresponds to full knowledge of the object.

Semantic breakdown also occurs along the abstractness/concreteness dimension. Normal subjects show an advantage for concrete words (e.g., Ref. 43), and it would not be surprising if brain damage magnified this effect. This is, in fact, the result that is most frequently reported. For example, repetition of abstract words is disproportionately impaired in deep dysphasia (e.g., Refs. 26 to 28), a pattern that also holds for oral reading in deep dyslexia (cf. Ref. 7). It is unlikely, however, that this effect simply reflects the greater difficulty of abstract words, as there are patients who show the reverse pattern, performing better on abstract than concrete words (e.g., Refs. 36, 44, and 45). There is some evidence that abstract word superiority is associated with differential impairment within the class of concrete words, specifically, worse performance on words denoting living things than those denoting artifacts.[32,36] This would suggest that both patterns reflect disproportionate loss of perceptual components of meaning, which are irrele-

vant to abstract words and more salient for some categories of concrete words than others.

Processing of Single Words: Production

Psycholinguists conceive of production as a multistage process that begins with a concept and ends with movement of the articulators (e.g., Refs. 11, 46, and 47). Here we will concern ourselves only with the processes exemplified in Fig. 15-1, which involve selection of a lexical entry (lemma) that corresponds to the concept to be communicated, followed by access to the phonologic form of the word. We will not review the evidence that supports the two-stage retrieval process here (see Refs. 11, 46, and 47), but consideration of the tip-of-the-tongue phenomenon—knowing that one knows a word without being able to encode it phonologically—suggests that there is a stage of lexicalization that precedes access to phonology. The second stage, phonologic encoding, is a complex process involving retrieval of a set of phonemes, arranging them in the correct serial order, and specifying their stress pattern (e.g., Ref. 11).

Although there is general agreement that word retrieval is a two-step process, the nature of the relationship between the two stages is controversial. Some theorists maintain that lemma selection precedes and is entirely uninfluenced by phonologic encoding (e.g., Ref. 11). Others view lexical retrieval as an interactive process, involving feedback from phonology as well as activation in the forward direction, with the result that phonology can affect lemma selection (e.g., Refs. 10 and 48). Observations that favor the latter account include the fact that mixed errors that bear both a semantic and a phonologic relationship to the target word (e.g., carrot → cabbage) are more frequent than would be expected by chance (e.g., Refs. 49 and 50). This finding suggests that phonologic feedback interacts with feedforward activation from semantics to promote the selection of alternatives that bear both a semantic and a phonologic relationship to the target.

Models of word production are based to a

large extent on normal speech error patterns (e.g., Refs. 46 and 47). It should be possible to account for aphasic speech errors within the same theoretical framework. The errors produced by normal speakers include word substitutions that are semantically (e.g., fork → spoon), or phonologically related to the target (e.g., index → insect) as well as the mixed errors referred to above. Semantic errors are common in aphasics, and, although the literature suggests that phonologically related word substitutions are rare (cf. Ref. 51), there are some patients who do produce high rates of these "formal paraphasias."[52,53] Perhaps the major difference between aphasic and normal speech errors (aside from the increase in overall rate of error production) is the frequency with which aphasics generate errors that are not words; these are referred to as phonemic paraphasias, or neologisms. Some of these errors bear a clear phonologic relationship to the target (e.g., scout → scut); others, sometimes referred to as abstruse neologisms (e.g., Ref. 54), do not.

Although patients generally produce both semantic and phonologic errors, there are cases in which one type of error dominates. For example, Caramazza and Hillis[55] describe a patient who produced only semantic errors, while Caplan and coworkers[56] report a case in which errors were exclusively phonologic. In general, the error patterns of aphasics are consistent with the two-stage model, with indications that semantic and phonologic processes can, on occasion, be disrupted independently.

Recently, there have been efforts to bring aphasic data to bear on the question of independent stage versus interactive models of lexical retrieval. As noted earlier, the interactive model predicts that mixed (semantic + phonologic) errors should exceed levels expected by chance; this prediction should hold for aphasics as well as for normals. Martin and coworkers[57] examined a corpus of errors elicited from aphasics in a picture-naming task and found that it does. Martin and her colleagues[53] were also able to simulate error patterns of a patient who produced a high rate of form-based word substitutions by altering parameter settings on an implemented version of an interactive computational model.[10]

Grammatical class is another important variable in lexical retrieval. It is not unusual to find patients who show significant differences in their ability to retrieve nouns versus verbs (e.g., Refs. 58 and 59). Case studies include those of McCarthy and Warrington[60] of a patient with a selective disturbance in verb production and comprehension and Zingeser and Berndt,[61] whose patient showed preservation of action naming relative to object naming. Different lesion sites have been implicated in these selective impairments—specifically, a frontal locus for verbs and a temporal locus for nouns (e.g., Ref. 62). But the functional basis for these grammatical class effects is not entirely clear. As grammatical class reflects a conceptual distinction, one might expect this factor to be operative early in word retrieval; indeed, the lemma is assumed to specify grammatical class (e.g., Ref. 11). However, Caramazza and Hillis[63] have argued that phonologic output from the lexicon is also organized with respect to grammatical class. This proposal follows from their study of two patients who showed selective deficits for verbs in a single modality—oral production in one case and written production in the other. They interpret these patterns to reflect selective impairment for verbs at the level of orthographic or phonologic encoding.

Sentence-Level Processing: Comprehension

As inspection of the sentences below will indicate, the meaning of a sentence is not solely a function of its lexical content. Failure to comprehend such sentences—interpreting sentence 1 to indicate that the cat was the chaser or that the dog was black—is not uncommon in aphasics, even when they understand all of the individual words. In an influential study, Caramazza and Zurif[64] demonstrated such an impairment in Broca's aphasics. Although their subjects had no difficulty understanding sentences like sentence 2, they performed at chance on sentences like sentence 1.

1. The cat that the dog chased was black.
2. The apple that the boy ate was red.

The difference between the two sentences, which have the same syntactic structure, is that the second one is semantically constrained (apples can't eat boys) while the first is not. In order to interpret sentence 1 correctly, it is necessary to recover the syntax of the sentence and to use this information to assign the nouns to the thematic roles specified by the verb (i.e., dog to the role of agent, or chaser, and cat to the role of theme, or the entity being chased). Caramazza and Zurif's experiment showed that the aphasics had difficulty utilizing syntactic information for this purpose, although they were clearly able to make use of semantic constraints. These authors showed, further, that performance was a function of syntactic complexity: although the patients did relatively well on simple active declarative sentences, their performance broke down on more complex structures, such as passives and object relatives (sentence 1, for example). Caramazza and Zurif interpreted this result to indicate that the patients were using heuristics such as "assign the preverbal noun the agent role and the postverbal noun the role of theme." Reliance on heuristics, together with semantic constraints, would account for the fact that sentence comprehension appears relatively preserved in Broca's aphasics.

Difficulty in sentence production—the pattern known as "agrammatism"—is also part of the symptom complex in Broca's aphasia. The fact that syntactic impairments in comprehension and production occurred in the same patients* gave rise to the hypothesis that the co-occurring deficits were due to a central syntactic deficit, character-

---

*The comprehension deficit is not, however, unique to Broca's aphasics. It is also demonstrated by conduction aphasics (e.g., Refs. 64 and 106), who, like Broca's, have little or no difficulty in comprehending single words. In fact, most aphasics tend to perform worse on semantically reversible sentences (e.g., The boy kissed the girl.); the critical point is that some patients are selectively impaired, performing virtually without error on nonreversible sentences.

ized as a loss of grammatical knowledge (e.g., Ref. 65). Another influential view was that both disturbances reflect impairment to the closed class vocabulary, consisting of elements such as prepositions and tense markers, which convey syntactic information (e.g., Ref. 66). Both hypotheses were subsequently challenged by two sources of evidence: reports of cases in which production was agrammatic but comprehension was intact (e.g., Ref. 67) and the demonstration that agrammatic Broca's aphasics with the "asyntactic" comprehension pattern described by Caramazza and Zurif[64] were able to detect grammatical violations such as those in sentences 3a and 3b.[68,69]

3a. How many did you see birds in the park?
3b. John was finally kissed Louise

These results, subsequently replicated in other laboratories (e.g., Refs. 70 and 71), present difficulty for both accounts of the agrammatic impairment. The ability to detect such violations requires knowledge of the grammar as well as sensitivity to the absence or presence and identity of the grammatical morphemes on which most of them depend.

What, then, is the basis for the "asyntactic" comprehension pattern? Linebarger and coworkers[68] suggested two possible accounts. The first of these is the limited capacity hypothesis. The patients have limited processing resources that will not suffice for parsing and interpretive operations; if they parse, they cannot interpret, and vice versa. Schwartz and coworkers[72] tested this hypothesis in a study in which patients judged the plausibility of sentences such as sentences 4a and 4b. The "padding" in sentence 6a should increase the difficulty of parsing relative to sentence 4b; on the limited capacity hypotheses, one might therefore expect worse performance on the padded sentences.

4a. The chicken killed the farmer.
4b. In the early part of the day, the chicken drank some water and then killed and ate the farmer.
4c. The farmer was killed by the chicken.

The results showed, however, that the effect of padding was negligible for the "asyntactic" comprehenders (though not for other aphasics); in contrast, the effect of the syntactic manipulation in sentence 4c, which involves movement of the nouns from their canonical (preverbal agent, postverbal theme) positions, was seriously detrimental. The second account is the mapping hypothesis. The patients are able to parse sentences but cannot carry out additional operations on the structures computed by the parser, such as mapping from a syntactic representation to thematic roles.

Interpretation of the "asyntactic" comprehension pattern remains controversial. The mapping and limited capacity hypotheses are still debated, as are other interpretations motivated by recent developments in linguistic theory (see Ref. 69 for discussion). The mapping hypothesis has led to the development of treatment programs directed at the mapping operation (see Refs. 73 and 74), which have produced gains in some chronic aphasics. The capacity limitation hypothesis has received support from studies conducted with normal subjects; it turns out that a variety of manipulations that might be expected to tax processing capacity (e.g., rapid serial visual presentation of the words in a sentence; divided attention; elimination of grammatical morphemes) result in comprehension patterns that mirror those of the aphasics (e.g., Refs. 75 to 77). However, this evidence in itself is not compelling. Assuming that it is the recovery of syntactic information and/or the mapping from syntactic to semantic structures that are most vulnerable under these conditions, one would expect other factors that contribute to sentence interpretation to be more influential; these include a tendency to assign the preverbal noun the role of agent, which it often is in English sentences (e.g., Ref. 78). Other proposals have come from linguists, who have attempted to interpret the asyntactic comprehension pattern in terms of constructs in linguistic theory (see Ref. 69 and other papers in that volume). To a large extent, these accounts emphasize the difficulty that these aphasics have in comprehending sentences with moved arguments; these structures are marked with "traces" (indicated by *t*) linked to the argument that has been moved, as in sentence 5:

5. The farmer was killed *t* by the chicken.

It is assumed that the necessity to link the moved argument (the farmer, in sentence 5) to the trace complicates sentence processing for the aphasics. Often ignored by proponents of these views, however, is the fact that "asyntactic" patients frequently have difficulty with sentences that (at least according to most theories) lack traces, such as the simple active declarative[79,80] and locative[79,81] sentences exemplified by sentences 6a and 6b.

6a. The boy follows the girl.

6b. The paper is on the book.

Thus, while the basic phenomena are well established, there is as yet no generally accepted interpretation of the "asyntactic" comprehension pattern.

Short-Term Memory and Sentence Processing

Other studies of aphasics have focused on the role of short-term memory (STM) in sentence processing. Although most aphasics show some degree of short-term verbal memory impairment (see Ref. 82 for review), there are cases in which STM capacity, as measured by digit and word span, is markedly deficient in the context of relatively preserved language abilities (e.g., Refs. 83 and 84). The STM deficit appears to reflect impairment of a phonologic component of STM (e.g., Ref. 8). Most STM patients have difficulty with sentence comprehension, demonstrating the performance pattern characteristic of agrammatic aphasics that was described above (e.g., Ref. 85). It has proved difficult, however, to specify the relationship between these two impairments. One complicating factor is that the two are not perfectly correlated; there are instances in which reduced memory span is not accompanied by impairment in comprehension (e.g., Refs. 86 and 87). Studies of normal sentence processing indicate, moreover, that syntactic and semantic encoding occur on line (e.g., Ref. 88), so that there would seem to be no need to maintain the input in phonologic form. But while phonologic memory may not be necessary for first-pass encoding operations, it may serve as a backup store that allows the listener to revise interpretations in light of information that comes later in the sentence (for discussion, see Refs. 89 and 90).

Sentence-Level Processing: Production

A schema for sentence production is outlined in Fig. 15-1. Although not explicitly represented in the diagram, most psycholinguists assume that sentence production involves retrieval of a syntactic frame that stipulates word order (e.g., determiner-noun-auxiliary-verb. . .) and serves as a template into which phonologically specified words are later inserted (e.g., Refs. 47 and 48). While there are other aphasics who are impaired in some aspects of sentence production (e.g., Ref. 91), it is the deficits of agrammatical Broca's aphasics that have drawn most attention. The production of such patients is characterized by the limited use of syntactic structures and the omission of grammatical morphemes, such as tense markers (e.g., -ed), determiners (e.g., the), and prepositions (e.g., to).* It seems likely that frame retrieval is seriously impaired in such patients, reflecting a reduction in the inventory of syntactic structures, their inaccessibility, or both (e.g., Ref. 92). The fact that patients occasionally produce utterances that are more complex than those constituting the bulk of their corpora suggests that inaccessibility of these structures is at least part of the problem (e.g., Ref. 93). In light of evidence from normals that use promotes further use,[94,95] it seems likely that a tendency to rely on a limited set of structures will render other structures progressively less accessible. There is some evidence that frame retrieval can be disrupted independently of access to grammatical morphology[67,96] and that bound (i.e., inflectional) and freestanding grammatical morphemes can be selectively affected.[97,98]

---

*Omission is common in English, which is not highly inflected. In other languages, such as Hebrew, substitution of grammatical morphemes is the dominant error pattern (e.g., Ref. 107).

NEW DIRECTIONS

Cognitive neuropsychology adopted the box-and-arrow information processing models that were favored by cognitive psychologists in the 1970s. The boxes stood for modules whose internal operations were largely unknown; the arrows symbolized the flow of information between them. More recently, cognitive theorists have turned to computer-implemented (neural network or "connectionist") models that specify more precisely how information is represented and processed (see Chap. 4). The models are networks of units that represent information; the informational significance of the units is either specified by the modeler (in "localist" models; e.g., Ref. 48) or acquired during learning trials (in parallel distributed processing, or PDP, models; e.g., Refs. 40 and 99). In the latter, inner layers of units are initially connected randomly to input and output layers in which units are specified for content. Thus, for example, models that learn to read aloud have input units that stand for individual letters or groups of letters and output units that stand for specific phonemes or groups of phonemes. Explorations of effects of "lesioning" these models (for example, by randomly eliminating units or altering the strength of connections between units) have revealed some interesting properties that have implications for fundamental assumptions in cognitive neuropsychology.

One major result of the simulation studies is that symptoms are not necessarily a direct reflection of the type of representation that is lesioned. For example, Shallice and colleagues[99,100] have developed a connectionist model of reading in which learning procedures are used to train graphemic units to activate units of meaning ("sememes" such as "brown," "has legs," etc.) which ultimately activate phoneme units. In other words, the model learns to pronounce written words by looking up their meanings. Lesioning this model can result in semantic errors (e.g., reading night as sleep) of the sort that are produced by patients with deep dyslexia. These errors were generally thought to reflect impairment at the semantic level (e.g., Ref. 101). The simulations on this model demonstrate, however, that semantic errors can be generated by lesions elsewhere in the network. A related point is made by data from a study by Farah and McClelland,[40] who lesioned a semantic network to simulate the disorders involving living and nonliving things. The model included two semantic subsystems, one representing functional properties and the other visual properties, which predominated for living things. As a result of the connectivity patterns within the network, damage to the visual subsystem rendered the functional properties of living things inaccessible. The "symptoms" therefore reflected perturbations that extended well beyond the subsystem targeted by the lesion. The implication of these findings is that the relationship between symptom and deficit may not be as direct as it is often taken to be (cf. Ref. 102).

Other simulation studies demonstrate that performance patterns that appear selective can be generated by "lesions" that are widespread. Employing a localist model of word retrieval,[10] which allows activation to feed back from phonemes to lemma to semantic units as well as to proceed in the forward direction, our group has shown that shifts in the dominant error types can be produced by altering different parameters of the model.[53,103] The two parameters are connection strength, which affects the ease with which activation flows (in both directions) from one level to another, and decay rate, which affects the persistence of activation within representational levels. Different error patterns result from connection weight and decay rate "lesions," both applied uniformly throughout the lexical system. A decrease in connection strength reduces the flow of activation to target-related units, resulting in an increase in nonword errors. Decay rate "lesions" have a different effect on the distribution of activation, shifting error production in the direction of semantic and formal substitutions. Lest it be thought that this is merely a formal exercise, manipulation of these two parameters closely simulated the individual error patterns of almost all (20/23) of the fluent aphasics that we tested.

How seriously should we take these demonstrations of nonlocal effects of lesions, and do they in any way invalidate the 20-year research program in cognitive neuropsychology? Computational modeling in the language domain is relatively new, and it is too soon to determine how useful this approach will prove to be. However, recent psycholinguistic studies indicate that normal language processing is characterized by a good deal of interaction among processing components (e.g., Refs. 10, 95, and 104). Interactive processing architectures complicate the task of inferring the locus of the deficit from a patient's performance. As Farah[102] has observed, the relationship between symptom and impaired process is no longer transparent; semantic errors, for example, need not necessarily reflect perturbation of a semantic process. But while it will be necessary to interpret new data more cautiously, and, perhaps, to reexamine earlier conclusions, the effort to tie phenomena of language breakdown to models of normal language function remains useful and valid. Neuropsychological data extend the database and testing ground for normative models, and the models, in turn, provide a coherent framework for the investigation and interpretation of clinical phenomena.*

ACKNOWLEDGMENT

Preparation of this chapter was supported by grant DC00191 from the National Institutes of Health.

REFERENCES

1. Goodglass H, Geschwind N: Language disorders (aphasia), in Carterette EC, Friedman MP (eds): *Handbook of Perception.* New York: Academic Press, 1976.
2. Caramazza A: The logic of neuropsychological

---

*One impediment to the clinical application of cognitive neuropsychological approaches to language disorders has been the dearth of appropriate diagnostic instruments. However, new tests that are intended to provide a psycholinguistic analysis of aphasic deficits are becoming available (e.g., Refs. 89 and 108).

research and the problem of patient classification in aphasia. *Brain Lang* 21:9–20, 1984.

3. Schwartz MF: What the classical aphasia categories can't do for us and why. *Cogn Neuropsychol* 21:3–8, 1984.

4. Marin OSM, Saffran EM, Schwartz MF: Dissociations of language in aphasia: Implications for normal function. *Ann NY Acad Sci* 280:868–884, 1976.

5. Caramazza A: On drawing inferences about the structure of normal cognitive systems from the analysis of patterns of impaired performance: The case for single-patient studies. *Brain Cogn* 5:41–66, 1986.

6. Shallice T: From neuropsychology to mental structure. Cambridge, England: Cambridge University Press, 1988.

7. Coltheart M, Patterson KE, Marshall JC (eds): *Deep Dyslexia.* London: Routledge, 1980.

8. Vallar G, Shallice T (eds): *Neuropsychological Deficits in Short-Term Memory.* Cambridge, England: Cambridge University Press, 1990.

9. Fodor JA: *The Modularity of Mind.* Cambridge, MA: MIT Press, 1983.

10. Dell GS, O'Seaghdha PG: Mediated and convergent lexical priming in language production: A comment on Levelt et al. *Psychol Rev* 98:604–614, 1991.

11. Levelt WJM. Accessing words in speech production: Stages, processes and representations. *Cognition* 42:1–21, 1992.

12. Mitchell DC: Sentence parsing, in Gernsbacher MA (ed): *Handbook of Psycholinguistics.* San Diego, CA: Academic Press, 1994.

13. Allport DA: Speech production and comprehension: One lexicon or two? in Prinz W, Sanders AF (eds): *Cognition and Motor Processes.* Berlin: Springer-Verlag, 1984.

14. Monsell S: On the relation between lexical input and output pathways for speech, in Allport A, MacKay D, Prinz W, Sheerer E (eds): *Language Perception and Production.* London: Academic Press, 1987.

15. Liberman AM, Studdert-Kennedy M: Phonetic perception, in Held R, Lebowitz H, Teuber H-L (eds): *The Handbook of Sensory Physiology: Perception.* Heidelberg: Springer-Verlag, 1978, vol 8, pp. 143–178.

16. Caramazza A, Berndt RS, Basili AG: The selective impairment of phonological processing: A case study. *Brain Lang* 18:128–174, 1983.

17. Albert ML, Bear D: Time to understand: A case study of word deafness with reference to the role of time in auditory comprehension. *Brain* 97:373–384, 1974.

18. Saffran EM, Marin OSM, Yeni-Komshian G: An analysis of speech perception in word deafness. *Brain Lang* 3:209–228, 1976.

19. Auerbach SH, Allard T, Naeser M, et al: Pure word deafness: Analysis of a case with bilateral lesions and defect at the prephonemic level. *Brain* 105:271–300, 1982.

20. Denes G, Semenza C: Auditory modality-specific anomie: Evidence from a case of pure word deafness. *Cortex* 14:41–49, 1975.

21. Tanaka Y, Yamadori A, Mori E: Pure word deafness following bilateral lesions. *Brain* 110:381–403, 1987.

22. Bramwell B: Illustrative cases of aphasia (case 11). *Lancet* 1:1256–1259, 1897. Reprinted with an introduction by AW Ellis in *Cogn Neuropsychol* 1:245–258, 1984.

23. Kohn SE, Friedman RB: Word-meaning deafness: A phonological semantic dissociation. *Cogn Neuropsychol* 3:291–308, 1986.

24. Schacter DL, McGlynn SM, Milberg WP, Church BA: Spared priming despite impaired comprehension: Implicit memory in a case of word-meaning deafness. *Neuropsychology* 7:107–118, 1993.

25. Franklin S, Howard D, Patterson K: Abstract word meaning deafness. *Cogn Neuropsychol* 11:1–34, 1994.

26. Howard D, Franklin S: *Missing the Meaning? A Cognitive Neuropsychological Study of Processing of Words by an Aphasic Patient.* Cambridge, MA: MIT Press, 1988.

27. Katz R, Goodglass H: Deep dysphasia: An analysis of a rare form of repetition disorder. *Brain Lang* 39:153–185, 1990.

28. Martin N, Saffran EM: A computational account of deep dysphasia: Evidence from a single case study. *Brain Lang* 43:240–274, 1992.

29. Berndt RS, Basili A, Caramazza A: Dissociation of functions in a case of transcortical sensory aphasia. *Cogn Neuropsychol* 4:79–101, 1987.

30. Martin N, Saffran EM: Factors underlying repetition and short-term memory in transcortical sensory aphasia. *Brain Lang* 37:440–479, 1990.

31. Warrington EK, Shallice T: Category specific semantic impairments. *Brain* 107:829–854, 1984.

32. Sirigu A, Duhamel J-R, Poncet M: The role of sensorimotor experience in object recognition. *Brain* 114:2555–2573, 1991.

33. Snowden JS, Goulding PJ, Neary D: Semantic dementia: A form of circumscribed cerebral atrophy. *Behav Neurol* 2:167–182, 1989.

34. Hodges JR, Patterson K, Oxbury S, Funnell E: Semantic dementia: Progressive fluent aphasia, with temporal lobe atrophy. *Brain* 115:1783–1806, 1992.

35. Saffran EM, Schwartz MF: Of cabbages and things: Semantic memory from a neuropsychological perspective—A tutorial review, in Umilta C, Moscovitch M (eds): *Attention and Performance: XV. Conscious and Nonconscious Processes.* Cambridge, MA: MIT Press, 1994.

36. Breedin SD, Saffran EM, Coslett HB: Reversal of the concreteness effect in a patient with semantic dementia. *Cogn Neuropsychol* 11:617–660, 1994.

37. Funnell E, Sheridan J: Categories of knowledge? Unfamiliar aspects of living and non-living things. *Cogn Neuropsychol* 9:135–154, 1992.

38. Stewart F, Parkin AJ, Hunkin NM: Naming impairments following recovery from herpes simplex encephalitis: Category specific? *Q J Exp Psychol* 44A:261–284, 1992.

39. Farah MJ, McMullen PA, Meyer MM: Can recognition of living things be selectively impaired? *Neuropsychologia* 29:185–193, 1991.

40. Farah MJ, McClelland JL: A computational model of semantic memory impairment: Modality specificity and emergent category. *J Exp Psychol (Gen)* 120:339–357, 1991.

41. Caramazza A, Hillis AE, Rapp B, Romani C: The multiple semantics hypothesis: Multiple confusion? *Cogn Neuropsychol* 7:161–189, 1990.

42. Allport DA: Distributed memory, modular subsystems and dysphasia, in Newman SK, Epstein R (eds.), *Current Perspectives in Dysphasia.* Edinburgh: Churchill Livingstone, 1985, pp 32–60.

43. Paivio A: Dual coding theory: Retrospect and current status. *Can J Psychol* 45:255–258, 1991.

44. Warrington EK: The selective impairment of semantic memory. *Q J Exp Psychol* 27:635–657, 1975.

45. Cipolotti L, Warrington EK: Semantic memory and reading abilities: A case report. *J Int Neuropsychol Soc* 1:104–110, 1995.

46. Fromkin VA: The non-anomalous nature of anomalous utterances. *Language* 47:27–52, 1971.

47. Garrett MF: Levels of processing in sentence production, in Butterworth B (ed): *Language Production.* New York: Academic Press, 1980, vol 1.

48. Dell GS: A spreading activation theory of retrieval in language production. *Psychol Rev* 93:283–321, 1986.

49. Dell GS, Reich PA: Stages in sentence production: An analysis of speech error data. *J Verb Learn Verb Behav* 20:611–629, 1981.

50. Martin N, Weisberg R, Saffran EM: Variables influencing the occurrence of naming errors: Implications for models of lexical retrieval. *J Mem Lang* 28:462–485, 1989.

51. Ellis AW: The production of spoken words, in Ellis AW (ed): *Progress in the Psychology of Language.* Vol 2. London: Erlbaum, 1985.

52. Blanken G: Formal paraphasias: A single case study. *Brain Lang* 38:534–554, 1990.

53. Martin N, Dell GS, Saffran EM, Schwartz MF: Origins of paraphasias in deep dysphasia: Testing the consequences of a decay impairment to an interactive spreading activation model of lexical retrieval. *Brain Lang* 47:609–660, 1994.

54. Schwartz MF, Saffran EM, Bloch DE, Dell GS: Disordered speech production in aphasic and normal speakers. *Brain Lang* 47:52–88, 1994.

55. Caramazza A, Hillis AE: Where do semantic errors come from? *Cortex* 26:95–122, 1990.

56. Caplan D, Vanier M, Baker C: A case study of reproduction conduction aphasia: I. Word production. *Cogn Neuropsychol* 3:99–128, 1986.

57. Martin N, Gagnon DA, Schwartz MF, et al: Phonological facilitation of semantic errors in normal and aphasic speakers. *Lang Cogn Process.* In press.

58. Miceh G, Silveri MC, Romani C, Caramazza A: On the basis for the agrammatic's difficulty in producing main verbs. *Cortex* 20:207–220, 1984.

59. Kohn SE, Lorch MP, Pearson DM: Verb finding in aphasia. *Cortex* 25:57–69, 1989.

60. McCarthy R, Warrington EK: Category specificity in an agrammatic patient: The relative impairment of verb retrieval and comprehension. *Neuropsychologia* 23:709–727, 1985.

61. Zingeser LB, Berndt RS: Retrieval of nouns and verbs in agrammatism and anomia. *Brain Lang* 39:14–32, 1990.

62. Daniele A, Giustolisi L, Silveri MC, et al: Evidence for a possible neuroanatomical basis for lexical processing of nouns and verbs. *Neuropsychologia* 32:1325–1341, 1994.

63. Caramazza A, Hillis AE: Lexical organization of nouns and verbs in the brain. *Nature* 349:788–790, 1991.

64. Caramazza A, Zurif EB: Dissociations of algorithmic and heuristic processes in language

comprehension: Evidence from aphasia. *Brain Lang* 3:572–582, 1976.

65. Caramazza A, Berndt RS: Semantic and syntactic processes in aphasia: A review of the literature. *Psychol Bull* 85:898–918, 1978.

66. Bradley DC, Garrett MF, Zurif EB: Syntactic deficits in Broca's aphasia, in Caplan D (ed): *Biological Studies of Mental Processes*. Cambridge, MA: MIT Press, 1980.

67. Miceli G, Mazzuchi A, Menn L, Goodglass H: Contrasting cases of Italian agrammatic aphasia without comprehension disorder. *Brain Lang* 19:65–97, 1983.

68. Linebarger MC, Schwartz MF, Saffran EM: Sensitivity to grammatical structure in so-called agrammatic aphasics. *Cognition* 13:641–662, 1983.

69. Linebarger MC: Agrammatism as evidence about grammar. *Brain Lang* 50:52–91, 1995.

70. Berndt RS, Salasoo A, Mitchum CC, Blumstein S: The role of intonation cues in aphasic patients' performance of the grammaticality judgment task. *Brain Lang* 34:65–97, 1988.

71. Shankweiler D, Crain S, Gorrell P, Tuller B: Reception of language in Broca's aphasia. *Lang Cogn Process* 4:1–33, 1989.

72. Schwartz MF, Linebarger M, Saffran EM, Pate DS: Syntactic transparency and sentence interpretation in aphasia. *Lang Cogn Process* 2:85–113, 1987.

73. Byng S: Sentence comprehension deficit: Theoretical analysis and remediation. *Cogn Neuropsychol* 5:629–676, 1988.

74. Schwartz MF, Saffran EM, Fink RB, et al: Mapping therapy: A treatment program for agrammatism. *Aphasiology* 8:19–54, 1994.

75. Miyake A, Carpenter PA, Just MA: A capacity approach to syntactic comprehension disorders: Making normal adults perform like aphasics. *Cogn Neuropsychol* 11:671–717, 1994.

76. Blackwell A, Bates E: Inducing agrammatic profiles in normals: Evidence for the selective vulnerability of morphology under cognitive resource limitation. *J Cogn Neurosci* 7:228–257, 1995.

77. Pulvermüller F: Agrammatism: Behavioral description and neurobiological explanation. *J Cogn Neurosci* 7:165–181, 1995.

78. Bever TG: The cognitive basis for linguistic structures, in Hayes JR (ed): *Cognition and the Development of Language*. New York: Wiley, 1970.

79. Schwartz MF, Saffran EM, Marin OSM: The word order problem in agrammatism: 1. Comprehension. *Brain Lang* 10:263–288, 1980.

80. Berndt RS, Mitchum CC, Haendiges AN: Comprehension of reversible sentences in "agrammatism." *Cognition*. In press.

81. Kolk H, Van Grunsven MJE: Agrammatism as a variable phenomenon. *Cogn Neuropsychol* 2:347–384, 1985.

82. Saffran EM: Short-term memory impairment and language processing, in Caramazza A (ed): *Advances in Cognitive Neuropsychology and Neurolinguistics*. Hillsdale, NJ: Erlbaum, 1990.

83. Saffran EM, Marin OSM: Immediate memory for word lists and sentences in a patient with deficient auditory short term memory. *Brain Lang* 2:420–433, 1975.

84. Vallar G, Baddeley AD: Phonological short-term store, phonological processing and sentence comprehension: A neuropsychological case study. *Cogn Neuropsychol* 1:121–142, 1984.

85. Saffran EM, Martin N: Short-term memory impairment and sentence processing, in Vallar G, Shallice T (eds): *Neuropsychological Impairments of Short Term Memory*. Cambridge, England: Cambridge University Press, 1990.

86. Butterworth B, Campbell R, Howard D: The uses of short-term memory: A case study. *Q J Exp Psychol* 38:705–737, 1986.

87. Martin RC: Articulatory and phonological deficits in short-term memory and their relation to syntactic processing. *Brain Lang* 32:159–192, 1987.

88. Marslen-Wilson W, Tyler LK: The temporal structure of spoken language understanding. *Cognition* 8:1–71, 1980.

89. Caplan D: *Language: Structure, Processing and Disorders*. Cambridge, MA: MIT Press, 1992.

90. Gathercole SE, Baddeley AD: *Working Memory and Language*. Hillsdale, NJ: Erlbaum, 1993.

91. Butterworth B, Howard D: Paragrammatisms. *Cognition* 26:1–38, 1987.

92. LaPointe S, Dell GS: A synthesis of some recent work on sentence production, in Tanenhaus MK, Carlson G (eds): *Linguistic Structure in Language Processing*. Dordrecht: Kluwer, 1988.

93. Menn L, Obler LK (eds): *Agrammatic Aphasia: A Cross-Language Narrative Sourcebook*. Philadelphia: John Benjamins, 1990.

94. Bock JK: Syntactic persistence in language production. *Cogn Psychol* 18:355–387, 1986.

95. Bock JK: Structure in language: Creating form in talk. *Amer Psychol* 45:1221–1236, 1990.

96. Saffran EM, Schwartz MF, Marin OSM: Evidence from aphasia: Isolating the components of a pro-

duction model, in Butterworth B (ed): *Language Production.* London: Academic Press, 1980, pp 221–240.

97. Nespoulous J-L, Dordain M, Perron C, et al: Agrammatism in sentence production without comprehension deficits: Reduced variability of syntactic structures and/or of grammatical morphemes? A case study. *Brain Lang* 33:273–295, 1988.

98. Saffran EM, Berndt RS, Schwartz MF: A scheme for the quantitative analysis of agrammatic production. *Brain Lang* 37:440–479, 1989.

99. Plaut D, Shallice T: Deep dyslexia: A case study of connectionist neuropsychology. *Cogn Neuropsychol* 10:377–500, 1993.

100. Hinton GE, Shallice T: Lesioning an attractor network: Investigations of acquired dyslexia. *Psychol Rev* 98:74–95, 1991.

101. Shallice T, Warrington EK: Single and multiple component central dyslexic syndromes, in Coltheart M, Patterson KE, Marshall JC (eds): *Deep Dyslexia.* London: Routledge, 1980, pp 119–145.

102. Farah MJ: Neuropsychological inference with an interactive brain: A critique of the "locality assumption." *Behav Brain Sci* 17:43–104, 1994.

103. Dell GS, Schwartz MF, Martin N, et al: Lesioning a connectionist model of lexical retrieval to simulate naming errors in aphasia. Presented at conference on Neural Modeling of Cognitive and Brain Disorders; June 9, 1995; College Park, MD.

104. MacDonald MC, Pearlmutter NJ, Seidenberg MS: Lexical nature of syntactic ambiguity resolution. *Psychol Rev* 101:676–703, 1994.

105. Howard D, Hatfield FM: Aphasia therapy: Historical and contemporary issues. Hillsdale, NJ: Erlbaum, 1987.

106. Heilman KM, Scholes RJ: The nature of comprehension errors in Broca's, conduction, and Wernicke's aphasics. *Cortex* 12:258–265, 1976.

107. Grodzinsky Y: The syntactic characterization of agrammatism. *Cognition* 16:99–120, 1984.

108. Kay J, Lesser R, Coltheart M: *Psycholinguistic Assessment of Language Processing in Aphasia (PALPA).* London: Erlbaum, 1992.

Chapter 16

ACQUIRED DISORDERS OF LANGUAGE IN CHILDREN

Maureen Dennis

Childhood-acquired language disorder, or *childhood-acquired aphasia,* refers to language impairment that is evident after a period of normal language acquisition and that is precipitated by a demonstrable form of brain insult. It may be differentiated from language acquisition disorders without clearly established brain pathology as well as from language deficits that emerge during initial language acquisition or afterwards in children with neurodevelopmental brain disorders evident at birth (see Chaps. 17 and 19).

EARLIER (BEFORE 1980) VERSUS RECENT (AFTER 1980) VIEWS OF CHILDHOOD-ACQUIRED APHASIA

The earlier era of research highlighted the apparent differences between adults and children with acquired aphasia. The reference point for judging whether a child was aphasic was adult aphasia syndromes rather than age-inappropriate language development. Childhood-acquired aphasia was largely defined by negative features, aphasic symptoms that were classically present in the aphasic adult but not evident in the aphasic child.

Using adult aphasia as the reference point, the earlier view[1,2] was that childhood-acquired aphasia involved nonfluent and transient language defects that arose from nonfocal and poorly lateralized brain mechanisms. In this perspective, childhood and adult-acquired aphasias differed with respect to language symptoms, rate of language recovery, lesion localization, and lesion laterality. More important, these differences between aphasic children and aphasic adults were attributed to the differing ages at onset of aphasia.

The recent view of childhood-acquired aphasia is different from the earlier view, and a variety of influences have shaped it, among them the burgeoning number of empirical studies since 1980, the publication of better benchmarks and assessment instruments for normal language development, and the increased availability and accessibility of brain imaging techniques for identifying side and site of aphasia-causing lesions. All of this has occurred in the context of emerging evidence about the sometimes greater cognitive morbidity in younger rather than older children as a result of brain tumors and head injury, which has led to a less sanguine view about the protective function for cognition of a young age at brain injury.[3]

In the earlier view, the child with acquired aphasia was advantaged over the adult aphasic by virtue of an earlier age at aphasia onset. It now appears that the advantage, if any, is short-lived and concerns the faster abatement of acute-stage aphasic symptoms. With respect to long-term language function, children with acquired aphasia often fare poorly. Age at aphasia-producing brain injury has proved to be less predictive of aphasic symptoms but more relevant to long-term language function than was previously thought. Given a similar brain injury, children and adults exhibit similar aphasic symptoms in the acute stage of acquired aphasia; however, while children show a faster resolution of aphasic symptoms than adults, their long-term language function may sometimes be poorer. These conclusions have emerged from studies conducted over the last 15 years, which have called into question all of the features once considered to define childhood-acquired aphasia.

Nonfluent Nature of Childhood-Acquired Aphasia

Historically, childhood-acquired aphasia was characterized by nonfluent and impoverished spontaneous speech,[4-6] ranging in severity from mutism to articulatory difficulties as well as by nonfluent language, often with simplified syntax, telegraphic speech, and word-finding difficulties (see Chap. 14 for a discussion of these aphasic signs). A period of mutism immediately postonset resolving to a nonfluent aphasia has long been reported in samples of childhood-acquired aphasia.[7-9] Even now, speech and language dysfluency is characteristic of many forms of childhood-acquired aphasia.[10]

One corollary of the traditional view of a primarily expressive deficit in childhood-acquired aphasia was that symptoms of adult fluent aphasia (logorrhea, verbal stereotypies, perseverations, neologisms, jargon, and paraphasias; see Chap. 14) would be absent in children with acquired language disorders.[8] More recent studies have shown that aphasic children do indeed exhibit fluent aphasia[11] that includes phonemic jargon, neologisms, and paraphasias.[12] In fact, there appear to be a large number of aphasic symptoms in children, more varied than previously thought.[13] Moreover, many adult aphasic syndromes have been described in children: jargon aphasia;[12,14] Wernicke's aphasia and transcortical sensory aphasia;[15] conduction aphasia;[16] transcortical sensory aphasia;[11,17] anomic aphasia;[18] and alexia without agraphia.[19 20] In short, most adult aphasic syndromes can be observed in children, albeit with different base frequencies.[21]

Many of the classic adult aphasic syndromes involve comprehension deficits, and these have also proved to be central to childhood-acquired aphasia. From its first description in 1957, the Landau-Kleffner syndrome (LKS),[22] whose defining feature is a severe and long-lasting verbal auditory agnosia for words and for sounds, became the paradigm of childhood-acquired aphasia.[23] Comprehension deficits are features of the long-term language function in several other childhood-acquired aphasic conditions and may even be more pronounced than in adults; for example, global aphasia from a childhood left middle cerebral artery infarct may resolve to a transcortical sensory aphasia characterized by poorer language comprehension than in comparable adult cases.[24] Thus, recent research has not confirmed the traditional idea that comprehension, especially auditory comprehension, is invariably preserved in childhood-acquired aphasia.

Transient Nature of Childhood-Acquired Aphasia

Recovery of aphasic symptoms in cases of childhood-acquired aphasia is often rapid,[25] although some 25 to 50 percent of cases still show aphasia 1 year postonset. More important is the observation that recovery of speech cannot be equated with recovery of language.[8]

Recent long-term follow-up studies have focused on recovery of language function rather than on abatement of aphasic symptoms. Considered in this manner, the consequences of childhood-acquired aphasia appear to be long-lasting and extend in time far beyond the disappearance of aphasic symptoms.[23] Although clinical signs of aphasia somewhat similar to those in the adult occur in the acute phase of childhood-acquired aphasia, long-term language outcome may still be poor after aphasic symptoms have resolved.[26] Even when clinical signs of aphasia abate, full and functional pragmatic language will not necessarily be acquired or restored.[27,28] And academic achievement in school-age children continues to be poor after clinical recovery from aphasic symptoms.[29-31] School difficulties—involving failure to accrue new learning[17]—may even become more pronounced with time, perhaps because of the escalating demands of academic work in the higher grades.[32]

Nonfocal Brain Bases of Childhood-Acquired Aphasia

The idea that childhood-acquired aphasia was based in nonfocal brain mechanisms arose for several reasons, among them the fact that early study groups of children with acquired aphasia had an overrepresentation of traumatic and infectious etiologies[7] and included patients with pathologic processes that appeared to be lateralized (on the basis of evidence of gross neurologic status, such as hemiplegia) but which actually affected functions bilaterally.[14] In addition, the early studies that shaped the traditional view of childhood-acquired aphasia could not include neuroimaging of the aphasia-producing lesions, resulting in inperfect information about lesion localization and extent.

In recent studies there has been increased recognition of the fact that child and adult aphasia-producing lesions may have different long-term effects on the brain. Some early lesions may leave little focal residual change,[33] with the result that the brain does not show characteristic gliotic changes but rather tissue shrinkage; thus, even with an initially focal insult, brain lesions in childhood may involve decreased brain volume.[34] This invalidates any simple comparison between children and adults at the point in time that aphasic symptoms are most florid.

Nonlateralized Brain Bases of Childhood-Acquired Aphasia

In the earlier view, language lateralization developed over the first decade of life in a gradual and linear manner. The question of whether cerebral dominance for language develops gradually or is innate, once considered so central to understanding childhood-acquired aphasia,[35] has in recent years come to seem less burning.[21] Perhaps more important, particular entailments of the view of a slowly-developing lateralization of language have been proven wrong, such as the idea that aphasia after right-sided lesions is more common in children than in adults.[14] If the left hemisphere has been damaged, the risk of acquired aphasia is approximately the same in right-handed children and right-handed adults;[25,36,37] evidently, child-

hood aphasia is no more uncommon than adult aphasia, given a unilateral lesion to the dominant hemisphere.[38] Further, left-sided lesions to the classic posterior language areas in childhood produce a fluent aphasia with many neologisms and paraphasias[39] of the sort observed in adults with similar brain lesions. And finally, recovery from childhood-acquired aphasia depends on the integrity of the left posterior language areas,[30] which suggests that a lateralized and focal language representation is well established by middle childhood and also that recovery from childhood-acquired aphasia depends on the intact areas of the left hemisphere rather than on a language shift to the nondominant hemisphere.[40]

Age-Related versus Etiologic Differences in Adult and Childhood-Acquired Aphasia

In the traditional view, the apparent better recovery from aphasia in the childhood aphasic versus the adult was attributed to the younger age of the child (and to the putative plasticity of the brain for which the younger age was a marker). Early research selected study groups on the basis of aphasia and combined heterogeneous pathologies in assessing outcome.[7] If subjects are accrued to a study because they show aphasic symptoms, any group of children will have an overrepresentation of traumatic and convulsive etiologies and an underrepresentation of vascular disorders in relation to an adult group. Differences in age at aphasia onset are thereby correlated with differences in etiology.

The consequences of the correlation between age and etiology have not been trivial for views of childhood-acquired aphasia. Because theories about acquired aphasia tend to be based on data from the most frequently described etiologies for any age group, the nature of adult-acquired aphasia has been shaped from arteritic stroke while that for childhood-acquired aphasia has been understood from head injury and convulsive disorders.

Childhood- and adulthood-acquired aphasias typically differ in both age and etiology,[31] and, indeed, recovery is different according to etiologic categories.[26] Perhaps the most important recent advance in understanding childhood-acquired aphasia has involved the specification of etiology to a greater extent than in an earlier research era, together with the increased recognition of the diversity of short- and long-term outcome as a function of etiology. One consequence of this recognition has been the increased attention in recent publications to the question of etiologic differences in childhood-acquired aphasia.[2,41] The analysis of childhood-acquired aphasia according to both etiology and age has challenged the assumption that language differences between childhood and adulthood aphasias are due to differences in age at onset of the aphasia.

PRINCIPAL ETIOLOGIES OF CHILDHOOD-ACQUIRED APHASIA

This section reviews the characteristics of the principal etiologies of childhood-acquired aphasia. For each etiology, some general issues are discussed, and, where sufficient evidence is available, cross-etiology comparisons are facilitated by Tables 16-1 through 16-4.

Seizure and Seizure-Related Disorders: The Landau-Kleffner Syndrome

Seizure disorders affect language function, and language symptoms have been observed both as part of clinical seizures[42] and as part of ictal speech automatisms. In addition, recurrent generalized seizures and medication may have diffuse effects that can confound the interpretation of otherwise focal lesions. The most studied aphasia-producing seizure disorder, however, is the LKS,[22] the characteristics of which are reviewed in Table 16-1.

Vascular Disorders

Vascular disorders involve interruptions to the blood supply within the brain as a result of occlusion (ischemic stroke) or rupture (hemorrhagic stroke). Most vascular diseases observed in the adult also occur in children, albeit with different base frequencies. Degenerative disorders like atherosclerosis are common in the middle-aged and elderly but rare in children, while vascular disorders associated with congenital heart disease occur principally in childhood[68] and may produce strokes by an embolism from the heart, from complications of heart surgery, or from hypoperfusion from prolonged hypotension. The characteristics of childhood-acquired aphasia from vascular diseases are reviewed in Table 16-2.

Traumatic Disorders

Traumatic head injury is a principal cause of childhood-acquired aphasia. Children exhibit a variety of aphasic symptoms and language disturbances after head injury.[76] The characteristics of childhood-acquired aphasia from traumatic disorders are reviewed in Table 16-3.

Brain Tumors

Brain tumors in children are not uncommonly associated with language disturbances.[11,79,95] For tumors above the tentorium, there are few data available on the type and localization of aphasia-producing lesions. Posterior fossa tumors occur with a high frequency in children relative to adults, with the result that this tumor type has provided the principal source of information about childhood brain tumors and language.[96] The characteristics of childhood-acquired aphasia from posterior fossa tumors are reviewed in Table 16-4.

Cancer Treatments

Radiotherapy and chemotherapy are often part of the treatment for such childhood cancers as acute lymphoblastic leukemia. Central nervous system (CNS) prophylaxis is known to cause structural and functional damage to the brain.[106,107] Children treated for cancer show a variety of deficits in speech and language,[108] including mutism, expressive aphasia, anomia, and problems with academic tasks. Much about these speech and language deficits remains to be understood, however, including the relation between degree of language impairment and prophylactic dose, the specificity of the language disorders within particular conditions, and the correlation between language function and neuropathology.

Infectious Conditions

Infectious diseases of the brain may involve viral, bacterial, spirochetal, and other microorganisms that infect the meninges (meningitis) and/or the brain (encephalitis). Infectious conditions are reported to produce childhood-acquired aphasia,[109] either as a primary effect of CNS involvement in conditions like herpes simplex encephalitis or as a secondary effect of sensorineural hearing loss in conditions such as bacterial meningitis or toxoplasmosis.

Studies of the effects of meningitis on language function have not provided clear information. While some studies have suggested that deficits in communication are an effect of meningitis, others have not.[109] Differences in research methods and assessment procedures for language may be responsible for the apparent inconsistency in results in studies of meningitis and language.

Commonly, aphasia is part of the morbidity of herpes simplex encephalitis,[15,29,40,110] even though antiviral medication in recent years has reduced the mortality associated with this condition. In the acute stage of encephalitis, there is a severe defect of comprehension similar to that seen in global aphasia following an initial period of mutism. The comprehension deficit involves a fluent aphasia with neologisms, semantic and phonemic paraphasias, stereotypies, and perseverations.[15,29,111] That a fluent form of aphasia is associated with herpes simplex encephalitis appears consistent with the fact that the herpesvirus has a tropism for the temporal lobes.[2]

Recovery from aphasia is especially poor after herpes simplex encephalitis.[109] Children with aphasia from this infection continue to show paraphasias and severe comprehension deficits in the recovery period as well as long-term difficulties in word finding.[15,29] The poor outcome may be related to the fact that, while some infections are unilateral, most have bilateral effects on the brain,[33] and also that the herpesvirus causes ne-

crotic brain lesions and significant neurologic sequelae.[112]

Hypoxic Disorders

Anoxia is a state in which the oxygen levels in the body fall below physiologic levels because oxygen supply is deficient or absent. Anoxia can come about from various causes—including severe hypotension, cardiac arrest, carbon monoxide poisoning, near-drowning, and suffocation—that involve a drop in the level of cerebral blood flow or the oxygen content of the blood. In turn, this results in cerebral anoxia, a prolonged period of which will produce permanent brain damage or anoxic encephalopathy, which is associated with a range of neurologic disorders, including language deficits.[113]

In children, anoxic encephalopathy produces short- and long-term language deficits. An initial mutism resolves into a variety of forms of language disorder, ranging from dysarthria, increased speech rate, problems initiating speech movements, and anomia.[29,114] Children who suffer a near-drowning episode show speech and language disorders that appear to recover in the longer term,[115,116] although that subset of children who initially present as comatose after a near-drowning episode may continue to be at risk for language disorders.[113]

The neuropathology of cerebral anoxia is fairly well known, although there have been few research studies in children that correlate language status and patterns of anoxic brain damage. In one study, subcortical lesions resulting from anoxic encephalopathy in adolescence have been related to motor speech disorders involving a progression from mutism to dysarthria.[114]

Metabolic Disorders

Systemic metabolic disorders that result in the accumulation of metabolites in the bloodstream cause structural alterations in the brain that may result in speech and language deficits. Some of the inborn errors of metabolism that have been shown to affect speech and language[117] include

Table 16-1
Childhood-acquired aphasia and the Landau-Kleffner syndrome

Definition

- Landau-Kleffner syndrome (LKS) involves acquired aphasia with convulsive disorder[22] occurring in normal children who acutely or progressively lose previously acquired language ability.
- A variety of typologies have been proposed.[43]
- It was originally claimed that pregnancy, birth, and early development were normal in LKS,[44] and, classically, LKS occurs after some period of normal language development. More recently, however, it has been found that a history of language pathology may precede the onset of language deterioration and loss,[45] with some 75 percent of cases exhibiting language disturbance before the aphasia.[46]
- Loss of language is associated with either clinical seizures (generalized, partial, partial complex, or absence) or with an electroencephalogram (EEG) showing unilateral or paroxysmal activity, sometimes more prominent in slow-wave sleep.[47]
- It has been argued that LKS overlaps with other epileptic conditions: rolandic epilepsy, electrical status epilepticus during sleep (ESES), and autistic regression and disintegrative disorder associated with unilateral or bilateral centrotemporal spike/spike-wave discharges.[21]

Core Features

- A severe comprehension defect[48] occurs, characteristically with severe verbal auditory agnosia, which may involve both common sounds (such as a dog barking, or a doorbell ringing) and words.[2,49]
- Epileptic seizures occur in 70 to 75 percent of cases.[50]
- Severe behavior disturbances occur in 75 percent of cases.[50] Long-term (>7 years) follow-up studies have reported mild behavior disturbance (hyperactivity, impulsivity, and oppositional behavior) that is chronologically linked with the language disturbances and follows their fluctuations.[51]
- Oral expression is typically poorer than written expression,[52,53] although severe impairment of written language and mathematical skills has been reported.[48]
- Neurologic examination is reported to be normal.[54]
- Nonverbal intelligence appears to be well preserved.[55]
- Half the published cases present first with comprehension disorder, the other half with seizures.[50]
- Most LKS patients have a mild form of epilepsy that responds to drug therapy.[56]
- There is a correlation between the aphasia and the seizure disorder, although both may fluctuate out of phase,[56] so that the relation is not obvious.[57]

Epidemiology, Demography, and Risk Factors

- Some 200 cases have been reported from 1957 to 1995.[50]
- The male : female ratio is 2 : 1.[50]
- There are currently no epidemiologic data in regard to geography, infectious disease, toxins, nutrition, or environmental exposures.[58]

Age-Related Factors

- Onset occurs from 3 to 8 years in 50 percent of cases.[50]
- Onset is rare after 8 years, although several cases have been reported with loss of language after age 9. Later-onset cases are more likely to have a primarily expressive aphasia with dysfluency and word-finding difficulties.[59]
- An age-prognosis relationship has been proposed, such that the younger the child, the poorer the recovery from the acquired aphasia, the reasoning being that newly acquired language skills are particularly vulnerable to bilateral brain pathology.[44] However, age-prognosis effects, such as the claim that recovery is worse with a diagnosis before age 5,[60] have not been replicated with more clearly defined case selection criteria.[51]

Table 16-1 (Continued)

Time-Related Factors

- Language impairments in LKS persist for months or even years.[49]
- Long-term language outcome is often poor. When studied 10 to 28 years after onset of acquired aphasia, more than half of an LKS sample continued to show language disorder.[47] In a long-term follow-up of at least 7 years—into the adolescent years—no individual with LKS fully recovered language.[51]
- Typically, seizures remit before adulthood and the aphasia subsides, although not necessarily in parallel.[44]
- The long-term outcome of the aphasia has been considered to be unpredictable with respect to medical history features,[47] despite the fact that both epilepsy and EEG abnormalities improve.[61] There is an unpredictable prognosis on an individual case basis, with a fluctuating course of remissions and exacerbations for both aphasia and EEG abnormalities.
- In a long-term (2- to 15-year) follow-up of LKS cases, it was found that, even when the EEG normalized in the long term, few individuals achieved normal language, and, further, that no individual with persisting EEG abnormalities recovered normal or near normal language.[46] Thus, persisting EEG abnormalities appear to be a risk factor for continuing aphasia.

Neuropathologic Substrate

- Initially, it was unclear whether the language disturbances in LKS was functional or due to an identifiable brain lesion. Proposals for the brain basis of LKS have ranged widely.
- It has been suggested that LKS might involve focal subclinical epileptogenic discharges involving the language areas. In this view, aphasic symptoms arise because persistent epileptic discharges cause functional ablation of the primary cortical language areas.[62]
- Because the course of the aphasia in LKS may be linked to the appearance and disappearance of ESES,[61] LKS has been considered related to ESES. However, few children with ESES have specific language disorders, and the characteristic EEG of ESES is infrequently found in LKS.[56]
- The mild to moderate elevation of cerebrospinal fluid proteins in some LKS cases[47,63] has been used to suggest a low-grade focal inflammation of the brain as the mechanism of LKS aphasia.[64]
- Cortical biopsies in some LKS cases have shown changes indicative of a slow virus infection, implying that a subacute viral encephalitis might produce both aphasia and seizures, either from a low-grade selective encephalitis[55] or a subchronic viral encephalitis affecting both hemispheres.[44]
- The finding of a positive autoimmune reaction to myelin during clinical deterioration of language in LKS patients has been used to suggest a disorder of myelin metabolism and to account for the positive effect of corticosteroids as immunosuppressive therapy.[65]
- Computed tomography and structural magnetic resonance imaging are typically normal.[64]
- Angiography has shown isolated arteritis of some branches of the carotid arteries, which implies that focal cerebral vasculitis may be involved in the pathogenesis of LKS.[64]
- Positron emission tomography has shown abnormal glucose utilization during sleep, with lower metabolic rates in subcortical than in cortical areas.[66]

Treatment

- There is no convincing evidence of empirically effective therapy.[58]
- Various drug treatments (antiepileptics, corticosteroids) have been tried, with success on an individual case basis.
- Under the view that focal vasculitis is responsible for LKS, calcium channel blockers have been proposed as a possible therapy.[64]
- Subpial resection has been proposed as therapy in some cases of LKS.
- Speech and language therapy has long been used in the rehabilitation of individuals with LKS, but there has been controversy about whether therapy should involve enhancing the residue of oral language; intensive training in the visual domain (gestures, communication boards, signing, computers); brief training in the visual domain with rapid transfer to oral language; or a more pragmatic, multimodal approach. A recent review[67] suggests that no single therapy program will work, that LKS patients are not like deaf individuals, and that any therapy will likely take several years to be effective.

Table 16-2
Language disturbances from vascular etiologies

Definition

- Acquired aphasia may be precipitated by a vascular brain lesion, occurring in children who acutely or progressively lose previously acquired language skills.
- Brain localization depends on the pathophysiology of the stroke. In children, most strokes are secondary to intracranial occlusive disease and are localized in the basal ganglia;[69] however, cortical vascular lesions in the left temporoparietal lobe that produce aphasia have been reported to occur from cerebral arteritis[39] and ruptured arteriovenous malformations.[70]

Core Features

- The type of aphasia depends on the localization of the lesion. Aphasia is fluent in form with lesions to the posterior left hemisphere cortical language areas[71] but nonfluent with predominantly subcortical pathology.[72,73]
- In the fluent form of aphasia, anomia, word finding deficits, paraphasias, and circumlocutions occur.[39,70]
- Reading and spelling may be relatively preserved with cortical lesions in the left-hemispheric posterior language areas, despite anomia,[39,70] which suggests poor phonologic representation of target words.
- Reading and writing disorders are common in both the acute and chronic stages of subcortical vascular lesions.[73]

Epidemiology, Demography, and Risk Factors

- Few cases have been reported.[71]

Age-Related Factors

- Onset at any point throughout childhood.

Time-Related Factors

- There is significant recovery from aphasic symptoms after vascular lesions,[73] although naming and word-finding problems persist into the chronic stage of recovery.[39,70]

Neuropathologic Substrate

- The laterality and localization of cortical lesions are similar to those of anomic aphasia in adults; damage occurs to the posterior left hemisphere cortical language areas.[39,70]
- Most subcortical vascular aphasias of childhood also appear to accord with the clinical-radiologic correlation observed in adults with subcortical aphasias.[72,73]
- Lesion laterality may be related to the pattern of impaired language comprehension. In a mixed group of brain-injured children—many with acquired lesions from vascular etiologies—children with left-sided lesions were unable to integrate pragmatic knowledge with syntactic constraints,[74] whereas those with right-sided lesions showed impairments in lexical-semantic and pragmatic knowledge.[74,75]

Treatment

- None specific.

Table 16-3

Language disturbances from head injury

Definition

- Acquired aphasia may occur after a head injury, typically a closed head injury.

- The aphasia is precipitated by injury to the brain, which includes both immediate impact injury (contusions, diffuse axonal damage) and secondary brain damage involving intracranial events (hematomas, brain swelling, infections, subarachnoid hemorrhages, hydrocephalus) and extracranial factors (hypoxia, hypotension).

- Focal brain contusions are common in the frontal and temporal lobes after head injury, whether or not the head has been struck in these particular regions.[77]

Core Features

- Children with acquired aphasia from head injury show a variety of aphasic symptoms in the acute stage.[7,78,79]

- Frank aphasia and adultlike aphasic syndromes occur infrequently.[76]

- Mutism or reduced verbal output and anomia are common in the short term after head injury.[76,80,81]

Epidemiology, Demography, and Risk Factors

- Head injury is the leading cause of childhood death in North America,[82] with an incidence of 200 per 10,000 per year.[83] Eighty percent of survivors of severe childhood head injury have learning difficulties, including problems in language-related skills.[84]

Age-Related Factors

- Onset occurs at any point throughout childhood.

- A younger age at onset may be associated with more deficits in expressive language in the recovery phase, around 8 months postinjury.[85]

- Injury before age 7 versus injury at an older age is associated with more long-term difficulties in understanding the linguistic-symbolic nature of facial expressions, in metalinguistic awareness, and in comprehension monitoring.[86,87]

Time-Related Factors

- Aphasic symptoms resolve over time in children with acquired aphasia from head injury.[7,78,79]

- Anomia and reduced verbal fluency are consistent deficits after childhood head injury, even 18 months postinjury.[37,88–90]

- One group of persisting problems for children after head injury involve what have been termed nonaphasic language disorders with nonliteral language, discourse, and inferencing.[91] In the long term, head-injured children show a variety of discourse deficits, not so much in the gross aspects of communication[92,93] as in telling a story,[27] using and understanding idiomatic or ambiguous statements, making knowledge-based inferences in social scripts, and producing speech acts appropriate to particular contexts.[28]

- In the long term, children with head injury have difficulty in comprehension–monitoring tasks requiring them to evaluate statements that violate semantic selection rules, grammatical structures, or pragmatic constraints.[86]

- In the long term, children who have had a head injury at a younger rather than an older age are poor at referential communication tasks requiring them to judge the relevance of an instruction, suggesting poor metacognitive function.[86]

- Children with head injury have long-term difficulties in understanding how language is used to serve social-communicative goals that include emotional deception. These children have difficulty understanding the linguistic-symbolic nature of facial displays, such as those involved in the deceptive expression of emotion (e.g., they have difficulty selecting a neutral or happy expression when told that a story character is feeling sad but has a reason for hiding that feeling from another character).[87]

- Academic abilities in language-related areas are poor in the long-term after childhood head injury.[80,81]

- Vocabulary tests may deteriorate with increasing time, because head-injured children are unable to acquire new language-based knowledge at an age-appropriate rate.[29]

Neuropathologic Substrate

- The degree of residual language impairment appears to be related to the severity of the head injury,[5,81] and children with mild head injury recover functional language faster than do children with more severe injuries.[90]

- The clinical-pathologic correlation of language disorders in childhood head injury is poorly understood, particularly as it concerns contusional damage to the frontal and temporal lobes. However, it is known that frontal contusions and left-sided contusions in children and adolescents with head injury are variously associated with problems in understanding the linguistic-symbolic nature of facial expressions, in metalinguistic awareness, and in oral comprehension monitoring.[86,87]

- Early frontal lobe injury particularly affects nonaphasic discourse disorders in the long term after a childhood head injury,[86,87] which is consistent with the importance of an intact frontal lobe system for the development of social awareness and social cognition.[94]

Treatment

- None specific.

Table 16-4
Language disturbances after posterior fossa brain tumors

Definition

- Acquired aphasia occurs secondary to astrocytomas, medulloblastomas, and ependymomas of the cerebellum, fourth ventricle, and/or brainstem, occurring in children who acutely or progressively lose previously acquired language skills.

Core Features

- Mutism occurs commonly in acute-stage cerebellar lesions of childhood.[97,98]
- The mutism is not tumor-specific in that it involves various tumor pathologies.[97]
- A syndrome of mutism and subsequent dysarthria (MSD) has been identified,[99] not obviously related to cerebellar ataxia but characterized by a complete but transient loss of speech resolving into dysarthria.
- Analysis of the dysarthria of posterior fossa tumors in children suggests that it shares some of the features of adult dysarthria—namely, imprecise consonants, articulatory breakdowns, prolonged phonemes, prolonged intervals, slow rate of speech, lack of volume control, harsh voice, pitch breaks, variable pitch, and explosive onsets.[100]
- There appears to be no adultlike pattern of fluent or nonfluent aphasia in children treated for posterior fossa tumors.[100] However, children with treated posterior fossa tumors, including medulloblastomas, show mild language impairments in oral expression and auditory comprehension.[101]

Epidemiology, Demography, and Risk Factors

- As of 1994, a total of 36 cases of MSD have been reported.[99]
- In children with posterior fossa tumors, risk factors for the development of MSD are hydrocephalus at the time of tumor presentation, ventricular localization of the tumor, and postsurgical edema of the pontine tegmentum.[99]

Age-Related Factors

- Some 90 percent of MSD patients are less than 10 years of age, and the condition has been described in children as young as age 2.[99]

Time-Related Factors

- In cases of MSD, recovery of dysarthria to normal speech seems to be related to the recovery of complex movements of the mouth and tongue.[99]
- A range of short- and long-term intellectual, neuropsychological, and academic difficulties have been identified in children with posterior fossa tumors,[102] including language-related difficulties. Academic failure occurs frequently in survivors of posterior fossa tumors, and the rate is higher in survivors of medulloblastoma than in survivors of cerebellar astrocytomas.[103,104]

Neuropathologic Substrate

- Mutism may occur with a midline location of the tumor combined with postoperative complications that involve destruction of the midline roof structures and penetration of the peduncles and/or lateral wall or ventricular floor parenchyma.[97]
- Mutism occurs particularly with posterior fossa tumors located in the midline or vermis of the cerebellum, and with tumors invading both cerebellar hemispheres or the deep nuclei of the cerebellum.[97,98]
- Isolated lesions in cerebellar structures are not sufficient to produce MSD. An additional ventricular location of the tumor and adherence to the dorsal brainstem are necessary, an idea supported by the frequent occurrence of pyramidal and eye-movement signs in children with MSD.[99]
- Localization of the brainstem dysfunction in MSD appears to be rostral to the medulla oblongata and caudal to the mesencephalon.[99]
- It has been proposed that the mutism of MSD is related to bilateral involvement of the dentate nuclei and that the subsequent dysarthric speech represents a recovering cerebellar mechanism.[105]

Treatment

- None specific to the language disorders, only the appropriate course of tumor treatment.

phenylketonuria (an absence of the liver enzyme phenylalanine), galactosemia (an inability to utilize the sugars galactose and lactose because of disordered carbohydrate metabolism), and Wilson disease (a progressive degenerative disorder of the brain and liver resulting from inability to process dietary copper). Congenital hypothyroidism also affects intellectual functions, including language.[117] In addition to these relatively direct metabolic effects on the brain, other hereditary metabolic diseases such as homocystinuria, a disorder of amino acid metabolism, may cause vascular occlusive disease when enzyme deficiencies damage blood vessels, leading to thrombosis and ischemic stroke.[68] The specificity of speech and language disorders and the relation between language and neuropathology are poorly understood in these various metabolic conditions.

CONCLUSIONS AND FUTURE DIRECTIONS

In studies conducted over the last 15 years, separation of the principal etiologic subgroups, together with fuller descriptions of the language profiles associated with these etiologies, has significantly advanced our understanding of childhood-acquired aphasia. Descriptive studies of etiologies have provided the basis of more systematic knowledge about childhood-acquired aphasia: specifically, about the language symptoms and type of aphasia, the demographic and incidence factors, and the course of recovery or resolution of language symptoms as evidenced by longitudinal evaluations. A better information base has made it possible to consider some core issues about childhood-acquired aphasia, including its symptom spectrum, its similarities and differences with adult-acquired aphasia, its neuropathologic substrate, and the factors that promote or retard abatement of aphasic symptoms and recovery of language function.

Children show a wide range of language symptoms after brain damage that precipitates acquired aphasia, and there is no single profile of language loss in the acquired aphasic conditions

of childhood. Various profiles of language loss are associated with different etiologies of childhood-acquired aphasias, ranging from the mutism of extensive cerebellar lesions through nonaphasic language disorders, pragmatic and social discourse impairments commonly observed in the long term after traumatic lesions.

While the types of symptoms manifest in the acute phase of childhood-acquired aphasia often differ according to etiology, it is also the case that some acquired aphasic symptoms are common to a range of etiologies while others occur in a more limited number of conditions. Many types of childhood-acquired aphasia, indeed, many types of brain injury in children,[118] resolve to anomic and word-finding deficits. The severe auditory agnosia commonly associated with LKS, however, has not been reported in other conditions.

Age-Related Issues: Similarities and Differences between Children of Different Ages and between Children and Adults

One age-related issue concerns the difference among children with acquired aphasia in relation to age at onset of language disorder. Language disturbances involving the use and understanding of mental states and social discourse are more common with an earlier rather than a later age at head injury.[86,87]

A second age-related issue concerns the consequences for language-related skills of the developmental timing of brain injury. If the onset of epilepsy coincides with beginning to read and write, it will impair the acquisition of written language.[42] In comparison with later prophylaxis, earlier treatment for acute lymphoblastic leukemia in childhood results in less utilization of phonemically based spelling strategies and, by inference, poorer phonemic awareness.[119] From data such as these, it has been proposed that the skills that are in a period of active development but not yet consolidated are more vulnerable to disruption than either less or more consolidated skills.

Aphasic mutism is of interest under the above model of heightened vulnerability for skills that are in the course of acquisition but not yet automatized. Mutism occurs more commonly in children than in adults, variously from a range of etiologies that include the acute phase of vascular, epileptogenic, traumatic, tumorigenic, and infectious conditions. The ubiquity of aphasic mutism in childhood-acquired aphasia over the age range of childhood suggests that the initiation of speech is a volatile language function during childhood, one that is easily disrupted by a range of aphasia-precipitating forms of brain damage; it suggests further that the initiation of speech is imperfectly automatized throughout much of childhood.

An important age-related issue concerns similarities and differences between childhood- and adulthood-acquired aphasia. Children and adults show more similarities in aphasic patterns than was earlier recognized. This is not to argue, however, that the aphasic symptoms and patterns are identical in children and adults; for one reason, the base frequencies of symptoms like mutism are higher in children than in adults, whereas the base frequencies of symptoms like neologisms are lower in children than in adults.

The neuroanatomy of childhood-acquired aphasia is both similar to and different from that of adulthood-acquired aphasia.[17] Only by comparing the same etiologies in childhood and in adulthood can the effect of age itself be evaluated; when the same etiology is compared in childhood and in adulthood, many language deficits prove to be similar. In children as well as in adults, a lesion in the left-hemispheric posterior cortical language areas produces a fluent aphasia and impaired comprehension;[95] specifically, the correlation between lesion site on computed tomography (CT) and aphasia in children duplicates the anatomic-clinical correlation in adults.[17] In accordance with these results, age does not predict recovery from aphasic symptoms when etiology is constant.[30]

To be sure, aphasic symptoms are not identical in children and adults with the same brain damage. Unlike adults, for example, children do not suffer speech disturbances from damage to the superior paravermal cortical regions associated with posterior fossa tumors.[99] It is also possible that differences in base rate and frequency of aphasic symptoms involve different underlying

neuropathologic substrates in children and adults. The neuroanatomy of superficially similar symptoms may prove to be different in children and adults in important ways.

The differences between acquired aphasia in children and in adults, once thought to concern short-term aphasic symptoms, now appear to relate more to long-term language function. With increasing time since aphasia, adult language improves, albeit at variable rates. Time does not always improve language function after childhood-acquired aphasia. Aphasic children may show an increasing inability to accrue a new verbal knowledge base, which results in chronic problems in reading and vocabulary development.[29,73]

Time-Related Issues and Their Importance for Theoretical Accounts and Taxonomies of Childhood-Acquired Aphasia

What seems to discriminate among the different etiologies of childhood-acquired aphasia is the time course of aphasic symptoms and recovery of language function. Aphasic symptoms arising from head injury resolve more quickly than do symptoms from infectious and vascular etiologies. Granted that abatement of symptoms varies according to etiology,[26] a continuing task in understanding childhood-acquired aphasia is to specify the time course of symptoms within conditions.

A better understanding of the time course and pattern of preserved and disrupted language skills is essential to establishing a more theoretically grounded account of the childhood-acquired aphasias. This is also relevant to the question of a taxonomy of childhood-acquired aphasic conditions.

At present, there are few plausible theories of the language disturbances underlying the principal forms of childhood-acquired aphasia. Certainly, no single theory is likely to be adequate to cover all the different etiologic manifestations of childhood aphasia. Even within a particular etiology, any theory must account for the vagaries of symptoms throughout the time course of the aphasia. For example, central receptive deficits have been proposed to be primary in LKS,[60] but a closer analysis of the time course in LKS cases with more slowly developing symptoms reveals a predominantly motor aphasia evident during a language deterioration phase,[45] which seems inconsistent with the idea of an exclusively receptive disorder at the core of this condition. Only by understanding patterns of language deficits that change over time is it possible to provide a theoretically motivated account of what distinguishes impaired from preserved language skills in childhood-acquired aphasia.

The neuroanatomy of symptom patterns over time is likely to provide important clues to the underlying mechanisms of language loss and hence to be part of any theory of acquired aphasia. It has been claimed that subcortical lesions in children may have similar long-term effects to cortical lesions; for example, one interpretation of the mutism from subcortical vascular lesions is that it arises from a transient frontal diaschisis secondary to subcortical damage.[73] Correlations between language and neuroimaging to allow a detailed comparison of cortical and subcortical lesions producing acquired aphasia have not yet been reported.

At present, the working hypothesis must be that the same acquired aphasic symptom may be produced by more than one neural mechanism. In support of this, the time course of resolution of aphasic mutism appears to be different with supratentorial and subtentorial lesions. In the case of posterior fossa tumors, the mutism resolves to dysarthria; with vascular subcortical lesions, however, the resolution of the mutism does not appear to include dysarthric symptoms.[72] This suggests a role for the cerebellum in the initiation and programming of speech, perhaps in keeping with recent concepts of its broader role in higher cognitive functions, including the timing of nonautomatized language operations.[120]

Without a theory of language disruption grounded in the time course of symptoms and long-term language function, there can be no workable taxonomy for childhood-acquired aphasia and its symptom patterns. For the most part, the loose descriptive taxonomy that exists among etiologies is based simply on frequency of reporting and aphasic symptoms for particular etiologies, with a condition like LKS somewhat over-represented in publications on childhood-acquired aphasia in relation to its frequency of occurrence.[2]

At present, neither the classic adult taxonomy of aphasia nor existing childhood language classification systems are adequate for describing childhood-acquired aphasia. When childhood-acquired aphasia cases are coded according to a taxonomy of adult aphasia,[121] some 30 to 50 percent of cases cannot be classified.[16,20,122,123] In fact, the majority of children with acquired aphasia cannot be classified in either the Goodglass adult taxonomy or a taxonomy devised for pediatric conditions.[124]

Existing taxonomies of childhood-acquired aphasia still seem to rely largely on models of adult aphasia rather than on cognitive-developmental paradigms of normal language development. Perhaps a productive approach to the issue of taxonomy would be one that used theory-driven paradigms of normal language development rather than a priori taxonomies. In recent reviews of childhood-acquired aphasia, there has been a more explicit awareness of the need for paradigms of normal language development.[54] At the same time, it has become apparent that any such paradigms must be complex and expressed as patterns of acquisition over very long time spans, because there are wide individual differences in the rate, strategy, and style of language acquisition in normally developing children, and brain damage affects language acquisition patterns in a number of different ways.[125]

Neuropathology of Language Disorders

One reason for the dearth of workable taxonomies of childhood-acquired aphasic conditions must be the limited number of clinical-pathologic correlations that would allow comparisons of patterns of neuropathology underlying language disorders. An important objective in studies of childhood-acquired aphasia has been to contrast the pathologic processes that produce acquired aphasia with those that do not.[33] Only noninvasive forms of neuroimaging make possible this endeavor; in recent years, structural and functional neuroimaging has provided information about the temporal and spatial extent of brain pathology, and hence information about the neuropathologic substrates of childhood-acquired aphasia. Of direct relevance are findings from functional neuroimaging studies suggesting what had long been suspected, that areas of brain dysfunction are much larger than the areas of structural lesion in some forms of aphasia-producing childhood vascular lesions.[126]

Studies that correlate language status with neuroimaging are able to identify the factors that produce poor recovery of language. Three such factors have been suggested: an infectious etiology, poor verbal comprehension, and involvement of Wernicke's area.[30] As a larger data base of such studies is accrued, it will become easier to understand the mechanism of recovery in cases of childhood-acquired aphasia.[10]

Because detailed structural and functional neuroimaging studies are of relatively recent origin, their potential value in shaping a taxonomy of childhood-acquired aphasia has not yet been exploited. It seems likely that the clinicopathologic correlation between language and neuroimaging will ground any taxonomy of childhood-acquired aphasic conditions.

ACKNOWLEDGMENTS

The author's research described in this paper was supported by project grants from the Ontario Mental Health Foundation and the Physicians' Services Incorporated Foundation. I thank Marcia Barnes for her critical comments on the text and Tamara Bashirullah-Abousleman for assistance with preparation of the manuscript.

REFERENCES

1. Collignon R, Hécaen H, Angelergues R: A propos de 12 cas d'aphasie acquise de l'enfant. *Acta Neurol Belg* 68:245–277, 1968.
2. Paquier P, Van Dongen HR: Current trends in acquired childhood aphasia: An introduction. *Aphasiology* 7:421–440, 1993.
3. Dennis M, Barnes MA: Developmental aspects of neuropsychology: Childhood, in Zaidel D (ed): *Handbook of Perception and Cognition: Neuropsychology*. New York: Academic Press, 1994, pp 219–246.
4. Freud S: Infantile cerebral paralysis (trans by LA Russin, 1968). Coral Gables, FL: University of Miami, 1897.
5. Assal G, Campiche R: Aphasie et troubles du langage chez l'enfant apres contusion cerebrale. *Neurochirurgie* 19(suppl 4):399–406, 1973.
6. Byers RK, McLean WT: Etiology and course of certain hemiplegias with aphasia in childhood. *Pediatrics* 29:376–383, 1962.
7. Guttmann E: Aphasia in children. *Brain* 65:205–219, 1942.
8. Alajouanine TH, Lhermitte F: Acquired aphasia in children. *Brain* 88:653–662, 1965.
9. Hécaen H: Acquired aphasia in children and the ontogenesis of hemispheric functional specialization. *Brain Lang* 3:114–134, 1976.
10. Satz P: Symptom pattern and recovery outcome in childhood aphasia: A methodological and theoretical critique, in Martins IP, Castro-Caldas A, Van Dongen HR, Van Hout A (eds): *Acquired Aphasia in Children*. Dordrecht, The Netherlands: Kluwer Academic, 1991, pp 95–114.
11. Van Dongen HR, Paquier P: Fluent aphasia in children, in Martins IP, Castro-Caldas A, Van Dongen HR, Van Hout A (eds): *Acquired Aphasia in Children*. Dordrecht, The Netherlands: Kluwer Academic, 1991, pp 125–141.
12. Visch-Brink EG, Van de Sandt-Koenderman M: The occurrence of paraphasias in the spontaneous speech of children with an acquired aphasia. *Brain Lang* 23:258–271, 1984.
13. Van Hout A: Characteristics of language in acquired aphasia in children, in Martins IP, Castro-Caldas A, Van Dongen HR, Van Hout A (eds): *Acquired Aphasia in Children*. Dordrecht, The Netherlands: Kluwer Academic, 1991, pp 117–124.
14. Woods BT, Teuber HL: Changing patterns of childhood aphasia. *Ann Neurol* 3:273–280, 1978.
15. Van Hout A, Evrard P, Lyon G: On the positive semiology of acquired aphasia in children. *Dev Med Child Neurol* 27:231–241, 1985.
16. Van Dongen HR, Loonen MCB, Van Dongen KJ: Anatomical basis for acquired fluent aphasia in children. *Ann Neurol* 17:306–309, 1985.
17. Cranberg LD, Filley CM, Hart EJ, Alexander MP: Acquired aphasia in childhood: Clinical and CT investigations. *Neurology* 37:1165–1172, 1987.
18. Hynd GW, Semrud-Clikeman M, Lorys AR, et al: Brain morphology in developmental dyslexia and

attention deficit disorder/hyperactivity. *Arch Neurol* 47:919–926, 1990.

19. Makino A, Soga T, Obayashi M, et al: Cortical blindness caused by acute general cerebral swelling. *Surg Neurol* 29:393–400, 1988.

20. Paquier P, Saerens J, Parizel PM, et al: Acquired reading disorder similar to pure alexia in a child with ruptured arteriovenous malformation. *Aphasiology* 3:667–676, 1989.

21. Rapin I: Acquired aphasia in children. *J Child Neurol* 10:267–270, 1995.

22. Landau WM, Kleffner FR: Syndrome of acquired aphasia with convulsive disorder in children. *Neurology* 7:523–530, 1957.

23. Paquier P, Van Dongen HR: Acquired childhood aphasia: A rarity? *Aphasiology* 7(suppl 5):417–419, 1993.

24. Ikeda M, Tanabe H, Yamada K, et al: A case of acquired childhood aphasia with evolution of global aphasia into transcortical sensory aphasia. *Aphasiology* 7(suppl 5):497–502, 1993.

25. Satz P, Bullard-Bates C: Acquired aphasia in children, in Sarno MT (ed): *Acquired Aphasia.* San Diego, CA: Academic Press, 1981, pp 399–426.

26. Loonen MCB, Van Dongen HR: Acquired childhood aphasia: Outcome one year after onset, in Martins IP, Castro-Caldas A, Van Dongen HR, Van Hout A (eds): *Acquired Aphasia in Children.* Dordrecht, The Netherlands: Kluwer Academic, 1991, pp 185–200.

27. Chapman SB, Culhane KA, Levin HS, et al: Narrative discourse after closed head injury in children and adolescents. *Brain Lang* 43:42–65, 1992.

28. Dennis M, Barnes MA: Knowing the meaning, getting the point, bridging the gap, and carrying the message: Aspects of discourse following closed head injury in childhood and adolescence. *Brain Lang* 3:203–229, 1990.

29. Cooper JA, Flowers CR: Children with a history of acquired aphasia: Residual language and academic impairments. *J Speech Hear Disord* 52:251–262, 1987.

30. Martins IP, Ferro JM: Recovery of acquired aphasia in children. *Aphasiology* 6(suppl 4):431–438, 1992.

31. Van Hout A: Outcome of acquired aphasia in childhood: Prognosis factors, in Martins IP, Castro-Caldas A, Van Dongen HR, Van Hout A (eds): *Acquired Aphasia in Children.* Dordrecht, The Netherlands: Kluwer Academic, 1991, pp 163–169.

32. Cross JA, Ozanne AE: Acquired childhood aphasia: Assessment and treatment, in Murdoch BE (ed): *Acquired Neurological Speech/Language Disorders in Childhood.* London: Taylor & Francis, 1990, pp 66–123.

33. Woods BT: Patient selection in studies of aphasia acquired in childhood, in Martins IP, Castro-Caldas A, Van Dongen HR, Van Hout A (eds): *Acquired Aphasia in Children.* Dordrecht, The Netherlands: Kluwer Academic, 1991, pp 27–34.

34. Taveras JM, Wood EH: *Diagnostic Neuroradiology,* 2d ed. Baltimore: Williams & Wilkins, 1976, vol 1.

35. Seron X: L'aphasie de l'enfant. *Enfance* 24:249–270, 1977.

36. Carter RL, Hohenegger MK, Satz P: Aphasia and speech organization in children. *Science* 218:797–799, 1982.

37. Hécaen H: Acquired aphasia in children: Revisited. *Neuropsychologia* 21:581–587, 1983.

38. Satz P, Lewis R: Acquired aphasia in children, in Blanken G, Dittmann J, Grimm H, Marshall JC, Wallesch C-W (eds): *Linguistic Disorders and Pathologies: An International Handbook.* Berlin: Walter de Gruyter, 1993, pp 646–659.

39. Dennis M: Strokes in childhood: I. Communicative intent, expression, and comprehension after left hemisphere arteriopathy in a right-handed nine-year-old, in Rieber R (ed): *Language Development and Aphasia in Children.* New York: Academic Press, 1980, pp 45–67.

40. Martins IP, Ferro JM: Recovery from aphasia and lesion size in the temporal lobe, in Martins IP, Castro-Caldas A, Van Dongen HR, Van Hout A (eds): *Acquired Aphasia in Children.* Dordrecht, The Netherlands: Kluwer Academic, 1991, pp 171–184.

41. Murdoch BE: *Acquired Speech and Language Disorders: A Neuroanatomical and Functional Neurological Approach.* London: Chapman & Hall, 1990.

42. Deonna T, Davidoff V, Roulet E: Isolated disturbance of written language acquisition as an initial symptom of epileptic aphasia in a 7-year old child: A 3-year follow-up study. *Aphasiology* 7(suppl 5):441–450, 1993.

43. Deonna T, Beaumanoir A, Gaillard F, Assal G: Acquired aphasia in childhood with seizure disorder: A heterogeneous syndrome. *Neuropadiatrie* 8:263–273, 1977.

44. Lou HC, Brandt S, Bruhn P: Aphasia and epilepsy in childhood. *Acta Neurol Scand* 56:46–54, 1977.

45. Marien P, Saerens J, Verslegers W, et al: Some

controversies about type and nature of aphasic symptomatology in Landau-Kleffner's syndrome: A case study. *Acta Neurol Belg* 93:183–203, 1993.

46. Soprano AM, Garcia EF, Caraballo R, Fejerman N: Acquired epileptic aphasia: Neuropsychologic follow-up of 12 patients. *Pediatr Neurol* 11(suppl 3):230–235, 1994.

47. MantoVani JF, Landau WM: Acquired aphasia with convulsive disorder. *Neurology* 30:524–529, 1980.

48. Papagno C, Basso A: Impairment of written language and mathematical skills in a case of Landau-Kleffner syndrome. *Aphasiology* 7:451–461, 1993.

49. Cooper JA, Ferry PC: Acquired auditory verbal agnosia and seizures in childhood. *J Speech Hear Disord* 43:176–184, 1978.

50. Appleton RE: The Landau-Kleffner syndrome. *Arch Dis Child* 72:386–387, 1995.

51. Dugas M, Gerard CL, Franc S, Sagar D: Natural history, course and prognosis of the Landau and Kleffner syndrome, in Martins IP, Castro-Caldas A, Van Dongen HR, Van Hout A (eds): *Acquired Aphasia in Children*. Dordrecht, The Netherlands: Kluwer Academic, 1991, pp 263–277.

52. Aicardi J: Syndrome of acquired aphasia with seizure disorder: Epileptic aphasia, Landau-Kleffner syndrome, and verbal auditory agnosia with convulsive disorder, in Aicardi J (ed): *Epilepsy in Children*. New York: Raven Press, 1986, pp 176–182.

53. Dugas M, Masson M, Le Heuzey MF, Regnier N: Aphasie "acquise" de l'enfant avec epilepsie (syndrome de Landau et Kleffner): Douze observations personnelles. *Rev Neurol* 138:755–780, 1982.

54. Martins IP: Introduction, in Martins IP, Castro-Caldas A, Van Dongen HR, Van Hout A (eds): *Acquired Aphasia in Children*. Dordrecht, The Netherlands: Kluwer Academic, 1991, pp 3–12.

55. Worster-Drought C: An unusual form of acquired aphasia in children. *Dev Med Child Neurol* 13:563–571, 1971.

56. Genton P, Guerrini R: The Landau-Kleffner syndrome or acquired aphasia with convulsive disorder. *Arch Neurol* 50:1009, 1993.

57. Van Dongen HR, De Wijngaert E, Wennekes MJ: The Landau-Kleffner syndrome: Diagnostic considerations, in Martins IP, Castro-Caldas A, Van Dongen HR, Van Hout A (eds): *Acquired Aphasia in Children*. Dordrecht, The Netherlands: Kluwer Academic, 1991, pp 253–261.

58. Landau WM: Landau-Kleffner syndrome. *Arch Neurol* 49:353, 1992.

59. Gerard C-L, Dugas M, Valdois S, Franc S, Lecendreux M: Landau-Kleffner syndrome diagnosed after 9 years of age: Another Landau-Kleffner syndrome? *Aphasiology* 7:463–473, 1993.

60. Bishop DVM: Age of onset and outcome in "acquired aphasia with convulsive disorder." *Dev Med Child Neurol* 27:705–712, 1985.

61. Paquier PF, Van Dongen HR, Loonen CB: The Landau-Kleffner syndrome or "acquired aphasia with convulsive disorder." *Arch Neurol* 49:354–359, 1992.

62. Shoumaker RD, Bennett DR, Bray PF, Curless RG: Clinical and EEG manifestations of an unusual aphasic syndrome in children. *Neurology* 24:10–16, 1974.

63. McKinney W, McGreal DA: An aphasic syndrome in children. *Can Med Assoc J* 110:637–639, 1974.

64. Pascual-Castroviejo I, Lopez Martin VL, Martinez Bermejo AM, Perez Higueras AP: Is cerebral arteritis the cause of the Landau-Kleffner syndrome? Four cases in childhood with angiographic study. *Can J Neurol Sci* 19:46–52, 1992.

65. Nevsimalova S, Tauberova A, Doutlik S, et al: A role of autoimmunity in the etiopathogenesis of Landau-Kleffner syndrome? *Brain Dev* 14:342–345, 1992.

66. Maquet P, Hirsch E, Dive D, et al: Cerebral glucose utilization during sleep in Landau-Kleffner syndrome: A PET study. *Epilepsia* 31:778–783, 1990.

67. De Wijngaert E, Gommers K: Language rehabilitation in the Landau-Kleffner syndrome: Considerations and approaches. *Aphasiology* 7(suppl 5):475–480, 1993.

68. Ozanne AE, Murdoch BE: Acquired childhood aphasia: Neuropathology, linguistic characteristics and prognosis, in Murdoch BE (ed): *Acquired Neurological Speech/Language Disorders in Childhood*. London: Taylor & Francis, 1990, pp 1–65.

69. Zimmerman RA, Bilaniuk LT, Packer RJ, et al: Computed tomographic-arteriographic correlates in acute basal ganglionic infarction in childhood. *Neuroradiology* 24:241–248, 1983.

70. Hynd GW, Leathem J, Semrud-Clikeman M, et al: Anomic aphasia in childhood. *J Child Neurol* 10:189–293, 1995.

71. Klein SK, Masur D, Farber K, et al: Fluent aphasia in children: Definition and natural history. *J Child Neurol* 7:50–59, 1992.

72. Aram DM, Rose DF, Rekate HI, Whitaker HA:

Acquired capsular/striatal aphasia in childhood. *Arch Neurol* 40:614–617, 1983.

73. Martins IP, Ferro JM: Acquired childhood aphasia: A clinicoradiological study of 11 stroke patients. *Aphasiology* 7(suppl 5):489–495, 1993.

74. Eisele JA: Selective deficits in language comprehension following early left and right hemisphere damage, in Martins IP, Castro-Caldas A, Van Dongen HR, Van Hout A (eds): *Acquired Aphasia in Children*. Dordrecht, The Netherlands: Kluwer, 1991, pp 225–238.

75. Eisele JA, Aram DM: Differential effects of early hemisphere damage on lexical comprehension and production. *Aphasiology* 7:513–523, 1993.

76. Jordan FM: Speech and language disorders following childhood closed head injury, in Murdoch BE (ed): *Acquired Neurological Speech/Language Disorders in Childhood*. London: Taylor & Francis, 1990, pp 124–147.

77. Ommaya AK, Grubb RL, Naumann RA: Coup and contrecoup injury: Observations on the mechanics of visible brain injuries in the rhesus monkey. *J Neurosurg* 35:503–516, 1971.

78. Van Dongen HR, Loonen MCB: Factors related to prognosis of acquired aphasia in children. *Cortex* 13:131–136, 1977.

79. Loonen MCB, Van Dongen HR: Acquired childhood aphasia: Outcome one year after onset. *Arch Neurol* 47:1324–1328, 1990.

80. Ewing-Cobbs L, Fletcher JM, Landry SH, Levin HS: Language disorders after pediatric head injury, in Darby JK (ed): *Speech and Language Evaluation in Neurology: Childhood Disorders*. San Diego, CA: Grune & Stratton, 1985, pp 97–111.

81. Ewing-Cobbs L, Fletcher JM, Levin HS, Eisenberg HM: Language functions following closed head injury in children and adolescents. *J Clin Exp Neuropsychol* 5:575–592, 1987.

82. Goldstein FC, Levin HS: Epidemiology of pediatric closed head injury: Incidence, clinical characteristics, and risk factors. *J Learn Disabil* 20:518–525, 1987.

83. Annegers JF: The epidemiology of head trauma in children, in Shapiro K (ed): *Pediatric Head Trauma*. Mt. Kisco, NY: Futura, 1983, pp 1–10.

84. Ewing-Cobbs L, Iovino I, Fletcher JM, et al: Academic achievement following traumatic brain injury in children and adolescents (abstr). *J Clin Exp Neuropsychol* 13:93, 1991.

85. Ewing-Cobbs L, Miner ME, Fletcher JM, Levin HS: Intellectual, motor, and language sequelae following closed head injury in infants and preschoolers. *J Pediatr Psychol* 14:531–547, 1989.

86. Dennis M, Barnes MA, Donnelly RE, et al: Appraising and managing knowledge: Metacognitive skills after childhood head injury. *Dev Neuropsychol* 12:77–103, 1996.

87. Dennis M, Wilkinson M, Humphreys RP: How children with head injury represent real and deceptive emotion in short narratives. *Brain Lang* 1996. In press.

88. Jordan FM, Ozanne AE, Murdoch BE: Long-term speech and language disorders subsequent to closed head injury in children. *Brain Inj* 2:179–185, 1988.

89. Jordan FM, Ozanne AE, Murdoch BE: Performance of closed head injury children on a naming task. *Brain Inj* 4:27–32, 1990.

90. Jordan FM, Murdoch BE: A prospective study of the linguistic skills of children with closed-head injuries. *Aphasiology* 7:503–512, 1993.

91. McDonald S: Viewing the brain sideways? Frontal versus right hemisphere explanations of nonaphasic language disorders. *Aphasiology* 7:535–549, 1993.

92. Campbell TF, Dollaghan CA: Expressive language recovery in severely brain-injured children and adolescents. *J Speech Hear Disord* 55:567–586, 1990.

93. Jordan FM, Murdoch BE: Linguistic status following closed head injury in children: A follow-up study. *Brain Inj* 4:147–154, 1990.

94. Grattan LM, Eslinger PJ: Frontal lobe damage in children and adults: A comparative review. *Dev Neuropsychol* 7:283–326, 1991.

95. Martins IP, Ferro JM: Type of aphasia and lesions' localization, in Martins IP, Castro-Caldas A, Van Dongen HR, Van Hout A (eds): *Acquired Aphasia in Children*. Dordrecht, The Netherlands: Kluwer Academic, 1991, pp 143–159.

96. Hudson LJ: Speech and language disorders in childhood brain tumours, in Murdoch BE (ed): *Acquired Neurological Speech/Language Disorders in Childhood*. London: Taylor & Francis, 1990, pp 245–268.

97. Humphreys RP: Mutism after posterior fossa tumor surgery. *Concepts Pediatr Neurosurg* 9:57–64, 1989.

98. Rekate HL, Grubb RL, Aram DL, et al: Muteness of cerebellar origin. *Arch Neurol* 42:697–698, 1985.

99. Van Dongen HR, Catsman-Berrevoets CE, Van Mourik M: The syndrome of "cerebellar" mutism

and subsequent dysarthria. *Neurology* 44:2040–2046, 1994.

100. Hudson LJ, Murdoch BE, Ozanne AE: Posterior fossa tumours in childhood: Associated speech and language disorders post-surgery. *Aphasiology* 3:1–18, 1989.

101. Hudson LJ, Murdoch BE: Language recovery following surgery and CNS prophylaxis for the treatment of childhood medulloblastoma: A prospective study of three cases. *Aphasiology* 6:17–28, 1992.

102. Dennis M, Spiegler BJ, Hetherington CR, Greenberg ML: Neuropsychological sequelae of the treatment of children with medulloblastoma. *J Neurooncol* 1996. In press.

103. Hirsch JF, Reiner D, Czernichow P, et al: Medulloblastoma in childhood: Survival and functional results. *Acta Neurochir* 48:1–15, 1979.

104. Johnson DL, McCabe MA, Nicholson HS, et al: Quality of long-term survival in young children with medulloblastoma. *J Neurosurg* 80:1004–1010, 1994.

105. Ammirati M, Mirzai S, Samii M: Transient mutism following removal of a cerebellar tumour: A case report and review of the literature. *Childs Nerv Syst* 5:12–14, 1989.

106. Withers HR: Biological basis of radiation therapy for cancer. *Lancet* 339:156–159, 1992.

107. Dropcho EJ: Central nervous system injury by therapeutic irradiation. *Neurol Clin* 9:969–988, 1991.

108. Hudson LJ, Buttsworth DL, Murdoch BE: Effect of CNS prophylaxis on speech and language function in children, in Murdoch BE (ed): *Acquired Neurological Speech/Language Disorders in Childhood.* London: Taylor & Francis, 1990, pp 269–307.

109. Smyth V, Ozanne AE, Woodhouse LM: Communicative disorders in childhood infectious diseases, in Murdoch BE (ed): *Acquired Neurological Speech/Language Disorders in Childhood.* London: Taylor & Francis, 1990, pp 148–176.

110. Paquier P, Van Dongen HR: Two contrasting cases of fluent aphasia in children. *Aphasiology* 5:235–245, 1991.

111. Van Hout A, Lyon G: Wernicke's aphasia in a 10-year-old boy. *Brain Lang* 29:268–285, 1986.

112. Kleiman MB, Carver DH: Central nervous system infections, in Black P (ed): *Brain Dysfunction in Children: Etiology, Diagnosis, and Management.* New York: Raven Press, 1981, pp 79–107.

113. Murdoch BE, Ozanne AE: Linguistic status following acute cerebral anoxia in children, in Murdoch BE (ed): *Acquired Neurological Speech/Language Disorders in Childhood.* London: Taylor & Francis, 1990, pp 177–198.

114. Murdoch BE, Chenery HJ, Kennedy M: Aphemia associated with bilateral striato-capsular lesions subsequent to cerebral anoxia. *Brain Inj* 3:41–49, 1989.

115. Pearn JM, DeBuse P, Mohay M, Golden M: Sequential intellectual recovery after near-drowning. *Med J Aust* 1:463–464, 1979.

116. Reilly K, Ozanne AE, Murdoch BE, Pitt WR: Linguistic status subsequent to childhood immersion injury. *Med J Aust* 149:225–228, 1988.

117. Ozanne AE, Murdoch BE, Krimmer HL: Linguistic problems associated with childhood metabolic disorders, in Murdoch BE (ed): *Acquired Neurological Speech/Language Disorders in Childhood.* London: Taylor & Francis, 1990, pp 199–215.

118. Dennis M: Word finding after brain-injury in children and adolescents. *Top Lang Disord* 13:66–82, 1992.

119. Kleinman SN, Waber DP: Neurodevelopmental bases of spelling acquisition in children treated for acute lymphoblastic leukemia. *Cog Neuropsychol* 9:403–425, 1992.

120. Schmahmann JD: An emerging concept: The cerebellar contribution to higher function. *Arch Neurol* 48:1178–1186, 1991.

121. Goodglass H, Kaplan E: *The Assessment of Aphasia and Related Disorders.* Philadelphia: Lea & Febiger, 1972.

122. Marshall JC: The description and interpretation of aphasic language disorder. *Neuropsychologia* 24:5–24, 1986.

123. Martins IP, Ferro JM: Acquired conduction aphasia in a child. *Dev Med Child Neurol* 29:529–540, 1987.

124. Lees JA: Differentiating language disorder subtypes in acquired childhood aphasia. *Aphasiology* 7(suppl 5):481–488, 1993.

125. Bates E, Thal D, Janowsky JS: Early language development and its neural correlates, in Boller F, Grafman J (eds): *Handbook of Neuropsychology.* Amsterdam: Elsevier Science, 1992, vol 7, pp 69–110.

126. Shahar E, Gilday DL, Hwang PA, et al: Pediatric cerebrovascular disease: Alterations of regional cerebral blood flow detected by TC 99m–HMPAO SPECT. *Arch Neurol* 47:578–584, 1990.

Chapter 17

SPECIFIC LANGUAGE IMPAIRMENTS

Karin Stromswold

DEFINITION AND DIAGNOSIS OF SPECIFIC LANGUAGE IMPAIRMENTS

Without any formal instruction, essentially all normal children who are exposed to it acquire language in a remarkably uniform, rapid, and essentially error-free manner.[1,2] Over the years, researchers have reported that some apparently normal children inexplicably have difficulty acquiring language. These children have been said to suffer from childhood aphasia, congenital aphasia, congenital auditory imperception, congenital word deafness, developmental aphasia, developmental dysphasia, developmental language disorders, dyslogia, or idioglosia.[3] Today, *specific language impairments* (SLI) is the generally accepted term for developmental disorders characterized by severe deficits in the production and/or comprehension of language that cannot be explained by hearing loss, mental retardation, motor deficits, neurologic or psychiatric disorders, or lack of exposure to language. In order to receive the diagnosis of SLI, a child must meet inclusionary and exclusionary criteria such as those given in Table 17-1.[4–10] Special care must be taken to distinguish between developmental and acquired language disorders (see Chap. 16). Thus, in order to receive the diagnosis of SLI, a child cannot have risk factors associated with acquired brain injury (e.g., meningitis, head injuries resulting in loss of consciousness, etc.) or a clinical history consistent with acquired language disorders (e.g., cessation or regression of language skills). Last, children with SLI who are unable to speak must be distinguished from those who choose not to speak (i.e., children with elective mutism).

TYPES OF SPECIFIC LANGUAGE IMPAIRMENT

Because SLI is a diagnosis of exclusion, SLI children are a very heterogeneous group. They vary in the degree to which expressive and/or receptive language skills are impaired and also in the degree to which the different subcomponents of language (i.e., syntax, semantics, morphology, phonology, pragmatics, and the lexicon) are affected. This heterogeneity can and does affect the outcome of behavioral and neurologic studies, with different studies frequently reporting different results, depending on how SLI subjects were selected. The heterogeneity of SLI is problematic not just for basic researchers who seek to discover the nature and etiology of SLI and for applied researchers who attempt to evaluate the efficacy of different types of therapeutic interventions but also for clinicians who must diagnose, evaluate, refer, and make prognoses about SLI children.

Researchers and clinicians have attempted to address this diversity by proposing classification systems for developmental language impairments (see Table 17-2). Developmental language disorders have been classified according to etiology,[11] language function (i.e., repetition, comprehension, production, etc.),[12–14] neuropsychological or

Table 17-1
Diagnostic criteria for specific language impairments

1. Severe language disorder (e.g., performance on standardized language tests at least 6 to 12 months below chronological or mental age)
2. Normal hearing (hearing threshholds below 25 dB between 250 and 6000 Hz)
3. Normal nonverbal intelligence (performance IQ no more than 1 SD below the mean)
4. No "hard" neurologic signs ("soft" neurologic signs allowed)
5. No disorders, diseases, or injuries affecting the central nervous system (e.g., Down syndrome, cerebral palsy, familial dysautonomia, meningitis, severe head injury)
6. Articulation skills commensurate with expressive language skills (i.e., articulation no more than 6 months behind expressive language skills)
7. No obvious structural or functional peripheral oral-motor abnormalities
8. No evidence of a frank psychiatric, emotional, or behavioral disorder (e.g., no severe behavioral or adjustment problems noted by parents or teachers)
9. No history of neglect or abuse
10. Adequate exposure to language
11. No evidence of acquired language disorder (i.e., no cessation or regression of language)

Source: Adapted from Stark and Tallal,[10] with permission.

neurolinguistic profile,[15-17] linguistic profile,[18,19] or some combination of the above.[20] Some of these classification systems are based on language-impaired children's patterns of performance on batteries of language tests,[13,15-17] and others are based on patterns of impairments clinically observed in language-impaired children.[12,19,20] However, none of these classification system has gained widespread acceptance in either clinical or research settings. Aram and colleagues[5] advocate that, given the lack of a widely accepted classification system and the varying degree of congruence between and among SLI populations identified by poor performance on standardized tests and those identified by clinical judgment, it is of paramount importance that clinicians and researchers describe in detail how SLI children are identified.

THE ETIOLOGY OF SPECIFIC LANGUAGE IMPAIRMENTS: WHAT IS THE UNDERLYING DEFICIT?

Until recently, most studies of SLI have been concerned with the etiology or risk factors associated with SLI (see Table 17-3). Despite this, the etiology of SLI remains uncertain.[21] Researchers have proposed that SLI children suffer from impoverished or deviant linguistic input,[22,23] transient, fluctuating hearing loss,[24-27] impairment in short-term auditory memory,[28-30] impairment in auditory sequencing,[31,32] impairment in rapid auditory processing,[33-35] general impairment in sequencing,[36] general impairment in rapid sensory processing,[37] general impairment in representational or symbolic reasoning,[38-40] general impairment in hierarchical planning,[41] impairments in language perception or processing (e.g., the inability to acquire aspects of language that are not phonologically salient[42-44]), impairments in underlying grammar (e.g., the lack of linguistic features such as tense and number,[45-48] the inability to use government to analyze certain types of syntactic relations,[49] the inability to form certain types of agreement relations,[50-52] etc.), or some combination of the above. Some researchers have even suggested that SLI is not a distinct clinical entity, and that SLI children just represent the low end of the normal continuum in linguistic ability.[8,53]

None of the proposed etiologies of SLI have received unambiguous empirical support. A problem for theories that propose relatively general impairments as the basis of SLI[36-41] is that, although such general impairments might well cause secondary linguistic deficits, they should also cause more pervasive behavioral deficits. Another major difficulty in ascertaining the underlying impairment in SLI is distinguishing whether the impairment under investigation is the *cause* of the linguistic deficit or the *result* of the linguistic deficit. For example, although results of several studies suggest that parents may speak differently to

SLI children than to normal children,[22,23,54] there are no convincing data to suggest that differences in parental input *cause* SLI.[55] Parents may speak differently to SLI children because they are compensating for their children's language impairments. In other words, SLI children's linguistic impairments may cause the differences in parental input, rather than vice versa. Results of a number of studies[26,56–59] indicate that, although there does seem to be a relationship between language delay and chronic otitis media, language delays tend to resolve once hearing impairments resolve and there is no convincing evidence that transient episodes of otitis media result in persistent language impairment (but see Ref. 27). Tallal and Piercy[33–35] have argued that SLI children's language disorders result from their general difficulty in processing auditory information that changes rapidly. They have shown, for example, that SLI children do not categorically perceive stop consonants (e.g., /b/ and /p/) in the same way that normal children do.[33–35] Although the inability to perceive consonants categorically could be the result of a disorder in rapid auditory processing, it is also possible that by virtue of their linguistic deficits, SLI children do not have normal exposure to the phonemes of their language. If this is the case, then it may be that SLI children do not perceive phonemes categorically for the same reason that adult Japanese speakers have difficulty perceiving /l/ and /r/ categorically:[60–62] neither SLI children nor Japanese adults have had enough exposure to the linguistic stimuli necessary to permit categorical perception of these speech sounds.

In many studies of SLI children's nonverbal abilities, SLI children must understand verbal instructions or respond verbally. For example, one of the studies most frequently cited as evidence that SLI children have a general representational deficit is a mental rotation study.[38] In this study, SLI and normal children had to decide whether pairs of geometric figures rotated 45, 90, and 135° were the same or were mirror images. In order to do this, the SLI children had to understand complex verbal instructions and they had to make subtle left/right judgments—two tasks that language-impaired children frequently have difficulty with.

Despite this, SLI children were just as accurate as normal children and differed only in the amount of time it took them to do the task. Even in studies that do not require verbal responses, having linguistic labels may be useful in performing the task.[41]

In summary, *the* cause of SLI is not known. Given the heterogeneity in the children diagnosed with SLI, it is extremely unlikely that all children with SLI suffer from the same underlying impairment. Furthermore, it is likely that in many cases, whether a child will have a clinically evident language impairment depends on multiple, interacting factors. For example, whereas transient, fluctuating hearing loss might have no noticeable effect on the linguistic development of children who are not at risk for SLI, it might have a devastating effect on the linguistic development of children who are at risk for SLI.[57] Similarly, whereas most children appear to be able to acquire language within a wide range of linguistic environments, children who are at risk for developing SLI might require an optimal linguistic environment in order to acquire normal language.

THE NEURAL BASIS OF SPECIFIC LANGUAGE IMPAIRMENTS

At the neural level, the cause of SLI is also uncertain. Prior to the advent of modern neuroimaging techniques, it was theorized that children with SLI had bilateral damage to the perisylvian cortical regions that subserve language in adults.[63] Contrary to the bilateral-damage theory, computed tomography (CT) and magnetic resonance imaging (MRI) scans of SLI children have failed to reveal the types of gross perisylvian lesions typically found in patients with acquired aphasia.[64–66] However, CT and MRI scans have revealed that the brains of SLI children often do not have the normal pattern of the left temporal plane being larger than the right temporal plane.[64–66] Results from dichotic listening[67–71] and auditory evoked response potential (AEP) experiments[72] suggest that at least some SLI children have aberrant functional lateralization for language, with language

Table 17-2
Classification systems for developmental language disorders

Aram and Nation (1975)[13]

Repetition strength
Nonspecific formulation-repetition deficit
Generalized low performance
Phonologic comprehension-formulation-repetition deficit
Comprehension deficit
Formulation-repetition deficit

Bishop and Rosenbloom (1987)[18]

Type of language disorder		Examples
Phonology		
Expressive	Immature	Cluster reduction, final consonant deletion, fronting (e.g., "k" pronounced as "t")
	Deviant	Initial consonant deletion
Receptive	Immature	?
	Deviant	?
Grammar		
Expressive	Immature	Simple, telegraphic sentences lacking grammatical markers (e.g., "me want cookie")
		Grammatical overregularization ("goed" for "went")
	Deviant	Restricted use of a single sentence frame
		Bizarre syntax (e.g., "me buy go sweets")
Receptive	Immature	Tendency to ignore inflectional endings
	Deviant	Systematic misunderstanding of some structures
Semantics		
Expressive	Immature	Overextension of word meanings
	Deviant	Frequent failure to produce words that are known
Receptive	Immature	Weak vocabulary
	Deviant	Confused if one word has different meanings
Pragmatic		
Expressive	Immature	Failure to use polite forms
	Deviant	Use of inappropriately stilted language
Receptive	Immature	Failure to recognize sarcasm
	Deviant	Tendency to respond to utterances literally

Bloom and Lahey (1978)[19]

Impairment in form (i.e., syntax, morphology, and phonology)
Impairment in content (i.e., semantics and the lexicon)
Impairment in use (i.e., pragmatics and discourse)

Curtiss and Tallal (1988)[14]

Expressive language disorder
Receptive language disorder
Mixed language disorder

Denckla (1981)[15]

Anomic disorder (impaired naming with intact comprehension and repetition)

Table 17-2

Classification systems for developmental language disorders (Continued)

Denckla (1981)[15]

Anomic disorder with repetition deficits
Dysphonemic sequencing disorder (phonemic substitutions and missequencing)
Verbal memory disorder
Mixed language disorder (impaired repetition, comprehension, and production)
Right hemisyndrome with mixed language disorder

DSM-IV (1994)[12]

Expressive language disorder
Mixed expressive/receptive language disorder
Phonologic disorder (developmental articulation disorder in DMS-IIIR)

Ingram (1969)[11]

Disorders of voicing (dysphonia)
Disorders of respiratory coordination (dysrhythmia)
Disorders of speech sound production (dysarthria)
Disorders of speech sound production secondary to other diseases or adverse environmental factors (e.g., mental retardation, deafness, psychiatric disorder, acquired dysphasias)
Developmental speech disorders—developmental expressive and receptive dysphasia

Korkman and Hakkinen-Rihu (1994)[16]

Specific dyspraxia subtype
Specific comprehension subtype
Specific dysnomia subtype
Global subtype

Rapin and Allen (1983)[20]

Phonologic syntactic syndrome (with or without oromotor dysfunction)
Severe expressive syndrome with good comprehension
Verbal auditory agnosia (phonetic decoding deficit)
Syntactic-pragmatic syndrome
Semantic-pragmatic syndrome without autism ("cocktail party" speech)
Mute autistic syndrome
Autistic syndrome with echolalia

Wilson and Risucci (1986)[17]

Auditory semantic comprehension disorder
Auditory and visual semantic comprehension disorder
Auditory semantic comprehension and auditory and visual short-term memory disorder
Expressive and/or receptive disorder
Global disorder
Auditory memory and retrieval disorder
Expressive disorder
No deficits

Table 17-3

Proposed etiologies and underlying impairments in specific language impairments

Disorders affecting adequate input
    Hearing loss
    Impoverished linguistic input

Disorders affecting adequate output
    Subtle structural or functional oral-motor disorders (e.g., oral motor dyspraxia)

Disorders affecting auditory processing
    Auditory short-term memory
    Auditory sequencing
    Rapid auditory processing

Non-modality-specific disorders
    Impairment in short-term memory/storage
    Impairment in sequencing
    Impairment in rapid sensory processing
    Impairment in representation/symbolic reasoning
    Impairment in hierarchical planning

Linguistic disorders
    Disorders of performance
    Disorders of competence

No disorder (SLI children represent the low end of normal continuum)

Multifactorial

either present bilaterally or predominantly in the right hemisphere. Single photon emission computed tomography (SPECT) studies of normal and language-impaired children have revealed hypoperfusion in the inferior frontal convolution of the left hemisphere (including Broca's area) in two children with isolated expressive language impairment,[73] hypoperfusion of the left temporoparietal region and the upper and middle regions of the right frontal lobe in 9 of 12 children with expressive and receptive language impairment,[73] and hypoperfusion in the left temporofrontal region of language-impaired children's brains.[74]

Because SLI is not a fatal disorder and people with SLI have normal life spans, only one brain of a possible SLI child has come to autopsy to date. Postmortem examination of this brain revealed atypical symmetry of the temporal planes and a dysplastic microgyrus on the inferior surface

of the left frontal cortex along the inferior surface of the sylvian fissure,[75] findings similar to those reported for dyslexic brains.[76–80] Although it is tempting to use the results of this autopsy to argue—as Geschwind and Galaburda[79] have for dyslexia—that SLI is the result of subtle anomalies in the left perisylvian cortex, the child whose brain was autopsied had a performance IQ of only 74 (verbal IQ 70); hence, the anomalies noted on autopsy may be related to the child's general cognitive impairment rather than to her language impairment.

GENETIC STUDIES OF SPECIFIC LANGUAGE IMPAIRMENTS

Genetic studies of SLI are important for several reasons. If SLI is genetically transmitted, family history can aid in diagnosis. Genetically homogeneous groups are also advantageous for both basic and applied research. Last, if SLI is heritable, this suggests that it is not caused by impoverished linguistic environments or other environmental insults. Table 17-4 summarizes the results of 12 epidemiologic studies of familial aggregation of developmental spoken language disorders.[81–92] All 12 studies found that a higher percentage of language-impaired children had a positive family history of language impairment (between 30 and 70 percent) than did normal (control) children (between 11 to 46 percent).[81–92] In all but one of the 12 studies,[92] the difference was significant. All 12 studies also revealed that a higher percentage of the relatives of language-impaired children were language-impaired (between 9 to 42 percent) than were the relatives of the control children (between 2 and 18 percent).[81–92] In all but one of the 12 studies,[92] the difference was significant. Although it is possible that children who have language-impaired parents or siblings are more likely to be linguistically impaired themselves because they are exposed to deviant language, the deviant linguistic environment (DLE) account is unlikely for a number of reasons. First, research on language acquisition reveals that within a fairly wide range, linguistic environment has little or no effect

Table 17-4

Family aggregation studies of language disorders

Authors	Sample size	Proband diagnosis	Other diagnoses counted for plus family history	Presence of positive family history in probands and controls	Frequency of impairment in relatives of probands and controls
Ingram (1959)	75 probands	Developmental speech and language disorders	None	24% positive parental history 32% positive sibling history	N.A.
Luchsinger (1970)	127 probands	Developmental speech retardation	None	36% probands	N.A.
Byrne, Willerman, and Ashmore (1974)	18 severely impaired, 20 moderately impaired	Delayed speech	None	17% "severe" probands 55% "moderate" probands[b]	N.A.
Neils and Aram (1986)	74 probands, 36 controls	Developmental language disorders	Dyslexia, stuttering, articulation	46% first-degree proband relatives 8% first-degree control relatives[d]	20% all proband relatives 3% all control relatives[c]
Lewis, Ekelman, and Aram (1989)	20 probands, 20 controls	Phonologic disorder	Dyslexia, stuttering, LD	N.A.	*LI:* 9% all proband relatives vs. 1% all control relatives[d] *All disorders:* 12% all proband relatives vs. 2% all control relatives[d]
Tallal, Ross, and Curtiss (1989)	62 probands, 50 controls	Specific language impairment	Dyslexia, LD, school problem	77% first-degree proband relatives 46% first-degree control relatives[c]	42% first-degree proband relatives vs. 19% first-degree control relatives[c]
Tomblin (1989)	51 probands, 136 controls	Receiving speech or language therapy	Stuttering, articulation	53% first-degree proband relatives Controls: N.A.	23% first-degree proband relatives vs. 3% first-degree control relatives[d]
Haynes and Naido (1991)	156 probands	Specific language impairment	None	54% all proband relatives 41% first-degree proband relatives	28% proband parents affected, 18% proband sibs affected
Tomblin, Hardy, and Hein (1991)	55 probands, 607 normal	Lowest 10th percentile on test (50) or clinical history (5)	+FH = 1 first-degree or >1 extended family member	35% of low language 17% of normals[c]	N.A.
Whitehurst et al. (1991)	62 probands, 55 controls	Isolated expressive language delay	Late talker, speech problem, school problem	N.A.	*Late-talker:* 12% first-degree proband vs. 7% first-degree control relatives, NS *Speech:* 12% first-degree proband relative vs. 8% first-degree control relatives, NS
Beitchman, Hood, and Inglis (1992)	136 probands, 138 controls	Speech, language, or voicing disorder or stuttering	Dyslexia, LD, articulation	47% all proband relatives vs. 28% all control relatives[c] 34% first-degree proband relatives vs. 11% first-degree control relative[d]	N.A.
Lewis (1992)	87 probands, 79 controls	Phonologic disorder	Dyslexia, LD, stuttering, hearing loss	N.A.	*LI:* 14% all proband relatives vs. 2% all control relatives[d] (26% vs 4% for first-degree[d]) Significant differences for dyslexia and LD but not stuttering or hearing loss.

Key: Statistical significance (one-tailed test): [a]$p < .05$, [b]$p < .01$, [c]$p < .001$, [d]$p < .0001$; FH = family history; LD = unspecified learning disability; LI = language impairment; NA = not available; NS = not significant.

Source: Adapted from Stromswold,[95] with permission.

on language acquisition by normal children.[1,2,93,94] In addition, the DLE makes a number of predictions that were not borne out in these studies.[95] For example, contrary to the DLE, the more severely impaired children did not systematically have families with higher incidence of language impairment, and parents with a history of spoken language impairment who were no longer impaired were significantly more likely to have SLI children than were parents with no such history.

Monozygotic (MZ) twins and dizygotic (DZ) twins share essentially the same pre- and postnatal environment, whereas MZ twins share 100 percent of their genetic material and, on average, DZ twins share only 50 percent of their genetic material.[96] Therefore if, for a particular trait, MZ twins are more similar to one another than are DZ twins, this suggests that genetic factors play a role in the expression of that trait. Table 17-5 summarizes the results of five twin studies of spoken and written language disorders.[97–101] In all four studies that investigated the concordance rates for language disorders in twins,[97–99,101] the concordance rates were significantly greater for MZ twins (between 51 and 84 percent) than for DZ twins (between 20

and 32 percent), indicating that genetic factors play a role in written and spoken language disorders. DeFries and Gillis[98] also performed a multiple regression analysis on their twins' scores on standardized reading tests. This analysis revealed that 50 percent of their subjects' reading deficits were attributable to heritable factors.[98] In a different type of study, Locke and Mather[100] compared the articulation errors of MZ and DZ twins and found that MZ twins were significantly more likely to mispronounce the same target words than were DZ twins. However, MZ twins were no more likely to mispronounce a word in exactly the same way than were DZ twins.[100]

Stromswold[95] reviewed nine twin studies of spoken and written language disorders and found that in all nine studies, the pairwise and probandwise concordance rates were greater for MZ than DZ twin pairs. Overall, the nine studies included 400 MZ twin pairs and 293 DZ twin pairs. The overall pairwise concordance rates were 66.0 percent for MZ twins and 29.7 percent for DZ twins (chi square(1) = 89.19, $p < .0000005$).[95] The overall probandwise concordance rates were 79.5 percent for MZ twins and 45.8 percent for DZ twins

Table 17-5

Twin studies of language

Study	MZ twins	DZ twins	Proband selection	MZ pairwise concordance rate	DZ pairwise concordance rate
Bakwin[97]	31 (19 male, 12 female)	31 (19 male, 12 female)	History of dyslexia	Overall, 84% Male, 84% Female, 83%	Overall, 29% [d] Male, 42% [b] Female, 8% [c]
Matheny, Dolan, and Wilson[101]	17 (sex N.A.)	10 (sex N.A.)	History of dyslexia or academic problems	76% concordant	20% concordant [b]
Locke and Mather[100]	13 (5 male, 8 female)	13 (5 male, 8 female)	Poor performance on TD articulation test (>15% errors)	82% of errors shared	56% of errors shared [a]
Lewis and Thompson[99]	32 (24 male, 8 female)	25 (18 male, 7 female)	History of spoken or written language disorder	Any disorder, 67% Articulation, 95% Learning disorder, 53% Delayed speech, 71%	Any disorder, 32% [c] Articulation, 22% [d] Learning disorder, 33% Delayed speech, 0%
DeFries and Gillis[98]	133 (58 male, 75 female)	98 (57 male, 41 female)	History of dyslexia *and* poor performance on word recognition, spelling, and comprehension PIAT	51% concordant	28% concordant [c]

Key: Statistical significance (one-tailed test): [a]$p < .05$, [b]$p < .01$, [c]$p < .001$, [d]$p < .0001$; MZ = monozygotic; DZ = dizygotic; PIAT = Peabody Individual Achievement Tests; TD articulation = Templin-Darley Screening Test of Articulation.

Source: Adapted from Stromswold,[95] with permission.

($z = 8.77$, $p < .00000005$). If spoken language disorders and written language disorders are distinct entities, including twins with both types of disorders in one analysis would be inappropriate and could either hide a significant difference or create a spuriously significant difference. Of the nine twin studies Stromswold[95] reviewed, five investigated written language disorders and four investigated spoken language disorders. Stromswold's[95] metaanalyses included 212 MZ and 199 DZ twins pairs in which at least one member of the twin pair had a written language disorder. For written language disorders, the overall pairwise concordancy rates were 59.9 percent for MZ twins and 27.1 percent for DZ twins (chi square(1) $= 44.73$, $p < .0000005$), and the overall probandwise concordancy rates were 74.9 percent for MZ twins and 42.7 percent for DZ twins ($z = 6.53$, $p < .00000005$).[95] Stromswold[95] metaanalysis included 188 MZ and 94 DZ twin pairs in which at least one member of the twin pair had a spoken language disorder. For spoken language disorders, the overall pairwise concordancy rates were 72.9 percent for MZ twins and 35.1 percent for DZ twins (chi square(1) $= 37.330$, $p < .0000005$), and the probandwise concordancy rates were 84.3 percent for MZ twins and 52.0 percent for DZ twins ($z = 5.14$, $p < .00000025$).[95]

If pedigree studies of large, multigeneration families reveal that the pattern of family members who are language-impaired and not language-impaired is consistent with particular modes of genetic transmission, this supports the notion that SLI is a genetic disorder. Pedigree analyses involve evaluating models of genetic transmission by *rejecting* possible modes of transmission based on which family members in a pedigree are affected.[102] Researchers have reported a number of kindreds with extremely large numbers of severely affected family members in which transmission seems to be autosomal dominant with variable expressivity and penetrance.[46–48,103–106] Samples and Lane[107] analyzed a family in which six of six siblings had a severe developmental language disorder and concluded that the mode of transmission in that family was a single autosomal recessive gene. Stromswold[108] analyzed a family

with severe verbal dyspraxia in which transmission appears to be either autosomal recessive or multifactorial. To date, only one published segregation study exists for probands with spoken language disorders other than stuttering.[109] In this study, pedigrees of 45 probands with a history of a moderate to severe speech or language disorder were analyzed and the results were most consistent with multifactorial transmission.[109] In summary, the results of genetic studies indicate that there is a strong genetic component to developmental language disorders and that SLI is probably a genetically heterogeneous disorder.

ARE THESE CHILDREN DEVIANT OR ARE THEY MERELY DELAYED?

One of the central questions in SLI research is whether the major (perhaps only) difference between SLI children and normal children is the rate of language acquisition or whether the course of language acquisition by SLI children is deviant.[9,40,46–48,110–116] Even within the restricted domain of inflectional morphology where researchers generally agree that many SLI children exhibit particular difficulty (having difficulty using inflectional morphemes such as the past tense morpheme *-ed*), there is debate about whether SLI children's morphologic impairments reflect deviant underlying grammars,[45–52,117–121] limitations in language processing,[42,43,122–124] limitations in sensory processing,[33–35,37] or protracted (though essentially normal) acquisition of language.[113,125]

LONGITUDINAL COURSE AND PROGNOSIS IN SPECIFIC LANGUAGE IMPAIRMENTS

Follow-up studies of children diagnosed as having a spoken language disorder in preschool generally indicate that 40 to 60 percent of these children continue to have difficulties in later years (e.g., see Refs. 126–128). Most of these children had difficulties with written language or academic subjects, but many continued to have trouble with spoken language. One study found that 50 percent of children who had both comprehension and production deficits at age 3 still had deficits at age 5, whereas only 13 percent of children who only had production deficits at age 3 still had language deficits at age 5 and only 4 percent of children who only had comprehension deficits at age 3 still had deficits at age 5.[129] A follow-up study of the same children at age 11 revealed that children diagnosed with a language delay at age 3 were more likely to have lower verbal and full-scale IQs and reading scores than were children who were not diagnosed as language-delayed at age 3.[130] At age 11, there were no significant differences in IQ for children who had isolated production or comprehension deficits at age 3, but children diagnosed with global language deficits at age 3 had significantly lower IQs than either group.[130] At age 11, children with isolated expressive or isolated receptive delays had reading levels 2 years behind children who were not language-delayed at 3, and children with global language delays had reading levels more than 2.5 years behind normal children.[130] A 10-year follow-up study of children diagnosed with a specific language impairment in preschool revealed that preschool scores on the nonverbal Leiter IQ test[131] were the best predictor of adolescent scores on standardized tests of spoken language, reading achievement, and placement in a regular classroom.[132] Preschool scores on the expressive section of the Northwest Syntax Screening Test[133] were also a strong predictor of adolescent language scores.[132]

RELATIONSHIP BETWEEN SPECIFIC LANGUAGE IMPAIRMENTS AND DYSLEXIA

There is a growing consensus that many reading disabilities are language-based in origin.[130,134-144] Prospective studies of kindergarten and preschool-age children who were later diagnosed as dyslexic have revealed that such children exhibit weaknesses in phonemic awareness,[140,145-149] phonologic production,[140,150] receptive and expressive vocabulary,[140,147,148,151] syntactic comprehension

and production,[140,147,152] and syntactic awareness.[153] Follow-up studies have generally shown that many children who had spoken language impairments when they were of preschool age later exhibit signs of written language disorders.[126-128,130,132] In one 10-year follow-up study, over 90 percent of children who had spoken language disorders in preschool later exhibited evidence of learning difficulties or disorders in reading, spelling, or mathematics.[132] In retrospective studies, parents report that dyslexic children were more likely to have had spoken language impairments than were children without dyslexia.[154,155] Results from genetic studies also suggest that dyslexia and SLI are related. For example, as part of a twin study, Johnston and coworkers[156] found that preschool language skill was the best predictor of reading ability, accounting for 33 percent of the variance in reading-age discrepancy. In a different twin study, phonologic coding deficits were revealed to be highly heritable and accounted for most of the heritable variance in word recognition, whereas orthographic coding deficits were not significantly heritable and accounted for much of the environmental variance in word recognition.[157] Last, studies suggest that children with developmental phonologic disorders have significantly more nuclear and extended family members with dyslexia than do control children.[85,86]

IMPLICATIONS OF SPECIFIC LANGUAGE IMPAIRMENTS FOR COGNITIVE SCIENCE AND LINGUISTICS

If language acquisition involves the development of specialized, modular structures and operations that have no counterparts in nonlinguistic domains, then it should be possible for a child to be cognitively intact and linguistically impaired. If, on the other hand, language acquisition involves the development of the same general symbolic structures and operations used in other cognitive domains, then dissociation of language and general cognitive development should not be possible. Thus, the existence of children with SLI supports the position that language is cognitively and neurally distinct (or modular) from general intellectual abilities. Genetic studies which show that SLI is heritable provide further support for the acquisition of language being the result of innate, linguistically specific structures and not the result of instruction and general cognitive and neural structures. To the extent that SLI children's language is markedly different from that of normal children, this is consistent with the cognitive and neural processes that SLI children use to generate language being qualitatively different from those used by normal children.

In many modern linguistic theories, the subcomponents of language (e.g., syntax, semantics, morphology, phonology, and the lexicon) are believed to be functionally distinct or modular from one another.[158] The existence of SLI children whose linguistic impairments preferentially involve the acquisition of some subcomponents of language but not others (e.g., the acquisition of morphology, but not the acquisition of lexical items) is consistent with modular linguistic theories. Modern linguistic theories (particularly generative theories of grammar) also frequently make a distinction between a person's knowledge of the rules of language (competence) and a person's actual use of language in real situations (performance).[158,159] Some researchers have argued that SLI children's impairments or limitations are at the level of competence,[46–49,51,119,121] whereas other researchers have argued that SLI children's limitations are at the level of performance.[42,122–124]

Just as analyses of adult aphasics' deficits have been used to test specific linguistic and psycholinguistic theories,[160–163] careful investigations of SLI children's linguistic deficits may be useful in testing specific linguistic and psycholinguistic theories. A number of researchers have argued that the patterns of impairment in SLI children's language are consistent with SLI children having very specific linguistic impairments. For example, van der Lely[49] has suggested that SLI children's linguistic impairments reflect their inability to use government to analyze certain types of syntactic relations. Clahsen[51] has argued that, within a parametric theory of language (in which all languages share a number of universal properties, but differ

in the settings chosen for certain parameters), SLI children's linguistic deficits could be the result of them having miss-set or missing parametric setting(s). Another possibility within a learning theoretic-parametric framework is that the *threshold* at which SLI children reset parameters is aberrant. If SLI children's parameter-setting thresholds are too high, this could result in SLI children staying in the normal stages of language acquisition for prolonged periods of time. If Rice and Wexler[121] are correct and SLI children have an extended optional infinitive stage, this could be the result of SLI children having abnormally high thresholds for setting parameters.

To get a sense of the types of specific linguistic and psycholinguistic accounts that have been proposed to explain SLI children's language impairments, consider the accounts recently offered for why SLI children have particular difficulty with certain aspects of morphology, such as tense, number, and case. Leonard[42,43,123,164] has proposed that SLI children have difficulty perceiving and processing brief, unstressed linguistic elements and that this directly affects their ability to build the morphologic paradigms that Pinker[165] proposes are a key component of normal language acquisition. As support for the phonological salience theory, Leonard and colleagues report that SLI children who are acquiring English and Italian have specific difficulty learning grammatical morphemes that are expressed as word final consonants, even though the syntactic and semantic functions of these grammatical morphemes frequently differ in the two languages.[42,43,123,164] Gopnik and colleagues have argued that children with SLI make frequent morphologic errors because they are missing certain abstract syntactic-semantic features such as number, tense, animacy, and aspect.[45–48] A number of researchers have proposed that SLI children's morphological errors result from a specific deficit or delay in the acquisition of functional categories.[117,119,120] Clahsen has proposed that SLI children have difficulty forming subject-verb agreement relationships and this causes them to make certain types of morphologic errors.[50,51] Recently, Rice and colleagues have suggested that SLI children's morphologic errors may be caused by specific difficulties with specifier-head agreement relations[52] or by SLI children remaining in the optional infinitive stage of language acquisition for an abnormally long period of time.[121]

SUMMARY

Despite decades of intensive and productive research on specific language impairments in children, the answers to a number of fundamental questions about SLI remain uncertain. Although clinicians and researchers generally agree that considerable diversity exists in the behavioral profiles and manifestations of children diagnosed with SLI and that it is important to distinguish between various subtypes of SLI, no system for classifying the different behavioral subtypes of SLI is generally accepted. Researchers disagree about the etiology or underlying impairment in SLI, and offer proposals ranging from a specific impairment in a circumscribed aspect of abstract linguistics to general cognitive/processing impairments to environmental causes. Researchers disagree about the nature of the linguistic manifestations of SLI (be they primary or secondary to some underlying cause). Researchers disagree whether language acquisition in SLI is deviant or merely a prolonged version of the normal course of language acquisition. Researchers also disagree about whether SLI represents an impairment in the underlying grammar (competence) or the use of that grammar (performance). Even among researchers who believe that SLI is an impairment of linguistic competence, there is disagreement about what aspect of the underlying grammar is impaired.

Structural and functional neuroimaging studies suggest that children with SLI may not have the pattern of left-right asymmetry that normally developing children and adults have, but this research is somewhat preliminary and it is possible that SLI children's aberrant asymmetries reflect their linguistic impairments rather than cause them. Although the vast majority of the genetic studies of developmental language impairments indicate that there is a heritable component to

written and spoken language disorders, we know relatively little about the mode(s) of transmission and gene(s) responsible for spoken language disorders. Studies generally show that many SLI children continue to exhibit language and learning difficulties, particularly with written language. However, estimates of the prevalence of later language and learning disabilities in preschool children diagnosed with SLI vary considerably and not all children with a history of spoken language impairments have difficulty learning to read.

ACKNOWLEDGMENTS

Preparation of this chapter was supported by grants to the author from the John Merck Foundation on the Biology of Developmental Disorders and the Johnson and Johnson Foundation.

REFERENCES

1. Pinker S: *The Language Instinct: How the Mind Creates Language.* New York: William Morrow, 1994.
2. Stromswold K: The cognitive and neural bases of language acquisition, in Gazzaniga M (ed): *The Cognitive Neurosciences.* Cambridge, MA: MIT Press, 1995, pp 855–870.
3. Myklebust HR: Childhood aphasia: An evolving concept, in Travis LE (ed): *Handbook of Speech Pathology and Audiology.* New York: Appleton-Century-Crofts, 1971, pp 1181–1202.
4. Aram DM: Comments on specific language impairment as a clinical category. *Lang Speech Hear Serv Schools* 22:84–87, 1991.
5. Aram DM, Morris R, Hall NE: Clinical and research congruence in identifying children with specific language impairment. *J Speech Hear Res* 36:580–591, 1993.
6. Dale PS, Cole KN: What's normal? Specific language impairment in an individual differences perspective. *Lang Speech Hear Serv Schools* 22:80–83, 1991.
7. Lahey M: Who shall be called language disordered? Some reflections and one perspective. *J Speech Hear Dis* 55:612–620, 1990.
8. Leonard L: Specific language impairment as a clin-

ical category. *Lang Speech Hear Serv Schools* 22:66–68, 1991.

9. Leonard LB: Language impairment in children. *Merrill-Palmer Q* 25:205–232, 1979.

10. Stark RE, Tallal P: Selection of children with specific language deficits. *J Speech Hear Dis* 46:114–122, 1981.

11. Ingram TTS: Disorders of speech development in childhood. *Br J Hosp Med* 4:1608–1625, 1969.

12. American Psychiatric Association: *Diagnostic and Statistical Manual of Mental Disorders,* 4th ed. Washington, DC: American Psychiatric Association, 1994.

13. Aram DM, Nation JE: Patterns of language behavior in children with developmental language disorders. *J Speech Hear Res* 18:229–241, 1975.

14. Curtiss S, Tallal P: Neurolinguistic correlates of specific developmental language impairment. *J Clin Exp Neuropsychol* 10:18–19, 1988.

15. Denkla MB: Minimal brain dysfunction and dyslexia: Beyond diagnosis by exclusion, in Blair ME, Rapin I, Kinsbourne M (eds): *Child Neurology.* New York: Spectrum, 1981.

16. Korkman M, Hakkinen-Rihu P: A new classification of developmental language disorders (DLD). *Brain Lang* 47:96–116, 1994.

17. Wilson B, Risucci D: A model for clinical-quantitative classification: Generation I: Application to language-disordered preschool children. *Brain Lang* 27:281–309, 1986.

18. Bishop D, Rosenbloom L: Childhood language disorders: Classification and overview, in Yule W, Rutter M (eds): *Language Development and Disorders.* Philadelphia: Lippincott, 1987, pp 16–41.

19. Bloom L, Lahey M: *Language Development and Language Disorder.* New York: Wiley, 1978.

20. Rapin I, Allen DA: Developmental language disorders: Nosological considerations, in Kirk U (ed): *Neuropsychology of Language, Reading, and Spelling.* New York: Academic Press, 1983, pp 155–183.

21. Bishop DVM: The underlying nature of specific language impairment. *J Child Psychol Psychiatry Allied Disc* 33:3–66, 1992.

22. Cramblit N, Siegel G: The verbal environment of a language-impaired child. *J Speech Hearing Dis* 42:474–482, 1977.

23. Lasky E, Klopp K: Parent-child interactions in normal and language-disordered children. *J Speech Hear Dis* 47:7–18, 1982.

24. Bishop DVM, Edmundson A: Is otitis media a major cause of specific developmental language disorders? *Br J Disord Commun* 21:321–338, 1986.

25. Gordon AG: Some comments on Bishop's annotation "Developmental dysphasia and otitis media." *J Child Psychol Psychiatry* 29:361–363, 1988.

26. Gravel JS, Wallace IF: Listening and language at 4 years of age: Effects of early otitis media. *J Speech Hear Res* 35:588–595, 1992.

27. Teele DW, Klein JO, Chase C, et al: Otitis media in infancy and intellectual ability, school achievement, speech, and language at age 7 years. *J Infect Dis* 162:685–694, 1990.

28. Graham NC: Response strategies in the partial comprehension of sentences. *Lang Speech* 17:205–221, 1974.

29. Graham NC: Short-term memory and syntactic structure in educationally subnormal children. *Lang Speech* 11:209–219, 1968.

30. Rapin I, Wilson BC: Children with developmental language disability: Neuropsychological aspects and assessment, in Wyke MA (ed): *Developmental Dysphasia.* London: Academic Press, 1978, pp 13–41.

31. Efron R: Temporal perception, aphasia and deja vu. *Brain* 86:403–424, 1963.

32. Monsee EK: Aphasia in children. *J Speech Hear Disord* 26:83–86, 1961.

33. Tallal P, Piercy M: Defects of non-verbal auditory perception in children with developmental dysphasia. *Nature* 241:468–469, 1973.

34. Tallal P, Piercy M: Developmental aphasia: Impaired rate of non-verbal processing as a function of sensory modality. *Neuropsychologia* 11:389–398, 1973.

35. Tallal P, Piercy M: Developmental aphasia: Rate of auditory processing as a selective impairment of consonant perception. *Neuropsychologia* 12:83–93, 1974.

36. Poppen R, Stark J, Eisenson J, et al: Visual sequencing performance of aphasic children. *J Speech Hear Res* 12:288–300, 1969.

37. Tallal P: Fine-grained discrimination deficits in language-learning impaired children are specific neither to the auditory modality nor to speech perception. *J Speech Hear Res* 33:616–621, 1990.

38. Johnston J, Weismer S: Mental rotation abilities in language-disordered children. *J Speech Hear Res* 26:397–403, 1983.

39. Kahmi A: Nonlinguistic symbolic and conceptual abilities in language-impaired and normally devel-

oping children. *J Speech Hear Res* 24:446–453, 1981.

40. Morehead D, Ingram D: The development of base syntax in normal and linguistically deviant children. *J Speech Hear Res* 16:330–352, 1973.

41. Cromer R: Hierarchical planning disability in the drawings and constructions of a special group of severely aphasic children. *Brain Cogn* 2:144–164, 1983.

42. Leonard LB: Language learnability and specific language impairment in children. *Appl Psycholing* 10:179–202, 1989.

43. Leonard LB: Some problems facing accounts of morphological deficits in children with specific language impairments, in Watkins RV, Rice ML (eds): *Specific Language Impairments in Children.* Baltimore: Brookes, 1994, pp 91–106.

44. Leonard LB, McGregor KK, Allen GD: Grammatical morphology and speech perception in children with specific language impairment. *J Speech Hear Res* 35:1076–1085, 1992.

45. Crago MB, Gopnik M: From families to phenotypes: Theoretical and clinical implications of research into the genetic basis of specific language impairment, in Watkins RV, Rice ML (eds): *Specific Language Impairments in Children.* Baltimore: Brookes, 1994, pp 35–52.

46. Gopnik M: Feature blindness: A case study. *Lang Acquis* 1:139–164, 1990.

47. Gopnik M: Feature-blind grammar and dysphasia. *Nature* 344:715, 1990.

48. Gopnik M, Crago MB: Familial aggregation of a developmental language disorder. *Cognition* 39:1–50, 1991.

49. van der Lely HKJ: Canonical linking rules: Forward versus reverse linking in normally developing and specifically language-impaired children. *Cognition* 51:29–72, 1994.

50. Clahsen H: *Child Language and Developmental Dysphasia: Linguistic Studies of the Acquisition of German.* Philadelphia: Benjamins, 1991.

51. Clahsen H: The grammatical characterization of developmental dysphasia. *Linguistics* 27:897–920, 1989.

52. Rice ML: Grammatical categories of children with specific language impairments, in Watkins RV, Rice ML (eds): *Specific Language Impairments in Children.* Baltimore: Brookes, 1994, pp 69–90.

53. Johnston JR: The continuing relevance of cause: A reply to Leonard's "Specific language impairment as a clinical category." *Lang Speech Hear Serv Schools* 22:75–79, 1991.

54. Conti-Ramsden G, Dykins J: Mother-child interactions with language-impaired children and their siblings. *Br J Disord Commun* 26:337–354, 1991.

55. Leonard L: Is specific language impairment a useful construct? in Rosenberg S (ed): *Advances in Applied Psycholinguistics: Disorders of First Language Development.* New York: Cambridge University Press, 1987, pp 1–39.

56. Friel-Patti S, Finitzo T: Language learning in a prospective study of otitis media with effusion in the first two years of life. *J Speech Hear Res* 33:188–194, 1990.

57. Hall DMB, Hill P: Does secretory otitis media affect language development? *Arch Dis Child* 61:42–47, 1986.

58. Paradise JL: Otitis media during early life: How hazardous to development? A critical review of the evidence. *Pediatrics* 68:869–873, 1981.

59. Paul R, Lynn T, Lohr-Flanders M: History of middle ear involvement and speech/language development in late talkers. *J Speech Hear Res* 36:1055–1062, 1993.

60. MacKain K, Best C, Strange W: Categorical perception of English /r/ and /l/ by Japanese bilinguals. *Appl Psycholing* 2:369–390, 1981.

61. Strange W, Dittman S: Effects of discrimination training on the perception of /r-l/ by Japanese adults learning English. *Percept Psychophys* 36:131–145, 1984.

62. Strange W, Jenkins JJ: Role of linguistic experience in the perception of speech, in Walk D, Pick Jr HJ (eds): *Perception and Experience.* New York: Plenum, 1978, pp 125–169.

63. Bishop DVM: The causes of specific developmental language disorder ("developmental dysphasia"). *J Child Psychol Psychiatry* 28:1–8, 1987.

64. Jernigan TL, Hesselink JR, Sowell E, Tallal PA: Cerebral structure on magnetic resonance imaging in language impaired and learning-impaired children. *Arch Neurol* 48:539–545, 1991.

65. Plante E, Swisher L, Vance R: Anatomical correlates of normal and impaired language in a set of dizygotic twins. *Brain Lang* 37:643–655, 1989.

66. Plante E, Swisher L, Vance R, Rapsak S: MRI findings in boys with specifically language impairment. *Brain Lang* 41:52–66, 1991.

67. Arnold G, Schwartz S: Hemispheric lateralization of language in autistic and aphasic children. *J Autism Dev Disord* 13:129–139, 1983.

68. Boliek CA, Bryden MP, Obrzut JE: Focused attention and the perception of voicing and place of articulation contrasts with control and learning-disabled children. The 16th Annual Meeting of the International Neuropsychological Society. New Orleans, LA, January 1988.

69. Cohen H, Gelinas C, Lassonde M, Geoffroy G: Auditory lateralization for speech in language-impaired children. *Brain Lang* 41:395–401, 1991.

70. Obrzut JE, Conrad PF, Boliek CA: Verbal and nonverbal auditory processing among left- and right-handed good readers and reading disabled children. 16th Annual Meeting of the International Neuropsychological Society. New Orleans, LA, 1988.

71. Obrzut JE, Conrad PF, Bryden MP, Boliek CA: Cued dichotic listening with right-handed, left-handed, bilingual and learning-disabled children. *Neuropsychologia* 26:119–131, 1988.

72. Dawson G, Finley C, Phillips S, Lewy A: A comparison of hemispheric asymmetries in speech-related brain potentials of autistic and dysphasic children. *Brain Lang* 37:26–41, 1989.

73. Denays R, Tondeur M, Foulon M, et al: Regional brain blood flow in congenital dysphasia studies with technetium-99m HM-PAO SPECT. *J Nuc Med* 30:1825–1829, 1989.

74. Lou HD, Henriksen L, Bruhn P: Focal cerebral dysfunction in developmental learning disabilities. *Lancet* 335:8–11, 1990.

75. Cohen M, Campbell R, Yaghmai F: Neuropathological abnormalities in developmental dysphasia. *Ann Neurol* 25:567–570, 1989.

76. Galaburda A: Neuropathologic correlates of learning disabilities. *Semin Neurol* 11:20–27, 1991.

77. Galaburda AM: Developmental dyslexia and animal studies: At the inferface between cognition and neurology. *Cognition* 50:133–149, 1994.

78. Geschwind N, Galaburda A: Cerebral lateralization: Biological mechanisms, associations, and pathology: I. *Arch Neurol* 42:428–459, 1985.

79. Geschwind N, Galaburda AM: *Cerebral Lateralization: Biological Mechanisms, Associations, and Pathology.* Cambridge, MA: MIT Press, 1987.

80. Livingstone MS, Rosen GD, Drislane FW, Galaburda AM: Physiological and anatomical evidence for a magnocellular defect in developmental dyslexia. *Proc Natl Acad Sci USA* 88:7943–7947, 1991.

81. Beitchman JH, Hood J, Inglis A: Familial transmission of speech and language impairment: A

preliminary investigation. *Can J Psychiatry* 37:151–156, 1992.

82. Byrne BM, Willerman L, Ashmore LL: Severe and moderate language impairment: Evidence for distinctive etiologies. *Behav Genet* 4:331–345, 1974.

83. Haynes C, Naidoo S: *Children with Specific Speech and Language Impairment.* London: MacKeith Press, 1991.

84. Ingram TTS: Specific developmental disorders of speech in childhood. *Brain* 82:450–467, 1959.

85. Lewis BA: Pedigree analysis of children with phonology disorders. *J Learn Disabil* 25:586–597, 1992.

86. Lewis BA, Ekelman BL, Aram DM: A familial study of severe phonological disorders. *J Speech Hear Res* 32:713–724, 1989.

87. Luchsinger R: Inheritance of speech deficits. *Fol Phoniatr* 22:216–230, 1970.

88. Neils J, Aram DM: Family history of children with developmental language disorders. *Percept Motor Skills* 63:655–658, 1986.

89. Tallal P, Ross R, Curtiss S: Familial aggregation in specific language impairment. *J Speech Hear Disord* 54:167–173, 1989.

90. Tomblin JB: Familial concentrations of developmental language impairment. *J Speech Hear Dis* 54:287–295, 1989.

91. Tomblin JB, Hardy JC, Hein HA: Predicting poor-communication status in preschool children using risk factors present at birth. *J Speech Hear Res* 34:1096–1105, 1991.

92. Whitehurst GJ, Arnold DS, Smith M, et al: Family history in developmental expressive language delay. *J Speech Hear Res* 34:1150–1157, 1991.

93. Heath SB: *Ways with Words: Language, Life and Work in Communities and Classrooms.* New York: Cambridge University Press, 1983.

94. Singleton JL, Morford JP, Goldin-Meadow S: Once is not enough: Standards of well-formedness in manual communication created over three different timespans. *Language* 69:683–715, 1993.

95. Stromswold K: The genetic basis of language acquisition, in Stringfellow A, Cahana-Amitay D, Hughes E, Zukowski A (eds): *Proceedings of the 20th Annual Boston University Conference on Language Development.* Somerville, MA: Cascadilla Press, 1996, vol 2, pp 736–747.

96. Falconer DS: *Introduction to Quantitative Genetics.* New York: Ronald Press, 1960.

97. Bakwin H: Reading disabilities in twins. *Dev Medic Child Neurol* 15:184–187, 1973.

98. DeFries JC, Gillis JJ: Genetics of reading disabil-

ity, in Plomin R, McClearn GE (eds): *Nature, Nurture, and Psychology.* Washington, DC: American Psychological Association, 1993, pp 121–145.

99. Lewis BA, Thompson LA: A study of developmental speech and language disorders in twins. *J Speech Hear Res* 35:1086–1094, 1992.

100. Locke JL, Mather PL: Genetic factors in the ontogeny of spoken language: Evidence from monozygotic and dizygotic twins. *J Child Lang* 16:553–559, 1989.

101. Matheny AP, Dolan AB, Wilson RS: Twins with academic learning problems: Antecedent characteristics. *Am J Orthopsychiatr* 46:464–469, 1976.

102. Pauls DL: Genetic analysis of family pedigree data: A review of methodology, in Ludlow CL, Cooper JA (eds): *Genetic Aspects of Speech and Language Disorders.* New York: Academic Press, 1983, pp 139–147.

103. Arnold GE: The genetic background of developmental language disorders. *Fol Phoniatr* 13:246–254, 1961.

104. Hurst JA, Baraitser M, Auger E, et al: An extended family with a dominantly inherited speech disorder. *Dev Med Child Neurol* 32:347–355, 1990.

105. Lenneberg EH: *Biological Foundations of Language.* New York: Wiley, 1967.

106. Lewis BA: Familial phonological disorders: Four pedigrees. *J Speech Hear Disord* 55:160–170, 1990.

107. Samples J, Lane V: Genetic possibilities in six siblings with specific language learning disorders. *Am Speech Lang Hear Assoc* 27:27–32, 1985.

108. Stromswold K: Language comprehension without language production: Implications for theories of language acquisition. Boston University Conference on Language Development. Boston, January 1994.

109. Lewis BA, Cox NJ, Byard PJ: Segregation analysis of speech and language disorders. *Behav Genet* 23:291–297, 1993.

110. Benedict H: Early lexical development: Comprehension and production. *J Child Lang* 6:183–200, 1979.

111. Bishop DV, Edmundson A: Specific language impairment as a maturational lag: Evidence from longitudinal data on language and motor development. *Dev Med Child Neurol* 29:442–459, 1987.

112. Camarata S, Gandour J: Rule invention in the acquisition of morphology by a language-impaired child. *J Speech Hear Dis* 50:4–45, 1985.

113. Curtiss S, Katz W, Tallal P: Delay versus deviance

114. Gibson D, Ingram D: The onset of comprehension and production in a language delayed child. *Appl Psycholing* 4:359–375, 1983.

115. Grimm H, Weinert S: Is the syntax development of dysphasic children deviant and why? New findings to an old question. *J Speech Hear Res* 33:220–228, 1990.

116. Kahmi A: Metalinguistic abilities in language impaired children. *Topics Lang Disord* 7:1–12, 1987.

117. Guilfoyle E, Allen S, Moss S: Specific language impairment and the maturation of functional categories. BU Conference of Language Development. Boston, Oct 19, 1991.

118. Oetting JB, Rice ML: Plural acquisition in children with specific language impairment. *J Speech Hear Res* 36:1236–1248, 1993.

119. Rice ML, Oetting JB: Morphological deficits of children with SLI: Evaluation of number marking and agreement. *J Speech Hear Res* 36:1249–1257, 1993.

120. Rice ML, Oetting JB: Morphological deficits of SLI children: A matter of missing functional categories? BU Conference on Language Development. Boston, October 1991.

121. Rice ML, Wexler K: Extended optional infinitive (EIO) account of specific language impairment, in MacLaughlin D, McEwen S (eds): *19th Annual Boston University Conference on Language Development.* Boston: Cascadilla Press, 1995, pp 451–462.

122. Bishop DVM: Grammatical errors in specific language impairment: Competence or performance limitations. *Appl Psycholing* 15:507–550, 1994.

123. Leonard LB, Bortolini U, Caselli MC, et al: Morphological deficits in children with specific language impairment: The status of features in the underlying grammar. *Lang Acquis* 2:151–179, 1992.

124. Leonard LB, Sabbadini L, Volterra V, Leonard JS: Some influences on the grammar of English- and Italian-speaking children with specific language impairment. *Appl Psycholing* 9:39–57, 1988.

125. Lahey M, Liebergott J, Chesnick M, et al: Variability in children's use of grammatical morphemes. *Appl Psycholing* 13:373–398, 1992.

126. Aram DM, Nation JE: Preschool language disorders and subsequent language and academic difficulties. *J Commun Disord* 13:159–170, 1980.

127. Hall P, Tombin J: A follow-up study of children

with articulation and language disorders. *J Speech Hear Disord* 43:227–241, 1978.

128. King RR, Jones C, Lasky E: In retrospect: A fifteen-year follow-up report of speech-language disordered children. *Lang Speech Hear Serv School* 13:24–32, 1982.

129. Silva PA: The prevalence, stability, and significance of developmental language delay in preschool children. *Dev Med Child Neurol* 22:768–777, 1980.

130. Silva PA, Williams S, McGee R: A longitudinal study of children with developmental language delay at age three: Later intelligence, reading and behavior problems. *Dev Med Child Neurol* 29:630–640, 1987.

131. Arthur G: *The Arthur Adaptation of the Leiter International Performance Scale.* Washington, DC: Psychological Service Center Press, 1952.

132. Aram DM, Eklelman BL, Nation JE: Preschoolers with language disorders: 10 years later. *J Speech Hear Res* 27:232–244, 1984.

133. Lee LL: The developmental sentence scoring (DSS) reweighted scores, in Lee LLA (ed): *Developmental Sentence Analysis.* Evanston, IL: Northwestern University Press, 1974, pp 6–7.

134. Bowey JA, Patel RK: Metalinguistic ability and early reading achievement. *Appl Psycholing* 9:367–383, 1988.

135. Catts HW, Hu C-F, Larrivee L, Swank L: Early identification of reading disabilities in children with speech-language impairments, in Watkins RV, Rice ML (eds): *Specific Language Impairments in Children.* Baltimore: Brookes, 1994, pp 145–160.

136. Kahmi AG: Causes and consequences of reading disabilities, in Kahmi AG, Catts HW (eds): *Reading Disability: A Developmental Language Perspective.* Boston: Little, Brown, 1989, pp 67–99.

137. Kahmi AG, Catts HW: *Reading Disabilities: A Developmental Language Perspective.* Boston: Little, Brown, 1989.

138. Kavanagh JF, Yeni-Komshian G: *Developmental Dyslexia and Related Reading Disorders.* Bethesda, MD: National Institute of Child Health and Human Development, 1985.

139. Perfetti CA: *Reading Ability.* New York: Oxford University Press, 1985.

140. Scarborough HS: Very early language deficits in dyslexic children. *Child Dev* 61:1728–1743, 1990.

141. Scarborough HS, Dobrich W: Development of

children with early language delay. *J Speech Hear Res* 33:70–83, 1990.

142. Snyder LS, Downey DM: The language-reading relationship in normal and reading-disabled children. *J Speech Hear Res* 34:129–140, 1991.

143. Stanovich KE: The right and wrong places to look for the cognitive locus of reading disability. *Ann Dyslexia* 38:154–177, 1988.

144. Vellutino FR: *Dyslexia: Theory and Research.* Cambridge, MA: MIT Press, 1979.

145. Bryant PE, Bradley L, Maclean M, Crossland J: Nursery rhymes, phonological skills, and reading. *J Child Lang* 16:407–428, 1989.

146. Mann VA, Ditunno P: Phonological deficiencies: Effective predictors of future reading problems, in Pavlides G (ed): *Perspectives on Dyslexia.* New York: Wiley, 1990, pp 105–131.

147. Share DL, Jorm AF, Maclean R, Matthews R: Sources of individual differences in reading acquisition. *J Educ Psychol* 76:1309–1324, 1984.

148. Stanovich KE, Cunningham AE, Cramer BB: Assessing phonological awareness in kindergarten children: Issues of task comparability. *J Exp Child Psychol* 38:175–190, 1984.

149. Stuart M, Coltheart M: Does reading develop in a sequence of stages? *Cognition* 30:139–181, 1988.

150. Silva PA, McGee R, Williams W: Some characteristics of 9-year-old boys with general reading backwardness or specific reading retardation. *J Child Psychol Psychiatry* 26:407–421, 1985.

151. Wolf M, Goodglass H: Dyslexia, dysnomia, and lexical retrieval: A longitudinal study. *Brain Lang* 28:154–168, 1986.

152. Butler SR, Marsh HW, Sheppard MJ, Sheppard JL: Seven-year longitudinal study of the early prediction of reading achievement. *J Educ Psychol* 77:349–361, 1985.

153. Tunmer WE, Herriman ML, Nesdale AR: Metalinguistic abilities and beginning reading. *Read Res Q* 23:134–158, 1988.

154. Ingram TTS, Mason AW, Blackburn I: A retrospective study of 82 children with reading disability. *Dev Med Child Neurol* 12:271–281, 1970.

155. Rutter M, Yule W: The concept of specific reading retardation. *J Child Psychol Psychiatry* 16:181–197, 1975.

156. Johnston C, Prior M, Hay D: Prediction of reading disability in twin boys. *Dev Med Child Neurol* 26:588–595, 1984.

157. Olson RK, Wise B, Conners F, et al: Specific deficits in component reading and language skills:

Genetic and environmental influences. *J Learn Disabil* 22(6):339–348, 1989.

158. Chomsky N: *Knowledge of Language: Its Nature, Origin, and Use.* New York: Praeger, 1986.

159. Chomsky N: *Syntactic Structures.* The Hague: Mouton, 1957.

160. Caramazza A, Laudanna A, Romani C: Lexical access and inflectional morphology. *Cognition* 28:297–332, 1988.

161. Garrett MF: Production of speech: Observations from normal and pathological language use, in Ellis A (ed): *Normality and Pathology in Cognitive Functions.* London: Academic Press, 1982.

162. Grodzinsky Y: *Theoretical Perspectives on Language Deficits.* Cambridge, MA: MIT Press, 1990.

163. Zurif E, Swinney D, Prather P, et al: An on-line analysis of syntactic processing in Broca's and Wernicke's aphasia. *Brain Lang* 45:448–464, 1993.

164. Leonard LB, Sabbadini L, Leonard JS, Volterra V: Specific language impairment in children: A cross-linguistic study. *Brain Lang* 32:233–252, 1987.

165. Pinker S: *Language Learnability and Language Development.* Cambridge, MA: Harvard University Press, 1984.

Chapter 18

ACQUIRED DYSLEXIA

H. Branch Coslett

The study of acquired dyslexia or disorders of reading dates at least to the contributions of Déjerine, who, in 1891 and 1892, described two patients with quite different patterns of reading impairment. Déjerine's first patient[1] developed an impairment in reading and writing subsequent to an infarction involving the left parietal lobe. Déjerine termed this disorder "alexia with agraphia" and attributed the disturbance to a disruption of the "optical image for words," which he thought to be supported by the left angular gyrus. In an account that in some respects presages contemporary psychological accounts, Déjerine concluded that reading and writing required the activation of these "optical images" and that the loss of the images resulted in an inability to recognize or write familiar words.

Déjerine's second patient[2] was quite different. This patient was unable to read aloud or for comprehension but could write, a disorder that Déjerine designated "alexia without agraphia" (also known as agnosic alexia and pure alexia). The patient had a right homonymous hemianopia from a left occipital lesion, which included the fibers carrying visual information from the right to the left hemisphere. Déjerine explained alexia without agraphia in terms of a "disconnection" between visual information confined to the right hemisphere and the left angular gyrus, which he assumed to be critical for the recognition of words.

After the seminal contributions of Déjerine, the study of acquired dyslexia languished for de-cades, during which the relatively few investigations that were reported focused primarily on the anatomic underpinnings of the disorders. The study of acquired dyslexia was revitalized, however, by the elegant and detailed investigation by Marshall and Newcombe,[3] demonstrating that by virtue of a careful investigation of the pattern of reading deficits exhibited by dyslexic subjects, distinctly different and reproducible types of reading deficits could be elucidated. These investigators described a patient (GR) who read approximately 50 percent of concrete nouns but was severely impaired in the reading of abstract nouns and all other parts of speech. The most striking aspect of GR's performance, however, was his tendency to produce errors that appeared to be semantically related to the target word (e.g., *speak* read as "talk"). Marshall and Newcombe[3] designated this disorder "deep dyslexia." These investigators also described two patients whose primary deficit appeared to be an inability to derive the pronunciation of irregularly spelled words, such as "yacht." This disorder was designated "surface dyslexia."

On the basis of these data, Marshall and Newcombe[3] concluded that the meaning of written words could be accessed by two separate and distinct procedures. The first was a lexical (whole-word) procedure whereby familiar words activated the appropriate stored representation (or visual word form), which, in turn, activated meaning; reading in deep dyslexia was assumed to involve this procedure, labeled A in Fig. 18-1.

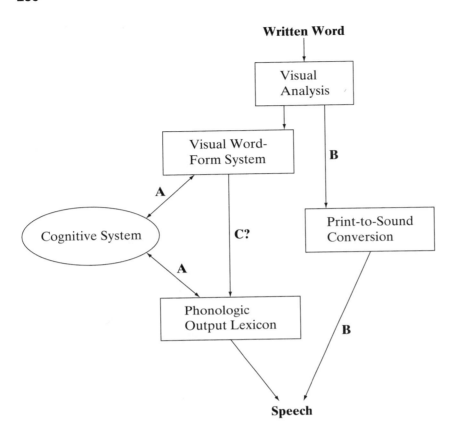

Written Word

Figure 18-1
A diagram of an information-processing model of reading incorporating three procedures for oral reading.

The second procedure was assumed to be a phonologically based process in which "grapheme-to-phoneme" (hereafter termed "print-to-sound") correspondences were employed to derive the appropriate phonology (that is, "sound out" the word); the reading of surface dyslexics was assumed to be mediated by this nonlexical procedure, labeled B in Fig. 18-1. Although a number of Marshall and Newcombe's specific hypotheses have been criticized, their argument that reading may be mediated by two distinct procedures has received considerable empirical support. Indeed, although it has occasionally been questioned,[4,5] the dual-route model of reading has provided the conceptual framework that has motivated most subsequent study of acquired dyslexias and animates the present discussion.

In this chapter we briefly summarize the clinical features and conceptual basis of the major types of acquired dyslexia. Additionally, the possible role of the right hemisphere in reading is briefly discussed. Finally, recent efforts to develop computational models of normal reading and acquired dyslexia are briefly described.

PERIPHERAL DYSLEXIAS

A useful starting point in the discussion of the dyslexias is the distinction offered by Shallice and Warrington[6] between "peripheral" and "central" dyslexias. The former are conditions characterized by a deficit in the processing of visual aspects of the stimulus that interfere with the matching of a familiar word to its stored orthographic representation or "visual word form."[6] Central dyslexias, in contrast, are attributable to an impairment of the "deeper" or "higher" reading functions by which visual word forms mediate access to meaning or speech production mechanisms. The major types of peripheral dyslexia are briefly described below.

Alexia without Agraphia (Pure Alexia)

The classic syndrome of alexia without agraphia or pure alexia is perhaps the prototypical peripheral dyslexia. As noted above, the traditional account[2,7] of this disorder attributes the syndrome to a "disconnection" of visual information, which is restricted to the right hemisphere, from the left-hemispheric word-recognition system.

Though these patients do not appear to be able to read in the sense of fast, automatic word recognition, many are able to use a compensatory strategy that involves naming the letters of the word in serial fashion; they read, in effect, letter by letter. Using the slow and inefficient letter-by-letter procedure, pure alexics typically exhibit significant effects of word length, requiring more time to read long as compared to short words. In contrast to the central dyslexias, performance is typically not influenced by linguistic factors such as parts of speech (e.g., noun versus functor), the extent to which the referent of the word is concrete (e.g., "table") or abstract (e.g., "destiny"), or whether the word is orthographically regular (that is, can be "sounded out").

A number of alternative accounts of the processing deficit in pure alexia have been proposed. Thus, some investigators have proposed that the impairment is attributable to a limitation in the transmission of letter identity information to the visual word system (e.g., Ref. 8), an inability to directly encode visual letters as abstract orthographic types,[9,10] or an inability to encode multiple visual shapes of any sort in rapid succession.[11,12] Other investigators have argued that the disorder is attributable to a disruption of the visual word-form system itself.[13,14]

Although most reports of pure alexia have emphasized the profound nature of the reading deficit, often stating that patients were utterly incapable of reading without recourse to a letter-by-letter strategy,[7,8] a number of investigators have reported data demonstrating that at least some pure alexic patients are able to comprehend words that they are unable to explicitly identify.[15–17] This capacity has been attributed by some investigators (e.g., Ref. 17) to the operation of a reading procedure based in the right hemisphere.

The anatomic basis of pure alexia has been extensively investigated. Although on rare occasions associated with lesions that "undercut" or disconnect the posterior perisylvian cortex on the left,[18] the disorder is typically associated with a lesion in the posterior portion of the dominant hemisphere, which compromises visual pathways in the dominant hemisphere as well white matter tracts (such as the splenium of the corpus callosum or forceps major) critical for the interhemispheric transmission of visual information.[19,20]

Neglect Dyslexia

Neglect dyslexia, which is most commonly encountered in patients with left-sided neglect, is characterized by a failure to explicitly identify the initial portion of a letter string. Interestingly, the performance of patients with neglect dyslexia is often influenced by the nature of the letter string; thus, patients with this disorder may fail to report the initial letters in nonwords (e.g., the "ti-" in a nonword such as "tiggle") but read real words (e.g., "giggle") correctly (Ref. 21; see also Refs. 22 and 23). The fact that performance is affected by the lexical status of the stimulus has been taken to suggest that neglect dyslexia is not attributable to a failure to register letter information but reflects an attentional impairment at a higher level of representation.

Although neglect dyslexia is generally seen in the context of the neglect syndrome (see Chaps. 10 and 11), it has occasionally been observed in isolation or even in the context of neglect of the opposite side of space.[24]

Attentional Dyslexia

Perhaps the least studied of the acquired dyslexias, attentional dyslexia is characterized by the relative preservation of single-word reading in the context of a gross disruption of reading when words are presented in text or in the presence of other words or letters.[25–28] Patients with this disorder may also exhibit difficulties identifying letters within words, even though the words themselves are read correctly[25] and be impaired in identifying words flanked by extraneous letters (e.g., "lboat"). We[28] have recently investigated a patient with attentional dyslexia secondary to autopsy-proven Alzheimer disease who produced frequent "blend" errors in which letters from one word of a two-word display intruded into the other word (e.g., "take lime" read as "tame"). Although several accounts for this disorder have been proposed, the disorder has been attributed by several investigators to an impairment in visual attention or a loss of location information. As visual attention may be critical to mapping the location of visually presented objects, these accounts are not clearly distinguishable.

CENTRAL DYSLEXIAS

In this section we briefly describe the clinical features and conceptual basis of the major types of central dyslexia including "deep," "phonologic," and "surface" dyslexia. Additionally, the phenomenon of "reading without meaning" is discussed.

Deep Dyslexia

Deep dyslexia, the most extensively investigated central dyslexia (see, for example, Coltheart and colleagues[29]) is in many respects the most compelling. The allure of deep dyslexia is due in large part to the intrinsically interesting hallmark of the syndrome, *semantic errors*. When shown the word *castle*, a deep dyslexic may respond "knight"; similarly, these interesting patients may read *bird* as "canary." At least for some deep dyslexics, it is clear that these errors are not circumlocutions and that the patients are not even aware that they have erred.

While semantic errors are typically regarded as essential for the diagnosis of deep dyslexia, the

frequency with which deep dyslexics produce them is quite variable; for some patients, semantic errors may represent the most frequent error type, whereas for others they constitute a small proportion of reading errors. These patients also produce a variety of other types of reading errors, including "visual" errors in which the response bears a clear visual similarity to the target (e.g., *skate* read as "scale") and "morphologic" errors, in which a prefix or suffix is added, deleted, or substituted (e.g., *scolded* read as "scolds"; *governor* read as "government").

Additional hallmarks of the syndrome include a greater success in reading words of high as compared to low imageability. Thus, words such as *table, chair, ceiling*, and *buttercup*, the referents of which are concrete or imageable, are read more successfully by deep dyslexics than words such as *fate, destiny, wish*, and *universal*, the referents of which are abstract.

Also characteristic of the syndrome is part-of-speech effect, such that nouns are read more reliably than modifiers (adjectives and adverbs), which are, in turn, read more accurately than verbs. Deep dyslexics manifest particular difficulty in the reading of functors (a class of words that includes pronouns, prepositions, conjunctions, and interrorogatives such as *that, which, they, because, under*, etc.). The striking nature of the part-of-speech effect is illustrated by the patient reported by Saffran and Marin[30] who correctly read the word *chrysanthemum* but was unable to read the word *the*! Many errors to functors involve the substitution of a different functor (*that* read as *which*) rather than the production of words of a different class, such as nouns or verbs.

As functors are, in general, less imageable than nouns, verbs, or adjectives, some investigators have claimed that the apparent effect of part of speech is in reality a manifestation of the pervasive imageability effect described above.[31] We have reported a patient,[32] however, whose performance suggests that the part-of-speech effect is not simply a reflection of a more general deficit in the processing of low-imageability words, as the difference remained after functors and content words were matched for imageability.

Finally, all deep dyslexics exhibit a substantial impairment in the reading of nonwords; when confronted with letter strings such as *flig* or *churt,* deep dyslexics are typically unable to employ print-to-sound correspondences to derive phonology; nonwords frequently elicit "lexicalization" errors (e.g., *flig* read as "flag"), perhaps reflecting a reliance on lexical reading in the absence of access to reliable print-to-sound correspondences.

How can deep dyslexia be accommodated by the model of reading depicted in Fig. 18-1? Several alternative explanations have been proposed. Most investigators agree that multiple processing deficits must be hypothesized to account for the full range of symptoms found in deep dyslexia. First, the strikingly impaired performance in reading nonwords and other tasks assessing phonologic function suggest that the print-to-sound conversion procedure is disrupted. Second, the presence of semantic errors and the effects of imageability (a variable usually thought to influence processing at the level of semantics) has been interpreted by many investigators as evidence that these patients also suffer from a semantic impairment; it should be noted in this context, however, that some deep dyslexic patients perform well on tests of comprehension with words they are unable to read aloud. Semantic errors in these patients have been attributed to a deficit in or access to representations in the output phonologic lexicon (Ref. 33; see also Ref. 6). Last, the production of visual errors has been interpreted by some to suggest that these patients suffer from an impairment in the visual word-form system. Other investigators (e.g., Coltheart;[34] Saffran and coworkers[35]) have argued that deep dyslexics' reading is mediated by a system not normally used in reading—that is, the right hemisphere. We will return to the issue of reading with the right hemisphere below.

Although deep dyslexia has occasionally been associated with posterior lesions, this disorder is typically encountered in association with large perisylvian lesions extending into the frontal lobe. As might be expected given the lesion data, deep dyslexia is usually associated with global or Broca's aphasia but may rarely be encountered in patients with fluent aphasia.

Phonologic Dyslexia: Reading without Print-to-Sound Conversion

First described in 1979 by Derouesne and Beauvois,[36] phonologic dyslexia is, perhaps, the "purest" of the central dyslexias in that the syndrome appears to be attributable to a selective deficit in the procedure mediating the translation from print to sound. Thus, although in many respects less arresting than deep dyslexia, phonologic dyslexia is of considerable theoretical import. It is of interest to note that the existence of this syndrome was *predicted* by dual-route accounts of reading similar to that proposed by Marshall and Newcombe[3] and subsequently identified when dyslexic patients were assessed with theoretically motivated tasks.

Phonologic dyslexia is a relatively mild disorder in which reading of real words may be only slightly impaired. Many patients with this disorder, for example, correctly read 85 to 95 percent of real words (e.g., Refs. 32, 36, 37). Some patients with this disorder read all different types of words with equal facility,[37–39] whereas other patients are relatively impaired in the reading of functors.[40,41] Unlike patients with surface dyslexia, described below, the regularity of print-to-sound correspondences is not relevant to the performance of phonologic dyslexics; thus, these patients typically pronounce orthographically irregular words such as *colonel* and words with standard print-to-sound correspondences such as *administer* with equal facility. Most errors in response to real words appear to have a visual basis, often involving the substitution of visually similar real words (e.g., *topple* read as "table").

The striking and theoretically relevant aspect of the performance of phonologic dyslexics is a substantial impairment in the oral reading of nonword letter strings. A number of investigators have described patients with this disorder, for example, who read more than 90 percent of real words of all types yet correctly pronounce only about 10 percent of nonwords.[32,36] Most errors in nonword reading involve the substitution of a visually similar real word (e.g., *phope* read as "phone") or the incorrect application of print-to-sound correspondences (e.g., *stime* read as "stim," rhyming with "him").

Within the context of the reading model depicted in Fig. 18-1, the account for this disorder is relatively straightforward. The patients' good performance with real words suggests that the processes involved in normal "lexical" reading—that is, visual analysis, the visual word-form system, semantics, and the phonologic output lexicon—are at least relatively preserved. The impairment in nonword reading suggests that the print-to-sound translation procedure is disrupted.

A final point of interest is that a number of phonologic dyslexics exhibit substantial deficits in processing morphologically complex words—that is, words with prefixes and suffixes.[37,41] The explanation for this association is not clear.

Phonologic dyslexia has been observed in association with lesions in a number of sites in the dominant perisylvian cortex and, on occasion, with lesions of the right hemisphere (e.g., Ref. 41). Damage to the superior temporal lobe and angular and supramarginal gyri in particular is found in most but not all patients with this disorder. Although quantitative data are lacking, the lesions associated with phonologic dyslexia appear to be smaller on average than those associated with deep dyslexia.

Just as there is variability with respect to the lesion site associated with phonologic dyslexia, there is variability with respect to the type and severity of aphasia observed in these patients. A phonologic dyslexic reported by Derouesne and Beauvois,[36] for example, did not exhibit a significant aphasia, whereas Funnell's patient WB[37] appears to have had a severe nonfluent aphasia.

Surface Dyslexia

Surface dyslexia is a disorder characterized by the inability to read words with "irregular" or exceptional print-to-sound correspondences. Patients with surface dyslexia are thus unable to read aloud words such as *colonel, yacht, island, have,* and *borough,* the pronunciation of which cannot be derived by phonologic or "sounding out" strategies. In contrast, these patients read words containing regular correspondences (e.g., *state, hand, mint, abdominal*) as well as nonwords (e.g., *blape*) quite well.

As noted above, normal subjects may read familiar words by matching the letter string to a stored representation of the word and retrieving the pronunciation by means of a mechanism linked to semantics (or, as discussed below, by means of a nonsemantic "direct" route). As this procedure involves the activation of stored representations, the pronunciation of the word is not computed by rules but is retrieved; consequently, the regularity of print-to-sound correspondences would not be expected to play a major role in performance.

In the context of a dual route model of reading, the sensitivity to the regularity of the print-to-sound correspondences provides prima facie evidence that the impairment in surface dyslexia is in the mechanism(s) mediating lexical reading. Similarly, the preserved ability to read regular words and nonwords provides compelling support for the claim that the procedures by which pronunciations are computed by the application of print-to-sound correspondences are at least relatively preserved.

Noting that there is substantial variability in the performance of surface dyslexics with respect to leading latencies as well as accuracy, Shallice and McCarthy[43] suggested that the syndrome of surface dyslexia be fractionated. Type 1 surface dyslexia, they suggested, is characterized by effortless and accurate reading of nonwords and regular words with poor performance with irregular words only. Type 2 surface dyslexia, in contrast, is characterized by slow, effortful reading; although these patients read irregular words less well than regular words and nonwords, they make errors with all types of stimuli. More recently, Shallice[44] suggested that at least for patients with type 2 surface dyslexia, the syndrome may reflect an attempt to compensate for damage to early stages of the reading process.

Other investigators have suggested that the syndrome may be fractionated even more. Thus, for example, surface dyslexia may be associated with disruption of the visual word-form system,[3] with a disruption of semantics (in conjunction with a deficit in the "direct" route),[45,46] or with a lesion involving the phonologic output lexicon.[47] Indeed, Coltheart and Funnell[48] proposed that within the context of a multiroute model of reading, surface dyslexia might be associated with as many as seven distinct types of impairment.

Finally, if as suggested above, patients with surface dyslexia are unable to access semantics by means of a direct lexical procedure, one might ask how these patients derive word meaning. At least for some surface dyslexics, access to a word's meaning appears to occur only after the phonologic form of the word has been derived. Thus, when presented the word *listen,* a patient described by Marshall and Newcombe[3] responded "Liston" and added "that's the boxer."

The anatomic correlate of surface dyslexia has not been well established. Indeed, in recent years the syndrome has been reported most frequently in the context of dementia.[46,49–54] Accordingly, surface dyslexia in demented patients is sometimes termed "semantic dyslexia." Many of these patients have exhibited brain atrophy most prominent in the temporal lobes (e.g., Refs. 50 and 53).

Reading without Meaning

In 1980, Schwartz and coworkers[45] reported a patient (WLP) who exhibited a profound loss of semantics in the context of dementia. Her performance was of particular interest because, unlike patients with surface dyslexia, she correctly read aloud both regular and irregular words that she was unable to comprehend. Thus, for example, when asked to sort written words into their appropriate semantic categories, she correctly classified only 7 of 20 animal names; critically, WLP correctly read aloud 18 of these animal names, including such orthographically ambiguous or irregular words such as *hyena* and *leopard.* The same basic phenomenon—that is, the ability to read aloud regular and irregular words that the patient does not understand—has subsequently

been reported by a number of investigators (see Refs. 55 and 56).

The pattern of performance exhibited by WLP and similar patients is of considerable theoretical interest. Recall that to this point, two procedures have been described by which written words may be pronounced. The first (labeled A in Fig. 18-1) involves the activation of an entry in the visual word-form system, access to semantic information, and ultimately activation of an entry in the phonologic output lexicon. The second (B in Fig. 18-1) involves the nonlexical print-to-sound translation process. Reading without semantics is of interest precisely because it cannot readily be accommodated by such an account. The fact that these patients do not comprehend the words they correctly pronounce indicates that their oral reading is not mediated by the semantically based reading procedure. Additionally, the fact that these patients can read irregular words suggests that they are not relying on a sublexical print-to-sound conversion procedure.

How, then, do these patients read aloud? Several explanations have been proposed. One response was to suggest that oral reading may be mediated by a third mechanism or route (e.g., Ref. 57). This mechanism was assumed to be lexically based, involving the activation of an entry in the visual word-form system and the "direct" activation of an entry in the phonologic output lexicon (C in Fig. 18-1); note that this procedure differs from the lexical procedure described above in that there is no intervening activation of semantic information. Based on the analysis of a phonologic dyslexic's performance across a variety of reading, writing, and repetition tasks, we[32] have reported data providing additional support for the existence of a lexical but nonsemantic reading procedure. An alternative hypothesis was proposed by Shallice and colleagues (Refs. 44 and 46; see also Ref. 58). These investigators attempted to explain reading without semantics within the context of a dual-route model by proposing that the phonologic reading procedure employs not only grapheme-to-phoneme correspondences but also correspondences based on larger units including syllables and even morphemes. Thus, on this account, WLP and similar patient are assumed to compute the pronunciation of irregular words they cannot understand by relying on the multiple levels of print-to-sound correspondences available in the phonologic system. Finally, Hillis and Caramazza[59] have suggested that the apparent ability to read without meaning is attributable to the fact that, while the patient is impaired, the semantic and phonologic reading procedures provide partial information that constrains the subject's responses. Thus, on this account, neither the semantic nor phonologic procedure is assumed to be capable of generating the correct response, but the combination of partial phonologic and incomplete semantic information is often sufficient to identify the stimulus.

READING AND THE RIGHT HEMISPHERE

One important and controversial issue regarding reading concerns the putative reading capacity of the right hemisphere. For many years investigators argued that the right hemisphere was "word blind."[2,6,7] In recent years, however, several lines of evidence have suggested that the right hemisphere may possess the capacity to read. One seemingly incontrovertible line of evidence comes from the performance of a patient who underwent a left hemispherectomy at age 15 for treatment of seizures caused by Rasmussen's encephalitis;[60] after the hemispherectomy, the patient was able to read approximately 30 percent of single words and exhibited an effect of part of speech; she was also utterly unable to use a print-to-sound conversion process. Thus, in many respects this patient's performance was similar to that of a person with deep dyslexia, a pattern of reading impairment that has been hypothesized to reflect the performance of the right hemisphere.[34,35]

The performance of some split-brain patients is also consistent with the claim that the right hemisphere is literate. These patients may, for example, be able to match printed words presented to the right hemisphere with an appropriate object.[61,62] Interestingly, the patients are apparently unable to derive sound from the words presented to the right hemisphere; thus, they are unable to determine if a word presented to the right hemisphere rhymes with an auditorially presented word.

Another line of evidence supporting the claim that the right hemisphere is literate comes from evaluation of the reading of patients with pure alexia and optic aphasia.[17,63] We reported data, for example, from four patients with pure alexia who performed well above chance on a number of lexical decision and semantic categorization tasks with briefly presented words that they could not explicitly identify. Three of the patients who regained the ability to identify rapidly presented words explicitly exhibited a pattern of performance consistent with the right-hemisphere reading hypothesis. These patients read nouns better than functors and words of high (e.g., *chair*) better than words of low (e.g., *destiny*) imageability. Additionally, both patients for whom data were available demonstrated a deficit in the reading of suffixed (e.g., *flowed*) as opposed to pseudo-suffixed (e.g., *flower*) words. These data are consistent with a version of the right-hemisphere reading hypothesis postulating that the right-hemisphere lexical-semantic system primarily represents high imageability nouns. On this account, functors, affixed words, and low imageability words are not adequately represented in the right hemisphere.

Finally, we reported data from an investigation with a patient with pure alexia in which transcranial magnetic stimulation (TMS) was employed to directly test the hypothesis that the right hemisphere mediates the reading of at least some patients with acquired dyslexia.[64] We reasoned that if the right hemisphere provides the neural substrate for reading, the transient, localized disruption of cortical processing caused by TMS of the right hemisphere would interfere with reading. An extensively investigated patient with pure alexia who exhibited the reading pattern described above was asked to read aloud briefly presented words, half of which were presented in association with TMS. Consistent with the hypothesis that his reading was mediated by the right hemisphere, stimulation of the right hemisphere interfered with oral reading, whereas left-hemisphere stimulation had no significant effect.

Although a consensus has not yet been achieved, there is mounting evidence that, at least for some people, the right hemisphere is not word-blind but may support the reading of some types of words. The full extent of this reading capacity and whether it is relevant to normal reading, however, remains unclear.

COMPUTATIONAL MODELS OF THE DYSLEXIAS

To this point, the discussion of acquired reading disorders has been motivated by a widely though not universally (see Refs. 4 and 5) accepted multiroute information processing model of reading. In recent years, however, computer-implemented parallel distributed processing (PDP) models of cognitive processing have made important contributions in many domains of cognitive science, including reading (see Chaps. 4 and 15). These models, which differ from traditional information processing models in that they offer (and in fact require) greater specification of the manner in which information is represented and processed, have called into question the necessity of hypothesizing two routes to account for the syndromes reviewed here. Although a detailed discussion of these models is beyond the scope of this chapter, several PDP accounts of reading are briefly summarized below.

Seidenberg and McClelland[65] have reported a PDP model of single-word reading in which the procedure for computing pronunciation directly from orthography (that is, without semantic mediation) is assumed to be mediated by a single network in which orthographic patterns are linked to phonologic representations by means of an intermediate "hidden layer."[65] In contrast to the information processing accounts described above, this model does not postulate a discrete "lexical" or word-representation procedure or distinct lexical and sublexical procedures for the computation of phonology. Of particular relevance in the present context is the fact that investigators have attempted to simulate the performance of dyslexic patients by modifying or "lesioning" this PDP model. Patterson and colleagues,[66] for example, have attempted to model the performance of surface dyslexics by eliminating a proportion of the connections or units at different "lesion" sites. Although the simulations do not appear to capture all of the characteristic features of the performance of surface dyslexics, the lesioned models generate data that are in many interesting and important respects similar to those of patients. More recently, Plaut and Shallice[67] have reported a series of simulations of different PDP architectures in an attempt to model the performance of patients with deep dyslexia.

Several investigators have developed explicit PDP models of single-word reading that incorporate several distinct procedures by which output phonology can be generated. Reggia and coworkers,[68] for example, reported a PDP model that incorporates both lexical and nonlexical procedures for the computation of phonology. This model, which employs a competitive distribution of activation to govern interaction between competing concepts, simulates many aspects of normal reading performance; "lesioning" of the model produces patterns of performance consistent in many respects with the syndromes of phonologic and surface dyslexia. Finally, Coltheart and coworkers[69] have developed a dual-route computational model of visual word recognition and reading aloud that accommodates many of the patterns of performance typical of normal reading. As with the model developed by Reggia and associates,[68] selective disruptions of the model have been demonstrated to simulate surface and phonologic dyslexia.

REFERENCES

1. Déjerine J: Sur en case de cecite verbal avec agraphie, suivi d'autopsie. *C R Seances Soc Biol* 3:197–201, 1891.
2. Déjerine J: Contribution a l'etude anatomo-

pathologique et clinique des differentes varietes de cecite verbale. *C R Seances Soc Biol* 4:61–90, 1892.

3. Marshall JC, Newcombe F: Patterns of paralexia: A psycholinguistic approach. *J Psycholing Res* 2:175–199, 1973.

4. Marcel AJ: Surface dyslexia and beginning reading: A revised hypothesis of the pronunciation of print and its impairments, in Coltheart M, Patterson KE, Marshall JC (eds): *Deep Dyslexia.* London: Routledge, 1980.

5. Van Orden GC, Pennington BF, Stone GO: Word identification in reading and the promise of sub-symbolic psycholinguistics. *Psychol Rev* 97:488–522, 1990.

6. Shallice T, Warrington EK: Single and multiple component central dyslexic syndromes, in Coltheart M, Patterson K, Marshall JC (eds): *Deep Dyslexia.* London: Routledge, 1980.

7. Geschwind N: Disconnection syndromes in animals and man. *Brain* 88:237–294, 585–644, 1965.

8. Patterson K, Kay J: Letter-by-letter reading: Psychological descriptions of a neurological syndrome. *Q J Exp Psychol* 34A:411–441, 1982.

9. Arguin M, Bub DN: Pure Alexia: Attempted rehabilitation and its implications for interpretation of the deficit. *Brain Lang* 47:233–268, 1994.

10. Arguin M, Bub DN: Single-character processing in a case of pure alexia. *Neuropsychologia* 31:435–458, 1993.

11. Kinsbourne M, Warrington EK: A disorder of si-multaneous form perception. *Brain* 85:461–486, 1962.

12. Farah MJ, Wallace MA: Pure alexia as a visual im-pairment: A reconsideration. *Cog Neuropsychol* 8:313–334, 1991.

13. Warrington EK, Shallice T: Word-form dyslexia. *Brain* 103:99–112, 1980.

14. Warrington EK, Langdon D: Spelling dyslexia: A deficit of the visual word-form. *J Neurol Neurosurg Psychiatry* 57:211–216, 1994.

15. Landis T, Regard M, Serrat A: Iconic reading in a case of alexia without agraphia caused by a brain tumor: A tachistoscopic study. *Brain Lang* 11:45–53, 1980.

16. Shallice T, Saffran EM: Lexical processing in the absence of explicit word identification: Evidence from a letter-by-letter reader. *Cog Neuropsychol* 3:429–458, 1986.

17. Coslett HB, Saffran EM: Evidence for pre-served reading in pure alexia. *Brain* 112:327–329, 1989.

18. Greenblatt SH: Subangular alexia without agraphia or hemianopia. *Brain Lang* 3:229–245, 1976.

19. Binder JR, Mohr JP: The topography of callosal reading pathways: A case-control analysis. *Brain* 115:1807–1826, 1992.

20. Damasio AR, Damasio H: The anatomic basis of pure alexia. *Neurology* 33:1573–1583, 1983.

21. Sieroff E, Pollatsek A, Posner MI: Recognition of visual letter strings following injury to the posterior visual spatial attention system. *Cog Neuropsychol* 5:427–449, 1988.

22. Behrman M, Moscovitch M, Black SE, Mozer M: Perceptual and conceptual mechanisms in neglect dyslexia. *Brain* 113:1163–1183, 1990.

23. Berti A, Frassinetti F, Umilta C: Nonconscious reading? Evidence from neglect dyslexia. *Cortex* 30:181–197, 1994.

24. Costello AD, Warrington EK: The dissociation of visual neglect and neglect dyslexia. *J Neurol Neuro-surg Psychiatry* 50:110–116, 1987.

25. Shallice T, Warrington EK: The possible role of se-lective attention in acquired dyslexia. *Neuropsy-chologia* 15:31–41, 1977.

26. Price CJ, Humphreys GW: Attentional dyslexia: The effects of co-occurring deficits. *Cog Neuropsy-chol* 6:569–592, 1993.

27. Warrington EK, Cipolotti L, McNeil J: Attentional dyslexia: A single case study. *Neuropsychologia* 31:871–886, 1993.

28. Saffran EM, Coslett HB: "Attentional dyslexia" in Alzheimer's disease: A case study. *Cog Neuropsy-chol.* In press.

29. Coltheart M, Patterson K, Marshall JC (eds): *Deep Dyslexia.* London: Routledge, 1980.

30. Saffran EM, Marin OSM: Reading without phonol-ogy: Evidence from aphasia. *Q J Exp Psychol* 29:515–525, 1977.

31. Allport DA, Funnell E: Components of the mental lexicon. *Phil Trans R Soc Lond B* 295:397–410, 1981.

32. Coslett HB: Read but not write "idea": Evidence for a third reading mechanism. *Brain Lang* 40:425–443, 1991.

33. Caramazza A, Hillis AE: Where do semantic errors come from? *Cortex* 26:95–122, 1990.

34. Coltheart M: Deep dyslexia: A right hemisphere hypothesis, in Coltheart M, Patterson K, Marshall JC (eds): *Deep Dyslexia.* London: Routledge, 1980.

35. Saffran EM, Bogyo LC, Schwartz MF, Marin OSM: Does deep dyslexia reflect right-hemisphere read-

ing? in Coltheart M, Patterson K, Marshall JC (eds): *Deep Dyslexia.* London: Routledge, 1980.

36. Derouesne J, Beauvois M-F: Phonological processing in reading: Data from alexia. *J Neurol Neurosurg Psychiatry* 42:1125–1132, 1979.

37. Funnell E: Phonological processes in reading: New evidence from acquired dyslexia. *Br J Psychol* 74:159–180, 1983.

38. Bub D, Black SE, Howell J, Kertesz A: Speech output processes and reading, in Coltheart M, Sartori G, Job R (eds): *Cognitive Neuropsychology of Language.* Hillsdale, NJ: Erlbaum, 1987.

39. Friedman RB, Kohn SE: Impaired activation of the phonological lexicon: Effects upon oral reading. *Brain Lang* 38:278–297, 1990.

40. Glosser G, Friedman RB: The continuum of deep/phonological dyslexia. *Cortex* 26:343–359, 1990.

41. Patterson KE: The relation between reading and psychological coding: Further neuropsychological observations, in AW Ellis (ed): *Normality and Pathology in Cognitive Functions.* London: Academic Press, 1982.

42. Friedman RB, Ween JE, Albert ML: Alexia, in Heilman KM, Valenstein E (eds): *Clinical Neuropsychology,* 3d ed. Oxford, England: Oxford University Press, 1993.

43. Shallice T, McCarthy R: Phonological reading: From patterns of impairment to possible procedures, in Patterson KE, Coltheart M, Marshall JC (eds): *Surface Dyslexia.* London: Erlbaum, 1985.

44. Shallice T: *From Neuropsychology to Mental Structure.* Cambridge, England: Cambridge University Press, 1987.

45. Schwartz MF, Saffran EM, Marin OSM: Dissociation of language function in dementia: A case study. *Brain Lang* 7:277–306, 1979.

46. Shallice T, Warrington EK, McCarthy R: Reading without semantics. *Q J Exp Psychol* 35A:111–138, 1983.

47. Howard D, Franklin S: Three ways for understanding written words, and their use in two contrasting cases of surface dyslexia (together with an odd routine for making "orthographic" errors in oral word production), in Allport A, Mackay D, Prinz W, Scheerer E (eds): *Language Perception and Production.* New York: Academic Press, 1987.

48. Coltheart M, Funnell E: Reading writing: One lexicon or two? in Allport DA, MacKay DG, Prinz W, Scheerer E (eds): *Language Perception and Production: Shared Mechanisms in Listening, Speaking,* *Reading and Writing.* London: Academic Press, 1987.

49. Warrington EK: The selective impairment of semantic memory. *Q J Exp Psychol* 27:635–657, 1975.

50. Hodges JR, Patterson K, Oxbury S, Funnell E: Semantic dementia: Progressive fluent aphasia with temporal lobe atrophy. *Brain* 115:1783–1806, 1992.

51. Patterson K, Hodges J: Deterioration of word meaning: Implications for reading. *Neuropsychologia* 30:1025–1040, 1992.

52. Graham KS, Hodges JR, Patterson K: The relationship between comprehension and oral reading in progressive fluent aphasia. *Neuropsychologia* 32:299–316, 1994.

53. Breedin SD, Saffran EM, Coslett HB: Reversal of the concreteness effect in a patient with semantic dementia. *Cog Neuropsychol* 11:617–660, 1994.

54. Cipolotti L, Warrington EK: Semantic memory and reading abilities: A case report. *J Int Neuropsychol Soc* 1:104–110, 1994.

55. Friedman RB, Ferguson S, Robinson S, Sunderland T: Dissociation of mechanisms of reading in Alzheimer's disease. *Brain Lang* 43:400–413, 1992.

56. Raymer AM, Berndt RS: Models of word reading: Evidence from Alzheimer's disease. *Brain Lang* 47:479–482, 1994.

57. Morton J, Patterson KE: A new attempt at an interpretation, or, an attempt at a new interpretation, in Coltheart M, Patterson K, Marshall JC (eds): *Deep Dyslexia.* London: Routledge, 1980.

58. McCarthy RA, Warrington EK: Phonological reading: Phenomena and paradoxes. *Cortex* 22:359–380, 1986.

59. Hillis AE, Caramazza A: Mechanisms for accessing lexical representations for output: Evidence from a category-specific semantic deficit. *Brain Lang* 40:106–144, 1991.

60. Patterson K, Vargha-Khadem F, Polkey CF: Reading with one hemisphere. *Brain* 112:39–63, 1989.

61. Zaidel E: Lexical organization in the right hemisphere, in Buser P, Rougeul-Buser A (eds): *Cerebral Correlates of Conscious Experience.* Amsterdam: Elsevier, 1978.

62. Zaidel E, Peters AM: Phonological encoding and ideographic reading by the disconnected right hemisphere: Two case studies. *Brain Lang* 14:205–234, 1981.

63. Coslett HB, Saffran EM: Preserved object recogni-

tion and reading comprehension in optic aphasia. *Brain* 12:1091–1110, 1989.

64. Coslett HB, Monsul N: Reading and the right hemisphere: Evidence from transcranial magnetic stimulation. *Brain Lang* 46:198–211, 1994.

65. Seidenberg MS, McClelland JL: A distributed, developmental model of word recognition and naming. *Psychol Rev* 96:522–568, 1989.

66. Patterson KE, Seidenberg MS, McClelland JL: Connections and disconnections: Acquired dyslexia in a computational model of reading processes, in Morris RGM (ed): *Parallel Distributed Processing: Implications for Psychology and Neurobiology.* Oxford, England: Oxford University Press, 1989.

67. Plaut D, Shallice T: Deep dyslexia: A case study of connectionist neuropsychology. *Cog Neuropsychol* 10:377–500, 1993.

68. Reggia J, Marsland P, Berndt R: Competitive dynamics in a dual-route connectionist model of print-to-sound transformation. *Complex Systems* 2:509–547, 1988.

69. Coltheart M, Langdon R, Haller M: Simulation of acquired dyslexias by the DRC model, a computational model of visual word recognition and reading aloud, in *Proceedings of the 1995 Workshop on Neural Modeling of Cognitive and Brain Disorders.* College Park, MD: University of Maryland, June 8–10, 1995.

Chapter 19

DEVELOPMENTAL READING DISORDERS

Maureen W. Lovett

For more than a century, it has been recognized that a sizable minority of otherwise intelligent, healthy children unexpectedly fail to learn to read. In 1895, Hinshelwood[1,2] described specific reading problems as *visual word blindness* and hypothesized that such difficulties were caused by damage to a visual memory center for words localized to the left angular gyrus. Early recognition of developmental learning disorders was influenced strongly by case studies of brain-damaged adults with acquired cognitive disorders.[3] In 1896, Morgan[4] suggested a parallel between cases of acquired and developmental reading disorder and drew attention to the fact that a congenital form of word blindness could exist in children with otherwise normal development. The most influential early student of reading disability was Samuel Orton,[5,6] who described a condition he labeled *strephosymbolia,* which he attributed to incomplete or delayed cerebral dominance. Orton suggested that developmental delay in specialization of the left hemisphere for language could cause the condition. Orton's work formed the basis for a number of early educational therapies for the disorder,[7,8] some of which remain popular today.[9]

Over 25 years ago, the World Federation of Neurology defined *specific developmental dyslexia* by exclusionary criteria as "a disorder manifested by difficulty in learning to read despite conventional instruction, adequate intelligence, and sociocultural opportunity." The disorder was attributed to "fundamental cognitive disabilities which are frequently of constitutional origin."[10] Some authors attributed dyslexia to a "well defined defect in any one of several specific higher cortical functions,"[11] drawing attention to the heterogeneous presentation of the accompanying cognitive deficits. Other authors observed that the majority of dyslexic children have accompanying, potentially precursive, speech and language concomitants to their reading disorder: In 1979, Denckla[12] described dyslexia as the "index symptom of a developmental language disorder too subtle to lead to referral of the child in preschool life" (p. 550), a view reiterated by other authors over the past decade.[13–16] Developmental dyslexia occurs relatively frequently, with prevalence rates conservatively estimated at 3 to 6 percent.[17–19]

Exclusionary definitions of dyslexia fostered diagnostic approaches based on defining a discrepancy between reading achievement and intellectual potential as measured by standardized psychometric tests. Regression formulas are used to classify as dyslexic those children who are reading significantly below IQ-based expectations. A discrepancy-based definition of dyslexia or developmental reading disability has dominated clinical practice and research for decades and has been legislated into eligibility requirements for special education services in parts of the United States and Canada.[20–23]

At the heart of the discrepancy-based approach is the assumption that aptitude-achievement discrepancies yield a more homogeneous—and more specific—diagnostic profile than that provided by definitions based on low achievement criteria alone. It was assumed that higher-IQ disabled readers experienced a more specific form of dyslexia characterized by a unique deviant pattern of development in reading-related cognitive processes, while low-IQ disabled readers were handicapped by developmental lags in many reading-related *and* -unrelated cognitive processes.[16,23] Some authors considered the discrepancy group more "purely" dyslexic and of potentially different (biologically driven?) etiology than the no-discrepancy group of "garden-variety" poor readers.[24]

Recent research has demonstrated, however, that disabled readers with and without aptitudeachievement discrepancies do not differ on the information processing subskills (phonologic and orthographic coding) that underlie word recognition. Word recognition deficiencies define the index symptom of reading disability; and all of the differences between these two groups of disabled readers lay outside the word-recognition module.[23] Similarly, recent epidemiologic evidence provides no support for specificity of cognitive deficits in relation to IQ-based discrepancies.[25] This evidence confirms that the principal correlate of reading disability is linguistic, with the most reliable predictors found in the phonologic processing domain. An assessment of intellectual potential, while useful in practice, is not essential to the definition of developmental reading disorders. Therefore the definition of dyslexia, or *developmental reading disability* (often used synonymously), is based on indications of severe difficulties in reading acquisition despite access to instructional, linguistic, and environmental opportunities.

CURRENT DEFINITIONS OF DEVELOPMENTAL READING DISABILITY

Current research defines the most reliable indicator of reading disability as a failure to acquire rapid, context-free word-identification skill.[16,19,24,26–30] Although disabled readers experience problems with decoding accuracy, reading rate, and comprehension when reading connected text, the index symptom of their disability involves severe developmental failures of word-recognition learning and deficiencies in component processes within the word-identification domain.

Reading disability is often accompanied by associated deficits in some aspect of speech and language development, although this is not invariably true. In the past 15 years, there has been converging evidence that the core linguistic deficit characterizing developmental reading disability is deficient phonologic awareness. Phonologic awareness can be defined as "the ability to reflect explicitly on the sound structure of spoken words,"[31] a multifaceted ability with different levels of analysis developing at different rates.[32] A certain degree of phonologic awareness and an ability to segment and blend individual speech sounds are considered prerequisites to learning grapheme-phoneme (letter-sound) correspondences and acquiring an alphabetic code.[33–35] Many aspects of phonologic awareness and phonologic processing skills have been reported deficient in dyslexic individuals, including difficulties segmenting individual sounds within words, blending individual speech sounds to produce a word, and using phonologic codes to facilitate working memory processes.[16,28,36–38] Phonologic processing abilities measured in kindergarten have been demonstrated to be the best predictors of reading ability and disability at the end of second grade.[39,40] Phonologic processing deficits have been demonstrated to persist into adulthood even when individuals with childhood diagnoses of dyslexia were shown to attain reasonable standards of literacy.[41]

Children with reading disability also have problems rapidly retrieving and accessing names for visually presented material.[42–48] The deficit in visual naming speed characterizes disabled readers from kindergarten[47] through adulthood,[49–51] has been documented in dyslexics of other languages,[52–54] and has been suggested to be causally implicated in failures to acquire rapid, context-free word-identification skill.[44,46]

Developmental reading disability, therefore, appears characterized by two highly specific deficits in separate aspects of speech, language, and visible language development: (1) problems in the ability to represent and access individual speech sounds in words and (2) difficulty in rapidly accessing and retrieving names for visual symbols. Both deficits interfere with language and visible language processing at the lexical level and are compatible with evidence that the defining feature of the dyslexic reading disability is a failure to acquire rapid, context-free word-identification skill.[55–57]

GENETIC AND NEUROBIOLOGICAL BASES OF DEVELOPMENTAL READING DISORDERS

The Genetics of Dyslexia

The biological bases of developmental reading disorders have attracted considerable scientific interest. Evidence of the familiality of the disorder was suggested in several early case reports and in a few early family and twin studies.[58–60] In 1970, an influential epidemiologic study on the Isle of Wight reported that dyslexia was identified with a frequency of 34 percent among the parents and siblings of reading-disabled children but was identified in only 9 percent of the families of control children.[61] Later comparison of results from four different family studies reported similar findings and strong evidence of the familiality of dyslexia: the median increase in the risk of dyslexia to a child having a dyslexic parent was approximately eight times the population prevalence figure of 5 percent, with sibling recurrence estimated at a rate between 38 and 43 percent.[62–65] Twin studies using multiple regression techniques to estimate heritable and common environmental contributions supported early speculation that familial aggregation is at least partly based on genetic transmission.[66] DeFries and his colleagues in the Colorado Family Reading Study estimated that approximately 30 percent of the cognitive phenotype in developmental dyslexia could be attributed to heritable factors; later heritability estimates for reading (44 percent), spelling (62 percent), and nonword reading (75 percent) were even higher.[63,66–68] Precise

mechanisms of transmission for dyslexia, however, are not suggested from these data.

In recent years, two major findings have been reported from large-scale genetic studies of developmental dyslexia. To evaluate mode of transmission, segregation analyses were conducted on four independently ascertained family samples (1698 individuals from 204 families): Pennington and colleagues found evidence of major gene transmission (dominant or additive) with sex-dependent penetrance (estimated as complete in males, incomplete in females) in three samples, and the suggestion of multifactorial-polygenic transmission in the fourth sample.[69] The investigators are careful to note, however, that genetic heterogeneity existed even in families selected for apparent dominant transmission. These segregation findings are interpreted as strong evidence for sex-influenced, major locus transmission in a large proportion of dyslexic families.[63]

Other investigators using segregation and linkage analysis techniques have concluded that their results indicate genetic heterogeneity in the transmission of dyslexia.[70,71] Earlier work in the 1980s had suggested evidence for linkage between dyslexia and chromosome 15 heteromorphisms in a minority of families with apparent autosomal dominant transmission.[72] Although at least one study failed to confirm linkage between dyslexia and chromosome 15 heteromorphisms,[73] further work by the Colorado group estimated that dyslexia may be linked to chromosome 15 in a minority (<20 percent) of families.[65]

The second critical recent finding is a report of a major dyslexia locus on chromosome 6 in the majority of affected families not linked to chromosome 15. Investigators have reported what is described as "compelling evidence" for a quantitative trait locus for reading disability on chromosome 6 within the human leukocyte antigen region.[74] Derived from interval mapping of genetic data from two independent samples of sibling pairs, this quantitative trait locus is suggested to have either a recessive or dominant mode of expression. The search was targeted to this region of chromosome 6 because of the association observed by some investigators between dyslexia and immune disorders,[75,76] and knowledge that specific fragments of chromosome 6 had been identified as containing genes that contribute to disorders like hay fever, migraine headaches, asthma, thyroid disease, and allergies. Many behavioral geneticists consider this finding confirmatory evidence that a majority of cases of dyslexia will be linked to a small specific part of the human genome, and that a gene for dyslexia may be found.

Although recent findings are the most provocative yet reported on the behavioral genetics of reading disability, the notion that a specific gene for dyslexia will be identified remains controversial. Pennington[63] cautions that behavioral genetics may not identify a single locus for the dyslexic disorder itself but rather a major locus effect relevant to the transmission of reading ability and disability. The familiality, heritability, and transmission results for normal variability in reading ability parallel those found for reading disability,[77] leading to speculation that a small number of quantitative trait loci may contribute to the transmission of both normal reading skill and dyslexia.[63] Dyslexics may have more unfavorable alleles at these loci and/or greater environmental risk: Pennington suggests that the locus or loci, therefore, are better described as "susceptibility" loci for reading disorders.

Plomin[78] is even more cautious, warning that applications of molecular biology to the study of behavior may be unproductive if it is assumed that one or two major genes will prove largely responsible for genetic variation: Plomin contends that there is generally scant evidence to suggest that genetic influence on behavior can be attributed to a few major genes. He recommends an alternative approach that allows the identification of multiple genes that account for small amounts of variance, with recognition of the fact that genetic variance typically does not account for half of observed behavioral variance and that nongenetic sources of variance are equally significant.

The Neurobiology of Dyslexia

Interest in defining the neuroanatomic substrates of developmental reading disability has been strong since Hinshelwood's localization of visual word memory to the left angular gyrus at the beginning of this century. Two types of investigations have been reported in the search for what is different in the brain morphology and brain function of dyslexic individuals. These include neuroimaging studies of dyslexic and matched control samples and postmortem studies of dyslexic and control brains. Until relatively recently, evidence from these two empiric approaches appeared to converge, suggesting a tentative model of structural differences in the brain development of dyslexic children that appeared grossly compatible with behavioral observations of core symptoms. Recent results appear far more divergent, however: both inconsistent findings and growing awareness of methodologic limitations suggest our current understanding of the neurobiologic correlates of dyslexia to be quite tentative.[79]

Because reading involves processing language in visible form and because of the speech-based concomitants of dyslexia, many attempts to study the neuroanatomy of dyslexia focused on brain systems believed to subserve language function, particularly those in the perisylvian association cortex of the left hemisphere.[80,81] Particular attention has been directed to bilateral measurement of the planum temporale (PT), a neuroanatomical landmark on the upper surface of the temporal lobe that contains several subdivisions of auditory cortex, has been implicated by left-sided lesions causing Wernicke's aphasia, and is thought to subserve auditory perception and association in the left hemisphere.[82–85] Early computed tomography (CT) and magnetic resonance imaging (MRI) studies reported increased symmetry for dyslexics in the regions of the planum temporale and the parietal-occipital cortex,[86,87] findings consistent with those from the first postmortem studies on dyslexia.[88] Most of these early neuroimaging studies were criticized on methodologic grounds by Hynd and Semrud-Clikeman,[89] however, for reliance on questionable criteria in the diagnosis of dyslexia and for their failure to include comparison groups with other diagnosed developmental and neurocognitive disorders. Although directed at studies conducted in the early 1980s, these methodologic concerns remain relevant to many current neuroimaging studies. Hynd and Semrud-Clikeman contended that without other well-defined clinical control groups, any differences between dyslexic and normal controls could not be considered evidence of neuroanatomic involvement specific to dyslexia.

In the past few years, greater access to MRI technologies has encouraged further research on brain morphology and dyslexia. Hynd and Semrud-Clikeman conducted an MRI study in an attempt to define syndrome-specific patterns of brain involvement in two different (although frequently comorbid) developmental disorders, dyslexia and attention deficit hyperactivity disorder (ADHD). They found that 70 percent of normal and ADHD children exhibited the expected pattern of left > right plana asymmetry, but only 10 percent of the dyslexic children did.[90] Both clinical groups had smaller right anterior width measurements than the normal controls, but these investigators concluded the significant increase in the incidence of plana symmetry or reversed asymmetry to be unique to dyslexia and they postulated a relationship to deviant patterns of corticogenesis.

Larsen and coworkers[91] reported somewhat similar MRI results, noting that among dyslexics with documented phonologic deficits none exhibited expected patterns of plana asymmetry. These investigators suggested asymmetry of the plana may be a prerequisite for normal language development in the phonological domain. The Larsen and colleagues[91] and Hynd and coworkers[90] results were not similar, however, at another level of analysis. Larsen's results indicated a reversal of the expected left asymmetry in the report of a *greater right* planum temporale length in dyslexic subjects. Rather than a greater right planum, Hynd and associates reported a *smaller left* planum compared to the right and a smaller insular region bilaterally.

These discrepancies are frequent among different neuroimaging results reported on dyslexia, a fact that Schultz and associates[81] and Filipek[79] attribute to both (1) wide variations in (and lack of attention to) subjects' age, sex, handedness, and diagnostic criteria validity in different studies and (2) inherent difficulties in accurately and reliably measuring structures like the planum temporale. In an attempt to replicate previous MRI results on dyslexia, Schultz and colleagues[81] found initial evidence of smaller left hemispheric structures in dyslexic brains: when analyses were conducted controlling for age and overall brain size, however, no reliable differences between dyslexics and normal controls were found on a range of measures including those of surface area and symmetry of the planum temporale. Sex, age, and overall brain size were all found to significantly influence specific morphometric measures of the brain, especially the surface area of the planum temporale. After reviewing all of the recent MRI studies on developmental dyslexia, Filipek[79] concluded that none of the planum temporale measurements in these studies were comparable, and that definition of the plana temporale remains one of the most difficult challenges for MRI-based work. Filipek concludes that, at present, no consistent morphologic correlates of developmental reading disorders can be identified from neuroimaging studies.

The second line of neuroanatomic evidence on dyslexia is provided through postmortem studies of dyslexic brains. The first autopsy study was reported by Drake,[92] detailing postmortem findings on a 12-year-old boy with multiple learning disabilities and a family history of dyslexia who died of a massive cerebellar hemorrhage. Several neurodevelopmental abnormalities were found that could not be attributed to brain damage, including an abnormal convolutional pattern bilaterally in the parietal lobes, a thinned corpus callosum, and ectopic neurons deep in the white matter. These findings suggested deviations in cellular migration during gestation.[93]

Subsequent studies by Galaburda and colleagues confirmed the presence of minor cortical malformations in four male dyslexic brains and alterations in the expected patterns of brain asymmetry in the language areas, particularly the planum temporale.[88] In all four autopsies, neurodevelopmental abnormalities were found primarily in the left frontal and left perisylvian region. Postmortem studies of three female dyslexic brains again revealed symmetry of the planum temporale and cortical abnormalities identical to those reported for the male brains.[94] The malformations were suggested to occur in the second trimester of pregnancy.[82]

Supported by experimental studies with animal models,[95-97] Galaburda speculates that a genetic defect may result in a tendency to small cerebral vascular accidents (CVAs) in fetal life, and that the sequelae of these events is abnormal neuronal migration and the establishment of abnormal neuronal circuits in brain areas typically devoted to language functions: the dyslexic brain is suggested to have too many neurons in the posterior language areas, particularly in the right hemisphere, rather than too few.[83] Based on Behan and Geschwind's[98] theory about the interrelationships between immune deficiencies and deviations in neuronal migration, Galaburda[99] speculates that the focal brain injury may even be mediated through allergic mechanisms.

Although not emphasized in the report, the focal ectopias and dysplasias revealed in the Galaburda and coworkers[88] work were bilateral in nature and involved both left and right frontal regions. As Hynd and Semrud-Clikeman[89] note, the bilateral involvement of the anterior cortex is very relevant behaviorally, and may support speculation that the language disturbances associated with developmental dyslexia may extend beyond left anterior-central structures to include right hemispheric systems.

Additional evidence on the neurobiology of dyslexia is found in combined neurophysiologic and neuroanatomic studies. In a controversial report, Lovegrove and colleagues[100] had identified a specific visual abnormality associated with dyslexia, abnormally slow flicker fusion rates (i.e., the fastest rate at which a contrast reversal of a stimulus can be seen) observed only at low spatial frequencies and at low contrasts. In evoked potentials studies, Livingstone and coworkers,[101] and Lehmkuhle and colleagues[102] found that the parvocellular pathway (the slow, more contrast-insensitive, and color-selective visual pathway) seemed to be functioning normally in a dyslexic sample, but that the visual pathway handling fast, low-contrast stimuli appeared abnormally slow. Fast stimuli are handled by the magnocellular

pathway, the two pathways being differentiated in the retina and separate through the lateral geniculate nucleus (LGN), the primary visual cortex, and higher order visual cortices.[82] Livingstone and colleagues[101] compared the magnocellular and parvocellular layers of the LGN in five dyslexic and five control brains and found that the magnocellular cells were smaller in the dyslexic brains but the parvocellular cells were not. In subsequent work, Galaburda and coworkers[103] reported abnormal asymmetry in the medial geniculate nuclei (MGN) of five dyslexic brains; unlike control brains which were symmetrical, left MGN neurons were smaller than right MGN neurons in dyslexic brains. This finding implicated parallel difficulties in the auditory system, and was hypothesized relevant to behavioral observations of left hemisphere–based phonologic processing deficits. Livingstone and colleagues speculate that other cortical systems may be subdivided into fast and slow subsystems and that dyslexics may prove selectively deficient in fast subsystem functions across modalities.[82,101,103,104]*

---

*The reports of slowed visual function, related to the magnocellular pathway, are controversial in the dyslexia literature for several reasons: First, these results have not been consistently replicated in independent studies (e.g., see Ref. 102 versus Refs. 105 and 106); second, the methodology has been criticized for vulnerability to artifactual effects;[107] and third, the results appear to contradict the bulk of evidence on phonological core deficits as characteristic of dyslexia.[23,108] The relevance of detailed examination of rapid temporal processing functions in visual, auditory, and motor domains is suggested, however, by existing evidence of auditory temporal processing deficits in language impaired children,[109,110] visual naming speed deficits in dyslexic children,[46,47] and impaired temporal resolution in bimanual motor coordination in dyslexic children.[111] Wolff[111] cautions against any simplistic attribution of the temporal resolution deficit of dyslexics to a single temporal behavioral variable or to specific regions of the central nervous system neuroanatomically: Wolff[111] suggests instead that some of the core dyslexic deficits may relate to problems assembling components of behavior into "temporally ordered larger ensembles," problems which may be associated with developmental difficulty in motor, language, and reading domains.

Postmortem observations on developmental dyslexia are necessarily limited by small sample sizes, significant heterogeneity in the individual histories of the cases, and retrospective and variable diagnostic and behavioral data. Despite the obvious methodologic shortcomings, the neuroanatomic data provided through both the postmortem and animal research studies of Galaburda and colleagues have provided evidence on potential biological etiologies for reading disability and yielded a rich source of neurobiological hypotheses. With the expanding technologies available for functional neuroimaging and new awareness of critical design controls in neuroimaging studies with pediatric and adult samples,[79,81,112] the next decade should witness significant advances in our understanding of the structural and functional bases of dyslexic disorders in the developing brain.

THE TREATMENT OF DEVELOPMENTAL READING DISORDERS

Many approaches to treating reading disorders have been advocated. Some methods aim to remediate the nonreading deficit or set of deficits presumed causal to the reading disability, and a great diversity of interventions have been attempted in this tradition. These include perceptual and perceptual-motor training programs of the 1960s and 1970s (e.g., Refs. 113 and 114), pharmacologic interventions of the 1980s and 1990s,[115,116] and mechanical devices like the "electronic ear," which remain popular.[117] None of these methods has proven effective in the remediation of reading disability despite controlled research on their efficacy.[118–122] The second type of treatment intervention for reading disorders attempts to remediate the deficient reading process directly and address the primary symptoms leading to referral. Consideration of this approach to treatment and what we learn of the core disorder through a systematic study of treatment response constitutes the remainder of this chapter.

Before the mid 1980s, there existed no reliable or credible evidence from well-controlled studies of the relative merit of any one intervention approach over another.[26,123–125] This dearth of

evidence led to inevitable questions about the amenability of the disorder to treatment. In the past decade, however, different investigators have reported positive findings from controlled intervention or training studies with samples of disabled readers.[33–35,126–134] Because the core deficit in phonologic awareness had been demonstrated to be a lifelong symptom, even with the attainment of some standard of literacy in adulthood,[41,135] reports of positive findings were particularly encouraging in demonstrating that children with developmental reading disability *are* able to benefit from some forms of literacy training.

The most recent treatment outcome data reveal the importance of addressing the core deficits defining the developmental reading disorder[127] rather than circumventing processing deficits and teaching to the child's "strengths." The best results appear with effective, well-directed treatment that remediates the basic phonologic and word-identification learning deficits. Both treatment successes and treatment failures from our intervention studies at the Hospital for Sick Children in Toronto have provided a window on the core acquisition deficits of children with developmental reading disability. Children with severe reading disabilities appear to have enormous difficulty abstracting grapheme-phoneme (letter-sound) pattern invariance. In one study, they failed to show significant transfer to uninstructed reading words even in situations where training on very similar instructed words had been clearly effective.[33] Despite their success on the training words, *line* and *mark,* for instance, dyslexic subjects were not reliably better after treatment in identifying *fine* and *dark.* In these studies, dyslexic subjects responded to intensive training by doubling their estimated reading vocabularies, yet they seemed to be acquiring specific lexical knowledge rather than systematic letter-sound knowledge that could facilitate their decoding of new, unknown words.

Transfer-of-Learning Issues

This pattern of dyslexic reading acquisition reflects basic difficulties in transfer of learning during the course of training. We have described these transfer-of-learning problems in the word-identification module and attributed them to difficulties in parsing syllables into subsyllabic units, a failure that limits dyslexic readers' acquisition of word recognition skill by preventing both large-unit (rime—i.e., the vowel and what comes after: the *ain* in *rain*) and smaller-unit (letter-sound, letter-cluster-sound) extraction of spelling-to-sound patterns when a new word is learned. We have attributed this difficulty to the phonemic awareness deficits known to characterize the most prevalent forms of developmental reading disability.[26,34] It has also been suggested that such difficulties may stem from the nature and/or accessibility of the lexical representations laid down in memory (e.g., Refs. 136 and 137) during learning.

Transfer-of-learning failures in reading acquisition are also exacerbated, however, by more general difficulties that many reading-disabled children experience in the metacognitive domain. The ability to identify new unknown words depends on age-appropriate phonologic processing skills, consolidated letter-sound knowledge, and also on effective and flexible strategies for identifying words and the child's ability to exert some metacognitive control over the decoding process. Children with reading disorders have been characterized as deficient and inefficient in the use of cognitive strategies.[138–142] Despite limitations in their phonemic awareness and letter-sound knowledge, disabled readers do not reliably use what they *do* know to help them decode what they do not.[127,143] Children with learning disorders have been characterized as lacking self-regulatory strategies, failing to self-monitor and self-correct the product of their efforts,[144–146] observations some authors have found suggestive of frontal lobe dysfunction.[147] Strategy acquisition, application, and monitoring is essential to any learning that extends beyond that which has been specifically taught; and strategy use and metacognitive knowledge are critical to achieving transfer of learning in many domains of functioning.[127,144,148]

Treating Transfer-of-Learning Failures

In a recent treatment outcome study, we have addressed two of the core deficits underlying devel-

opmental dyslexia and attempted to ameliorate transfer-of-learning difficulties in word-identification learning. Children with severe developmental reading disability were randomly assigned to two forms of word-identification training, both designed to promote transfer of learning, or to a study skills control program. One program addressed phonologic awareness and subsyllabic segmentation deficits through direct, intensive phonological training and direct instruction of letter-sound correspondences (PHAB/DI for Phonological Analysis and Blending/Direct Instruction).* The other program provided a metacognitive focus, training disabled readers in the acquisition, use, and monitoring of four metacognitive decoding strategies (WIST for Word Identification Strategy Training).† The two programs addressed subsyllabic segmentation with different-sized units, the phonologic program training the smallest units of spelling-to-sound mapping (letter-sound) and the metacognitive program dealing with larger spelling-to-sound units (i.e., the rime).

Results provided positive evidence of transfer of learning in the treatment of developmental reading disability.[127] Both intervention programs were associated with large positive effects, transfer attained on several different measures, and generalized achievement gains on standardized measures. Children who before training stumbled over high-frequency one-syllable words like *way*, *left*, and *put* were able (albeit slowly) after training to decode multisyllabic words like *unintelligible, mistakenly,* and *disengaged.* A critical finding of this research was the demonstration that the deficient phonologic processing skills of dyslexic children *are* amenable to treatment and that

---

*The PHAB/DI Program used direct instructional materials developed by Engelmann and colleagues at the University of Oregon[149–151] to train phonologic analysis, phonologic blending, and letter-sound association skills.

†The WIST Program was developed in our laboratory classrooms at the Hospital For Sick Children. This program is based in part on the Benchmark School Word Identification/Vocabulary Development Program developed by Gaskins and coworkers.[152]

phonologic segmentation, blending, and letter-sound learning abilities can be improved with effective and focused intervention methods. Both speech- and print-based phonologic skills of this impaired sample, although not normalized after 35 h of training, were significantly improved and closer to age-appropriate expectations. Different patterns of transfer were observed following the two different interventions, the phonologic program resulting in greater transfer across the phonologic domain, and the metacognitive program resulting in broader-based transfer for real English words (i.e., regular and exception words).

The success of both programs suggests that different routes of subsyllabic segmentation are possible in the remediation of reading disability: both the letter-sound (PHAB/DI) and the letter cluster-sound (WIST) approaches were associated with improved word identification and decoding skills. Some level of segmentation within the syllable, however, is essential to allow transfer from a just-learned word to a similarly spelled word: without subsyllabic segmentation that is explicitly trained and practiced, disabled readers will fail to transfer new word learning and be prevented from becoming independent readers.

In this study, both metacognitive and phonologically based training proved to be of merit in the remediation of developmental reading disability. These results are interpreted as evidence that only systematic deficit-directed remediation will allow severely disabled readers to overcome transfer-of-learning failures in the course of reading acquisition. Effective remediation of children with reading disabilities must address the problem of transfer of learning in every remedial lesson, and provide intensive remediation of the core processing deficits contributing to reading acquisition failure.[127]

SUMMARY COMMENTS

Developmental reading disability has been recognized as a specific developmental disorder for over a century. The term is usually reserved for those 3 to 6 percent of otherwise normally developing children who experience significant, often unexpected, difficulties in acquiring basic literacy skills. Once considered only to describe children reading below IQ-based predictions (i.e., those with higher IQs and lower reading achievement), the disorder is now recognized to affect children with a range of intellectual abilities and to be attributable to the same core processing deficits irrespective of a child's estimated intellectual potential.

Reading disorders are often accompanied by two highly specific deficits in separate aspects of speech and language development: (1) problems in the ability to represent and rapidly access individual speech sounds in words and (2) difficulty rapidly accessing and retrieving names for visual symbols. Both deficits have been found to persist into adulthood. Many reading-disabled children also appear generally deficient and inefficient in the use and monitoring of cognitive strategies, a tendency that exacerbates the difficulties attributable to their core processing deficits and makes it particularly hard for them to profit from remedial instruction. Our recent treatment results described severely reading-disabled children as experiencing basic problems with transfer of learning during the course of word-identification learning. Taught to read the words *rain* and *car,* these children could not reliably identify *pain* or *far,* a transfer failure we attribute to phonologically based difficulties in subsyllabic segmentation and a lack of effective decoding strategies.

The most recent treatment results with reading-disabled samples are encouraging in demonstrating that two of the above core deficits are amenable to treatment with systematic, intensive, and focused remediation: two different remedial teaching approaches were identified which allowed severely dyslexic children to improve their word identification and nonword decoding skills and demonstrate significant transfer of learning to a variety of words, nonwords, and reading tasks. While not completely ameliorated, the pervasive and persistent phonologic processing deficits of these children were significantly improved following intensive phonologic training. Similarly, children who stumbled over one-syllable words before treatment acquired the ability to decode difficult multisyllabic words following a metacognitive approach to literacy training. These results demonstrate that systematic deficit-directed remediation will allow severely dyslexic children to overcome transfer-of-learning problems: Effective remedial techniques are available to address the deficits contributing to reading acquisition failure in these children.

There are a number of neurobiological explanations advanced in research on the potential etiology of dyslexia. The possible heritability of dyslexia was recognized decades ago, with recognition that the disorder tended to familial aggregation. Although evidence for genetic heterogeneity is strong even for specially selected family samples, there is very recent evidence of a possible dyslexia locus on a specific region of chromosome 6. The search for neuroanatomic and neurophysiologic substrates of dyslexia has implicated areas of the left hemisphere specialized for language function but has also demonstrated evidence of bilateral frontal ectopias and other abnormalities in dyslexic brains. It has been speculated that deviations in neuronal pruning and neuronal migration in the second trimester of pregnancy result in too many neurons in the posterior language areas rather than too few, particularly in the right hemisphere. These deviations in fetal brain development have been attributed by different authors to possible viral infection in the mother,[153] small cerebrovascular accidents mediated through allergic mechanisms, or to conditions mediated by genetic predisposition.

Significant advances have been made in the definition, diagnosis, and treatment of developmental reading disabilities. At the same time, technical capabilities for functional neuroimaging research have expanded, and there is increasing commitment to methodologic rigor in the pursuit of a neurobiological perspective on reading, language, and their developmental disorders. With the wealth of interdisciplinary data now available, and the potential for new conceptualizations of developing brain and behavioral systems and their interrelationships, developmental dyslexia may become a model for examining development and developmental variability in this decade of the brain.

REFERENCES

1. Hinshelwood J: Word blindness and visual memories. *Lancet* 2:1566–1570, 1895.
2. Hinshelwood J: *Congenital Word Blindness.* London: Lewis, 1917.
3. Spreen O, Tupper D, Risser A, et al: *Human Developmental Neuropsychology.* New York: Oxford University Press, 1984.
4. Morgan WP: A case of congenital word-blindness. *Br Med J* 2:1378, 1896.
5. Orton ST: "Word-blindness" in school children. *Arch Neurol Psychiatry* 14:581–615, 1925.
6. Orton ST: Specific reading disability—Strephosymbolia. *J Am Med Assoc* 90:1095–1099, 1928.
7. Gillingham A, Stillman BW: *Remedial Training for Children with Specific Disability in Reading, Spelling, and Penmanship.* Cambridge, MA: Educators Publishing Service, 1960.
8. Orton ST: *Reading, Writing, and Speech in Children.* New York: Norton, 1937.
9. Ansara A: The Orton-Gillingham approach to remediation, in Malatesha RN, Aaron PG (eds): *Reading Disorders: Varieties and Treatment.* New York: Academic Press, 1982, pp 409–433.
10. Critchley M: *The Dyslexic Child.* Springfield, IL: Charles C Thomas, 1970.
11. Mattis S: Dyslexia syndromes: A working hypothesis that works, in Benton AL, Pearl D (eds): *Dyslexia: An Appraisal of Current Knowledge.* New York: Oxford University Press, 1978.
12. Denckla MB: Childhood learning disabilities, in Heilman KM, Valenstein E (eds): *Clinical Neuropsychology.* New York: Oxford University Press, 1979.
13. Bishop DVM, Adams C: A prospective study of the relationship between specific language impairment, phonological disorders and reading retardation. *J Child Psychol Psychiatry* 31:1027–1050, 1990.
14. Gathercole SE, Baddeley AD: The processes underlying segmental analysis. *Eur Bull Cogn Psychol* 7:462–464, 1987.
15. Scarborough HS: Very early language deficits in dyslexic children. *Child Devel* 61:1728–1743, 1990.
16. Stanovich KE: Annotation: Does dyslexia exist? *J Child Psychol Psychiatry* 55:579–595, 1994.

17. Hynd GW, Cohen M: *Dyslexia: Neuropsychological Theory, Research, and Clinical Differentiation.* New York: Grune & Stratton, 1983.

18. Rutter M: Prevalence and types of dyslexia, in Benton A, Pearl D (eds): *Dyslexia: An Appraisal of Current Knowledge.* New York: Oxford University Press, 1978.

19. Stanovich KE: Matthew effects in reading: Some consequences of individual differences in the acquisition of literacy. *Read Res Q* 21:360–407, 1986.

20. Frankenberger W, Fronzaglio K: A review of state's criteria and procedures for identifying children with learning disabilities. *J Learn Disabil* 24:495–500, 1991.

21. Frankenberger W, Harper J: State's criteria and procedures for identifying learning disabled children: A comparison of 1981/82 and 1985/86 guidelines. *J Learn Disabil* 20:118–121, 1987.

22. Satz P, Fletcher J: Minimal brain dysfunctions: An appraisal of research, concepts, and methods, in Rie HE, Rie ED (eds): *Handbook of Minimal Brain Dysfunctions: A Critical Review.* New York: Wiley, 1980, pp 669–714.

23. Stanovich KE, Siegel LS: Phenotypic performance profile of children with reading disabilities: A regression-based test of the phonological-core variable-difference model. *J Educ Psychol* 86:24–53, 1994.

24. Gough PB, Tunmer WE: Decoding, reading, and reading disability. *Remed Special Educ* 7:6–10, 1986.

25. Fletcher JM, Shaywitz SE, Shankweiler DP, et al: Cognitive profiles of reading disability: Comparisons of discrepancy and low achievement definitions. *J Educ Psychol* 86:6–23, 1994.

26. Lovett MW: Developmental dyslexia, in Rapin I, Segalowitz SJ (eds): *Handbook of Neuropsychology.* Amsterdam: Elsevier Science, 1992, pp 163–185.

27. Perfetti CA: *Reading Ability.* New York: Oxford University Press, 1985.

28. Stanovich KE: Changing models of reading and reading acquisition, in Rieben L, Perfetti CA (eds): *Learning to Read: Basic Research and Its Implications.* Hillsdale, NJ: Erlbaum, 1991, pp 19–31.

29. Vellutino FR: *Dyslexia: Theory and Research.* Cambridge, MA: MIT Press, 1979.

30. Wolf M, Vellutino F: A psycholinguistic account of the reading process, in Berko-Gleason J, Bernstein-Ratner N (eds): *Psycholinguistics.* New York: Macmillan, 1993, pp 352–391.

31. Snowling M, Hulme C: Developmental dyslexia and language disorders, in Blanken G, Dittmann J, Grimm H, et al (eds): *Linguistic Disorders and Pathologies: An International Handbook.* New York: Walter de Gruyter, 1993, pp 724–732.

32. Goswami U, Bryant PE: *Phonological Skills and Learning to Read.* Hillsdale, NJ: Erlbaum, 1990.

33. Lovett MW, Warren-Chaplin PM, Ransby MJ, Borden SL: Training the word recognition skills of reading disabled children: Treatment and transfer effects. *J Educ Psychol* 82:769–780, 1990.

34. Lovett MW: Reading, writing, and remediation: Perspectives on the dyslexic learning disability from remedial outcome data. *Learn Indiv Diff* 3:295–305, 1991.

35. Vellutino FR, Scanlon DM: Phonological coding, phonological awareness, and reading ability: Evidence from a longitudinal and experimental study. *Merrill-Palmer Q* 33:321–363, 1987.

36. Liberman IY, Shankweiler D: Phonology and the problems of learning to read and write. *Remed Spec Educ* 6:8–17, 1985.

37. Mann V: Why some children encounter reading problems, in: Torgesen J, Wong B (eds): *Psychological and Educational Perspectives on Learning Disabilities.* New York: Academic Press, 1986, pp 133–159.

38. Wagner RK, Torgesen JK: The nature of phonological processing and its causal role in the acquisition of reading skills. *Psychol Bull* 101:192–212, 1987.

39. Wagner RK, Torgesen JK, Laughon P, et al: Development of young readers' phonological processing abilities. *J Educ Psychol* 85:83–103, 1993.

40. Wagner RK, Torgesen JK, Rashotte CA: Development of reading-related phonological processing abilities: New evidence of bidirectional causality from a latent variable longitudinal study. *Dev Psychol* 30:73–87, 1994.

41. Bruck M: Persistence of dyslexics' phonological awareness deficits. *Dev Psychol* 28:874–886, 1992.

42. Bowers PG, Steffy RA, Tate E: Comparison of the effects of IQ control methods on memory and naming speed predictors of reading disability. *Read Res Q* 23:204–319, 1988.

43. Bowers PG, Swanson LB: Naming speed deficits in reading disability: Multiple measures of a singular process. *J Exp Child Psychol* 51:195–219, 1991.

44. Bowers PG, Wolf M: Theoretical links between naming speed, precise mechanisms, and ortho-

graphic skill in dyslexia. *Reading Writing* 5:69–85, 1993.

45. Wolf M: The word retrieval process and reading in children and aphasics, in Nelson K (ed): *Children's Language.* Hillsdale, NJ: Erlbaum, 1982, pp 473–493.

46. Wolf M: Naming speed and reading: The contribution of the cognitive neurosciences. *Read Res Q* 26:123–141, 1991.

47. Wolf M, Bally H, Morris R: Automaticity, retrieval processes, and reading: A longitudinal study in average and impaired readers. *Child Dev* 57:988–1000, 1986.

48. Wolf M, Obregon M: Early naming deficits, developmental dyslexia, and a specific deficit hypothesis. *Brain Lang* 42:219–247, 1992.

49. Felton RH, Brown IS: Phonological processes as predictors of specific reading skills in children at risk for reading failure. *Reading Writing* 2:39–59, 1990.

50. Wolff P, Michel G, Ovrut M: Rate variables and automatized naming in developmental dyslexia. *Brain Lang* 39:556–575, 1990.

51. Wolff P, Michel G, Ovrut M, Drake C: Rate and timing precision of motor coordination in developmental dyslexia. *Dev Psychol* 26:349–359, 1990.

52. Novoa L: *Word Retrieval Process and Reading Acquisition and Development in Bilingual and Monolingual Children.* Cambridge, MA: Harvard University Press, 1988.

53. Wolf M, Pfeil C, Lotz R, Biddle K: Towards a more universal understanding of the developmental dyslexias: The contribution of orthographic factors, in Berninger VW (ed): *The Varieties of Orthographic Knowledge, I.* Dordrecht: Kluwer, 1994, pp 137–171.

54. Yap R, Van der Liej A: Word processing in dyslexia: An automatic coding deficit? *Reading Writing* 5:261–279, 1993.

55. Bowers PG: Re-examining selected reading research from the viewpoint of the double-deficit-hypothesis. Society for Research in Child Development. Indianapolis, April 1995.

56. Lovett MW: Remediating dyslexic children's word identification deficits: Are the core deficits of developmental dyslexia amenable to treatment? Society for Research in Child Development. Indianapolis, April 1995.

57. Wolf M: The double deficit hypothesis for developmental reading disorders. Society for Research in Child Development. Indianapolis, April 1995.

58. Hinshelwood J: Four cases of congenital word-blindness occurring in the same family. *Br Med J* 2:1229–1232, 1907.

59. Hinshelwood J: Two cases of hereditary word-blindness. *Br Med J* 1:608–609, 1911.

60. Stephenson S: Six cases of congenital word-blindness affecting three generations of one family. *Ophthalmoscope* 5:482–484, 1907.

61. Rutter M, Tizard J, Whitmore K: *Education, Health, and Behavior.* New York: Krieger, 1970.

62. Gilger JW, Pennington BF, DeFries JC: Risk for reading disabilities as a function of parental history of learning problems: Data from three samples of families demonstrating genetic transmission. *Reading Writing* 3:205–217, 1991.

63. Pennington BF: Genetics of learning disabilities. *J Child Neurol* 10:S69–S77, 1995.

64. Vogler GP, DeFries JC, Decker SN: Family history as an indicator of risk for reading disability. *J Learn Disabil* 18:419–421, 1985.

65. Pennington BF: The genetics of dyslexia. *J Child Psychol Psychiatry* 31:193–201, 1990.

66. DeFries JC, Fulker DW, LaBuda MC: Reading disability in twins: Evidence for a genetic etiology. *Nature* 329:537–539, 1987.

67. DeFries JC, Stevenson J, Gillis JJ, Wadsworth SJ: Genetic etiology of spelling deficits in the Colorado and London twin studies of reading disability. *Reading Writing* 3:271–283, 1991.

68. Olson RK, Gillis JJ, Rack JP, et al: Confirmatory factor analysis of word recognition and process measures in the Colorado reading project. *Reading Writing* 3:235–248, 1991.

69. Pennington BF, Gilger JW, Pauls D, et al: Evidence for major gene transmission of developmental dyslexia. *JAMA* 26:1527–1534, 1991.

70. Lewitter FI, DeFries JC, Elston RC: Genetic models of reading disability. *Behav Genet* 10:9–30, 1980.

71. Smith SD, Pennington BF, Kimberling WJ, Ing PS: Familial dyslexia: Use of genetic linkage analysis to define subtypes. *J Am Acad Child Psychiatry* 29:204, 1990.

72. Smith SD, Kimberling WJ, Pennington BF, Lubs MA: Specific reading disability: Identification of an inherited form through linkage analysis. *Science* 219:1345–1347, 1983.

73. Bisgaard ML, Eiberg H, Moller N, Niebuhr E, et al: Dyslexia and chromosome 15 heteromorphism: Negative lod score in a Danish material. *Clin Genet* 32:118–119, 1987.

74. Cardon LR, Smith SD, Fulker FW, et al: Quantitative trait locus for reading disability on chromosome 6. *Science* 266:276–279, 1994.

75. Geschwind N, Behan P: Left-handedness: Association with immune disease, migraine, and developmental learning disorder. *Proc Natl Acad Sci USA* 79:5097–5100, 1982.

76. Pennington BF, Smith SR, Kimberling WJ, et al: Left-handedness and immune disorders in familial dyslexics. *Arch Neurol* 44:634–639, 1987.

77. Harris EL: The contribution of twin research to the study of the etiology of reading disability, in Smith SD (ed): *Genetics and Learning Disabilities.* San Diego, CA: College Hill Press, 1986, pp 3–19.

78. Plomin R: The role of inheritance in behavior. *Science* 248:183–188, 1990.

79. Filipek PA: Neurobiologic correlates of developmental dyslexia: How do dyslexics' brains differ from those of normal readers? *J Child Neurol* 10:S62–S69, 1995.

80. Caplan D: *Language: Structure, Processing, and Disorders.* Cambridge, MA: MIT Press, 1992.

81. Schultz RT, Cho NK, Staib LH, et al: Brain morphology in normal and dyslexic children: The influence of sex and age. *Ann Neurol* 35:732–742, 1994.

82. Galaburda AM: Neurology of developmental dyslexia. *Curr Opin Neurol Neurosurg* 5:71–76, 1992.

83. Galaburda AM: Neuroanatomic basis of developmental dyslexia. *Neurol Clin* 11:161–173, 1993.

84. Galaburda AM, Sanides F: Cytoarchitectonic organization of the human auditory cortex. *J Comput Neurol* 190:597–610, 1980.

85. Luria AR: *Higher Cortical Functions in Man.* New York: Basic Books, 1980.

86. Haslam RH, Dalby JT, Johns RD, Rademaker AW: Cerebral asymmetry in developmental dyslexia. *Arch Neurol* 38:679–682, 1981.

87. Rumsey JM, Dorwart R, Vermess M, et al: Magnetic resonance imaging of brain anatomy in severe developmental dyslexia. *Arch Neurol* 43:1045–1046, 1986.

88. Galaburda AM, Sherman GF, Rosen GD, et al: Developmental dyslexia: Four consecutive patients with cortical anomalies. *Ann Neurol* 18:222–233, 1985.

89. Hynd GW, Semrud-Clikeman M: Dyslexia and brain morphology. *Psychol Bull* 106:447–482, 1989.

90. Hynd GW, Semrud-Clikeman M, Lorys AR, et al: Brain morphology in developmental dyslexia and attention deficit disorder/hyperactivity. *Arch Neurol* 47:919–926, 1990.

91. Larsen JP, Hoien T, Lundberg I, Odegaard H: MRI evaluation of the size and symmetry of the planum temporale in adolescents with developmental dyslexia. *Brain Lang* 39:289–301, 1990.

92. Drake WE: Clinical and pathological findings in a child with a developmental learning disability. *J Learn Disabil* 1:486–502, 1968.

93. Hynd GW, Semrud-Clikeman M: Dyslexia and neurodevelopmental pathology: Relationships to cognition, intelligence, and reading skill acquisition. *J Learn Disabil* 22:204–220, 1989.

94. Humphreys P, Kaufmann WE, Galaburda AM: Developmental dyslexia in women: Neuropathological findings in three cases. *Ann Neurol* 28:727–738, 1990.

95. Humphreys P, Rosen BD, Press DM, et al: Freezing lesions of the developing rat brain: A model for cerebrocortical microgyria. *Neuropathol Exp Neurol* 50:145–160, 1991.

96. Sherman GF, Galaburda AM, Geschwind N: Cortical anomalies in brains of New Zealand mice: A neuropathologic model of dyslexia? *Proc Natl Acad Sci USA* 82:8072–8074, 1985.

97. Sherman GF, Galaburda AM, Behan PO, Rosen GD: Neuroanatomical anomalies in autoimmune mice. *Acta Neuropathol* 74:239–242, 1987.

98. Behan PO, Geschwind N: Dyslexia, congenital anomalies, and immune disorders: The role of the fetal environment. *Ann NY Acad Sci* 457:13–18, 1985.

99. Galaburda AM: Developmental dyslexia. *Buffalo Branch Orton Dyslexia Soc News* 5–11, 1993.

100. Lovegrove WJ, Garzia RP, Nicholson SB: Experimental evidence for a transient system deficit in specific reading disability. *J Am Optom Assoc* 61:137–146, 1990.

101. Livingstone MS, Rosen GD, Drislane FW, Galaburda AM: Physiological and anatomical evidence for a magnocellular defect in developmental dyslexia. *Proc Natl Acad Sci USA* 88:7943–7947, 1991.

102. Lehmkuhle S, Garzia RP, Turner BS, et al: A defective visual pathway in children with reading disability. *N Engl J Med* 328:989–996, 1993.

103. Galaburda AM, Menard MT, Rosen GD: Evidence for aberrant auditory anatomy in developmental dyslexia. *Proc Natl Acad Sci USA* 91:8010–8013, 1994.

104. Galaburda AM, Livingstone M: Evidence for a

magnocellular defect in developmental dyslexia. *Ann NY Acad Sci* 68:70–82, 1993.

105. Hayduk S, Bruck M, Cavanagh P: Low level processing skills of adults and children with dyslexia: A critical evaluation. *Cogn Neuropsychol.* In press.

106. Smith A, Early F, Grogan S: Flicker masking and developmental dyslexia. *Perception* 15:473–482, 1986.

107. Badcock D, Sevdalis E: Masking by uniform field flicker: Some practical problems. *Perception* 16: 641–647, 1987.

108. Hulme C: The implausibility of low-level visual deficits as a cause of children's reading difficulties. *Cogn Neuropsychol* 5:369–374, 1988.

109. Tallal P, Stark RE, Mellits D: The relationship between auditory temporal analysis and receptive language development: Evidence from studies of developmental language disorder. *Neuropsychologia* 23:527–534, 1985.

110. Tallal P, Stark RE, Mellits D: Identification of language-impaired children on the basis of rapid perception and production skills. *Brain Lang* 25:314–322, 1985.

111. Wolff PH: Impaired temporal resolution in developmental dyslexia. *Ann NY Acad Sci* 682:87–103, 1993.

112. Shaywitz BA, Shaywitz SE, Pugh KR, et al: Sex differences in the functional organization of the brain for language. *Nature* 373:607–609, 1995.

113. Delacato CH: *Neurological Organization and Reading.* Springfield, IL: Charles C Thomas, 1966.

114. Frostig M: *Move, Grow, Learn.* Chicago, IL: Follet, 1969.

115. Wilsher CR, Bennett D, Chase CH, et al: Piracetam and dyslexia: Effects on reading tests. *J Clin Psychopharmacol* 7:230–237, 1987.

116. Levinson HN: *A Solution to the Riddle Dyslexia.* New York: Springer-Verlag, 1980.

117. Tomatis A: *Education and Dyslexia.* France-Quebec: Les Editions, 1978.

118. Di Ianni M, Wilsher C, Blank MS, et al: The effects of piracetam in children with dyslexia. *J Clin Psychopharmacology* 5:272–278, 1985.

119. Gittelman R, Feingold I: Children with reading disorders: I. Efficacy of reading remediation. *J Child Psychol Psychiatry* 24:167–191, 1983.

120. Kershner JR, Cummings RL, Clarke KA, et al: Evaluation of the Tomatis Listening Training Program with learning disabled children. *Can J Special Educ* 2:1–32, 1986.

121. Kershner JR, Cummings RL, Clarke KA, et al: Two-year evaluation of the Tomatis Listening Training Program with learning disabled children. *Learn Disabil Q* 13:43–53, 1990.

122. Robinson HM: Visual and auditory modalities related to methods for beginning readers. *Reading Res Q* 8:7–39, 1972.

123. Gittelman R: Treatment of reading disorders, in Rutter M (ed): *Developmental Neuropsychiatry.* New York: Guilford Press, 1983, pp 520–541.

124. Hewison J: The current status of remedial intervention for children with reading problems. *Dev Med Child Neurol* 24:183–186, 1982.

125. Johnson DL: Remedial approaches to dyslexia, in Benton AL, Pearl D (eds): *Dyslexia: An Appraisal of Current Knowledge.* New York: Oxford University Press, 1978, pp 397–421.

126. Lovett MW, Barron RW, Forbes JE, et al: Computer speech-based training of literacy skills in neurologically-impaired children: A controlled evaluation. *Brain Lang* 47:117–154, 1994.

127. Lovett MW, Borden SL, DeLuca T, et al: Treating the core deficits of developmental dyslexia: Evidence of transfer-of-learning following phonologically- and strategy-based reading training programs. *Dev Psychol* 30:805–822, 1994.

128. Lovett MW, Ransby MJ, Barron RW: Treatment, subtype, and word type effects in dyslexic children's response to remediation. *Brain Lang* 34: 328–349, 1988.

129. Lovett MW, Ransby MJ, Hardwick N, et al: Can dyslexia be treated? Treatment-specific and generalized treatment effects in dyslexic children's response to remediation. *Brain Lang* 37:90–121, 1989.

130. Olson RK, Wise BW: Reading on the computer with orthographic and speech feedback. *Reading Writing* 4:107–144, 1992.

131. Olson RK, Wise B, Conners F, Rack J: Organization, heritability, and remediation of component word recognition and language skills in disabled readers, in Carr T, Levy BA (eds): *Reading and Its Development: Component Skills Approaches.* San Diego, CA: Academic Press, 1990, pp 261–322.

132. Roth SF, Beck IL: Theoretical and instructional implications of the assessment of two microcomputer word recognition programs. *Reading Res Q* 22:197–218, 1987.

133. Wise BW, Olson R, Anstett M, et al: Implementing a long-term computerized remedial reading program with synthetic speech feedback: Hard-

ware, software, and real world issues. *Behav Res Meth Instr Comput* 21:173–180, 1989.

134. Wise BW, Olson RK: Remediating reading disabilities, in Obrzut JE, Hynd GW (eds): *Neuropsychological Foundations of Learning Disabilities: A Handbook of Issues, Methods, and Practice.* San Diego, CA: Academic Press, 1991, pp 631–658.

135. Bruck M: The adult functioning of children with specific learning disabilities: A follow-up study, in Siegel IE (ed): *Advances in Applied Developmental Psychology.* Norwood, NJ: Ablex, 1985, pp 91–129.

136. Lemoine HE, Levy BA, Hutchinson A: Increasing the naming speed of poor readers: Representations formed across repetitions. *J Exp Child Psychol* 55:297–328, 1993.

137. Perfetti CA: Representations and awareness in the acquisition of reading competence, in Rieben L, Perfetti CA (eds): *Learning to Read: Basic Research and Its Implications.* Hillsdale, NJ: Erlbaum, 1991, pp 33–44.

138. Borkowski JG, Estrada MT, Milstead M, Hale CA: General problem-solving skills: Relations between metacognition and strategic processing. *Learn Disabil Q* 12:57–70, 1989.

139. Gaskins IW, Elliot TT: *Implementing Cognitive Strategy Training Across the School: The Benchmark Manual for Teachers.* Cambridge, MA: Brookline Books, 1991.

140. Kavale KA: The reasoning abilities of normal and learning disabled readers on measures of reading comprehension. *Learn Disabil Q* 3:34–45, 1980.

141. Meltzer L: Problem-solving strategies and academic performance in learning-disabled students: Do subtypes exist? in Feagans LV, Short EJ, Meltzer LJ (eds): *Subtypes of Learning Disabilities: Theoretical Perspectives and Research.* Hillsdale, NJ: Erlbaum, 1991, pp 163–188.

142. Paris SG, Oka ER: Strategies for comprehending text and coping with reading difficulties. *Learn Disabil Q* 12:32–42, 1989.

143. Gaskins IW, Downer MA, Anderson RC, et al: A metacognitive approach to phonics: Using what you know to decode what you don't know. *Remed Special Educ* 9:36–41, 66, 1988.

144. Meltzer LJ: Assessment of learning disabilities: The challenge of evaluating the cognitive strategies and processes underlying learning, in Lyon GR (ed): *Frames of Reference for the Assessment of Learning Disabilities: New Views on Measurement Issues.* Baltimore: Brookes, 1994, pp 571–606.

145. Pressley M: Can learning-disabled children become good information processors? How can we find out? in Feagans LV, Short EJ, Meltzer LJ (eds): *Subtypes of Learning Disabilities: Theoretical Perspectives and Research.* Hillsdale, NJ: Erlbaum, 1991, pp 137–161.

146. Pressley M, Harris KR, Marks B: But good strategy instructors are constructivists! *Educ Psychol Rev* 4:3–33, 1992.

147. Levin BE: Organizational deficits in dyslexia: Possible frontal lobe dysfunction. *Dev Neuropsychol* 6:95–110, 1990.

148. Harris KR, Graham S, Pressley M: Cognitive-behavioral approaches in reading and written language: Developing self-regulated learners, in Singh NN, Beale IL (eds): *Learning Disabilities: Nature, Theory, and Treatment.* New York: Springer-Verlag, 1992, pp 415–451.

149. Engelmann S, Bruner EC: *Reading Mastery I/II Fast Cycle: Teacher's Guide.* Chicago: Science Research Associates, 1988.

150. Engelmann S, Carnine L, Johnson G: *Corrective Reading, Word Attack Basics, Decoding A.* Chicago: Science Research Associates, 1988.

151. Engelmann S, Johnson G, Carnine L, et al: *Corrective Reading: Decoding Strategies, Decoding B1.* Chicago: Science Research Associates, 1988.

152. Gaskins IW, Downer MA, Gaskins RW: *Introduction to the Benchmark School Word Identification/ Vocabulary Development Program.* Media, PA: Benchmark School, 1986.

153. Livingston R, Adam BS, Bracha HS: Season of birth and neurodevelopmental disorders: Summer birth is associated with dyslexia. *J Am Acad Child Adolesc Psychiatry* 32:612–616, 1993.

Chapter 20

AGRAPHIA

David P. Roeltgen

Agraphia is traditionally defined as an acquired disorder of writing, although current usage also includes disorders of spelling.[1] Breakdown in writing may occur at any level of production, including the paragraph and sentence level. However, agraphia has typically been studied at the word level. At this level, dysfunction may be the result of either linguistic or motor disturbances. These disturbances may either be unique to the writing or spelling systems (pure agraphia) or more generalized, with associated neuropsychological dysfunction.

HISTORICAL BACKGROUND

Remote History

In 1865, Benedict[2] applied the term *agraphia* to disorders of writing, and many of the current concepts and controversies in the study of writing disorders are actually reflected in the nineteenth-century literature. Ogle[3] found that although aphasia and agraphia usually occur together, they are occasionally separable. He concluded that centers for writing may be separable from centers for speaking. Ogle classified agraphia into two types, amnemonic agraphia and atactic agraphia, a distinction that is still in use today. *Amnemonic agraphia* refers to writing by patients who produce well-formed but incorrect letters. In current terms, this is a linguistic disorder of writing. *Atac-*

tic agraphia is writing by patients who produce poorly formed letters. In current terms, this is a motor disorder of writing. It is rarely appreciated that the nineteenth-century literature even contains descriptions of different linguistic abilities, that, when dysfunctional, may lead to agraphia. In anticipation of dual route models of coding and writing, Dejerine[4] and Pitres[5] proposed that orthographic or visual word images were important for proper spelling, whereas Grashey[6] and Wernicke[7] postulated that the translation of sound units into letters was important for production of correct spelling. Last, there has always been an interest in the localization of functions for the production of writing. Beginning in the nineteenth century, the angular gyrus[4,5,8–10] and the frontal motor center for writing, "Exner's area,"[8–11] are the areas that have been emphasized the most.

Recent History

In the past decades, two basic approaches have been used in describing agraphias. One of these may be termed the neurologic approach. This emphasizes traditional neurologic disorders and their association with agraphia. These disorders include aphasia, limb apraxia, constructional apraxia, confusion, Parkinson's disease, callosal lesions, and dementia. The second may be termed the neuropsychological or cognitive approach. This approach attempts to examine cognitive processing breakdowns underlying the agraphias.

NEUROLOGIC MODEL

Agraphia and Aphasia

Table 20-1 lists the classic aphasias and their associations with agraphia. Typically, the agraphia is described as being similar to the aphasia.[15] Therefore, the nonfluent agraphias consist of sparse output with effortful processing and agrammatism, while the fluent agraphias consist of normal output, easy production, and normal sentence length. The nonfluent agraphias are usually associated with clumsy calligraphy and the fluent agraphias with well-formed letters.[15] However, some studies[16] have described patients with Broca's aphasia and noted that their agraphia more closely resembled the agraphia of patients with Wernicke's aphasia than the agraphias of other patients with Broca's aphasia. This reflects the dissociation of aphasia and agraphia first described by Ogle.[3]

Agraphia and Alexia

The association between agraphia and alexia has also been noted since the previous century.[4] Benson and Cummings[15] indicate that the agraphia usually resembles that of fluent aphasia and agraphia. Agraphia with alexia has also been called parietal agraphia. Patients with agraphia and alexia who do not have significant aphasia frequently have parietal lobe lesions.[13] However, the category appears to be heterogeneous, and different descriptions of this disorder have been presented. Benson and Cummings's patients produced well-formed letters, while Kaplan and Goodglass's[13] typically made poorly formed letters.

Agraphia and Praxic or Spatial Disturbances

Apraxic agraphia is described as difficulty in writing letters, writing spontaneously, and writing to dictation.[2,12,17,18] Copying or oral spelling are usually less impaired. The lesions causing apraxic agraphia are usually in the parietal lobe, especially the superior parietal lobule[19] opposite the preferred hand (dominant parietal lobe). In contrast, lesions in the parietal lobe ipsilateral to the preferred hand (nondominant parietal lobe) are traditionally associated with spatial agraphia. Patients with this disorder typically duplicate strokes and have spatial disturbances in their writing. This includes trouble writing on a horizontal line and writing only on the right side of the paper. It is frequently associated with the neglect syndrome.[12,17,20,21] With spatial agraphia, there may also be letter omissions or additions within orthographic groupings (e.g., syllables or morphologic units).

Agraphia and Parkinson Disease

Many patients with Parkinson disease have micrographia. This may be one of the earliest findings in Parkinson disease. The writing is not only small but diminishes in size as the patients write across the line. Abnormal kinetics with slower speed and varying force of motor production are associated with this.[22] The micrographia frequently improves with pharmacologic treatment of the parkinsonian patient.[23]

Agraphia and Confusion

Patients with acute confusional states frequently have agraphia.[24] Chedru and Geschwind found agraphia in 33 of 34 cases of acute confusion. Their patients had disruption of linguistic performance with spelling and syntactical disturbances. They also had motor impairment and spatial impairment with poorly formed and improperly placed letters.

Table 20-1
Agraphia and the aphasias

Nonfluent agraphia
    Agraphia and Broca's aphasia[12,13]
        Poor grapheme production
        Agrammatism
    Agraphia and transcortical motor aphasia[14]
Fluent agraphia
    Agraphia and conduction aphasia[12]
    Agraphia and Wernicke's aphasia[12,13]
    Agraphia and anomia[15]

Table 20-2
Callosal agraphias

Callosal region damaged	Type of functional disruption	Type of agraphia
Genu	Verbal motor engrams	Unilateral apraxic agraphia with inability to type
Body	Visual kinesthetic engrams	Unilateral apraxic agraphia with ability to type
Splenium	Linguistic information	Unilateral aphasic agraphia (incorrect spellings)

Agraphia and Callosal Lesions

Spelling and written letter-production systems can access the right hemisphere via the neocommissures. This allows the left hand in a right-handed person with left hemispheric language to write with the left hand. Callosal agraphia occurs when patients have this interhemispheric transfer disrupted. This results in a unilateral agraphia.[25–33] The resultant agraphia from a callosal lesion is, to a degree, variable among patients. Watson and Heilman[33] suggested a model to help explain these variabilities. Some patients may have an apparent apraxic agraphia and inability to type,[27] some may have an apraxic agraphia with preserved ability to type,[33] and others have an agraphia more typical of aphasic agraphia with some preserved ability to produce letters.[26] Watson and Heilman suggested that this related to the location of the callosal lesion and to the subsequent type of information transfer that is disrupted by the callosal lesion (Table 20-2).

Agraphia and Dementia

Agraphia is common in patients with Alzheimer disease.[34–40] Such patients may have a loss of lexical specificity and make semantic errors, such as writing *pencil* for *paper,* or they may have an impaired semantic access to written output, again producing semantic errors or, as frequently tested, homophone errors.[40] (These patients will write *night* when asked to write *knight,* as in "he is a *knight* in shining armor.") Patients may also have a spelling impairment consistent with lexical

breakdown, producing lexical agraphia (see below),[41] and impairment of attentional mechanisms, producing errors consistent with disruption of the graphemic buffer (see below).[42,43] Patients with Alzheimer disease have also been described who produce illegible words and poor spacing, consistent with a spatial agraphia.[44] The findings in patients with Alzheimer disease are consistent with the other cognitive disturbances typically found in Alzheimer patients, including semantic disruption, lexical disruption, and visuospatial dysfunction.

Isolated or Pure Agraphia

This is a writing disorder without other significant language disturbance. These patients produce well-formed letters but make different types of spelling errors that may be dependent upon the lesion location. Multiple lesion sites have been implicated in pure agraphia, including the second frontal gyrus (Exner's area).[12,13,17,45,46] These patients appear to make predominantly linguistic errors.

A second lesion site that has been associated with pure agraphia is the superior parietal lobe.[47–49] Dysfunction from lesions in this region produce varying types of agraphia. The posterior perisylvian region has also been implicated.[50,51] These patients appear to produce predominantly spelling errors. Other lesions that have been associated with pure agraphia are the left occipital lobe,[52] posterior insula and posterior putamen,[50] basal ganglia,[50,53] and left centrum semiovale.[54]

COGNITIVE AND NEUROPSYCHOLOGICAL MODELS

An alternate approach to the neurologic models comprises attempts to analyze the patterns of breakdown in terms of the underlying cognitive processes required for normal performance. This has led to the development of information processing models of writing and its breakdown. Occasionally authors have attempted to assess localization[2,51] or to assess the type of breakdown in specific disorders, such as Alzheimer disease.[40–43] In part, based on studies by Beauvois and Derouesne[55] and Shallice,[56] Ellis[57] developed one of the first information processing models. Others have followed.[16]

A Neuropsychological Model

One model has been described and developed by the author over the past decade[2,16,58] (Fig. 20-1). It divides agraphias into linguistic agraphias and motor agraphias, similar to the classic differentiations. The linguistic agraphias include phonologic agraphia, lexical agraphia, and semantic agraphia. The peripheral agraphias, which are primarily motor, include graphemic buffer agraphia, agraphia from impaired graphemic representations (disruption of graphic programming and disruption of allographic mechanisms), and agraphia from impaired spatial orientation.

Linguistic Agraphias

Phonologic Agraphia Phonologic agraphia is due to a disruption of sound-letter translation.[59] The hallmark of phonologic agraphia is loss of the ability to spell pronounceable nonsense words (i.e., nud) with preserved ability to spell real words, including words that are orthographically irregular (do not correspond to simple sound-letter relationships—i.e., island).[56] Most patients with phonologic agraphia have some impairment of real word spelling (and writing) as well,[59–67] although isolated or pure phonologic agraphia has been described.[55,68] Some patients with impaired non-word-writing ability have additional deficits

including production of semantic paragraphias (i.e., writing *airplane* for *propeller*). This pattern of dysfunction is termed deep agraphia,[59,62,69–73] analogous to deep dyslexia (see Chap. 18). Phonologic agraphia has been associated with midperisylvian lesions, including the insula and the anterior inferior supramarginal gyrus.[58,59,65]

Lexical Agraphia In contrast to phonologic agraphia, lexical agraphia includes preserved ability to spell or write nonsense words but impaired ability to spell irregular words.[55] Patients with this type of dysfunction will regularize irregular words, such as spelling *island* as *iland*.[61,65,74–80] Lexical agraphia appears to be associated with nonperisylvian lesions in multiple sites within the left hemisphere.[58] It has also been described in Alzheimer disease.[41]

Semantic Agraphia Semantic agraphia is due to a disruption of semantic influence on spelling output.[81] Patients with this disorder have trouble incorporating meaning into spelling and writing.[82,83] The error made by these patients is most commonly that of homophone confusions, such as writing *knight* when asked to write *night*, as in "The moon comes out at *night*." Lesion sites associated with semantic agraphia include those regions typically associated with transcortical aphasias with impaired comprehension.[58,77] This type of agraphia also occurs in and may be one of the earliest linguistic disruptions of many Alzheimer disease patients.[40]

Peripheral Agraphias

Graphemic Buffer Agraphia The graphemic buffer is thought to be a temporary working memory store of abstract letters. It was conceptually defined before patients with proposed disruption of this store were described.[57] Disorders within this system produce errors that are not affected by linguistic factors (i.e., words or nonsense words). Errors include letter omissions, substitutions, insertions, and transpositions. The patients usually produce correctly formed letters. There is usually

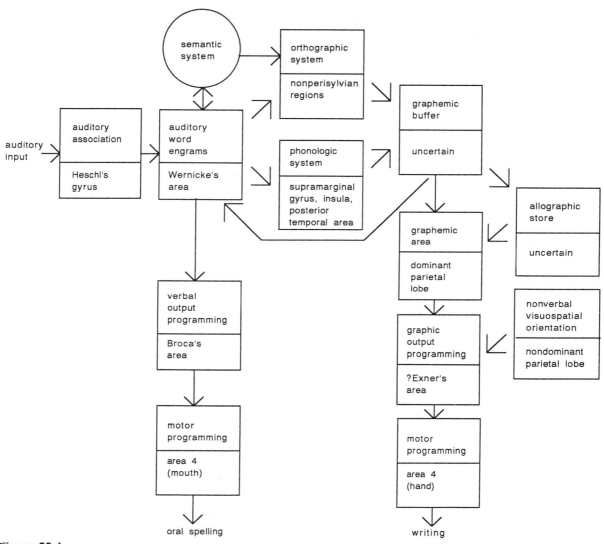

Figure 20-1
A neuropsychological model of writing and spelling. (From Roeltgen,[2] with permission.)

a significant influence of word length, with longer words being written less well than shorter words. Patients with both focal lesions[84–86] and Alzheimer disease[42,43] produce this type of agraphia. Lesion sites associated with impaired attention appear to be associated with this type of agraphia.

Apraxic Agraphia Apraxic agraphia has been described in patients with apraxia as well as in those without apraxia. In the latter case, this has also been termed ideational agraphia. Subjects with apraxic agraphia produce poorly formed letters, spell aloud better than they write, and improve their performance when copying.[87,88] They are usually able to type or use anagram letters.[89] Baxter and Warrington[90] used the term *ideational agraphia* to describe their patient, who produced poor letters but had good praxis and visuospatial skills. A similar patient has been described by Croisile and coworkers.[75]

Allographic Agraphia Patients with agraphia due to disruption of the allographic store spell aloud better than they write, have normal praxis, normal visuospatial ability, and normal letter form, but they make frequent case (lower versus upper) and style (print versus script) errors. Ellis[57] hypothesized the existence of the allographic store on the basis of errors made by normal subjects. Since then, there have been a few reports of patients with apparent disruption of this type.[91–93] The anatomic location of the allographic store is unclear.

Spatial Agraphia In information processing models, this disorder is similar to the agraphia from spatial disturbances described previously in this chapter.

Impaired Oral Spelling The mechanisms for oral spelling are not well defined. Rare patients have been described with good writing but impaired oral spelling.[94] Since oral spelling is not a common behavior and is infrequently examined, further delineation of this potential disorder is difficult.

AGRAPHIAS AND THEIR ASSESSMENT

As indicated previously, agraphia can occur at the paragraph, sentence, and word levels. Spontaneous writing is the most sensitive test for examining all levels of breakdown. With spontaneous writing, both form and content can be judged. However, having the patient write to dictation affords the examiner better control of the stimuli. Using the possible dysfunctions in the models described previously, the dictated stimuli can be varied (short word or long word, real word or nonsense

word) and the errors analyzed. The error analyses include both spelling and letter form. The patients can also be asked to copy and spell aloud. The approach to assessment usually produces sufficient information that the examiner can have an understanding of the agraphia type and its relationship to other neurologic or neuropsychological deficits.[2]

REFERENCES

 1. Benedikt M: Uber Aphasie, Agraphie und verwandte pathologische Zustande. *Wien Med Pr* 6:1865.
 2. Roeltgen DP: Agraphia, in Heilman KM, Valenstein E (eds): *Clinical Neuropsychology.* 3d ed. New York: Oxford University Press, 1993, pp 63–89.
 3. Ogle JW: Aphasia and agraphia. *Report of the Medical Research Counsel of St. George's Hospital (London)* 2:83–122, 1867.
 4. Dejerine J: Sur un cas de cecite verbale avec agraphie, suivi d'autopsie. *Mem Soc Biol* 3:197–201, 1891.
 5. Pitres A: *Rapport sur la question des agraphies.* Bordeaux: Congres Francais de Medecine Interne, 1894.
 6. Grashey H: Uber aphasie und ihre beziehungen zur wahrnehmung, *Arch Psychiatrie Nervenkrankh* 16:654–688, 1885. De Bleser R (trans). *Cogn Neuropsychol* 6:515–546, 1989.
 7. Wernicke C: Nervenheilkunde: Die neueren Arbeiten uber Aphasie. *Fortschr Med* 4:463–482, 1886. De Bleser R (trans). *Cogn Neuropsychol* 6:547–569, 1989.
 8. Henschen SE: *Klinische und Anatomische Beitrage zur Pathologie des Gehirns: VII. Uber motorische Aphasie und Agraphie.* Stockholm: Nordiska Bokhandel, 1922.
 9. Nielsen JM: *Agnosia, Apraxia, Aphasia: Their Value in Cerebral Localization.* New York: Hoeber, 1946.
10. Pick A: Aphasie, in Bumke O, Foerster O (eds): *Handbuch der Normalen und Pathologischen Physiologie.* Berlin: Springer, 1931, vol xv.
11. Exner S: Untersuchungen uber die Lokalization der Funktionen, in *Der Grosshirnrinde des Menschen.* Wien: Wilhelm Braumuller, 1881.
12. Marcie P, Hecaen H: Agraphia, in Heilman KM, Valenstein (eds): *Clinical Neuropsychology.* New York: Oxford University Press, 1979, pp 92–127.
13. Kaplan E, Goodglass H: Aphasia-related disorders,

in Sarno MT (ed): *Acquired Aphasia*. New York: Academic Press, 1981, pp 303–325.

14. Rubens AB: Transcortical motor aphasia, in Whitaker H, Whitaker HA (eds): *Studies in Neurolinguistics*. New York: Academic Press, 1976, vol 1, pp 293–303.

15. Benson DF, Cummings JL: Agraphia, in Vinken PJ, Bruyn GW, Klawans HL, Frederiks JAM (eds): *Clinical Neuropsychology*. New York: Elsevier, 1985, vol 45, pp 457–472.

16. Roeltgen DP, Heilman KM: Review of agraphia and proposal for an anatomically-based neuropsychological model of writing. *Appl Psycholing* 6:205–230, 1985.

17. Hecaen H, Albert ML: *Human Neuropsychology*. New York: Wiley, 1978.

18. Leischner A: The agraphias, in Vinken PJ, Bruyn GW (eds): *Disorders of Speech, Perception and Symbolic Behavior*. Amsterdam: North-Holland, 1969, pp 141–180.

19. Alexander MP, Fischer RS, Friedman R: Lesion localization in apraxic agraphia. *Arch Neurol* 49:246–251, 1992.

20. Ardila A, Rosselli M: Spatial agraphia. *Brain Cogn* 22:137–147, 1993.

21. Benson DF: *Aphasia, Alexia and Agraphia*. New York: Churchill Livingstone, 1979.

22. Margolin DI, Wing A: Agraphia and micrographia: Clinical manifestations of motor programming and performance disorders. *Acta Psychol* 54:263–283, 1983.

23. McLennan JE, Nakano K, Tyler HR, Schwab RS: Micrographia in Parkinson's disease. *J Neurol Sci* 15:141–152, 1972.

24. Chedru F, Geschwind N: Writing disturbances in acute confusional states. *Neuropsychologica* 10:343–354, 1972.

25. Bogen JE: The other side of the brain: I. Dysgraphia and dyscopia following cerebral commissurotomy. *Bull LA Neurol Soc* 34:3–105, 1969.

26. Gersh F, Damasio AR: Praxis and writing of the left hand may be served by different callosal pathways. *Arch Neurol* 38:634–636, 1981.

27. Geschwind N, Kaplan EF: A human cerebral disconnection syndrome. *Neurology* 12:675–685, 1962.

28. Levy J, Nebes RD, Sperry RW: Expressive language in the surgically separated minor hemisphere. *Cortex* 71:49–58, 1971.

29. Liepmann H, Maas O: Fall von Linksseitger agraphie und apraxie bei rechtsseitiger lahmung. *J Psychol Neurol* 10:214–227, 1907.

30. Rubens AB, Geschwind N, Mahowald MW, Mastri A: Posttraumatic cerebral hemispheric disconnection syndrome. *Arch Neurol* 34:750–755, 1977.

31. Sugishita M, Toyokura Y, Yoshioka M, Yamada R: Unilateral agraphia after section of the posterior half of the truncus of the corpus callosum. *Brain Lang* 9:212–225, 1980.

32. Watson RT, Heilman KM: Callosal apraxia. *Brain* 106:391–404, 1983.

33. Yamadori A, Osumi Y, Ikeda H, Kanazawa Y: Left unilateral agraphia and tactile anomia. Disturbances seen after occlusion of the anterior cerebral artery. *Arch Neurol* 37:88–91, 1980.

34. Bayles KA, Tomoeda CK: Caregiver report of prevalence and appearance order of linguistic symptoms in Alzheimer's patients. *Gerontologist* 31:210–216, 1991.

35. Henderson VW, Buckwalter JG, Sobel E, et al: The agraphia of Alzheimer's disease. *Neurology* 42:776–784, 1992.

36. Horner J, Heyman A, Dawson D, Rogers H: The relationship of agraphia to the severity of dementia in Alzheimer's disease. *Arch Neurol* 45:760–763, 1988.

37. Neils J, Boller F, Gerdeman B, Cole M: Descriptive writing abilities in Alzheimer's disease. *J Clin Exp Neuropsychol* 11:692–698, 1989.

38. Neils J, Roeltgen DP: Does lexical dysgraphia occur in early Alzheimer's disease? *J Med Speech Lang Pathol* 2:281–289, 1994.

39. Glosser G, Kaplan E: Linguistic and nonlinguistic impairments in writing: A comparison of patients with focal and multifocal CNS disorders. *Brain Lang* 37:357–380, 1989.

40. Neils J, Roeltgen DP, Constantinidou F: Decline in homophone spelling associated with loss of semantic influence on spelling in Alzheimer's disease. *Brain Lang* 49:27–49, 1995.

41. Rapcsak SZ, Arthur SA, Bliklen DA, Rubens AB: Lexical agraphia in Alzheimer's disease. *Arch Neurol* 46:65–68, 1989.

42. Croisile B, Brabant M, Carmoi T, et al: Comparison between oral and written spelling in Alzheimer's disease. *Brain Lang.* In press.

43. Neils J, Roeltgen DP, Grier A: Spelling and attention in early Alzheimer's disease: Evidence for impairment of the graphemic buffer. *Brain Language* 49:241–262, 1995.

44. LaBarge E, Smith DS, Dick L, Storandt M: Agraphia in dementia of the Alzheimer type. *Arch Neurol* 49:1151–1156, 1992.

45. Aimard G, Devick M, Lebel M, et al: Agraphie pure (dynamique?) origine frontale. *Rev Neurol* 7:505–512, 1975.

46. Vernea JJ, Merory J: Frontal agraphia (including a case report). *Proc Aust Assoc Neurol* 12:93–99, 1975.

47. Auerbach SH, Alexander MP: Pure agraphia and unilateral optic ataxia associated with a left superior parietal lobule lesion. *J Neurol Neurosurg Psychiatry* 44:430–432, 1981.

48. Basso A, Taborielli A, Vignolo LA: Dissociated disorders of speaking and writing in aphasia. *J Neurol Neurosurg Psychiatry* 41:556–563, 1978.

49. Kinsbourne M, Rosenfeld DB: Agraphia selective for written spelling, an experimental case study. *Brain Lang* 1:215–225, 1974.

50. Rosati G, De Bastiani P: Pure agraphia: A discreet form of aphasia. *J Neurol Neurosurg Psychiatry* 44:266–269, 1981.

51. Roeltgen DP: Prospective analysis of a model of writing, anatomic aspects. Presented at the Academy of Aphasia, October 1989, Sante Fe, NM.

52. Kapur N, Lawton NF: Dysgraphia for letters: A form of motor memory deficit. *J Neurol Neurosurg Psychiatry* 46:573–575, 1983.

53. Laine TN, Marttila RJ. Pure agraphia: A case study. *Neuropsychologia* 19:311–316, 1981.

54. Croisile B, Laurent B, Michel D, Trillet M: Pure agraphia after deep left hemisphere haematoma. *J Neurol Neurosurg Psychiatry* 53:263–265, 1990.

55. Beauvois MF, Derouesne J: Lexical or orthographic agraphia. *Brain* 104:21–49, 1981.

56. Shallice T: Phonological agraphia and the lexical route in writing. *Brain* 104:412–429, 1981.

57. Ellis AW: Spelling and writing (and reading and speaking), in Ellis AW (ed): *Normality and Pathology in Cognitive Functions.* London: Academic Press, 1982, pp 113–146.

58. Roeltgen DP, Rapcsak SZ: Acquired disorders of writing and spelling, in Blanken G, Dittmann J, Grimm H (eds): *Linguistic Disorders and Pathologies: An International Handbook.* Berlin: De Gruyter, 1993, pp 262–278.

59. Roeltgen DP, Sevush S, Heilman KM: Phonological agraphia: Writing by the lexical-semantic route. *Neurology* 33:733–757, 1983.

60. Baxter DM, Warrington EK: Category specific phonological dysgraphia. *Neuropsychologia* 23:653–666, 1985.

61. Bolla-Wilson K, Speedie LJ, Robinson RG: Phonologic agraphia in a left-handed patient after a right-hemisphere lesion. *Neurology* 35:1778–1981, 1985.

62. Goodman-Schulman R, Caramazza A: Patterns of dysgraphia and the nonlexical spelling process. *Cortex* 23:143–148, 1987.

63. Hatfield FM: Visual and phonological factors in acquired dysgraphia. *Neuropsychologia* 23:13–29, 1985.

64. Morton J: The logogen model and orthographic structure, in Frith U (ed): *Cognitive Processes in Spelling.* London: Academic Press, 1980, pp 117–133.

65. Nolan KA, Caramazza A: Modality-independent impairments in word processing in a deep dyslexic patient. *Brain Lang* 16:236–264, 1982.

66. Roeltgen DP, Heilman KM: Lexical agraphia, further support for the two-system hypothesis of linguistic agraphia. *Brain* 107:811–827, 1984.

67. Roeltgen DP, Rothi LJG, Heilman KM: Isolated phonological agraphia from a focal lesion. Presented at the Academy of Aphasia, October 1982, New Paltz, NY.

68. Roeltgen DP: Prospective analysis of writing and spelling: Part II. Results not related to localization. *J Clin Exp Neuropsychol* 13:48, 1991.

69. Assal G, Buttet J, Jolivet R: Dissociations in aphasia: A case report. *Brain Lang* 13:223–240, 1981.

70. Bub D, Kertesz A: Deep agraphia. *Brain Lang* 17:146–165, 1982.

71. Marshall J, Newcombe F: Syntactic and semantic errors in paralexia. *Neuropsychologica* 4:169–176, 1966.

72. Saffran EM, Schwartz MF, Marin OSM: Semantic mechanisms in paralexia. *Brain Lang* 13:255–265, 1981.

73. Van Lancker D: A case of deep dysgraphia attributed to right hemispheric function. Presented at the Academy of Aphasia, October 1990, Baltimore, MD.

74. Alexander MP, Friedman R, LoVerso F, Fischer R: Anatomic correlates of lexical agraphia. Presented at the Academy of Aphasia, October 1990, Baltimore, MD.

75. Croisile B, Trillet M, Laurent B, et al: Agraphie lexicale par hematome temporo-parietal gauche. *Rev Neurol (Paris)* 145:287–292, 1989.

76. Friedman RB, Alexander MP: Written spelling agraphia. *Brain Lang* 36:503–517, 1989.

77. Hatfield FM, Patterson KE: *Phonological spelling.* *Q J Exp Psychol* 35A:451–468, 1983.

78. Rapcsak SZ, Arthur SA, Rubens AB: Lexical

agraphia from focal lesion of the left precentral gyrus. *Neurology* 38:1119–1123, 1988.

79. Rapcsak SZ, Rubens AB, Laguna JF: From Letters to words: Procedures for word recognition in letter-by-letter reading. *Brain Lang* 38:504–514, 1990.

80. Rothi LJG, Roeltgen DP, Kooistra CA: Isolated lexical agraphia in a right-handed patient with a posterior lesion of the right cerebral hemisphere. *Brain Lang* 30:181–190, 1987.

81. Roeltgen DP, Rothi LG, Heilman KM: Linguistic semantic agraphia. *Brain Lang* 27:257–280, 1986.

82. Patterson K: Lexical but nonsemantic spelling? *Cogn Neuropsychol* 3:341–367, 1986.

83. Rapcsak SZ, Rubens AB: Disruption of semantic influence on writing following a left prefrontal lesion. *Brain Lang* 38:334–344, 1990.

84. Badecker W, Hillis A, Caramazza A: Lexical morphology and its role in the writing process: Evidence from a case of acquired dysgraphia. *Cognition* 35:205–243, 1990.

85. Caramazza A, Miceli G, Villa G, Romani C: The role of the graphemic buffer in spelling: Evidence from a case of acquired dysgraphia. *Cognition* 26:59–85, 1987.

86. Hillis AE, Caramazza A: The graphemic buffer and attentional mechanisms. *Brain Lang* 36:208–235, 1989.

87. Heilman KM, Coyle JM, Gonyea EF, Geschwind N: Apraxia and agraphia in a left hander. *Brain* 96:21–28, 1973.

88. Heilman KM, Gonyea EF, Geschwind N: Apraxia and agraphia in a right hander. *Cortex* 10:284–288, 1974.

89. Valenstein E, Heilman KM: Apraxic agraphia with neglect-induced paragraphia. *Arch Neurol* 67:44–56, 1979.

90. Baxter DM, Warrington EK: Ideational agraphia: A single case study. *J Neurol Neurosurg Psychiatry* 49:369–374, 1986.

91. Black SE, Bass K, Behrmann M, Hacker P: Selective writing impairment: A single case study of a deficit in allographic conversion. *Neurology* 37:174, 1987.

92. De Bastiani K, Barry C: A cognitive analysis of an acquired dysgraphic patient with an "allographic" writing disorder. *Cogn Neuropsychol* 6:25–41, 1989.

93. Yopp KS, Roeltgen DP: Case of alexia and agraphia due to a disconnection of the visual input to and the motor output from an intact graphemic area. *J Clin Exp Neuropsychol* 9:42, 1987.

94. Kinsbourne M, Warrington EK: A case showing selectively impaired oral spelling. *J Neurol Neurosurg Psychiatry* 28:563–566, 1965.

Part IV
MEMORY

Chapter 21

AMNESIA I: NEUROANATOMIC AND CLINICAL ISSUES

Stuart Zola

A BRIEF HISTORY OF IDEAS ABOUT LOCALIZATION OF MEMORY

Ideas about the localization of memory in the brain can be divided roughly into three eras. The first era spans the period from antiquity to about the second century A.D. During this era, debate focused not on the issue of memory explicitly but on the location of the soul—i.e., what bodily organ was the source of all mental life. As recounted in Chap. 1, the two leading contenders were the heart and brain. By the time of Galen, in the second century A.D., the brain had been widely accepted as the organ of the mind. From the second to the eighteenth centuries, the issue was whether cognitive functions were localized either in the ventricular system of the brain or in the brain matter itself. Ventricular hypotheses had the support of the church, as the empty spaces of the ventricular system could contain ethereal spirits, and mind-brain dualism could therefore be maintained. Eventually, however, empirical science upheld the alternative view, according to which brain tissue itself was the material substrate of the mind. The third and current era of ideas about localization of brain function ranges from the nineteenth century to the present time. During this era, the debate has focused on how mental activities are organized in the brain. An early idea, which came to be known as the localizationist view, was that specific mental functions were carried out by specific parts of the brain. An alternative idea was that all parts of the brain were equally involved in all mental activity and there was no specificity of function with respect to particular brain areas. This idea became known as the equipotential view.

Some of the most influential ideas about localization of brain function came from early-nineteenth-century localizationist Franz Joseph Gall (for a recent review of Gall's contributions to understanding brain organization, see Ref. 6). Two assumptions made by Gall are germane to the present discussion. They were that (1) the brain is the organ of all faculties, tendencies, and feelings ("the organ of the soul")[7] and (2) the brain is composed of as many particular organs as there are faculties, tendencies, and feelings. According to Gall, for a particular individual, the specific regions of the brain associated with especially prominent behaviors were enlarged, and these brain enlargements could be detected by prominences on the individual's cranium. Memory and other higher cognitive functions, for example, were located in the anterior portion of the brain (Fig. 21-1). As it turned out, Gall was wrong about most or all of the details regarding the regions of the brain associated with particular cognitive functions. He was correct, however, in his fundamental idea that specific parts of the brain support specific functions. A substantial portion of contemporary neuroscientific research and neuropsychological practice continues to be guided by this fundamental idea.

Nearly 100 years after Gall proposed that particular regions of the brain were specialized for processing particular kinds of information,

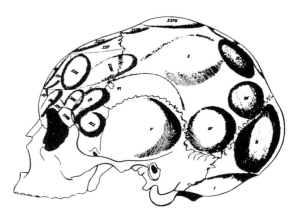

Figure 21-1
Gall's system of organology seen from the left side of the head. The organs were, for the most part, bilateral. Gall's 27 organs representing specific functions of the mind were divided into two groups. There were 19 organs common to humans and animals. Organ 11, the memory of things, memory of facts, refers to the ability to recall specific details of an event or item that distinguishes it from another event or item. Overall, Gall viewed memory not as a separate and fundamental faculty, but as secondary to each of the 27 faculties and organs. (From Zola-Morgan,[6] with permission.)

evidence began to accumulate that linked a particular region of the brain, the medial temporal lobe, to memory function. Von Bechterew (1900)[8] presented postmortem neuropathologic findings from the brain of a 60-year-old man who had memory problems during the last part of his life. The patient's brain showed pathologic changes in the medial temporal lobe, including the hippocampal formation.

Following von Bechterew's finding, several other case studies were published that linked defects in memory to damage in the medial temporal lobe (e.g., Refs. 9 and 10). One of the best-known of these cases, that of patient H. M., was published during the 1950s.[11,12] Patient H. M. developed severe impairment in new learning following bilateral removal of the medial temporal lobe regions of his brain in order to treat intractable seizures. He has been studied extensively during the last 40 years. During this interval, his memory impair-

ment has remained stable, and work with this patient has contributed substantially to our understanding of how memory is organized in the brain. Recent findings from magnetic resonance imaging studies of H. M. (at the age of 66) have determined that the bilateral lesion does not extend as far posteriorly as originally supposed; nevertheless, substantial portions of the hippocampal formation together with perirhinal cortex and entorhinal cortex are damaged bilaterally.[13]

NEUROPSYCHOLOGICAL ASPECTS OF AMNESIA

The impairment of new learning, or *anterograde amnesia*, is a defining attribute of organic amnesia. Severe anterograde amnesia will prevent patients from learning the facts of their hospitalization, the names and faces of clinical staff, and the routes linking their rooms and other locations around the hospital. Yet amnesic patients may have intact intellect as measured by standard psychometric tests (other than memory tests). Recently, it has also been established that certain forms of learning may be intact in amnesic patients, although conscious, explicit recollection is impaired. In addition to anterograde amnesia, most amnesic patients have some degree of *retrograde amnesia*, that is, impairment for memories acquired before their brain damage. The retrograde component of amnesia is most often temporally graded, with recently acquired memories more vulnerable than remote memories. The following chapter includes discussion of the nature of the information processing impairment in amnesia, including the nature of preserved learning in the anterograde component of amnesia and the temporal gradient in the retrograde component.

Assessment of memory impairment normally includes tests of verbal and nonverbal memory, which may be differentially affected in patients with unilateral lesions. Tests of new learning of verbal information generally take the form of lists that must be recalled or recognized (e.g., the California Auditory Verbal Learning Test[14]) or stories that must be recalled (e.g., the Logical

Memory subtest of the Wechsler Memory Scale—Revised[15]). Visual learning is generally tested with either recall (by drawing) or multiple choice recognition of abstract designs (e.g., Benton Visual Retention Test[16]). For a fuller discussion of neuropsychological assessment of memory, see Ref. 17.

Development of an Animal Model of Human Amnesia

In 1978, an important study by Mishkin (1978)[18] signaled the development of a model of human amnesia in nonhuman primates. Work with the animal model has allowed us to identify with certainty structures within the medial temporal lobe that are important for memory and to begin to determine systematically how individual structures within the medial temporal lobe contribute to memory function.[19–22] In parallel with this work in monkeys, extensive neuropathologic information has recently been obtained from several well-studied amnesic patients whose damage was limited to the medial temporal lobe. The remainder of this chapter describes the findings from work in monkeys as well as from amnesic patients with medial temporal lobe damage and presents the implications of these findings for the organization of memory in the medial temporal lobe. The role in memory of other regions of the brain (e.g., the diencephalon) has recently been reviewed[23] and is not addressed here. In addition, findings from work with rats have been recently reviewed[24,25] and are also not addressed here.

In monkeys, bilateral lesions of the medial temporal lobe, intended to reproduce the surgical lesion sustained by amnesic patient H. M., produced many of the features of memory impairment in human amnesia.[22] As in human amnesia, the memory deficit in monkeys with damage to the medial temporal lobe occurred in both visual and tactual modalities,[26,27] and the deficit was exacerbated by distracting the animals during the retention interval.[28] Moreover, as in human amnesia, the monkeys with bilateral medial temporal lobe lesions showed certain preserved learning abilities.[29]

Trial-Unique Delayed Nonmatching-to-Sample Task   The work with monkeys has depended on several tasks known to be sensitive to human amnesia,[22] including retention of simple object discriminations and the simultaneous learning of multiple pairs of objects (eight-pair concurrent discrimination learning). The most widely used memory task has been trial-unique delayed nonmatching to sample.[30] In this test of recognition memory, the monkey first sees a sample object. Then, after a delay, the original object and a novel object are presented together, and the monkey must displace the novel object to obtain a food reward. New pairs of objects are used on each trial.

The validity of this task as a test of recognition memory was recently questioned, on the grounds that medial temporal lesions seemed to affect performance as much at short delays as at long delays (whereas a memory impairment should be manifest primarily at long delays).[31] However, this conclusion was not based on studies designed to compare short and long retention intervals. When appropriate experimental designs are used, the impairment is indeed confined to long-delay conditions, consistent with the memory performance of amnesic patients.[31a,31b]

Identification of a Memory System in the Medial Temporal Lobe

A difficulty in the work with both monkeys and humans has been a long-standing imprecision with respect to the terminology used to describe the components of the medial temporal lobe. In particular, the term *hippocampus* is sometimes used interchangeably to refer to the cell fields of the hippocampus proper and sometimes to a more extensive region that includes the hippocampus proper as well as the dentate gyrus or the subicular complex. In the present chapter, the following terminology is used in reference to particular components of the medial temporal lobe memory system in both monkeys and humans: The term *hippocampus* includes the cell fields of the hippocampus proper and the dentate gyrus; the term *hippocampal region* includes the hippocampus proper, the dentate gyrus, and the subicular region; and the term *hippocampal formation* includes the hippocampal region and the entorhinal cortex.

Research in monkeys and humans has identified a system of anatomically related structures in the medial temporal lobe that is important for memory (for reviews, see Refs. 19, 21, 23, 32). The medial temporal lobe system is necessary for establishing long-term declarative memory—i.e., the capacity for conscious recollection of facts and events[33] (another term used to describe this kind of memory is *explicit memory*). This system is not required for short-term memory or for a variety of nondeclarative (or implicit) forms of learning, whereby acquired information is expressed through performance (see Chap. 22). This system comprises the hippocampal region and cortical areas adjacent to the hippocampal region (Fig. 21-2). The cortex adjacent to the hippocampal region includes the entorhinal, perirhinal, and parahippocampal cortices. All of these cortical areas are anatomically related to the hippocampal region.[34–39] In particular, the perirhinal cortex and the parahippocampal cortex provide nearly two-thirds of the cortical input to the entorhinal cortex.[38,39] The entorhinal cortex, in turn, provides the major source of cortical projections to the hippocampus and dentate gyrus.[35,39]

The following sections briefly review the findings that have led to three important and interrelated ideas about the role of the medial temporal lobe system in memory function: (1) the severity of memory impairment depends on the locus and extent of damage within the medial temporal lobe memory system, (2) the hippocampal region is itself important for memory, and (3) the cortical regions of the medial temporal lobe memory system (i.e., the entorhinal, perirhinal, and parahippocampal cortices) themselves play an essential role in memory.

1.　Relation between severity of memory impairment and the locus and extent of damage within the medial temporal lobe memory system.

Work with monkeys and humans has led to the idea that the severity of memory impairment increases as more components of the medial temporal lobe memory system are damaged. This idea has been supported by a large number of individual studies in monkeys where performance on memory tasks by groups of monkeys with varying damage to the medial temporal lobe has been compared (for example, see Refs. 18, 40, and 41). We recently took advantage of cumulated data from more than 10 years of testing monkeys to examine the relationship between severity of memory impairment and extent of damage in the medial temporal lobe.[42] The memory performance in three groups of monkeys with differing extents of damage to the medial temporal lobe memory system was compared to the memory performance in a group of 10 normal monkeys (Fig. 21-3). All of the monkeys had completed testing on our standard memory battery, and all monkeys had

Figure 21-2

A schematic view of the medial temporal lobe memory system. The entorhinal cortex is the major source of projections to the hippocampal region. Nearly two-thirds of the cortical input to the entorhinal cortex originates in the adjacent perirhinal and parahippocampal cortices, which, in turn, receive projections from unimodal and polymodal areas in the frontal, temporal, and parietal lobes. The entorhinal cortex also receives other direct inputs from orbital frontal cortex, cingulate cortex, insular cortex, and superior temporal gyrus. All these projections are reciprocal. (From Zola-Morgan et al.,[42] with permission.)

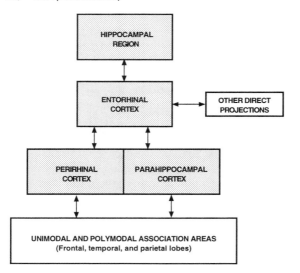

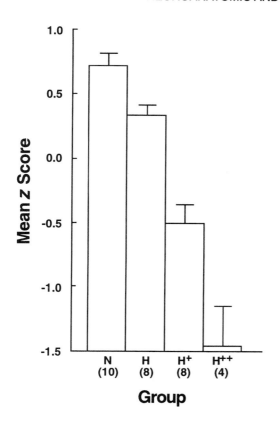

Figure 21-3

Mean z scores based on the data from four measures of memory for 10 normal monkeys (group N); 8 monkeys with damage limited to the hippocampus proper, the dentate gyrus, and the subicular complex (group H); 8 monkeys with damage that also included the adjacent entorhinal and parahippocampal cortices (group H+); and 4 monkeys in which the H+ lesion was extended forward to include the anterior entorhinal cortex and the perirhinal cortex (group H++). As more components of the medial temporal lobe were included in the lesion, the severity of memory impairment increased. All between-group comparisons were statistically significant. Group H consisted of monkeys from two different studies, i.e., 4 monkeys with ischemic damage limited to the hippocampal region[47] and 4 monkeys with stereotaxic radiofrequency lesions limited to the hippocampal region.[41] Both groups exhibited significant and long-lasting memory impairment when evaluated in their respective studies using our standard battery of memory tasks; both groups performed better overall than the H+ group, and the two H groups were not statistically different from each other.[42] Error bars indicate standard errors of the mean. (From Zola-Morgan et al.,[42] with permission.)

been tested on the tasks in the same order. Performance measures from each of the 30 monkeys were converted to z scores, so that different performance measures could be averaged together.

The main finding was that the severity of memory impairment depended on the locus and extent of damage within the medial temporal lobe memory system (Fig. 21-3). Damage limited to the hippocampal region (group H) caused significant memory impairment. More severe memory impairment occurred following H damage that included the adjacent entorhinal and parahippocampal cortex (group H+). The severity of impairment was greater still following H damage that also included all the adjacent cortical regions—i.e., the perirhinal, entorhinal, and parahippocampal cortices (group H++).

The finding that monkeys with damage that included the hippocampal region together with adjacent cortical regions (groups H+ and H++) ex-

hibited more severe impairment than monkeys with damage limited to the hippocampal region (group H) emphasizes the importance for memory function of the adjacent cortical regions. Indeed, the damage to these cortical regions likely contributes substantially to the severe memory impairment produced by medial temporal lobe lesions in monkeys and in humans.[23] It is important to note that the findings just described cannot be attributed to a principle like mass action.[43] That is, the severity of memory impairment exhibited by the monkeys with H++ lesions was not simply due to the fact that they had more damage overall than the monkeys with H+ lesions. When the H+ lesion was extended forward to include the amygdala (the H+A lesion), the memory impairment associated with the H+ lesion was not increased.[57] Thus, it is not just the extent of damage in the medial temporal lobe that is critical but which specific structures are damaged.[41]

2. The role in memory of the hippocampal region.

In the retrospective study just described, the finding of impairment in monkeys in group H supports the view that the hippocampus itself is critical for memory function. The finding of impaired memory following bilateral damage limited to the hippocampal region in monkeys is consistent with findings from human amnesia. As described later in this chapter, during the last several years, postmortem material from four well-studied cases of human amnesia associated with damage limited to the hippocampal region or damage limited to the hippocampal formation (i.e., the hippocampal region together with the entorhinal cortex) have become available.[44–46a]

An important issue about ischemic or anoxic damage is whether the damage indentifiable in histopathologic examination provides an accurate estimate of direct neural damage. For instance, additional direct damage might be present that is sufficient to disrupt neuronal function in areas important for memory and sufficient to impair behavioral performance but not sufficient to progress to cell death and to be detectable in histopathology. In our work with monkeys we have been able to address this issue directly by developing an animal model of cerebral ischemia in the monkey using a noninvasive technique that involves 15 min of carotid occlusion together with pharmacologically induced hypotension. This procedure reliably produced detectable damage only in the CA1 and CA2 cell fields of the hippocampus and in the hilar region of the dentate gyrus. There was no detectable damage elsewhere in the brain.[47] The behavioral result was that the ischemic group performed similarly to a group with a known surgical lesion of the hippocampal region (the H lesion) and significantly better than the H[+] and H[++] lesion groups. Thus, the available data do not support the idea that covert damage occurs sufficiently following global ischemia to contribute to memory impairment. The data suggest instead that the severity of memory impairment in monkeys and humans with ischemic damage is about what would be predicted from the damage that can be detected histopathologically and can be comparable to the impairment that results from histopathologically similar neurosurgical lesions.

The finding of impaired memory following bilateral damage limited to the hippocampal region and the hippocampal formation has also been reported for rats (for reviews see Refs. 25 and 48). Accordingly, the finding from rats, monkeys, and humans, are in good correspondence.[33] Damage limited to the hippocampal region and the hippocampal formation in all three species can produce significant and long-lasting memory impairment.

3. Memory and the entorhinal, perirhinal, and parahippocampal cortices.

Work with monkeys has led to the idea that the cortical regions of the medial temporal lobe (i.e., the perirhinal, entorhinal, and parahippocampal cortices), either separately or together, must themselves contribute to memory function, presumably by virtue of their extensive reciprocal connections with widespread regions of neocortex.[35–37,39,49] Straightforward evidence for the possible importance of the cortical regions came from studies in which direct circumscribed damage has been caused to the perirhinal, entorhinal, or parahippocampal cortices, either separately or in combination.[27,40,50–53] For example, monkeys with combined lesions of the perirhinal and parahippocampal cortices (the PRPH lesion) exhibited severely impaired performance on both a visual[27,40] and tactual[27] version of the delayed nonmatching-to-sample task. Moreover, the monkeys with PRPH lesions continued to exhibit impaired performance when retested on the visual version of the delayed nonmatching-to-sample task approximately 2 years after surgery.[27]

More limited lesions of the cortical regions also produce memory impairment. Monkeys with bilateral lesions limited to the perirhinal cortex exhibit impaired memory.[52,54] Moreover, damage to perirhinal cortex can produce more substantial impairment on the delayed nonmatching-to-sample task than damage to any other single component of the medial temporal lobe memory system.[52,53] In addition, the memory impairment following perirhinal lesions is long-lasting.[54]

Monkeys with bilateral lesions limited to the entorhinal cortex exhibited impaired memory,[50,52,53] and the impairment occurred in both visual and tactile modalities.[50] Overall, however, the impairment following entorhinal damage was less severe than that following perirhinal damage. In addition, the impairment following entorhinal damage is transient. Monkeys with bilateral entorhinal lesions were impaired on the delayed nonmatching-to-sample task when tested postoperatively, but they were not impaired when they were retested on the same task 9 to 14 months after surgery.[53] This finding suggests that while entorhinal cortex may normally participate in tasks that are dependent on the medial temporal lobe system, entorhinal cortex might not, in itself, be essential for the kinds of memory tasks used in the studies just described—e.g., the delayed nonmatching-to-sample task.

The effects in monkeys of damage limited to the parahippocampal cortex have not yet been systematically studied. Preliminary work from monkeys with bilateral parahippocampal cortex lesions has suggested that the parahippocampal cortex might not play an important role in object-recognition memory as measured by the delayed nonmatching-to-sample task or in other visual memory tasks.[54,55]

It is useful to note that the findings from monkeys with circumscribed lesions of the cortical regions need to be evaluated in the context of their neuroanatomic connectivity. That is, it is reasonable to suppose that the individual cortical regions might make different contributions to memory. This idea follows from the fact that information from neocortex enters the medial temporal lobe memory system at different points. For example, perirhinal cortex, unlike parahippocampal cortex, receives rather strong projections from unimodal visual area TE.[39,56] Parahippocampal cortex, but not perirhinal cortex, receives inputs from parietal cortex.[31,39] In this sense it could be supposed that perirhinal cortex might play a greater role than

parahippocampal cortex in visual memory, while parahippocampal cortex might play a greater role than perirhinal cortex in spatial memory.

By this view, the finding that lesions of the perirhinal cortex have thus far been reported to have a greater disruptive effect on memory than lesions of the entorhinal or parahippocampal cortex must be tempered by the fact that most of the tasks that have been used to evaluate the effects of damage to the cortical regions have been tasks of visual object memory. While recent findings point to the importance of the cortical regions adjacent to the hippocampal region, it will be important to evaluate the effects of damage to these cortical regions using a variety of tasks in addition to visual object memory.

It is instructive at this point to address the role of two additional brain regions that have been linked to memory function, i.e., the amygdala and the temporal stem. A major point of view during the last decade was that both the hippocampal formation and the amygdala had to be damaged conjointly to produce severe and long-lasting memory impairment in human and monkeys (e.g., Ref. 18). During the last decade, a different conclusion has been reached, based on experimental work.[21,32] A key breakthrough was the development of a procedure for making circumscribed bilateral lesions of the amygdala by a stereotaxic approach that spared surrounding cortex (i.e., the entorhinal and perirhinal cortices). Complete bilateral lesions of the amygdala made by this method did not impair performance on four different memory tasks, including delayed non-matching to sample.[57] Moreover, extending a lesion of the hippocampal formation forward to include circumscribed damage to the amygdala did not exacerbate the memory impairment that followed lesions of the hippocampal formation alone.[57]

These findings showed that severe memory impairment, of the kind exhibited in human amnesia, depends on damage to the hippocampal formation and adjacent anatomically related cortex (specifically, the perirhinal, entorhinal, and parahippocampal cortices; see Fig. 21-2). One or more of these cortical regions had always been damaged in the earlier studies during the surgical approach ordinarily used to remove the amygdala. A consensus has now been reached about the role of the amygdala.[23,32] (It is also important to note that this consensus is compatible with the idea that the amygdala plays an important role in certain kinds of memory, including conditioned fear and other forms of affective memory.[58-62])

Separate studies in monkeys have also evaluated the effects on memory of separate lesions of the "temporal stem," a fiber system that lies superficial to the hippocampal region. This fiber system links temporal neocortex with subcortical regions, and it had been proposed to be the critical structure damaged in temporal lobe amnesia.[63] However, monkeys with lesions of the temporal stem were not amnesic.[64] Moreover, the recent imaging study of patient H.M.[13] indicates that the temporal stem was not damaged, as originally supposed.[65]

New Cases of Human Amnesia with Lesions Limited to the Hippocampal Formation

As described previously, the findings from formal memory testing of patient H. M., as well as from other patients with less extensive bilateral medial temporal lobe removal, led to the view that damage to the medial temporal lobe and, in particular, the region of the hippocampus was responsible for the amnesia.[66] Damage to the hippocampus was also linked to memory impairments associated with a variety of neurologic conditions, including viral encephalitis,[67,68] posterior cerebral artery occlusion,[69] and hypoxic ischemia.[70] In addition, several single case studies had attributed impaired memory to hippocampal damage (e.g., Refs. 71–75). However, in these cases memory function was sometimes not assessed in a systematic way, and damage often extended beyond the hippocampus and involved other medial temporal lobe regions. Thus, although these cases in humans substantiated the importance in memory functions of the medial temporal lobe, they left some uncertainty as to whether lesions limited to the hippocampus were sufficient to cause amnesia. In the following

sections, several new case studies are described where damage has been limited either to the hippocampal region or to the hippocampal formation.

Damage Restricted Primarily to the Hippocampal Region   In 1986, we reported a case of amnesia in a patient (R.B.) who developed memory impairment following an episode of ischemia associated with cardiac surgery.[76] Following this episode, patient R. B. exhibited a marked anterograde memory impairment that remained unchanged until his death 5 years later. He showed minimal retrograde amnesia and no signs of cognitive impairment other than memory. Thorough histologic examination revealed that the only damage that could reasonably be associated with the memory defect was a circumscribed bilateral lesion involving the entire CA1 field of the hippocampus. This was the first reported case of amnesia following a lesion limited to the hippocampus in which extensive neuropathologic and neuropsychological information was available.

Recently, an additional case of amnesia with damage limited to the CA1 field of the hippocampus has become available (patient G.D.[45,46,46a]). Patient G. D. became amnesic in 1983 at the age of 43. The event that precipitated his amnesia was a hypotensive episode that occurred during major surgery. Patient G. D., like patient R. B., had damage restricted primarily to the CA1 region of the hippocampus (Fig. 21-4, top right panel). Patient G. D. was studied for 9.5 years until his death from congestive heart failure.

Patients R. B. and G. D. exhibited about the same degree of memory impairment in the anterograde domain. Their scores were similar across a range of anterograde memory tasks, including paired associate learning, where subjects were given three consecutive trials to learn 10 unrelated word pairs (maximum score = 30; R. B. = 1, G.D. = 5; and control subjects = 22) and diagram recall where subjects first copied a complex figure and then, without forewarning, were asked to reproduce it from memory 10 to 20 min later (maximum score for delay test = 36; R. B. = 3; G. D. = 7; and control subjects = 20.6).

Retrograde memory—i.e., memory for

events that occurred before the onset of amnesia—was also evaluated in the patients. Descriptions of the tests of retrograde memory and the data for the patients described here have been published previously.[76,77–81] Overall, patients R. B. and G. D. exhibited little evidence of retrograde amnesia.[45,46,46a,76]

Finally, Victor and Agamanolis reported another case of amnesia which developed after a series of generalized seizures, the lesion involved all the fields of the hippocampus and the dentate gyrus.[81] Little neuropsychological data concerning anterograde and retrograde deficits were provided for this case, but the severity of memory impairment described in the report seemed greater than that observed in patients R.B and G.D.

Damage Involving the Hippocampal Formation Patient L. M. became amnesic in 1984 at the age of 54.[46,46a,47] The precipitating event was a series of closely occurring generalized seizures and associated respiratory distress and respiratory acidosis. Patient L. M. had more extensive damage to the hippocampal region than did patients R. B. or G. D. His lesion involved all of the CA fields of the hippocampal region as well as the dentate gyrus (Fig. 21-4, lower left panel). In addition, patient L. M. evidenced some loss of cells in entorhinal cortex. Patient L. M. was studied for 6 years following the onset of his amnesia until his death from lung cancer.

Patient L.M.'s performance on individual tests of anterograde memory was similar to the performance of the other two patients (paired associate learning = 5; delay test for diagram recall = 6). However, because patient G. D. had the least education and a low IQ, it was not possible to rank order with confidence the severity of anterograde amnesia in R. B., G.D., and L.M.

On tests of retrograde amnesia, patient L. M. showed a clearly different pattern of performance than the other two patients. While patients R. B. and G. D. evidenced little retrograde memory impairment, patient L. M. demonstrated extensive retrograde amnesia. For example, in a test of autobiographical memory where memories were produced in response to 75 single-word

cues,[78] patient G. D. produced episodes from both recent and remote decades in a pattern similar to the responses of normal subjects and showed no evidence of retrograde amnesia. Patient L. M., however, produced mostly episodes from before 1950, and he had very few recollections from the 1960s to the 1980s. The findings from this test and other tests of retrograde memory indicate that patient L. M. had extensive, temporally graded retrograde amnesia (i.e., his memory was poorer for events close to the time of the onset of his amnesia and better for events more remote from the time of onset of amnesia), and his retrograde memory deficit extended back for at least 15 years.[45,46,46a]

Patient W. H. became amnesic during several days in March 1985 at the age of 63.[46,46a] The precise etiology of his amnesia is not clear. The damage in patient W. H. was more extensive than in the previously described patients and involved all of the components of the hippocampal region including the subicular complex (Fig. 21-4, lower right panel). In addition, W.H.'s entorhinal cortex sustained some cell loss. W. H. was studied for 7.5 years until he developed end-stage emphysema in 1993.

Patient W.H.'s anterograde memory impairment was somewhat greater than that of the other patients. On paired associate learning, he obtained a score of 0, and on the delay test of diagram recall he obtained a score of 1. On tests of retrograde memory, patient W. H. performed like patient L. M. That is, he had a severe retrograde memory deficit, and he demonstrated temporally graded retrograde amnesia that extended back at least 15 years.[45,46,46a]

Anterograde Amnesia: The Relationship between Severity of Impairment and Extent of Damage in the Medial Temporal Lobe

Figure 21-5 summarizes the neuropsychological and the neuropathologic information for patients R.B., G.D., L.M., and W.H. The findings from these patients make two important points with respect to anterograde amnesia. First, the findings from patients R.B., G.D., and L.M. underscore the fact that damage limited mainly to the hippocampal region is sufficient to produce clinically significant and long-lasting anterograde memory impairment. (L.M. did have some cell loss in entorhinal cortex.) As described in previous sections, significant memory impairment has also been shown in monkeys and rats when damage is limited to the hippocampal region.[41,47,48] These findings, therefore, support the long-standing idea that the hippocampal region itself is important for memory.

Second, patients R.B., G.D., and L.M., with damage limited primarily to the hippocampal region, demonstrated less severe memory impairment overall than patient W.H. or patient H.M., both of whom sustained additional damage. In the case of W.H., the additional damage involved the subicular complex; in the case of H.M., the additional damage involved the entorhinal and perirhinal cortices.[65] The findings from work with amnesic patients, like the findings in work with monkeys with medial temporal lobe lesions,[42] indicate that memory impairment can be exacerbated when damage includes cortical regions adjacent to the hippocampal region. Thus, findings from the work with amnesic patients are consistent with ideas that have been developed from work with monkeys—i.e., that the severity of memory impairment depends on the locus and extent of damage to the medial temporal lobe and that the cortical regions adjacent to the hippocampal region are themselves important for memory.[42,82]

Retrograde Amnesia: The Relationship between Severity of Impairment and Extent of Damage in the Medial Temporal Lobe

It has rarely been possible to study retrograde amnesia in patients with selective, histologically confirmed damage. The findings from the several patients described here provide important information about several aspects of retrograde amnesia. With respect to the relationship between severity of retrograde amnesia and the extent of damage in the medial temporal lobe, it appears that damage limited to the CA1 field does not produce severe or temporally graded retrograde amnesia (patients R.B. and D.G.). When the damage involves more than the CA1 field, however, extensive, temporally graded retrograde amnesia can occur (patients L.M., W.H., and the case report of Victor and Agamanolis,[81] as well as case H.M.[12]).

The findings from the patients described here also begin to address long-standing questions about the relationship between retrograde amnesia and anterograde amnesia. The impairments in the patients presented here as well as findings from

---

Figure 21-4

(Top left panel) *Coronal section through the left hippocampal region of a normal human brain stained for Nissl bodies.* (Top right panel) *Coronal section through the left hippocampal region of patient G. D. The lesion includes most of the cells in the CA1 region* (marked by arrowheads). *The subiculum sustained slight cell loss bilaterally.* (Bottom left panel) *Coronal section through the right hippocampal region of patient L. M. Note the complete loss of CA3 pyramidal cells and the nearly complete loss of CA1 pyramidal cells. The CA2 field is partially intact* (arrowheads). *There was also extensive loss of cells in the hilar region of the dentate gyrus* (arrows), *and the entorhinal cortex demonstrated some cell loss.* (Bottom right panel) *Coronal section through W.H.'s right hippocampal region. Extensive pyramidal cell loss is evident in cell fields CA1 and CA3. Less substantial cell loss occurred in field CA2. The dentate gyrus appears very abnormal, with dispersion of the granule cells and complete loss of polymorphic cells. Patchy cell loss is evident in the subiculum and there was patchy cell loss in the entorhinal cortex as well.* Abbreviations: *CA1, CA2 CA3 = cell fields of the hippocampus; DG = dentate gyrus; EC = entorhinal cortex; gl = granular layer; ml = molecular layer; PaS = parasubiculum; pl = polymorphic layer; PrS = presubiculum; S = subiculum.*

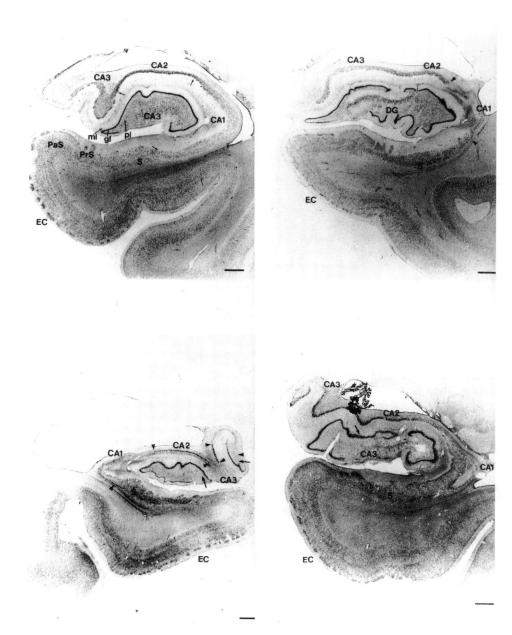

Figure 21-5
(Left panel) *Summary of over-all findings from patients R. B., G.D., L. M., and W. H. on tests of anterograde memory (anterograde amnesia) and retrograde memory (retrograde amnesia).* (Right panel) *Summary of brain damage in the medial temporal lobe for each patient.*

	Anterograde Amnesia	Retrograde Amnesia	Damage to the Hippocampal Formation
RB	moderate	minimal	CA1 field
GD	moderate	minimal (?)	CA1 field
LM	moderate	extensive	CA1, CA2, CA3 fields, dentate gyrus (entorhinal cortex)
WH	severe	extensive	CA1, CA2, CA3 fields, dentate gyrus, subiculum, entorhinal cortex

other amnesic patients suggest that retrograde amnesia and anterograde amnesia can be caused by damage to the same region—i.e., the hippocampal formation. While anterograde and retrograde memory are both normally dependent on the integrity of the hippocampal formation, it appears that anterograde memory can be more easily disrupted than retrograde memory (e.g., a lesion of the CA1 field is sufficient to produce significant anterograde memory impairment). As described above, retrograde amnesia, like anterograde amnesia, can vary in its severity as a function of the extent of damage to the hippocampal formation.

Finally, the finding that very remote memories are typically preserved in amnesic patients means that the site of permanent memory storage cannot be the hippocampal formation or any of the other damaged structures in the medial temporal lobe. Thus, while the hippocampal formation is critically involved in the formation of new memories, it has been supposed that the hippocampal formation and related structures must have only a temporary role in memory storage.[23,33,83] That is, the medial temporal lobe memory system has only a temporary role in the formation and maintenance of declarative memory. After learning, memory is gradually reorganized over time. It is initially dependent on this system, but its role diminishes as more permanent memory is established elsewhere, presumably in neocortex.[83]

It is important to note that some memory-impaired patients have extensive retrograde amnesia with no evidence of a temporal gradient.[84] In such cases, remote memory appears to be severely and similarly impaired across all time periods. One possibility is that severe and ungraded retrograde amnesia requires damage in addition to (or different from) that to the medial temporal lobe structures associated with circumscribed amnesia. This additional damage might impair performance on remote memory tests without contributing proportionally to anterograde amnesia. Additional neuropsychological and anatomic information will be needed to identify the determinants of ungraded retrograde amnesia and to confirm that ungraded forms of retrograde amnesia are dissociable from anterograde memory impairment.

OVERVIEW

In concluding, it is useful to underscore that work in monkeys (specifically, the finding that the severity of memory impairment increases as more components of the medial temporal lobe memory system are damaged) is fully consistent with findings from human amnesia. The moderately severe memory impairment in the patients described above who had damage limited to the hippocampal formation can be contrasted with the more severe memory impairment observed in patient H. M., who sustained bilateral resection of the medial temporal lobe, including the hippocampal region and adjacent cortical regions.[65]

For the last 100 years, amnesia has been associated with damage to several regions of the brain. Among these are the amygdala, hippocampal region, and cortex adjacent to the hippocampal region in the medial temporal lobe, and the mammillary nuclei and medial thalamus in the diencephalon. Until recently, it has remained unclear, however, whether damage confined to any of these structures would produce a clinically significant memory impairment. At the present time, the findings from work in three species—rats, monkeys, and humans—share many points of correspondence with the findings from monkeys with medial temporal lobe lesions. In particular, the findings show that circumscribed bilateral lesions limited to the hippocampal region are sufficient to produce amnesia. Additional findings indicate that the cortical regions adjacent to and anatomically linked to the hippocampal region—i.e., the perirhinal, entorhinal, and parahippocampal cortices—are also important for memory function.

ACKNOWLEDGMENTS

This work was supported by the Medical Research Service of the Department of Veterans Affairs and NIH Grant 19063. I thank Larry R. Squire for his contributions to this work.

REFERENCES

1. McHenry LC Jr: *Garrison's History of Neurology.* Springfield, IL, Charles C Thomas, 1969.
2. Finger S: *Origins of Neuroscience: A History of Explorations into Brain Function.* New York, Oxford University Press, 1994.
3. Gross CG: Early history of neuroscience, in Edelman G (ed): *Encyclopedia of Neuroscience.* Boston, Birkhauser, 1987.
4. Baader J: Observationes medicae, incisionibus cadaverum anatomicis illustrae, in Sandifort E (ed): *Thesaurus Dissertationum* 3:1–62, 1762 (in Latin).
5. Clendening L: *Source Book of Medical History.* New York, Dover, 1942.
6. Zola-Morgan S: Localization of brain function: The legacy of Franz Joseph Gall (1758–1828). *Annu Rev Neurosci* 18:359–383, 1995.
7. Gall FJ: *Sur les Fonctions du Cerveau.* Paris, Shoell, 1822 (in French).
8. von Bechterew W: Demonstration eines Gehirns mit Zerstörung der vorderen und inneren Theile der Hirnrinde beider Schlaffenlappen. *Neurol Zentralb* 19:990–991, 1900.
9. Grunthal E: Über das klinische Bild nach umschriebenem beiderseitigam Ausfall der Ammonshornrinde. *Monatsschr Psychiatrie Neurol* 113:1–16, 1947.
10. Glees P, Griffith HB: Bilateral destruction of the hippocampus (cornu ammonis) in a case of dementia. *Psychiatry Neurol Med Psychol (Leipz)* 123:193–204, 1952.
11. Scoville WB: The limbic lobe and memory in man. *J Neurosurg* 11:64, 1954.
12. Scoville WB, Milner B: Loss of recent memory after bilateral hippocampal lesions. *J Neurol Neurosurg Psychiatry* 20:11–21, 1957.
13. Corkin S, Amaral DG, Johnson KA, Kyman BT: H.M.'s MRI scan shows sparing of the posterior half of the hippocampus and parahippocampal gyrus. *J Neurosci.* In press.
14. Deus DC, Kramer JH, Kaplan E, Ober BA: *California Verbal Learning Test Manual.* San Antonio, The Psychological Corporation, 1987.
15. Wechsler D: *Wecshsler Memory Scale—Revised.* New York, The Psychological Corporation, 1987.
16. Benton AL: *The Revised Visual Retention Test,* 4th ed. New York, The Psychological Corporation, 1974.
17. Lezak MD: *Neuropsychological Assessment,* 2d ed. New York, Oxford University Press, 1987.
18. Mishkin M: Memory in monkeys severely impaired by combined but not separate removal of the amygdala and hippocampus. *Nature* 273:297–298, 1978.
19. Mishkin M: A memory system in the monkey. *Phil Trans R Soc Lond* 98:85–95, 1982.
20. Mahut H, Moss M: Consolidation of memory: The hippocampus revisited, in Squire LR, Butters N (eds): *Neuropsychology of Memory.* New York, Guilford, 1984, pp 297–315.
21. Squire LR, Zola-Morgan S: The medial temporal lobe memory system. *Science* 253:1380–1386, 1991.
22. Squire LR, Zola-Morgan S, Chen K: Human amnesia and animal models of amnesia: Performance of amnesic patients on tests designed for the monkey. *Behav Neurosci* 11:210–221, 1988.
23. Zola-Morgan S, Squire LR: Neuroanatomy of memory. *Annu Rev Neurosci* 16:547–563, 1993.
24. Eichenbaum H, Otto T, Cohen NJ: The hippocampus—What does it do? *Behav Neural Biol* 57:2–36, 1992.

25. Jarrard LE: On the role of the hippocampus in learning and memory in the rat. *Behav Neural Biol* 60:9–26, 1993.

26. Murray EA, Mishkin M: Severe tactual as well as visual memory deficits follow combined removal of the amygdala and hippocampus in monkeys. *J Neurosci* 4:2565–2580, 1984.

27. Suzuki WA, Zola-Morgan S, Squire LR, Amaral DG: Lesions of the perirhinal and parahippocampal cortices in the monkey produce long-lasting memory impairment in the visual and tactual modalities. *J Neurosci* 13:2430–2451, 1993.

28. Zola-Morgan S, Squire LR: Medial temporal lesions in monkeys impair memory on a variety of tasks sensitive to human amnesia. *Behav Neurosci* 99:22–34, 1985.

29. Zola-Morgan S, Squire LR: Preserved learning in monkeys with medial temporal lobe lesions: Sparing of motor and cognitive skills. *J Neurosci* 4:1072–1085, 1984.

30. Mishkin M, Delacour J: An analysis of short-term visual memory in the monkey. *J Exp Psychol* 1:326–334, 1975.

31. Ringo JL: Memory decays at the same rate in macaques with and without brain lesions when expressed in d' or arcsine terms. *Behav Brain Res* 42:123–134, 1991.

31a. Alvarez-Royo P, Zola-Morgan S, Squire LR: Impairment of long-term memory and sparing of short-term memory in monkeys with medial temporal lobe lesions: A reply to Ringo. *Behav Brain Res* 52:1–5, 1992.

31b. Alvarez-Royo P, Zola-Morgan S, Squire LR: The animal model of human amnesia: Long-term memory impaired and short-term memory intact. *Proc Nat Acad Sci* 91:5637–5641, 1994.

32. Murray EA: Medial temporal lobe structures contributing to recognition memory: The amygdaloid complex versus the rhinal cortex, in Aggleton JP (ed): *The Amygdala: Neurobiological Aspects of Emotion, Memory, and Mental Dysfunction.* New York, Wiley-Liss, 1992, pp 453–470.

33. Squire LR: Declarative and nondeclarative memory: Multiple brain systems supporting learning and memory. *J Cogn Neurosci* 4:232–243, 1992.

34. Van Hoesen G: The parahippocampal gyrus: New observations regarding its cortical connections in the monkey. *Trends Neurosci* 5:345–350, 1982.

35. Van Hoesen GW, Pandya DN: Some connections of the entorhinal (area 28) and perirhinal (area 35) cortices of the rhesus monkey: I. Temporal lobe afferents. *Brain Res* 95:1–24, 1975.

36. Van Hoesen GW, Pandya DN: Some connections of the entorhinal (area 28) and perirhinal (area 35) cortices of the rhesus monkey. III. Efferent connections. *Brain Res* 95:39–59, 1975.

37. Van Hoesen GW, Pandya DN, Butters N: Some connections of the entorhinal (area 28) and perirhinal (area 35) cortices of the rhesus monkey. II. Frontal lobe afferents. *Brain Res* 95:25–38, 1975.

38. Insausti R, Amaral DG, Cowan WM: The entorhinal cortex of the monkey: II. Cortical afferents. *J Comp Neurol* 264:356–395, 1987.

39. Suzuki WA, Amaral DG: Perirhinal and parahippocampal cortices of the macaque monkey: Cortical afferents. *J Comp Neurol* 350:497–533, 1994.

40. Zola-Morgan S, Squire LR, Amaral DG, Suzuki WA: Lesions of perirhinal and parahippocampal cortex that spare the amygdala and hippocampal formation produce severe memory impairment. *J Neurosci* 9:4355–4370, 1989.

41. Alvarez P, Zola-Morgan S, Squire LR: Damage limited to the hippocampal region produces long-lasting memory impairment in monkeys. *J Neurosci* 15:3796–3807, 1995.

42. Zola-Morgan S, Squire LR, Ramus SJ: Severity of memory impairment in monkeys as a function of locus and extent of damage within the medial temporal lobe memory system. *Hippocampus* 4:483–494, 1994.

43. Lashley KS: *Brain Mechanisms and Intelligence: A Quantitative Study of Injuries to the Brain.* Chicago, University of Chicago Press, 1929.

44. Zola S, Squire LR: Human amnesia and the medial temporal lobe, in Kato N (ed): *Functions and Clinical Relevance of the Hippocampus.* New York, Elsevier, 1996.

45. Rempel-Clower NL, Zola-Morgan S, Squire LR: Damage to the hippocampal region in human amnesia: Neuropsychological and neuroanatomical findings from two new cases. *Soc Neurosci Abstr* 24:1975, 1994.

46. Rempel-Clower NL, Zola-Morgan S, Squire LR: Importance of the hippocampal region and entorhinal cortex in human memory: Neuropsychological and neuropathological findings from a new patient. *Soc Neurosci Abstr* 25:1493, 1995.

46a. Rempel-Clower N, Zola-Morgan S, Squire LR, Amaral DG: Three cases of enduring memory impairment following bilateral damage limited to the hippocampal formation. *J Neurosci* Submitted.

47. Zola-Morgan S, Squire LR, Rempel NL, et al: Enduring memory impairment in monkeys after ischemic damage to the hippocampus. *J Neurosci* 9:4355–4370, 1992.

48. Jaffard R, Meunier M: Role of the hippocampal formation in learning and memory. *Hippocampus* 3:203–217, 1993.

49. Witter MP, Groenewegen HJ, Lopes da Silva FH, Lohman AHM: Functional organization of the extrinsic and intrinsic circuitry of the parahippocampal region. *Prog Neurobiol* 33:161–254, 1989.

50. Moss M, Mahut H, Zola-Morgan S: Concurrent discrimination learning of monkeys after hippocampal, entorhinal, or fornix lesions. *J Neurosci* 1:227–240, 1981.

51. Gaffan D, Murray EA: Monkeys (*M. fascicularis*) with rhinal cortex ablations succeed in object discrimination learning despite 24-hour intertrial intervals and fail at matching to sample despite double sample presentation. *Behav Neurosci* 106:30–38, 1992.

52. Meunier M, Bachevalier J, Mishkin M, Murray EA: Effects on visual recognition of combined and separate ablations of the entorhinal and perirhinal cortex in rhesus monkeys. *J Neurosci* 13:5418–5432, 1993.

53. Leonard BW, Amaral DG, Squire LR, Zola-Morgan S: Transient memory impairment in monkeys with bilateral lesions of the entorhinal cortex. *J Neurosci* 15:5637–5659, 1995.

54. Ramus SJ, Zola-Morgan S, Squire LR: Effects of lesions of perirhinal cortex or parahippocampal cortex on memory in monkeys. *Soc Neurosci Abstr* 24:1074, 1994.

55. Horel JA, Pytko-Joiner E, Voytko ML, Salsbury K: The performance of visual tasks while segments of the inferotemporal cortex are suppressed by cold. *Behav Brain Res* 23:29–42, 1991.

56. Webster MJ, Ungerleider LG, Bachevalier J: Connections of inferior temporal areas TE and TEO with medial temporal-lobe structures in infant and adult monkeys. *J Neurosci* 11:1095–1116, 1991.

57. Zola-Morgan S, Squire LR, Amaral DG: Lesions of the amygdala that spare adjacent cortical regions do not impair memory or exacerbate the impairment following lesions of the hippocampal formation. *J Neurosci* 9:1922–1936, 1989.

58. Davis M: Pharmacological and anatomical analysis of fear conditioning using the fear-potentiated startle paradigm. *Behav Neurosci* 100:814–824, 1986.

59. Gallagher M, Graham PW, Holland P: The amygdala central nucleus and appetitive Pavlovian conditioning: Lesions impair one class of conditioned behavior. *J Neurosci* 10:1906–1911, 1990.

60. Kesner RP: Learning and memory in rats with an emphasis on the role of the amygdala, in Aggleton J (ed): *The Amygdala*. New York, Wiley, 1992, pp 379–400.

61. LeDoux J: Emotion, in Brookhart JM, Mountcastle VB (eds): *Handbook of Physiology: The Nervous System: V. Higher Functions of the Nervous System*, 5th ed. Bethesda, MD, American Physiological Society, 1987, pp 419–460.

62. McGaugh JL: Involvement of hormonal and neuromodulatory systems in the regulation of memory storage. *Annu Rev Neurosci* 12:255–287, 1989.

63. Horel JA: The neuroanatomy of amnesia. *Brain* 101:403–445, 1978.

64. Zola-Morgan S, Squire LR, Mishkin M: The neuroanatomy of amnesia: Amygdala-hippocampus versus temporal stem. *Science* 218:1337–1339, 1982.

65. Corkin S, Amaral DG, Johnson KA, Hyman BT: HM's MRI scan shows sparing of the posterior half of the hippocampus and parahippocampal gyrus. *J Neurosci*. In press.

66. Scoville WB, Milner B: Loss of recent memory after bilateral hippocampal lesions. *J Neurol Neurosurg Psychiatry* 20:11–21, 1957.

67. Damasio AR, Eslinger PJ, Damasio H, et al: Multimodal amnesic syndrome following bilateral temporal and basal forebrain damage. *Arch Neurol* 42:252–259, 1985.

68. Rose FC, Symonds CP: Persistent memory defect following encephalitis. *Brain* 83:195–212, 1960.

69. Benson DF, Marsden CD, Meadows JC: The amnesic syndrome of posterior cerebral artery occlusion. *Acta Neurol Scand* 50:133–145, 1974.

70. Volpe BT, Hirst W: The characterization of an amnesic syndrome following hypoxic ischemic injury. *Arch Neurol* 40:436–440, 1983.

71. Cummings JL, Tomiyasu U, Read S, Benson DF: Amnesia with hippocampal lesions after cardiopulmonary arrest. *Neurology* 34:679–681, 1984.

72. DeJong RN, Itabashi HH, Olson JR: "Pure" memory loss with hippocampal lesions: A case report. *Trans Am Neurol Assoc* 93:31–34, 1968.

73. Duyckaerts C, Derouesne C, Signoret JL, et al: Bilateral and limited amygdalohippocampal lesions causing a pure amnesic syndrome. *Ann Neurol* 18:314–319, 1985.

74. Muramoto O, Kuru Y, Sugishita M, Toyokura Y: Pure memory loss with hippocampal lesions: A

pneumoencephalographic study. *Arch Neurol* 36: 54–56, 1979.

75. Woods BT, Schoene W, Kneisley L: Are hippocampal lesions sufficient to cause lasting amnesia? *J Neurol Neurosurg Psychiatry* 45:243–247, 1982.

76. Zola-Morgan S, Squire LR, Amaral DG: Human amnesia and the medial temporal region: Enduring memory impairment following a bilateral lesions limited to field CA1 of the hippocampus. *J Neurosci* 6:2950–2967, 1986.

77. Squire LR, Haist F, Shimamura AP: The neurology of memory: Quantitative assessment of retrograde amnesia in two groups of amnesic patients. *J Neurosci* 9:828–839, 1989.

78. MacKinnon DF, Squire LR: Autobiographical memory and amnesia. *Psychobiology* 17:247–256, 1989.

79. Salmon DP, Lasker BR, Butters N, Beatty WW: Remote memory in a patient with circumscribed amnesia. *Brain Cogn* 7:201–211, 1988.

80. Beatty WW, Salmon DP, Bernstein N, Butters N: Remote memory in a patient with amnesia due to hypoxia. *Psychol Med* 17:657–665, 1987.

81. Victor M, Agamanolis D: Amnesia due to lesions confined to the hippocampus: A clinico-pathologic study. *J Cogn Neurosci* 2:246–257, 1990.

82. Mishkin M, Murray EA: Stimulus recognition. *Curr Opin Neurobiol* 4:200–206, 1994.

83. Alvarez P, Squire LR: Memory consolidation and the medial temporal lobe: A simple network model. *Proc Nat Acad Sci USA* 91:7041–7045, 1994.

84. Squire LR, Alvarez P: Retrograde amnesia and memory consolidation: A Neurobiological perspective. *Curr Opin Neurobiol* 5:169–177, 1995.

Chapter 22

AMNESIA II: COGNITIVE NEUROPSYCHOLOGICAL ISSUES

Tim Curran
Daniel L. Schacter

Research in cognitive neuroscience has inspired the view that distinct neural systems are differentially involved in various aspects of memory. While most or all information processing systems in the brain are capable of using past information to influence current behavior, there is a great deal of functional heterogeneity in the aspects of learning and memory that are supported by different neural mechanisms. This chapter provides an overview of cognitive neuroscience research on the principal brain mechanisms of memory. We start with a discussion of research that has attempted to evaluate the contribution of the medial temporal lobe and related structures to memory by investigating the amnesic syndrome. This research has inspired new perspectives on the storage and retrieval of information in long-term memory. Findings of preserved learning and memory in amnesic patients have suggested that some brain mechanisms support forms of memory that can operate unconsciously (implicit memory) and have also pointed toward distinct short-term forms of memory (working memory). Finally, the contribution of the prefrontal cortex to long-term memory and working memory are discussed.

AMNESIA AND MEDIAL TEMPORAL LOBE FUNCTION: COGNITIVE NEUROPSYCHOLOGICAL PERSPECTIVES

Patients with organic amnesia show profound learning and memory impairments that are typi-cally attributable to medial temporal lobe and/or diencephalic damage (see Chap. 21) for a review of these impairments). Research investigating the functional deficit(s) underlying organic amnesia have been strongly influenced by theories of normal learning and memory. Models of human memory that posit a distinction between short- and long-term memory[1] generally have been supported by the finding that amnesic patients show normal retention of small amounts of information (about seven items) across short temporal durations (less than about 30 s). As discussed below, short-term or working memory is supported by neurocognitive processes that are separable from long-term forms of retention. We now consider the component processes of long-term retention that may be compromised in organic amnesia.

Cognitive psychologists generally distinguish between three different information processing stages of memory: encoding, storage, and retrieval. The integrity of each of these stages has been investigated in order to understand the memory impairment resulting from organic amnesia. The observation that amnesic patients can show normal levels of memory when certain retrieval cues are provided (e.g., a three-letter word stem, *tru,* to cue memory for *truck*) led to the hypothesis that amnesia results from a retrieval deficit. Because interference, or competition among similar memories, is considered to be a primary determinant of retrieval failure in normal subjects, retrieval-deficit theories predicted abnormally high levels of interference in amnesic patients. Contrary to this prediction, direct tests of this hypothesis found that amnesic and control subjects were similarly susceptible to interference.[2,3]

Retrieval-deficit theories of amnesia suffered from another, more fundamental flaw that does not relate to interference. The ability to retrieve information encountered prior to the onset of amnesia can remain intact (especially if the information was learned long before the onset of amnesia) despite profound impairments in retaining new information[4] (see Chap. 21). That is, anterograde amnesia can exist without retrograde amnesia. If amnesia involved only a general retrieval deficit, it should affect the retrieval of old and new information equally. The separability of anterograde and retrograde amnesia suggests that the amnesic deficit is likely attributable (at least in part) to an impairment at the time of learning. For this reason among others, encoding deficit theories of amnesia have been proposed.

The levels-of-processing framework[5] has greatly influenced cognitive psychologists' ideas about the manner in which information is encoded into memory. Simply stated, this framework describes the fact that information is remembered more accurately when semantic rather than superficial aspects of stimuli are encoded. Thus, amnesic patients' memory impairments have been hypothesized to reflect a deficit in encoding to-be-remembered information at a semantic level. Semantic coding deficit theories received initial support when Korsakoff's amnesics failed to show a normal levels-of-processing effect,[6] but subsequent studies have found normal levels-of-processing effects with other amnesic patients.[7] Other studies suggested that amnesic patients did not spontaneously use semantic information to organize and encode information in memory[8] but that they could encode semantic aspects of stimuli when properly instructed.[9] Ultimately, semantic coding deficits cannot entirely explain the memory deficit of patients with anterograde amnesia. Besides the evidence that amnesics can properly encode semantic attributes, any theory that focuses purely on encoding processes has difficulty explaining the differential effectiveness of different retrieval cues or the fact that anterograde amnesia is typically associated with some retrograde memory loss.[4]

Cognitive theories of encoding (e.g., levels-of-processing) and retrieval (e.g., interference theory) have generally been unsuccessful in explaining the amnesic syndrome. Storage-deficit theories, rather than being directly borrowed from cognitive psychology, exemplify how neuropsychological evidence has influenced the evolution of psychological theories. In particular, cognitive neuroscience research on amnesia has revolutionized our ideas about the storage process known as consolidation. Consolidation was originally conceptualized as the process by which information is transferred from short- to long-term memory. More recent theories posit that consolidation is a longer-term process by which memories are integrated with existing knowledge over a time course that lasts from minutes to years. According to consolidation theories,[4,10] memories initially depend on an interaction between the temporal lobe/diencephalon and the cerebral cortex. Over time, the learned representations become integrated with other knowledge in the cerebral cortex and no longer depend on the medial temporal lobe or diencephalon. Evidence for this view is derived from the observation that (1) retrograde and anterograde amnesia are typically correlated and (2) retrograde amnesia follows a temporal gradient. The temporal gradient of retrograde amnesia refers to the finding that retrograde amnesia is typically most severe for information that was encountered immediately prior to the onset of amnesia but is progressively less severe for remote events[4] (see Chap. 21). According to consolidation theories, remote memories have already been completely consolidated with information in the cerebral cortex, so they are no longer dependent on the brain regions affected in amnesia (i.e., medial temporal lobes and/or diencephalon). More recent memories, for which retrograde amnesia is most severe, have not been consolidated, so they are most likely to be lost upon the onset of amnesia.

Another proposed function of the medial temporal lobes—related to consolidation—is the binding of distinct memory attributes that are represented in distributed cortical areas.[10,11] By this view, different stimulus attributes are ultimately represented and stored in dedicated cortical areas: visual features in occipitotemporal cortex, spatial information in parietal cortex, auditory information in superior temporal cortex, and so on. Medial temporal lobe mechanisms interact with these cortical representations to bind them into a coherent memory of the remembered episode. Through consolidation, these cortical representations become directly associated with each other and are no longer dependent upon medial temporal lobe binding.

The previously discussed theories of the amnesic deficit can be collectively referred to as process theories because they try to relate medial temporal lobe function to a particular memory process (e.g., encoding, binding, consolidation, retrieval). Another general class of theories, content theories, have posited that the memory deficits of amnesic patients involve only certain types of information. One example of such a theory posits that amnesics' memory for information about individual items is normal, but amnesics' deficit is specific to contextual or associative information. Other theories hold that the performance of amnesic patients is impaired on tests that require conscious recollection of a previous episode ("explicit memory") but is spared on tasks in which memory influences behavior without conscious recollection ("implicit memory"). As will be seen, these dichotomies (item information versus contextual/associative information, explicit versus implicit) are orthogonal to the process theories, and it is reasonable to combine the two approaches. That is, if amnesics' memory deficits are confined to associative information, this associative-memory deficit could be attributable to a certain stage of information processing. Furthermore, these content dichotomies are not mutually exclusive, so, for example, it is important to consider implicit memory for item information as well as implicit memory for associative information.

Context-memory deficit hypotheses suggest that memory for individual stimuli is spared by organic amnesia, but memory for contextual information (e.g., time, place, and so on) within the learning episode is impaired.[12] A related idea holds that damage to medial temporal lobe structures has little effect on memory for individual stimuli but impairs the ability to remember complex associative or relational information about multiple stimuli.[13,14] A central issue in evaluating context-memory deficit theories is whether or not amnesics' recognition abilities (i.e., the ability to discriminate studied from nonstudied items) is relatively spared in comparison with free or cued recall. The importance of recall versus recognition performance is derived from the fact that recall is typically more context-dependent than recognition. Some studies have found that recognition is spared relative to recall in patients with organic amnesia[15] but others have shown that recall and recognition are similarly impaired.[16] Even if amnesics do show a greater deficit on recognition than recall, context-deficit theories have difficulty explaining the fact that recognition—though better than recall—is not normal in amnesic patients. Such an explanation requires more detailed theories of the conditions in which context-memory influences item recognition.

There is an important relationship between content theories positing an amnesic deficit in associative/contextual memory and process theories positing that the medial temporal lobes act as a binding mechanism. The ability to remember associations between stimuli or to remember the episodic context in which a stimulus was encountered clearly depends on the associative binding of information in memory. Theories that posit a medial temporal lobe (and diencephalic) contribution to consolidation and binding appear to be very promising. Below, we discuss the capacity for other types of learning and memory that do not depend on these mechanisms.

IMPLICIT MEMORY

In considering evidence for retrieval-deficit theories of amnesia, we discussed the finding that amnesic patients' memory can appear normal when tested with appropriate cues like word stems. Graf and coworkers[17] showed that the instructions given to subjects may be just as important as the physical retrieval cue in determining how the memory performance of amnesic patients will compare to that of control subjects. When subjects were asked to intentionally recall a studied word that completes the stem (a direct test of explicit memory), control subjects outperformed amnesic patients. However, when subjects were simply asked to respond with the first correct completion that came to mind (an indirect test of implicit memory), amnesic and control subjects performed equivalently. Both groups of subjects showed superior completion rates for studied compared to nonstudied words (this effect is typically called "priming"), so it is clear that both groups were being influenced by memory for the studied words. This finding of spared priming on implicit tasks has been well replicated (for reviews, see Refs. 18 and 19). Thus, implicit memory does not seem to depend on the medial temporal and diencephalic brain areas that are damaged in organic amnesia.

Implicit memory is observed in tasks in which previous experience can influence behavior in the absence of conscious recollection (for review, see Ref. 20). Research on normal subjects has distinguished between two types of implicit memory tasks: (1) perceptual tasks in which the retrieval cue is perceptually related to the target item (e.g., stem completion, *tru—*) and (2) conceptual tasks in which the retrieval cue is conceptually related to the target item (e.g., category exemplar generation, *vehicle-?*). We will focus on perceptual forms of priming because more is known about the underlying brain mechanisms. In general, performance on perceptual implicit memory tasks is unaffected by semantic variables that greatly influence explicit memory. For example, in our discussion of encoding theories of amnesia, we noted that explicit memory normally benefits from semantic encoding compared to an encoding strategy that emphasizes physical characteristics of the studied stimulus.[5] In contrast, perceptual priming shows little benefit from semantic encoding. Unlike explicit memory, perceptual priming is sensitive to the perceptual compatibility between study and test conditions. On a visual stem completion task, for example, priming is superior

when the study list is presented visually rather than auditorally.[21]

The semantic independence and perceptual sensitivity of implicit memory has suggested that it reflects the influence of previous experience on presemantic brain mechanisms that are normally involved in perception. Cognitive neuroscience studies of perception indicate that different cortical areas are involved in the perception of different kinds of stimuli, such as visual words, auditory words, or visual objects (see Chaps. 6, 15, and 18). For example, evidence from neuropsychology and neuroimaging has converged on the idea that perception of visual words relies on mechanisms in occipitotemporal cortex.[22]

Schacter[23] has suggested that implicit memory is driven by modality-specific perceptual systems. This view has been supported by positron emission tomography (PET; see Chap. 3) studies of the functional anatomy of stem-completion priming.[24,25] Activation by PET in bilateral occipitotemporal regions was stronger when word stems were completed with nonstudied words compared to previously studied words. This is consistent with the idea that priming reflects an influence of previous experience on the mechanisms that underlie visual word perception such that word perception is made easier by previously studying the word. Other PET evidence suggests that similar conclusions apply in the domain of visual object processing.[26]

Converging evidence for a contribution of visual cortical areas to implicit memory has been provided by a study of memory and priming in a patient, M. S., who had most of his right occipital lobe removed in order to alleviate intractable epilepsy.[27] M. S. showed normal explicit memory on a variety of tests but impaired perceptual priming on word-stem completion and word-identification tasks. Further evidence for the visuoperceptual nature of his priming impairment was obtained by demonstrating normal priming when words were studied auditorally rather than visually and normal priming on a conceptual test of implicit memory.

In summary, neuropsychological and neuroimaging studies of visual word priming have strongly implicated visual perceptual mechanisms in occipitotemporal cortex. Other evidence suggests that distinct perceptual mechanisms contribute to implicit memory for auditory words and visual objects.[23] Similarly, brain areas controlling perceptuomotor coordination can implicitly learn information that helps to guide subsequent behavior (often referred to as "procedural learning").[28] These results support the general conclusion that implicit learning and memory reflect the effects of experience on the brain mechanisms that normally support perception and guide behavior. These same information processing mechanisms likely form the cortical storage sites that are bound by medial temporal lobe mechanisms to support explicit recollection of coherent memory episodes. In this light, it is interesting to note that memory for novel associations between multiple stimuli cannot be implicitly retrieved by amnesic patients except under conditions of very extensive training.[29] This is consistent with the notion that conscious recollection and associative binding are dependent on the medial temporal lobe, but unbound cortical memories can still have an unconscious influence on behavior.

PREFRONTAL CONTRIBUTIONS TO LONG-TERM MEMORY

Neuropsychological studies of patients with frontal lobe damage have traditionally suggested that prefrontal cortex plays only a subsidiary role in normal memory functioning. This view has been derived from the observation that patients with frontal lesions typically show memory deficits only for certain types of information (e.g., source memory and memory for temporal context). The term *source amnesia* refers to cases in which a person can normally remember some previously learned information yet cannot remember the source of that information (where or when it was learned or who taught it).[30] For example, Janowsky and colleagues[31] taught subjects some new trivia facts (e.g., "The name of the dog on the Cracker Jack box is Bingo"). Patients with frontal lobe lesions were able to answer correctly questions based on

the newly learned information (e.g., "What is the name of the dog on the Cracker Jack box?") as well as control subjects, yet they showed an impaired ability to remember where they learned the information or when they had most recently encountered it. Impaired memory for temporal information has been demonstrated in experiments in which subjects are asked to remember the order in which items appeared on a studied list. Patients with frontal lobe lesions can demonstrate normal recognition memory but impaired temporal memory for the same stimuli.[32]

Other evidence suggests that the prefrontal cortex is more intimately involved with normal memory functioning than merely supporting memory for circumscribed types of information such as temporal or source memory. Explicit memory studies using PET have found that activity in the right prefrontal cortex is consistently associated with the retrieval of information from memory (for review, see Ref. 33). These results suggest that prefrontal mechanisms may play a more central role in memory retrieval than previously believed.

Recent neuropsychological work has sought to better understand the contribution of prefrontal cortex to memory retrieval. Shimamura and colleagues[34,35] have suggested that patients with frontal lobe lesions have difficulty disregarding or inhibiting irrelevant information. Shimamura and coworkers[34] had subjects learn consecutive lists with competing paired associates (e.g., *lion-hunter* in list 1 and *lion-circus* in list 2). Patients with frontal lobe lesions showed impaired memory when asked to recall the list 2 associations (*lion-?*) because of high levels of interference from the pairs in list 1.

Unlike patients with the classic amnesic syndrome, patients with memory problems associated with frontal lobe damage often confabulate.[34] Confabulation can be characterized as "honest lying,"[36] in which patients present inaccurate and sometimes bizarre "memories" of previous events. Other patients with frontal lobe lesions, who do not spontaneously confabulate about their life experiences, exhibit an intriguing form of false memory on recognition tests.[37–39] For example, one patient with a right frontal lesion, B.G., has been tested in a large number of recognition memory experiments in our laboratory.[39] He classifies nonstudied test items as "studied" at a rate that consistently exceeds the false recognition of control subjects. Furthermore, like other frontal patients exhibiting false recognition, he shows an abnormally high degree of confidence in the accuracy of his false memories.

One experiment was particularly informative for understanding the possible basis of B.G.'s false recognition and shedding some light on prefrontal contributions to memory (Ref. 39, experiment 7). B.G. studied a list of pictures that were selected from a limited number of categories (e.g., furniture, tools, and so on). In the recognition test, nonstudied pictures were either members of the studied categories or not members of categories that were tested (e.g., animals). Figure 22-1 shows the percentage of times that subjects called pictures "studied" in each condition. The error bars represent the range of eight control subjects. As seen in Fig. 22-1, B. G. shows a heightened sensitivity to the category membership of the nonstudied pictures. His false recognition rate was near normal when nonstudied pictures were taken from nonstudied categories but was drastically higher when they were taken from studied categories. This suggests that B. G. may be more reliant on a general match between study-list characteristics and test items than are normal subjects. Hence, his right frontal lesion may make him less able to retrieve item-specific information from memory and force him to depend more on general representations of the target episode.[40] This pattern might also be interpreted within Shimamura's[34,35] theory that patients with frontal lobe lesions have difficulty suppressing interfering information—the categorical structure of the list may indiscriminately bring all members of the studied categories to mind, but he may be unable to pick out the pictures that were actually studied.

Other theories of prefrontal contributions to memory emphasize its general involvement in the high-level control of cognition and behavior. Such high-level, or executive, control processes are thought to guide memory functioning just as they

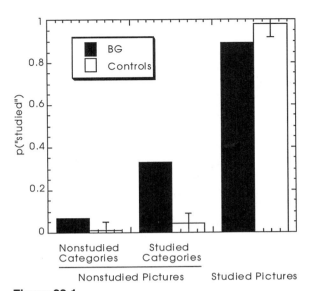

Figure 22-1
Recognition memory performance of patient B. G., who has a right frontal lobe lesion. The dependent measure is the proportion of pictures that subjects classified as "studied" from each condition. Subjects studied a list of pictures from six distinct categories (e.g., furniture, tools, etc.), followed by a recognition test with nonstudied pictures from different categories (left bars), nonstudied pictures from the studied categories (middle bars), and studied pictures (right bars). Error bars represent the range of eight control subjects. The results indicate that B. G. has an abnormal tendency to falsely recognize nonstudied pictures that are categorically consistent with studied pictures.

guide other cognitive processes. Executive processes may strategically guide memory search processes, or they may be used to monitor the information that is retrieved from memory and verify its accuracy.[41,42] Either of these proposals could potentially account for the false recognition pattern exhibited by patient B. G. B.G. may falsely recognize pictures that are related to actually studied pictures because he fails to search for memory attributes that will successfully discriminate between studied and nonstudied pictures. In addition, B. G. may have a deficit in verifying the information that is retrieved from memory in order to avoid false recognition.[38]

WORKING MEMORY

Baddeley[43,44] has hypothesized that an executive control process (the "central executive") forms the centerpiece of a tripartite working memory system that allows for the temporary maintenance and manipulation of information. In addition to the central executive (similar to the frontal executive processes discussed above), two modality-specific slave systems—the "phonological loop" and "visuospatial scratch pad"—are hypothesized to temporally store and manipulate speech-based and visuospatial information respectively. Working memory is typically normal in patients with the amnesic syndrome discussed at the opening of this chapter, so it is considered to be independent from the medial temporal lobe and diencephalic memory system that is required for normal long-term memory. In addition, phonologic and visuospatial working memory appear to be functionally and neuroanatomically distinct, because brain-injured patients with working memory deficits have shown impairments for either speech-based or visuospatial information but never both. In general, these modality-specific subsystems appear to operate in conjunction with the brain mechanisms that are involved in the perception of speech and visuospatial information.

A number of patients have been described who show impaired verbal short-term memory but normal long-term memory (for review, see Ref. 45). The possibility of normal long-term with impaired short-term memory contradicted early information-processing models of memory, which supposed that normal short-term memory processing is a necessary antecedent of normal long-term memory.[1] Such patients may have a phonologic loop impairment, and their lesions are typically near the left supramarginal gyrus (inferior parietal lobe). A recent PET study has also found activation of the supramarginal gyrus in a phonologic working memory task.[46]

Other neuropsychological patients appear to have deficits in visuospatial working memory but preserved verbal working memory (for review, see Ref. 47). The anatomic origins of these impairments have not been well localized beyond the predominance of right-hemispheric damage. Better information about the functional anatomy of visuospatial working memory has been provided by a PET study of visuospatial working memory.[48] Consistent with the existing neuropsychological evidence, activity related to visuospatial working memory was confined to the right-hemispheric regions, including prefrontal, premotor, parietal, and occipital cortices. A prefrontal contribution to spatial working memory has also been suggested by single-unit recording in monkeys performing a task that requires short-term memory of visuospatial stimuli.[49] Within the framework of Baddeley's working memory model, it is unclear whether this prefrontal activity reflects the central executive or the visuospatial scratch pad (see Chap. 25 for further discussion of the choice between central executive and working memory accounts of prefrontal function). Given the well-established role of the parietal and occipital cortices in processing spatial and visual information, it seems clear that activity in these areas uniquely reflects the maintenance of visuospatial information—much like the hypothesized visuospatial scratch pad.

SUMMARY

Cognitive neuroscience research has inspired the view that memory is supported by multiple neural systems. Research on implicit memory and perceptual priming suggests that cortical information-processing modules are capable of some rudimentary forms of learning and memory. Experience shapes the operation of these perceptual mechanisms in a manner that can influence subsequent behavior without conscious recollection. The medial temporal lobe acts to bind information from these diverse cortical modules into a coherent memory episode that can be consciously recollected. Over time, these bound representations become consolidated into a distributed memory trace that is integrated with other information in long-term memory and is no longer dependent upon medial temporal lobe binding. Mechanisms of the prefrontal cortex interact with these core memory mechanisms in a manner that is just beginning to be elucidated. Prefrontal mechanisms may be necessary for establishing effective retrieval strategies, monitoring the quality of retrieved information, and inhibiting irrelevant information. More generally, the prefrontal cortex may act as a central executive that allows for strategic control of long-term memory systems as well as control of modality-specific working memory mechanisms that temporarily hold and manipulate information.

REFERENCES

1. Atkinson RC, Shiffrin RM: Human memory: A proposed system and its control processes, in Spence KW, Spence JT (eds): *The Psychology of Learning and Motivation.* New York: Academic Press, 1968, vol 2, pp 89–105.
2. Kinsbourne M, Winocur G: Response competition and interference effects in paired-associate learning by Korsakoff's amnesics. *Neuropsychologia* 18:541–548, 1980.
3. Warrington EK, Weiskrantz L: Further analysis of prior learning on subsequent retention in amnesic patients. *Neuropsychologia* 16:169–177, 1978.
4. Squire LR: Memory and the hippocampus: A synthesis of findings with rats, monkeys, and humans. *Psychol Rev* 99:195–231, 1992.
5. Craik FIM, Lockhart RS: Levels of processing: A framework for memory research. *J Verbal Learn Verbal Behav* 11:671–684, 1972.
6. Cermak LS, Reale L: Depth of processing and retention of words by alcoholic Korsakoff's patients. *J Exp Psychol Hum Learn Mem* 4:165–174, 1978.
7. Myers A, Meudell P, Neary D: Do amnesics adopt inefficient encoding strategies with faces and random shapes? *Neuropsychologia* 18:527–540, 1980.
8. Cermak LS, Butters N, Moreines J: Some analyses of the verbal encoding deficit of alcoholic Korsakoff patients. *Brain Lang* 1:141–150, 1974.
9. Winocur G, Kinsbourne M, Moscovitch M: The effect of cueing on release from proactive interference in Korsakoff amnesic patients. *Exp Psychol Hum Learn Mem* 7:56–65, 1981.
10. McClelland JL, McNaughton BL, O'Reilly RC: Why there are complimentary learning systems in the hippocampus and neocortex: Insights from the successes and failures of connectionist models of learning and memory. *Psychol Rev* 102:419–457, 1995.
11. Squire LR: Declarative and nondeclarative memory: Multiple brain systems supporting learning and memory, in Schacter DL, Tulving E (ed): *Memory Systems 1994.* Cambridge, MA: MIT Press, 1994, pp 203–231.
12. Mayes AR, Meudell PR, Pickering A: Is organic amnesia caused by a selective deficit in remembering contextual information? *Cortex* 21:167–202, 1985.
13. Cohen NJ, Eichenbaum H: Memory, amnesia, and the hippocampal system. Cambridge, MA: MIT Press, 1993.
14. Rudy JW, Sutherland RJ: The memory-coherence problem, configural associations, and the hippocampal system, in Schacter DL, Tulving E (ed): *Memory Systems 1994.* Cambridge, MA: MIT Press, 1994, pp 119–146.
15. Hirst W, Johnson MK, Phelps EA, Volpe BT: More on recognition and recall in amnesics. *J Exp Psychol Learn Mem Cogn* 14:758–762, 1988.
16. Haist F, Shimamura AP, Squire LR: On the relationship between recall and recognition memory. *J Exp Psychol Learn Mem Cogn* 18:691–702, 1992.
17. Graf P, Squire LR, Mandler G: The information that amnesic patients do not forget. *J Exp Psychol Learn Mem Cog* 10:164–178, 1984.
18. Moscovitch M, Vriezen E, Goshen-Gottstein Y: Implicit tests of memory in patients with focal lesions or degenerative brain disorders, in Spinnler H, Boller F (ed): *Handbook of Neuropsychology.* Amsterdam: Elsevier, 1993, vol 8, pp 133–173.
19. Schacter DL, Chiu CYP, Ochsner KN: Implicit memory a selective review. *Annu Rev Neurosci* 16:159–182, 1993.
20. Roediger HL, McDermott KB: Implicit memory in normal human subjects, in Spinnler H, Boller F (eds): *Handbook of Neuropsychology.* Amsterdam: Elsevier, 1993, vol 8, pp 63–131.
21. Graf P, Shimamura AP, Squire LR: Priming across the modalities and priming across category levels: Extending the domain of preserved function in amnesia. *J Exp Psychol Learn Mem Cogn* 11:386–396, 1985.
22. Posner MI, Carr TH: Lexical access and the brain: Anatomical constraints on cognitive models of word recognition. *Am J Psychol* 105:1–26, 1992.
23. Schacter DL: Priming and multiple memory systems: Perceptual mechanisms of implicit memory, in Schacter DL, Tulving E (eds): *Memory Systems 1994.* Cambridge, MA: MIT Press, 1994, pp 233–268.

24. Buckner RL, Peterson SE, Ojeman JG, et al: Functional anatomical studies of explicit and implicit memory retrieval tasks. *J Neurosci* 15:12–29, 1995.

25. Schacter DL, Alpert N, Savage C, et al: Conscious recollection and the human hippocampal formation: Evidence from positron emission tomography. Proceedings of the *National Academy of Sciences*. In press, 1996.

26. Schacter DL, Reiman E, Uecker A, et al: Brain regions associated with the retrieval of structurally coherent information. *Nature* 376:587–590, 1995.

27. Gabrieli JDE, Fleischman DA, Keane MM, et al: Double dissociation between memory systems underlying explicit and implicit memory in the human brain. *Psychol Sci* 6:76–82, 1995.

28. Willingham DB: Systems of motor skill, in Squire LR, Butters N (eds): *Neuropsychology of Memory.* New York: Guilford Press, 1992, pp 166–178.

29. Bowers J, Schacter DL: Priming of novel information in amnesic patients: Issues and data, in Graf P, Masson M (eds): *Implicit Memory.* Hillsdale, NJ: Erlbaum, 1993, pp 303–326.

30. Schacter DL, Harbluk JL, McLachlan DR: Retrieval without recollection: An experimental analysis of source amnesia. *Verbal Learn Verbal Behav* 23:593–611, 1984.

31. Janowsky JS, Shimamura AP, Squire LR: Source memory impairments in patients with frontal damage. *Neuropsychologia* 27:1043–1056, 1989.

32. Milner B, Corsi P, Leonard G: Frontal-lobe contribution to recency judgments. *Neuropsychologia* 29:601–618, 1991.

33. Buckner RL, Tulving E: Neuroimaging studies of memory: Theory and recent PET results, in Boller F, Grafman J (eds): *Handbook of Neuropsychology.* Amsterdam: Elsevier, 1995, vol 10, pp 439–466.

34. Shimamura AP, Jurica PJ, Mangels JA, et al: Susceptibility to memory interference effects following frontal damage: Findings from tests of paired-associate learning. *J Cog Neurosci* 7:144–152, 1995.

35. Shimamura AP: Memory and frontal lobe function, in Gazzaniga MS (ed): *The Cognitive Neurosciences.* Cambridge: MIT Press, 1995, pp 803–813.

36. Moscovitch M: Confabulation, in Schacter DL, Coyle JT, Fischbach GD, et al (eds): *Memory Distortion.* Cambridge, MA: Harvard University Press, 1995, pp 226–251.

37. Delbecq-Derouesné J, Beauvois MF, Shallice T: Preserved recall versus impaired recognition. *Brain* 113:1045–1074, 1990.

38. Parkin AJ, Bindschaedler C, Harsent L, Metzler C: Verification impairment in the generation of memory following ruptured aneurysm of the anterior communicating artery. *Brain Cog.* In press.

39. Schacter DL, Curran T, Galluccio L, et al: False recognition and the right frontal lobe: A case study. *Neuropsychologia.* In press, 1996.

40. Norman KA, Schacter DL: Implicit memory, explicit memory, and false recognition: A cognitive neuroscience perspective, in Reder L (ed): *Implicit Memory and Metacognition.* In press.

41. Moscovitch M: Memory and working with memory: Evaluation of a component process model and comparisons with other models, in Schacter DL, Tulving E (eds): *Memory Systems 1994.* Cambridge, MA: MIT Press, 1994, pp 269–310.

42. Shallice T: *From Neuropsychology to Mental Structure.* Cambridge, England: Cambridge University Press, 1988.

43. Baddeley A: *Working Memory.* Oxford, England: Claredon Press, 1986.

44. Baddeley A: Working memory: The interface between memory and cognition, in Schacter DL, Tulving E (ed): *Memory Systems 1994.* Cambridge, MA: MIT Press, 1994, pp 351–367.

45. Vallar G, Shallice T: *Neuropsychological Impairments of Short-Term Memory.* Cambridge, England: Cambridge University Press, 1990.

46. Paulesu E, Frith CD, Frackowiak RSJ: The neural correlates of the verbal component of working memory. *Nature* 362:342–345, 1993.

47. Della Sala S, Logie RH: When working memory does not work: The role of working memory in neuropsychology, in Boller F, Grafman J (eds): *Handbook of Neuropsychology.* Amsterdam: Elsevier, 1993, vol 8, pp 1–62.

48. Jonides J, Smith EE, Koeppe RA, et al: Spatial working memory in humans as revealed by PET. *Nature* 363:623–625, 1993.

49. Goldman-Rakic PS: Cellular and circuit basis of working memory in prefrontal cortex of nonhuman primates, in Uylings HBM, Van Eden CG, De Bruin JPC, et al (eds): *Progress in Brain Research.* Amsterdam: Elsevier, 1990, vol 85, pp 325–336.

Chapter 23

SEMANTIC MEMORY IMPAIRMENTS

Martha J. Farah
Murray Grossman

The term *semantic memory* refers to our general knowledge of the objects, people, and events of the world.[1] The facts that Paris is the capital of France, birds have feathers, and a desk is a piece of furniture are examples of semantic memory. More particular knowledge, tied to an individual's personal experience, is considered *episodic memory* rather than semantic memory. Examples of the latter include the facts that you bought this book at a certain store or ate a certain food for breakfast this morning. Neurologic disease and damage can affect semantic memory disproportionately. In this chapter the different forms of semantic memory impairment are reviewed, with attention to their etiologies, major behavioral features, and implications for the neural substrates and functional organization of semantic memory in the normal brain.

GENERALIZED IMPAIRMENT OF SEMANTIC MEMORY

Warrington[2] first documented a pattern of preserved and impaired performance indicative of semantic memory impairment in a series of three patients suffering from progressive degenerative brain disease. Her subjects were relatively preserved on most measures of language and cognitive function but did poorly on tasks dependent on semantic memory, including confrontation naming, word-picture matching, and a verification task in which subjects were shown pictures or words and asked questions such as "Is it a bird?" or "Is it heavy?" In subsequent years a number of similar cases were reported, and the term *semantic dementia* was coined in the context of one such report.[3] Hodges and coworkers[4] presented a wide-ranging study of five new cases of semantic dementia, reviewed the literature, and drew a number of useful generalizations concerning the condition. A summary of their conclusions is presented here.

Semantic dementia may present initially as a language disorder whose most prominent feature is vocabulary loss, both expressive and receptive. Naming is minimally aided by phonemic cues, and naming errors tend to share a semantic relation with the correct name (e.g., *violin* for *accordion*, or *animal* for *fox*). In production, category fluency is severely impaired, and word definitions are impoverished or wrong. Such patients have sometimes been described as having a fluent form of primary progressive aphasia (see Chaps. 14 and 15), but additional language testing and nonverbal semantic memory testing suggest that the underlying impairment is one of semantic memory knowledge rather than language. Syntax and phonology tend to be preserved, whereas entirely pictorial tasks that depend on knowledge of the depicted objects, such as sorting together semantically related objects or distinguishing real from imaginary objects, are failed. Although the formal assessment of episodic memory is difficult because of the loss of knowledge of word and picture meanings, Hodges and coworkers[4] observe that at least some patients show significant preservation of autobiographical memories and practical day-to-day memory. The neuropathologic changes in semantic dementia are focused in the temporal lobes, often affecting the left more than the right. A small number of brains have come to autopsy with Pick's disease.

Another degenerative condition affecting semantic memory is Alzheimer disease[5–10] (AD), although semantic memory is just one of many aspects of cognition impaired in AD, and initially some cases may present with only episodic memory impairment. To the extent that semantic memory is impaired in AD, pathologic changes in temporal cortex are responsible.

In sum, semantic memory is at least partially dissociable from other forms of memory, language, and cognition, generally as a result of degenerative diseases. It appears to depend on temporal cortex, with some degree lateralization to the left suggested.

SELECTIVE IMPAIRMENTS OF SEMANTIC MEMORY

In addition to the generalized impairments of semantic memory described above, particular aspects of semantic memory can be disproportionately impaired. These disorders are potentially informative about the internal organization of semantic memory in the brain, although their proper interpretation and even their existence have been issues of controversy.

Category-Specific Semantic Memory Impairment

In some cases it appears that knowledge from certain semantic categories is disproportionately impaired, suggesting that the neural bases of semantic memory are subdivided by semantic category. Category-specific semantic memory impairments are sometimes confused with category-specific impairments in name retrieval and visual recognition. The "fruit and vegetable" impairment observed in two cases[11,12] affects naming only; the face-specificity of prosopagnosia (see Chap. 7) af-

fects visual recognition only. In contrast, category-specific semantic memory impairments are manifest in all tasks that require knowledge of the object, whether they involve vision, language, or other modalities of stimulus and response. The most common category-specific semantic memory impairment affects knowledge of living things.

The first report of impaired knowledge of living things was made by Warrington and Shallice,[13] who described three patients who had survived herpes encephalitis. Although the patients were impaired across the board at tasks such as picture naming and defining words, they were dramatically worse when the pictures or words represented animals and plants than when they represented artifacts. In subsequent years numerous other reports appeared of similar cases, generally suffering damage to temporal cortex from herpes encephalitis, closed head injury or, less frequently, cerebrovascular or degenerative disease. Category-specific disorders of semantic memory are distinct from the disorders described in the previous section, despite the implication of temporal brain regions in both, as neither semantic dementia[4] nor Alzheimer disease[14] routinely affect knowledge of living things more than nonliving.

The idea that certain brain regions are specialized for representing knowledge about living things has naturally aroused some skepticism and prompted a search for alternative explanations of apparently impaired knowledge of living things. The simplest alternative explanation is that the impairment is an artifact of the greater difficulty of retrieving knowledge about living things. It has been suggested that when difficulty is equated across living and nonliving test items, the selectivity of the semantic memory impairment disappears.[15,16] However, the selectivity has also been shown to be reliable in two cases when multiple measures of difficulty are accounted for,[17] and the null results in other controlled studies are likely due to insufficient statistical power, as our reliable findings disappeared when we reduced our data set to the size of the other studies' data sets.[18]

Cases of impaired knowledge of nonliving things with relatively spared knowledge of living things are rarer but have also been described.[19–23] The lesions in these cases are confined to the left hemisphere. A precise intrahemispheric localization is not possible, as the lesions are typically large and relatively few cases have been reported, although the left temporal region again seems involved.[23] These patients provide the other half of a double dissociation with impaired knowledge of living things, thus adding further support to the hypothesis that category-specific semantic memory impairments are not simply due to the differential difficulty of particular categories.

Building on the hypothesis of Allport,[24] that semantic memory is subdivided into different sensorimotor modalities (e.g., visual knowledge, tactile knowledge, and motor knowledge; see Fig. 23-1 for an illustration of this idea), Warrington and Shallice[13] proposed a different kind of alternative explanation for category-specific knowledge deficits. They suggested that living and nonliving things may differ from one another in their reliance on knowledge from different sensorimotor modalities, with living things being known predominantly by their visual and other sensory attributes. Impaired knowledge of living things could result from an impairment of visual knowledge. Similarly, nonliving things might be known predominantly by their function, an abstract form of motoric representation, and impaired knowledge of nonliving things could result from an impairment of functional knowledge. This interpretation has the advantage of parsimony, in that it invokes a type of organization already known to exist in the brain—modality-specific organization—rather than invoking an organization based on semantic categories such as aliveness. A computer simulation of semantic memory and its impairments has shown that a modality-specific organization can account for category-specific impairments, even the finding that functional knowledge of living things is impaired after visual semantic damage.[25] The latter finding is explained by the need for a certain "critical mass" of associated knowledge to help activate collaterally any one part of a distributed representation; if most of the representation of living things is visual and visual

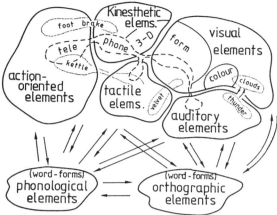

Figure 23-1

A modality-specific organization for semantic memory. Rather than hypothesize a store of knowledge in the brain separate from the various sensorimotor modalities used in perception and action, semantic memory is hypothesized to consist of representations in sensorimotor systems themselves. (From Allport,[24] with permission.)

knowledge is damaged, then the remaining functional knowledge cannot be activated.

Modality-Specific Semantic Memory Impairment

There is a second way in which the phrase *modality-specific semantic memory* has been used in neuropsychology, and that is for components of semantic memory that are accessed *through* a particular input or output modality. According to this usage, visual semantics refers not to semantic knowledge of the visual appearance of objects but to the semantic knowledge of appearance, function, and so on that is accessed when an object is seen. Whether semantic memory has a modality-specific organization in this sense is not clear, although such an organization has been hypothesized for purposes of explaining "optic aphasia."

Optic aphasia is a puzzling disorder, consisting of an impairment in naming visually presented stimuli in the face of relatively preserved naming of nonvisual stimuli and relatively preserved nonverbal demonstrations of visual recognition. It seems reasonable to assume that visual confrontation naming requires three major stages of processing: vision, semantics, and lexical retrieval. That is, it requires seeing the object clearly enough to access semantic knowledge of it, and using that semantic knowledge of what the object is to retrieve its name. Paradoxically, the preserved nonvisual naming and nonverbal recognition performance of optic aphasics seem to exonerate all three stages.

A variety of attempts have been made to explain how an anomia could exist for visual stimuli only, although none has been thoroughly tested or gained wide support (see Ref. 26 for a review). One of these accounts invokes a modality-specific semantic memory system in which visual semantics (i.e., the semantic knowledge accessed by visual inputs) has been disconnected from verbal semantics (i.e., the semantic knowledge necessary to access a verbal output).[27,28] This hypothesis was formulated to explain the major features of optic aphasia and is successful in so doing, although converging evidence from other sources is now desirable.

REFERENCES

1. Tulving E: Episodic and semantic memory, in Tulving E, Donaldson W (eds): *Organization of Memory.* New York: Academic Press, 1972.
2. Warrington EK: The selective impairment of semantic memory. *Q J Exp Psychol* 27:635–657, 1975.
3. Snowden JS, Goulding PJ, Neary D: Semantic dementia: A form of circumscribed cerebral atrophy. *Behav Neurol* 2:167–182, 1989.
4. Hodges JR, Patterson K, Oxbury S, Funnell E: Semantic dementia. *Brain* 115:1783–1806, 1992.
5. Martin A, Fedio P: Word production and comprehension in Alzheimer's disease: The breakdown of semantic knowledge. *Brain Lang* 19:124–141, 1983.
6. Bayles KA, Tomoeda CK, Trosset MW: Naming and categorical knowledge in Alzheimer's disease: The process of semantic memory deterioration. *Brain Lang* 39:498–510, 1990.
7. Chertkow H, Bub D: Semantic memory loss in dementia of Alzheimer's type: What do various measures measure? *Brain* 113:397–417, 1990.
8. Hodges JR, Salmon DP, Butters N: Semantic memory impairment in Alzheimer's disease: Failure of access of degraded knowledge? *Neuropsychologia* 30:301–314, 1992.
9. Nebes RD: Cognitive dysfunction in Alzheimer's disease, in Craik FIM, Salthouse TA (eds): *The Handbook of Aging and Cognition.* Hillsdale, NJ: Erlbaum, 1992.
10. Grossman M, Mickanin J: Picture comprehension and probable Alzheimer's disease. *Brain Cogn* 26:43–64, 1994.
11. Hart J, Berndt RS, Caramazza A: Category-specific naming deficit following cerebral infarction. *Nature* 316:439–440, 1985.
12. Farah MJ, Wallace MA: Semantically bounded anomia: Implications for the neural implementation of naming. *Neuropsychologia* 30:609–621, 1992.
13. Warrington EK, Shallice T: Category specific semantic impairments. *Brain* 107:829–854, 1984.
14. Tippett LJ, Grossman M, Farah MJ: The semantic memory deficit of Alzheimer's disease: Category-specific? *Cortex* 31, 1995.
15. Funnell E, Sheridan J: Categories of knowledge? Unfamiliar aspects of living and non-living things. *Cogn Neuropsychol* 9:135–154, 1992.
16. Stewart F, Parkin AJ, Hunkin NM: Naming impairments following recovery from herpes simplex encephalitis: Category specific? *Q J Exp Psychol* 44A:261–284, 1992.
17. Farah MJ, McMullen PA, Meyer MM: Can recognition of living things be selectively impaired? *Neuropsychologia* 29:185–193, 1991.
18. Farah MJ, Meyer MM, McMullen PA: The living/nonliving dissociation is not an artifact: Giving an a priori implausible hypothesis a strong test. *Cogn Neuropsychol* 13:137–154, 1996.
19. Warrington EK, McCarthy R: Category specific access dysphasia. *Brain* 106:859–878, 1983.
20. Warrington EK, McCarthy R: Categories of knowledge: Further fractionations and an attempted explanation. *Brain* 110:1273–1296, 1987.
21. Hillis A, Caramazza C: Category-specific naming and comprehension impairment: A double dissociation. *Brain* 114:2081–2094, 1991.
22. Sacchett C, Humphreys GW: Calling a squirrel a squirrel but a canoe a wigwam: A category-specific deficit for artifactual objects and body parts. *Cogn Neuropsychol* 9:73–86, 1992.

23. Tippett LJ, Glosser G, Farah MJ: A category-specific naming deficit after temporal lobectomy. *Neuropsychologia.* 34:139–146, 1996.

24. Allport DA: Distributed memory, modular subsystems and dysphasia, in Newman S, Epstein R (eds): *Current Perspectives in Dysphasia.* Edinburgh: Churchill Livingstone, 1985.

25. Farah MJ, McClelland JL: A computational model of semantic memory impairment: Modality-specificity and emergent category-specificity. *J Exp Psychol Gen* 120:339–357, 1991.

26. Farah MJ: *Visual Agnosia: Disorders of Object Recognition and What They Tell Us about Normal Vision.* Cambridge, MA: MIT Press/Bradford Books, 1990.

27. Beauvois MF: Optic aphasia: A process of interaction between vision and language. *Philos Trans R Soc Lond* B298:35–47, 1982.

28. Shallice T: Impairments of semantic processing: Multiple dissociations, in Coltheart M, Sartori G, Job R (eds): *The Cognitive Neuropsychology of Language.* London: Erlbaum, 1987.

Part V
OTHER HIGHER FUNCTIONS

Chapter 24

FRONTAL LOBES I: CLINICAL AND ANATOMIC ISSUES

D. Frank Benson
Bruce L. Miller

FRONTAL LOBES: CLINICAL AND ANATOMIC ASPECTS

For over a century, the frontal lobes have been an enigma to brain scientists. Significant progress has been made in the past several decades, but many anatomic and functional aspects remain mysterious. The frontal lobes, particularly in humans, are massive in relation to other, better understood cortical areas, and it was long considered that the frontal lobes were the seat of human intelligence. This proved untrue, at least as intelligence is defined by psychometric testing. The functions of the frontal lobes in human behavior remain a mystery.

In 1973 the great Russian psychologist A. R. Luria[1] proposed a simple outline of brain functions. He suggested that subcortical structures, particularly the midbrain and diencephalon, functioned to produce *tonic regularity*. He further stated that the posterior cortex—the premotor and motor aspects of the frontal lobe and all cortex posterior to these areas—carried out primary *sensorimotor functions,* and that the comparatively massive prefrontal cortex functioned to *regulate* mental activities. This tripartite description of mental functions was further elaborated by Albert,[2] who suggested the terms *fundamental, instrumental,* and *superordinate* to define the activities of the brainstem, posterior cortex, and prefrontal cortex respectively.

Classic neuroanatomy divides the cortical surface of the frontal lobes into three major segments: (1) *motor*—the narrow strip of cortical tissue located just anterior to the rolandic fissure; (2) *premotor*—the larger area of frontal tissue anterior to the motor strip that acts as a motor association cortex (Brodmann areas 6 and 8); and (3) *prefrontal*—the vast amount of frontal cortex anterior to the premotor cortex, including a significant amount of the anterior/lateral cortex, most of the medial frontal cortex, and the entire orbital frontal cortex. In the classification suggested by Luria,[1] the motor and premotor areas of the frontal lobes would be included in the sensorimotor division and the prefrontal cortex would carry out the regulatory activities. The motor functions of the frontal lobes are adequately reviewed in many neuroanatomy texts. The prefrontal regulatory functions are important for psychology and are the topic of this chapter.

Of considerable significance in discussion of the neural basis of prefrontal psychological functions are the connections of frontal cortex with other brain areas. The prefrontal cortex receives direct or indirect input from most ipsilateral cortical areas and from the opposite hemisphere via callosal connections. In addition, prefrontal cortex receives strong input from a number of significant subcortical sources: (1) the limbic system, (2) the reticular system, (3) the hypothalamus, and (4) neurotransmitter systems. Prefrontal cortex is the only cortical area that receives strong sensorimotor, limbic, and reticular input. Additional input of hypothalamic and autonomic data and the effects of many neurotransmitters place prefrontal cortex in a strong position to monitor both intrinsic and extrinsic stimuli and to exert regulatory control of brain functions.

PREFRONTAL FUNCTIONS

Behavioral functions performed by the prefrontal cortex have proved difficult to delineate. To date, almost all information has been derived from behavioral aberrations seen following frontal brain damage. In the past several decades some psychological tests aimed directly at the assessment of prefrontal function have been devised (see Chapter 25), and, more recently, psychological testing has been combined with functional brain imaging techniques to provide valuable insights. In general, however, psychological tests of prefrontal function demand inferences from data obtained through primary sensorimotor functions, which themselves may be impaired.[3]

A second problem in studying prefrontal function is a lack of clearly delineated neuropathology. Frontal brain tumors tend to become massive, affecting both posterior ipsilateral tissues and tissues in the opposite frontal lobe, before diagnosis can be made. The only vascular lesion confined to prefrontal cortex involves the anterior cerebral artery, a vessel with considerable collaterals; consistent vascular lesions are rare. Prefrontal leukotomies provided clean, relatively precise prefrontal lesions but were performed only in individuals with significant behavioral abnormality; postsurgical testing was often frustrated by the inherent mental disorder.

Perhaps because of these problems, the underlying impairment in frontally damaged patients has yet to be satisfactorily established. A review of current attempts at characterizing prefrontal function and its impairment is presented in the following chapter. Here we note some of the more common effects of prefrontal damage in terms of their clinical manifestations.

Personality changes following frontal lobe lesions are of two main types. One type could be called pseudoretarded or pseudodepressed, and is characterized by apathy, lethargy, little spontane-ity of behavior, unconcern, reduced sexual interest, little overt emotion, and reduced ability to plan ahead. Although such patients appear retarded, their IQs may be normal or near normal. The other type could be called pseudopsychopathic and is characterized by inappropriate social behavior, lack of concern for others, increased motor activity, sexual disinhibition, and *Witzelsucht,* an inappropriately puerile, jocular attitude. There is some suggestion of differential localization for these two types of personality change, the former being associated with dorsolateral lesions and the latter with orbitofrontal lesions. However, because of the nonfocal effects of many frontal lesions, mentioned above, patients will frequently manifest an almost paradoxical mixture of both personality types.

The cognitive impairments of patients with prefrontal damage are apparent in a variety of tasks, some of which are reviewed in the following chapter. The domains affected include complex motor behavior (see also Chap. 27), planning and sequencing, attention, memory, and language (see discussions of Broca's aphasia and transcortical motor aphasia in Chap. 14). Often patients can perform well on standard tests of intelligence but fail miserably in less constrained real-life situations calling for planning and flexibility.

CONDITIONS THAT INFLUENCE FRONTAL LOBE FUNCTION

Vascular

Ischemic Infarction   The vascular territory for the frontal lobes comes from the anterior cerebral artery (ACA) and middle cerebral arteries (MCA), both of which are branches of the internal carotid artery.[4] The anterior and medial portions of the frontal lobes are supplied by the ACA, while the anterior branch of the MCA supplies most of the lateral dorsal frontal cortex. With ACA infarctions (see Fig. 24-1), the eyes tend to deviate toward the injured hemisphere. This conjugate eye deviation occurs following injury to the frontal eye fields in Brodmann area 8 and is ac-

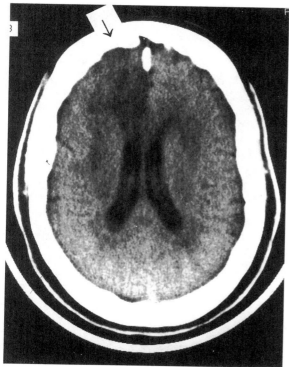

Figure 24-1
Computed tomography scan showing findings of a large anterior cerebral artery infarction involving the medial frontal cortex.

companied by frontal neglect. Conjugate deviation following from injury to area 8 tends to disappear after a few days, while the frontal neglect often persists. Because the medial portions of the motor strip of the frontal cortex contain fibers for the leg, weakness and sensory loss associated with these infarctions is greatest in the leg, with relative sparing of motor and sensory function in the arm and face. Also, involvement of the supplementary motor area leads to a forced grasp of the contralateral hand. Transcortical motor aphasia is the most common aphasia syndrome seen with ACA occlusion of the dominant hemisphere.[5] Following these infarcts, common behavioral abnormalities include profound apathy and loss of executive control. A manic syndrome may follow acute injury, particularly when the infarction involves the

right hemisphere. Conversely, depression, though more common with left frontal stroke, can occur with injury to either side. Rarely, a single ACA supplies both medial frontal lobes; ACA occlusion can produce bifrontal infarction leading to an akinetic mute state.

Strokes of the dominant hemisphere involving the MCA lead to paralysis of the face and arm on the contralateral side with eyes deviated toward the side of infarction (away from the paralysis). When the stroke is restricted to the anterior MCA branch of the dominant hemisphere, Broca's aphasia occurs; in contrast, complete MCA strokes lead to global aphasia. Loss of sequencing ability and disturbed executive control may be persistent problems. Forced grasp is not a feature of MCA stroke. Neglect may occur following either right- or left-sided MCA occlusion, but denial of illness is more common with right-sided lesions.

Other Vascular Lesions   Other types of vascular injury can also produce frontal dysfunction. A common site for aneurysms is the anterior communicating artery; following rupture, ischemia or infarction within the territory of the ACA often occurs. The sagittal sinus lies adjacent to the medial portions of the frontal lobes, and thrombus formation in this sinus can produce variations on anterior artery syndromes, although seizures and alterations in consciousness are more common with sinus thrombosis than simple arterial infarction. This disease is often idiopathic, although hypercoagulable states are known to cause this disorder.[6]

Trauma

The poles of the frontal lobes lie adjacent to frontal bone while the basal (orbital) frontal regions sit upon the skull's cribriform plate. The frontal lobe's intimate association with bone makes this area particularly prone to injury following trauma (see Fig. 24-2). Patients often recover from the motor and sensory deficits that follow a head injury, only to be left with profound behavioral abnormalities such as disinhibition, apathy, and loss of executive control. Behavioral disinhibition

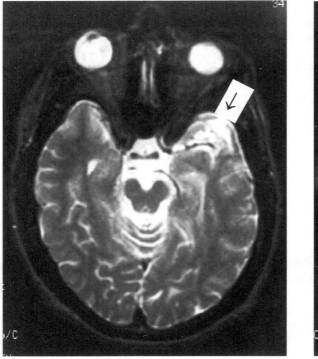

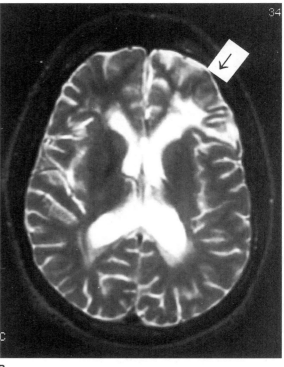

A   B

Figure 24-2
*These T$_2$-weighted MRI scans from the anterior temporal (A) and anterior frontal (B)
lobes demonstrate loss of tissue secondary to trauma. The patient was a sexually and
verbally disinhibited male with profound frontal-systems deficits on neuropsychological
testing.*

associated with head trauma is often also associated with injury of frontal orbitobasal regions; the loss of executive control is a sequela of more widespread frontal damage.[3] Neuropsychological batteries that focus upon executive function can help to identify a frontal injury. When the injury occurs to basofrontal regions, however, neuropsychological test results may be normal, even when there is profound behavioral disinhibition.[7] In these patients, careful questioning and recording of the insights of the family, along with systematic observations by the physician, help delineate the presence and severity of the frontal syndrome.

Documentation of the severity of frontal dysfunction associated with head injury is important,

as therapy for these patients is difficult. A rigidly structured environment can help patients with frontal injury cope with routine daily activities. Unfortunately, current therapies and management of therapies for apathy and loss of executive control have only limited efficacy. Antidepressant medications may help to relieve the depressions that follow frontal injury; tegretol and propranolol have limited efficacy for disinhibition, violence, and irritability.

Tumors

Tumors either intrinsic or extrinsic to the frontal lobes can produce frontal lobe symptomatology.

The most common extrinsic tumors are meningiomas, which typically compress the frontal lobes in either the parasagittal (see Fig. 24-3) or the cribriform plate regions.[8] Parasagittal meningiomas affect the medial aspects of the frontal lobes, so that bilateral leg weakness is a common finding. Once these tumors become sufficiently large, apathy, loss of executive control, or disinhibition can occur. Loss of the sense of smell is a common finding because of the close association of midline frontal tumors to the olfactory nerves. Cribriform plate meningiomas affect the basofrontal lobes, and behavioral disinhibition is common.

Primary brain tumors (gliomas, oligodendrogliomas, etc.) and metastases that involve the frontal lobes also alter frontal function. In current practice, these lesions are easily detected with computed tomography (CT) or magnetic resonance imaging (MRI) and effective surgical and medical therapies can be administered. However, diagnosis is often preceded by vague behavioral alterations that, in retrospect, were caused by frontal dysfunction.

Figure 24-3

This T$_1$-weighted gadolinium-enhanced MRI scan demonstrates a large parasagittal frontal meningioma.

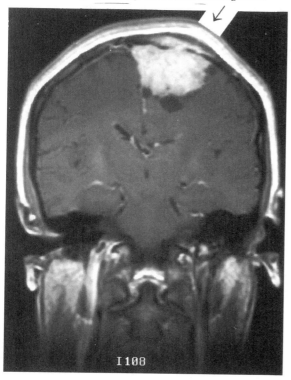

I108

Hydrocephalus

Abnormal absorption of cerebrospinal fluid (CSF) via the arachnoid granulation can cause "normal-pressure hydrocephalus" (NPH). The classic triad of hydrocephalus includes memory disturbance, urinary incontinence, and gait apraxia. Other common findings are profound apathy and even akinetic states. Magnetic resonance imaging typically shows the panventricular dilatation (see Fig. 24-4) as well as extravasated periventricular fluid. Treatment of obstructive hydrocephalus (including NPH) is by shunting CSF from the ventricles to a distant area for absorption. Unfortunately, this therapy is effective in only a minority of cases, and complications of shunt therapy can be troublesome.

Infections

Many infectious processes can involve frontal cerebral tissues. Bacterial, tuberculous, fungal, and toxoplasmal abscesses can selectively penetrate the frontal regions. Now rare, tertiary syphilis, or "general paresis of the insane" (GPI), showed a predilection to involve the frontal regions.[10] One of the clinical syndromes associated with GPI was characterized by disinhibition and grandiose manic syndromes. Another was characterized by disinterest and slowed cognitive processing. An apathetic frontal lobe syndrome is the most characteristic clinical feature of dementia due to human immunodeficiency virus (HIV). This is probably based on involvement of both subcortical and frontal structures.[11] Often, HIV-dementia responds at least transiently to antiviral therapy.

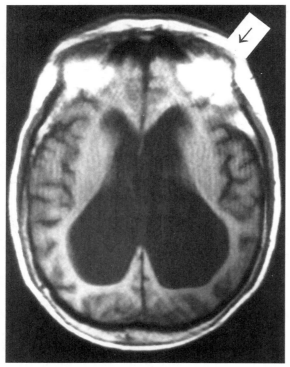

Figure 24-4
A T₁-weighted MRI scan demonstrating hydrocephalus with enlarged frontal and posterior ventricles. There is no periventricular extravasation of fluid.

Degenerative Dementias

Frontotemporal Dementia Although all degenerative brain disorders probably produce frontal dysfunction eventually, several entities show early and selective involvement of the frontal lobes. The frontotemporal dementias (FTDs) are a group of disorders that cause focal degeneration of prefrontal cortex. These are probably the second most common presenile degenerative dementias, ranking only behind Alzheimer disease. The disorders (there are probably several causes) have a mean age of onset in the sixth decade and are slowly progressive; the time from onset to death is typically 7 to 10 years.[12–14] Approximately 50 percent of subjects with FTD have a family history suggesting that FTD is transmitted as an autoso-

mal dominant trait. In some subjects, amyotrophic lateral sclerosis (ALS) occurs, either preceding or following signs of frontal dysfunction. A linkage with chromosome 17 has been demonstrated.[15] Misdiagnosis is common, but the clinical and imaging features of FTD clearly distinguish FTD from other degenerative dementias, and diagnostic accuracy should be over 90 percent. Initially some mixture of social withdrawal and behavioral disinhibition occurs; as the disease progresses, apathy becomes the dominant finding. Higher cortical deficits include decreased speech output and deficits in judgment, insight, and executive control functions. Antisocial conduct occurs in nearly half of all FTD subjects. Excessive eating and compulsions are common. In the later stages, parkinsonian features and eye-movement abnormalities occur, reflecting degeneration in the midbrain. Eventually profound apathy supervenes and most subjects enter a mute, akinetic state. Visuospatial skills and calculation remain normal or near normal, reflecting the relative sparing of parietal cortex with FTD. Focal presentations of FTD may occur; patients with predominantly left-sided degeneration show progressive aphasia or apraxia, while those with right-sided degeneration suffer profound alterations of social skills. In most FTD patients, MRI shows frontal and anterior temporal atrophy, but generalized atrophy or even normal MRIs may be seen. Functional studies (e.g., single photon emission tomography, or SPECT, and positron emission tomography, or PET) invariably show focal frontal or temporal deficits (see Fig. 24-5).

Histologic studies reveal neuronal loss and gliosis, greatest in the frontal and anterior temporal regions. In about 20 percent of FTD patients, cellular inclusions, so-called Pick bodies, are found. Midbrain cell loss is common, with more variable findings of gliosis in the thalamus and basal ganglia. Severe pre- and postsynaptic deficits in brain serotonin have been reported and may be correlated with the clinical findings of weight gain and compulsions.

Other Degenerative Dementias Most of the degenerative dementias eventually involve the

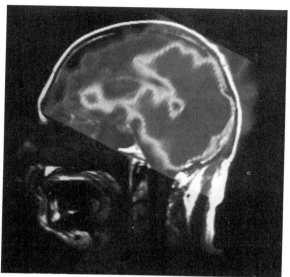

Figure 24-5
This is a xenon-133–corrected-HMPAO SPECT coregistered upon a T_2-weighted MRI scan from a patient with frontotemporal dementia. There is profound frontal hypoperfusion.

frontal lobes, even though primary pathology is elsewhere. A few disorders appear to have a selective influence upon frontal lobe function.

Progressive Supranuclear Palsy   In this degenerative disorder the primary pathology is located in the midbrain. Extensive frontal connections with midbrain may explain the combination of midbrain and frontal lobe findings. Primary frontal degeneration has not, however, been ruled out. The classical clinical findings in progressive supranuclear palsy (PSP) include frequent falls, axial rigidity, pseudobulbar palsy, dementia, and a loss of vertical gaze. On SPECT, frontal hypoperfusion is seen.[16]

Metachromatic Leukodystrophy   This degenerative disorder selectively injures white matter underlying the frontal cortex. A progressive frontal dementia occurs; diagnosis is made by demonstration of an enzymatic abnormality in arylsul-

fatase. Although most cases occur in childhood and early adolescence, late-life onset can occur.[17]

Alcohol   Many toxins can affect cerebral cortex, but the symptom picture most often suggests diffuse (toxic) rather than focal abnormalities. The concept of alcohol-induced dementia remains somewhat controversial; in some individuals, chronic alcohol abuse appears to be associated with selective dysfunction of the frontal lobes (apathy and cognitive slowing). In some instances, the frontal symptoms disappear or are considerably improved following abstinence from alcohol; in other cases, permanent dementia seems to develop.[18] The pathology of this dementia is poorly understood, but the presence of frontal symptoms is consistent.

REFERENCES

1. Luria AR: *The Working Brain: An Introduction to Neuropsychology* (Haig B, trans). New York, Basic Books, 1973.
2. Albert ML: Subcortical dementia, in Katzman R, Terry RD, Bick KI (eds): *Alzheimer's Disease, Senile Dementia and Related Disorders.* New York, Raven Press, 1978, pp 173–180.
3. Stuss DT, Benson DF: *The Frontal Lobes.* New York, Raven Press, 1986.
4. Gauthier JC, Mohr JP: Intracranial internal carotid artery disease, in Barnett HJM, Mohr JP, Stein BM, Yatsu FM (eds): *Stroke.* New York, Churchill Livingstone, 1986, pp 337–350.
5. Benson DF: *Aphasia, Alexia, and Agraphia.* New York, Churchill Livingstone, 1979.
6. Tsai FY, Higashida RT, Matovich V, Alrieri K: Acute thrombosis of the intracranial dural sinus: Direct thrombolytic treatment. *Am J Neuroradiol* 13:1137–1141, 1992.
7. Damasio AR: The frontal lobes, in Heilman KM, Valenstein E (eds): *Clinical Neuropsychology.* New York, Oxford University Press, 1979, pp 360–412.
8. Adams RD, Victor M: *Principles of Neurology,* 5th ed. New York, McGraw-Hill, 1993.
9. Hakim S: Biomechanics of hydrocephalus, in Harbert JC (ed): *Cisternography and Hydrocephalus.* Springfield, IL, Charles C Thomas, 1972, pp 22–25.

10. Cummings JL, Benson DF: *Dementia: A Clinical Approach.* Boston, Butterworth-Heinemann, 1992.

11. Price RW, Brew B, Sidtis J, et al: The brain in AIDS: Central nervous system HIV-1 infection and AIDS dementia complex. *Science* 239:286–292, 1988.

12. Brun A: Frontal lobe degeneration of non-Alzheimer type: I. Neuropathology. *Arch Gerontol Geriatr* 6:193–208, 1987.

13. Neary D, Snowden JS, Northen B, Goulding PJ: Dementia of frontal lobe type. *J Neurol Neurosurg Psychiatry* 51:353–361, 1988.

14. Miller BL, Cummings JL, Villanueva-Meyer J, et al: Frontal lobe degeneration: Clinical, neuropsychological and SPECT characteristics. *Neurology* 41:1374–1382, 1991.

15. Wilhelmsen K, Lynch T, Pavlou E, et al: Localization of disinhibition-dementia-parkinsonism-amyotrophy complex to 17q21-22. *Am J Hum Genet* 55:1150–1165, 1994.

16. Johnson KA, Sperling RA, Holman BL, et al: Cerebral perfusion in progressive supranuclear palsy. *J Nucl Med* 33:704–709, 1992.

17. Austin J, Armstrong D, Fouch S, et al: Metachromatic leukodystrophy (MLD). *Arch Neurol* 18:225–240, 1968.

18. Lishman WA: Cerebral disorder in alcoholism: Syndromes of impairment. *Brain* 104:1–20, 1981.

Chapter 25

FRONTAL LOBES II: COGNITIVE ISSUES

Daniel Y. Kimberg
Mark D'Esposito
Martha J. Farah

As the previous chapter makes clear, prefrontal cortex plays a crucial role in normal intelligent behavior. However, a more precise characterization of the functions of prefrontal cortex has been elusive. In this chapter we provide a brief review of some of the cognitive impairments that often follow prefrontal damage and survey current theoretical claims about the role of the frontal lobes in cognition.

COGNITIVE IMPAIRMENTS FOLLOWING PREFRONTAL DAMAGE

A wide range of tasks have been found to be sensitive to prefrontal damage. Some of the best known are described here for the purpose of illustrating the range and variety of abilities that depend on prefrontal cortex.

Wisconsin Card Sorting Test

In the Wisconsin Card Sorting Test (WCST),[1] patients are given a series of cards and asked to sort them by placing each into one of four piles. The cards vary according to three attributes: the number of objects drawn on the card, the shape of the objects, and their color. The piles are to be started beneath four reference cards, which also vary along these same dimensions, so that each possible value of each attribute will be represented in exactly one pile. The subject is given a deck of cards and asked to place each, in sequence, into one of the four piles. The only feedback given to the subject is the word *right* or *wrong* after each card. Initially, color is the correct sorting category, and the subject is given positive feedback only if the card is placed in the pile of the same color. For example, if the card is red, the subject must place the card next to the reference card that has red objects. However, whenever the subject sorts 10 consecutive cards correctly, the category changes. Only sorts according to the new category will result in positive feedback. The category first changes to shape, then to number, and then repeats in the same order, starting from color. The subject must learn to change sorting categories according to feedback. The test ends after 128 cards or after 6 categories are achieved. Scoring of the test includes two measures: the number of perseverative errors, or failures to change sorting strategy after negative feedback, and the number of categories achieved.

Milner[2,3] tested a variety of neurosurgical patients on the WCST and found that as compared to patients with lesions elsewhere in the brain, patients with damage to the dorsolateral prefrontal cortex made an unusually high number of errors and achieved fewer categories. These differences can be attributed mainly to perseveration. While the dorsolateral prefrontal group committed nonperseverative errors at rates similar to those of the control groups, their rates of perseverative errors were significantly higher. Also striking is Milner's analysis comparing those patients with the smallest dorsolateral frontal lobe removals and those with the largest removals elsewhere (five with parietal-temporal removals and seven with orbito-frontal removals). Whereas the groups performed similarly preoperatively, the dorsolateral prefrontal group performed significantly worse postoperatively, due largely to an increase in perseverative errors. Thus, although patients with many different loci of damage may perform poorly at the WCST, damage to the dorsolateral prefrontal cortex seems closely tied to perseveration at this test. A number of other studies have confirmed the basic finding that the WCST is particularly sensitive to frontal damage[4,5] (but see Ref. 6).

Sequencing Tasks

The term *sequencing* can describe anything from concrete motor sequences, such as sequences of hand motions, to more abstract behavioral sequences, such as the morning routine of preparing to go to work. Of the sequencing errors made by frontal-damaged patients, many but not all are perseverative in nature.[7,8] A number of studies of simple manual and oral movement sequences have indicated that frontal lesions are most disruptive of these abilities.[9–11] Anecdotal reports suggest that the problem extends to the sequencing of more abstract kinds of actions. For example, Penfield and Evans[12] describe a patient who could perform all the individual actions necessary to prepare a meal but could not actually prepare the meal without someone to tell her the order in which to do things.

Tasks that require planning of a sequence in advance may also depend on the frontal areas. Shallice[13] tested frontal-damaged patients on the Tower of London test, a variant of the Tower of Hanoi game, designed specifically to require subjects to use advance planning. Left-frontal-damaged patients showed a disproportionate impairment at this task.

Verbal Fluency

Asked to produce words beginning with a particular letter, frontal-damaged patients (even those with no overt aphasic signs) will typically produce few unique responses, often repeating earlier responses. This frequently reported clinical finding has been supported by a variety of experimental studies.

An early study by Milner[3] demonstrated that patients with left frontal damage were impaired at a written test of verbal fluency when compared to a group with temporal lobe excisions. Benton[14] later confirmed the relative importance of the left frontal areas in the now more common oral version of the test. More recently, Janowsky and coworkers[15] compared verbal fluency in frontal-damaged patients with a variety of control groups and found that patients with left or bilateral frontal lesions but not right frontal lesions were impaired at verbal fluency.

Other fluency tasks have also been found to be sensitive to frontal pathology. Jones-Gotman and Milner[16] have found deficits in design fluency, a nonverbal analogue of the fluency task, in patients with right frontal removals. Similarly, Jason[9] found deficits in gesture fluency in frontal-damaged groups.

Neuroimaging studies have tended to confirm the importance of prefrontal areas in fluency tasks. Parks and coworkers[17] used positron emission tomography (PET) to compare the brain activity of subjects performing a verbal fluency task with controls in a resting state and found increases in activation bilaterally in both the frontal and temporal lobes. Frith and coworkers[18,19] performed PET studies of word finding, comparing the fluency condition to a lexical decision task. They found that "intrinsic" (subject-initiated) generation of a word was associated with increased activity in Brodmann area 46.

Context Memory

Although most frontal-damaged patients are not amnesic, they have nevertheless been found to have impairments on certain memory tasks. The most widely documented impairments involve memory for contextual information, either the source of a correctly recalled fact or its temporal context. Schacter[20] has applied the term *spatio-*

temporal context to the type of memory that is impaired in frontal-damaged patients.

Janowsky and colleagues[15] investigated memory for recently learned facts and memory for the source of the facts in a group of frontal-damaged patients. Although the patients were normal in their ability to recall the facts, they frequently attributed the facts to incorrect sources. Shimamura and coworkers[21] found that frontal-damaged patients, while unimpaired at recall and recognition of words printed on cards, were impaired at placing the cards in their original sequence of presentation. They also tested the same patients on a similar test of famous events (from 1941 to 1985), also finding that frontal-damaged patients recognized the events but were impaired at judging the decade in which the events occurred.

Similarly, frontal-damaged patients have difficulty identifying which of two items has been presented more recently in a recognition task. Milner and coworkers[22,23] found that left-frontal-damaged patients were most impaired at making recency judgments with verbal materials, while right-frontal-damaged patients were most impaired with nonverbal materials.

Additional support for the role of the frontal lobes in memory for spatiotemporal context comes from studies in which patients with Korsakoff syndrome are compared to non-Korsakoff amnesics. Because Korsakoff syndrome is often accompanied by frontal atrophy, differences between patients with Korsakoff syndrome and those with other amnesias can be used to infer frontal contributions to memory. Disproportionately impaired context memory has been found in this group.[24,25]

Go–No-Go Tasks

In tasks designed to elicit false-alarm motor responses, frontal-damaged patients often seem unable to inhibit inappropriate responses. This widely reported clinical sign was confirmed by Drewe,[26] using a version of this test in which subjects were trained to hit a key in response to either of two lights (red and blue). They were then given a test in which they were asked to hit a key only when they thought it would turn the light off. The key was effective only for the red light, so subjects were supposed to learn not to hit the key in response to the blue light. Drewe reported that frontal-damaged patients made more errors than non-frontal damaged patient controls and in particular that they made more false-positive responses.

Self-Ordered Tasks

Given a series of cards with multiple stimuli and asked to point to a different item of their choosing on each card, epileptic patients with frontal excisions make more errors than other epileptic patients with temporal lobe excisions,[27] thus failing to monitor a series of self-generated choices. Lesions placed in the mid-dorsolateral prefrontal cortex of nonhuman primates will markedly impair their ability to recall which one of a set of objects they had previously chosen, a process that is critical for successful performance of the self-ordered task.[28] Furthermore, Petrides and colleagues have shown that performance at these self-ordered tasks in normal human subjects activates this same region of the mid-dorsolateral frontal cortex.[29]

Conditional Associative Learning

Frontal-damaged patients are impaired at learning and associating between a set of stimuli (e.g., colored lights) and a set of available responses (e.g., a set of abstract designs).[30,31] Lesions placed in the posterior dorsolateral prefrontal cortex of nonhuman primates (an area adjacent and posterior to the lesions causing impairments in self-ordered tasks) will markedly impair performance on conditional association learning tasks in which the monkey must perform different responses conditional upon the presence of a particular stimulus.[32] Furthermore, Petrides and colleagues have shown that performance of a conditional associative learning task in normal human subjects activates this same region of posterior dorsolateral frontal cortex.[29]

Stroop Task

In this task devised by Stroop,[33] subjects are presented with an array of color names printed in different-colored inks and asked either to name the ink colors or to read the words. Reaction time can be measured either for individual stimuli or for the reading of an entire array. There is a congruent condition, in which the word and the color always agree, and a conflict condition, in which the word and the color always disagree. In addition, control conditions in which the words are replaced with X's or color patches (color-naming control) or in which the words are printed in black ink (word-naming control) are usually used. The general finding is that when naming the color, a conflicting word creates a significant amount of interference, while a congruent word provides a smaller but still notable amount of facilitation.[34] When subjects are reading the word, a similar pattern exists in the reaction times, although the differences between conditions are much smaller.

Perret[35] reported the performance of several patient groups on the Stroop task and found that left-frontal-damaged patients had disproportionate difficulty in the conflict condition, when the dominant response to the word ordinarily causes interference with the color-naming task. Other researchers have replicated this finding.[36,37]

Delayed-Response Tasks

Evidence from infants, monkeys, and adult human subjects using a variety of methodologies has converged to indicate the importance of the prefrontal areas in performing delayed-response tasks (see Ref. 38 for a review). In a typical delayed-response task, the subject is shown some reward (e.g., food for monkeys or a toy for infants) that is placed in one of two locations. The two possible locations are both obscured during a delay period of several seconds, after which the subject is allowed to select one of the two locations (usually by reaching). Many variants of this basic paradigm have been found to depend on the prefrontal cortex.

Jacobsen[39] first established a connection between delayed-response performance and the prefrontal cortex, and the basic facts established in his studies have been well supported by subsequent findings. In his classic study, monkeys with bilateral prefrontal removals were found to be impaired at delayed-response tasks (as well as de-

layed-alternation tasks) but intact at simple visual discriminations. The result has since been confirmed and refined in a variety of studies.[40,41] Evidence from other methodologies has been consistent. Fuster[42] has provided evidence from a variety of methods, including single-unit recording[43,44] and cooling techniques,[45] which converge to implicate the prefrontal areas in the performance of delayed-response tasks.

Freedman and Oscar-Berman[46] found a delayed-response deficit in patients with bilateral frontal lobe lesions as compared to amnesic and alcoholic control groups. And Diamond and Goldman-Rakic[41] have argued that maturation of the prefrontal cortex in human infants underlies the development of competence at delayed-response tasks.

THEORIES OF FRONTAL LOBE FUNCTION

Unified versus Multicomponent Theories

Theories of frontal lobe function vary in the breadth of phenomena they are intended to explain. In some cases they are aimed at explaining performance in just one task, whereas in others they are intended to account for most or all of the cognitive changes that follow prefrontal damage. In this chapter we focus on theories intended to account for more than one isolated phenomenon.

Given the diversity of tasks affected by prefrontal damage, from the execution of simple manual sequences to the sorting of cards according to abstract categories, it might seem unlikely that prefrontal cortex has a single underlying cognitive function. In addition, performance deficits in the "frontal" tasks reviewed above are dissociable. Although most patients who are impaired at one task will also be impaired at some others, across-the-board impairment is rare. Prospects for a unified theory of frontal lobe function seem even slimmer when the known functional anatomy of the frontal lobes is considered. Prefrontal cortex alone includes the frontal eye fields, which are implicated in the control of voluntary eye movements, and Broca's area, which is implicated in language processes. Dorsolateral prefrontal damage is more closely associated with cognitive deficits, while orbitofrontal damage seems to be related to more obvious changes in personality. Consistent and reliable differences in function have been found even between different areas within the dorsolateral areas (e.g., Ref. 29). Finally, hemispheric asymmetries have been widely noted. The left frontal lobe is more strongly and more often implicated in tasks that involve verbal materials, while the right is most clearly implicated in some tasks involving nonverbal materials.[14,16,22,35,47]

Nevertheless, despite the diversity of cognitive changes following frontal damage, their dissociability, and the heterogeneity of the known functional neuroanatomy, unified theories of frontal lobe function are still being sought. What makes the unified theory so irresistible is the sense that many of the distinct and dissociable deficits described above have some underlying commonality. In the eloquent words of Hans-Lukas Teuber:[48] "I started out by trying to find a unitary concept, but as I moved along, it became clear that no single-factor hypothesis could carry one far enough to cover all the manifestations of frontal lesions. And yet the thing that is so tempting to me after this symposium is to think that there may be a family resemblance among symptoms, even among those which seem in part dissociable."

In some cases, the basis of the resemblance is clear. For instance, frontal-damaged patients seem to show perseveration at a variety of tasks, ranging from concrete motor tasks to the sorting of cards into abstract categories.[7,8] The impulsivity that characterizes these patients' failures on the "go–no-go" task is also at times shockingly apparent in their everyday behavior. Impulsivity could also possibly explain their increased susceptibility to interference on the Stroop test. The challenge for unified theories of frontal lobe function is to capture the intuitive commonalities among these signs of frontal damage in an explicit, mechanistic account of frontal lobe function.

Abstract Thinking

Goldstein[49,50] proposed that the frontal lobes were especially important for abstract thought and that the "abstract attitude" could not be adopted by patients with extensive frontal damage. Although it may well be true that many frontal-damaged patients think concretely, this hypothesis does not explain many of the central phenomena of frontal damage. Patients who fail the Wisconsin Card Sorting Test, for example, are often able to describe verbally the different abstract categories into which stimuli might be sorted, but they nevertheless perseverate in using the same categories even after negative feedback.[2] Walsh[51] reports this as well, noting one subject who, after perseverating in grouping several objects according to shape even when asked to form a new grouping, was shown a grouping by color. The subject described the grouping as "one of each shape in each group"—an extremely abstract description—while remaining unable to recognize the new scheme. While not every patient who perseverates on the card sort will produce this kind of behavior, this observation does show that impaired performance on this classic frontal task cannot be attributed to difficulty with abstract thinking. Furthermore, most of the tasks reviewed above do not seem particularly dependent on abstract thought (e.g., sequencing tasks, Stroop, go–no-go, context memory).

Error Utilization

Luria[52,53] suggested that frontal patients are impaired in the utilization of errors to guide their behavior. Performance on the WCST is a perfect example of this. While a normal subject would take negative feedback as a cue to switch categories, frontal-damaged patients perseverate in their errors. Another example described by Luria is that frontal patients often fail to concentrate their study time on previously missed items in a memory task. However, most of the tasks reviewed above do not seem to tax error utilization in particular.

Planning

Many authors have attributed a planning function to the frontal lobes,[13,14,53] and Duncan[54] has framed this idea in terms of recent cognitive science models of problem solving. He proposes that human purposive activity requires a list of goals and a set of action structures resembling scripts. Goal-directed behavior is produced by a process similar to that of Newell and Simon's[55] means-end analysis. In effect, the goals inhibit those action structures that are not relevant to their achievement. The authors suggest that a defect in the use of the goal list to constrain behavior is responsible for the behavior of frontal-damaged patients. This account can explain failure on many but not all of the tasks reviewed earlier. For example, it does not explain context memory difficulties. Furthermore, if the notion of goal lists is extended to account for failures in such simple tasks as go–no-go or fluency, then it seems to predict failure at virtually any cognitive task, contrary to the evidence.

Inhibition

The theory that the frontal lobes serve an inhibitory function, suppressing dominant action tendencies in favor of more goal-appropriate behavior, has been proposed recently to account for a variety of data, including normal human development and physiologic experiments with monkeys. Diamond[56] has argued, from the development of reaching behaviors of infants and infant monkeys, that the prefrontal cortex serves such a function in inhibiting inappropriate reaches to formerly rewarded locations. She also suggests that this explanation may generalize to explain frontal deficits at the WCST as well as "capture" behavior, the intrusion of familiar but contextually inappropriate actions that have sometimes been noted after frontal damage. Similarly, Dempster[57] has proposed that inhibitory functions in the frontal cortex, in particular the suppression of irrelevant stimuli or associations, may account for a wide variety of patterns in both cognitive development and cognitive aging as well as data from frontal-damaged patients. And Roberts and coworkers[58] argue that frontal inhibitory processes (as well as working memory) underlie patterns of performance in normal and patient groups at antisaccade tasks. At some level, theories of inhibition are descriptively correct—when a subject produces an inappropriate response, it is true that the response should have been inhibited (at least implicitly). However, since a complex process must underlie the decision to inhibit a prepotent response, it is not clear why the locus of the impairment must be in an inhibitory component. Attributing apparent errors of disinhibition to a malfunctioning inhibitory mechanism raises the equally puzzling question of how the system knows when to inhibit and when to allow a prepotent response. And, as with the other theories so far reviewed, this one fails to explain a number of the phenomena associated with frontal damage in humans (e.g., context memory, self-ordered tasks).

Supervisory Attentional System

According to Shallice,[13,59,60] the frontal lobes instantiate a supervisory attentional system (SAS). Although this system is not needed for routine action, which is controlled by learned associations between stimuli in the environment and possible action, it serves to override these associations when stimuli or goals are novel. Thus, frontal-damaged patients, in whom the SAS is damaged, are no longer able to exert goal-directed control over their actions but simply respond to stimuli. This theory accords well with much of the observed behavior of frontal-damaged patients. For instance, it predicts that they should behave more normally in familiar situations than in unfamiliar ones. It also accords with the slow learning evidenced by many patients in the WCST, as their behavior seems very much like the slow learning of an associative module combined with the tendency of more familiar, routinized responses to emerge even when inappropriate (as in Stroop and go–no-go tasks). However, a number of the other tasks listed earlier do not seem particularly dependent on breaking out of routine action patterns (e.g., verbal fluency, context memory, and conditional associative responses). In addition, compared to the other theories, the SAS could be viewed as less parsimonious in that it represents a new component of the cognitive architecture over and above the components that carry out the tasks, whose sole function is to guide the use of those other components. Last, an impairment to a truly central executive would seem to imply that all frontal signs should always co-occur, which is certainly not the case.

Working Memory

"Working memory" is a form of short-term memory (see Chap. 22) that is often described when the writer wishes to emphasize that the information is being held on line for the purpose of performing computations on it (analogous to a mental scratch pad). Fuster[61,62] provided the first detailed account of the role of working memory in prefrontal processes. He describes the role of the prefrontal cortex as that of integrating temporally distributed information, a complex process which he attributed partly to short-term working memory. Contrasting this view with SAS-like executive accounts of prefrontal function, he writes: "The prefrontal cortex would not superimpose a steering or directing function on the remainder of the nervous system, but rather, by expanding the temporal perspectives of the system, it would allow it to integrate longer, newer, and more complex structures of behavior" (Ref. 62, page 172).

Goldman-Rakic[63] has also proposed a working-memory account of frontal lobe function on the basis of extensive research with nonhuman primates. Building on the well-established relationship between the prefrontal cortex and delayed-response tasks, she argues that the prefrontal cortex is responsible for maintaining information ("representational memory") that is later used to guide action. Funahashi and colleagues[44,64] have carried out a variety of lesion studies and single-unit recording studies to establish the role of prefrontal cortex in working memory, primarily with monkeys trained to perform spatial working-memory tasks. Neuroimaging studies in humans[65–68] suggest that similar working-memory processes are located prefrontally in the human brain. Goldman-Rakic[63] has suggested that the association between prefrontal cortex and working memory can in principle explain a range of human cognitive impairments following focal frontal lesions as well as other nonfocal pathologies affect-

ing prefrontal cortex (e.g., schizophrenia, Huntington disease, Parkinson disease).

The proposal that a working memory impairment could underlie the range of cognitive changes seen after prefrontal damage first found direct support in the work of Cohen and Servan-Schreiber.[69] They built a computational model of some of the cognitive and linguistic tasks that are characteristically failed by schizophrenic patients, including the Stroop task, lexical disambiguation, and the Continuous Performance Test. When the model's representation of context—held in working memory—is degraded, the model simulates the behavior of schizophrenic patients in these tasks.

Kimberg and Farah[70] selected four seemingly disparate tasks from those discussed in the previous section and modeled their performance computationally. When the strength of working memory associations was attenuated, the model perseverated on the WCST, made perseverative and nonperseverative sequencing errors on a simple motor sequencing task, showed source amnesia with relatively preserved recognition memory, and tended to read words rather than name colors in the Stroop task.

We favor working-memory accounts of prefrontal function for a number of reasons. First, they are parsimonious, in that working-memory theories contain only the individual processing components needed to perform the task without needing a central executive (such as the SAS) to coordinate these components (and to serve as the locus of damage when explaining patient behavior). Second, they have proven capable of explaining a wider range of seemingly disparate impairments than other nonexecutive theories.[69,70] Third, they are supported by a wealth of evidence from monkey neurophysiology[42,44,63,64] and, increasingly, from neuroimaging studies in humans.[65–68] Fourth, they suggest a way of resolving what is perhaps the central problem of the neuropsychology of frontal lobe function: the paradox of dissociable impairments with an untuitively compelling "family resemblance." If we assume that working memory is compartmentalized in prefrontal cortex according to what is being represented in memory (for which evidence exists—see

Refs. 66, 71, and 72), then performance in different tasks can be impaired or spared depending on which types of working memory have been damaged. Nevertheless, according to working-memory accounts, there is an underlying commonality among the tasks sensitive to prefrontal damage—namely, their dependence on working memory.

REFERENCES

1. Grant AD, Berg EA: A behavioral analysis of reinforcement and ease of shifting to new responses in a Weigl-type card sorting. *J Exp Psychol* 38:404–411, 1948.
2. Milner B: Effects of different brain lesions on card sorting. *Arch Neurol* 9:90–100, 1963.
3. Milner B: Some effects of frontal lobectomy in man, in Warren J, Akert K (eds): *The Frontal Granular Cortex and Behavior.* New York: McGraw-Hill, 1964.
4. Drewe EA: The effect of type and area of brain lesion on Wisconsin Card Sorting Test performance. *Cortex* 10:159–170, 1974.
5. Nelson HE: A modified card sorting test sensitive to frontal lobe defects. *Cortex* 12:313–324, 1976.
6. Anderson SW, Damasio H, Jones RD, Tranel D: Wisconsin card sorting test performance as a measure of frontal lobe damage. *J Clin Exp Neuropsychol* 13:909–922, 1991.
7. Luria AR: Two kinds of motor perseveration in massive injury of the frontal lobes. *Brain* 88:1–10, 1965.
8. Sandson J, Albert M: Varieties of perseveration. *Neuropsychologia* 22:715–732, 1984.
9. Jason GW: Manual sequences learning after focal cortical lesions. *Neuropsychologia* 23:483–496, 1985.
10. Kimura D: Left-hemisphere control of oral and brachial movements and their relation to communication. *Philos Trans R Soc Lond B* 298:135–149, 1982.
11. Kolb B, Milner B: Performance of complex arm and facial movements after focal brain lesions. *Neuropsychologia* 19:491–503, 1981.
12. Penfield W, Evans J: The frontal lobe in man: A clinical study of maximum removals. *Brain* 58:115–133, 1935.
13. Shallice T: Specific impairments of planning. *Philos Trans R Soc Lond B* 298:199–209, 1982.
14. Benton AL: Differential behavioral effects of frontal lobe disease. *Neuropsychologia* 6:53–60, 1968.
15. Janowsky JS, Shimamura AP, Squire LR: Source memory impairment in patients with frontal lobe lesions. *Neuropsychologia* 27:1043–1056, 1989.
16. Jones-Gotman M, Milner B: Design fluency: The invention of nonsense drawings after focal cortical lesions. *Neuropsychologia* 15:653–674, 1977.
17. Parks RW, Loewenstein DA, Dodrill KL, et al: Cerebral metabolic effects of a verbal fluency test: A PET scan study. *J Clin Exp Neuropsychol* 10:565–575, 1988.
18. Frith CD, Friston KJ, Liddle PF, et al: A PET study of word finding. *Neuropsychologia* 29:1137–1148, 1991.
19. Friston KJ, Frith CD, Liddle PF, et al: Investigating a network model of word generation with positron emission tomography. *Proc R Soc Lond B Biol Sci* 244:101–106, 1991.
20. Schacter DL: Memory, amnesia, and frontal lobe dysfunction. *Psychobiology* 15:21–36, 1987.
21. Shimamura AP, Janowsky JS, Squire LR: Memory for the temporal order of events in patients with frontal lobe lesions and amnesic patients. *Neuropsychologia* 28:803–813, 1990.
22. Milner B, Corsi P, Leonard G: Frontal-lobe contribution to recency judgements. *Neuropsychologia* 29:601–618, 1991.
23. McAndrews MP, Milner B: The frontal cortex and memory for temporal order. *Neuropsychologia* 29:849–859, 1991.
24. Schacter DL, Harbluk JL, McLachlan DR: Retrieval without recollection: An experimental analysis of source amnesia. *J Verb Learn Verb Behav* 23:593–611, 1984.
25. Squire LR: Comparisons between forms of amnesia: Some deficits are unique to Korsakoff's syndrome. *J Exp Psychol Learning, Memory, Cognition* 8:560–571, 1982.
26. Drewe EA: Go–no-go learning after frontal lobe lesions in humans. *Cortex* 11:8–16, 1975.
27. Petrides M, Milner B: Deficits on subject-ordered tasks after frontal- and temporal-lobe lesions in man. *Neuropsychologia* 20:249–262, 1982.
28. Petrides M: Monitoring of selections of visual stimuli and the primate frontal cortex. *Proc R Soc Lond B Biol Sci* 246:293–298, 1991.
29. Petrides M, Alivisatos B, Evans AC, Meyer E: Dissociation of human mid-dorsolateral from posterior dorsolateral frontal cortex in memory processing. *Proc Natl Acad Sci USA* 90:873–877, 1993.

30. Petrides M: Deficits on conditional associative learning tasks after frontal- and temporal-lobe lesions in man. *Neuropsychologia* 23:601–614, 1985.
31. Petrides M: Nonspatial conditional learning impaired in patients with unilateral frontal but not unilateral temporal-lobe excisions. *Neuropsychologia* 28:137–149, 1990.
32. Petrides M: Deficits in non-spatial conditional associative learning after periarcuate lesions in the monkey. *Behav Brain Res* 16:95–101, 1985.
33. Stroop JR: Studies of interference in serial verbal reactions. *J Exp Psychol* 18:643–662, 1935.
34. MacLeod CM: Half a century of research on the Stroop effect: An integrative review. *Psychol Bull* 109:163–203, 1991.
35. Perret E: The left frontal lobe of man and the suppression of habitual responses in verbal categorical behavior. *Neuropsychologia* 12:323–330, 1974.
36. Regard M: Cognitive Rigidity and Flexibility: A Neuropsychological Study. Unpublished doctoral dissertation: University of Victoria, British Columbia.
37. Stuss DT, Benson DF: Neuropsychological studies of the frontal lobes. *Psychol Bull* 95:3–28, 1984.
38. Oscar-Berman M, McNamara P, Freedman M: Delayed-response tasks: Parallels between experimental ablation studies and findings in patients with frontal lesions, in Levin HS (ed): *Frontal Lobe Function and Dysfunction.* New York: Oxford University Press, 1991, pp 230–255.
39. Jacobsen CF: Studies of cerebral functions in primates: I. The function of the frontal association areas in monkeys. *Comp Psychol Monogr* 13:1–60, 1936.
40. Goldman PS, Rosvold HE: Localization of function within the dorsolateral prefrontal cortex of the rhesus monkey. *Exp Neurol* 27:291–304, 1970.
41. Diamond A, Goldman-Rakic PS: Comparison of human infants and rhesus monkeys on Piaget's AB task: Evidence for dependence on dorsolateral prefrontal cortex. *Exp Brain Res* 74:24–40, 1989.
42. Fuster JM: *The Frontal Lobes.* New York: Raven Press, 1989.
43. Fuster JM, Alexander GE: Neuron activity related to short-term memory. *Science* 173:652–654, 1971.
44. Funahashi S, Bruce CJ, Goldman-Rakic PS: Mnemonic coding of visual space in the monkey's dorsolateral prefrontal cortex. *J Neurophysiol* 61:331–349, 1989.
45. Bauer RH, Fuster JM: Delayed-matching and delayed-response deficit from cooling dorsolateral prefrontal cortex in monkeys. *J Comp Physiol Psychol* 90:293–302, 1976.
46. Freedman M, Oscar-Berman M: Bilateral frontal lobe disease and selective delayed response deficits in humans. *Behav Neurosci* 100:337–342, 1986.
47. Petrides M, Alivisatos B, Meyer E, Evans AC: Functional activation of the human frontal cortex during the performance of verbal working memory tasks. *Proc Natl Acad Sci USA* 90:878–882, 1993.
48. Teuber H-L: The riddle of frontal lobe function in man, in Warren JM, Akert K (eds): *The Frontal Granular Cortex and Behavior.* New York: McGraw-Hill, 1964.
49. Goldstein K: Mental changes due to frontal lobe damage. *J Psychol* 17:187–208, 1944.
50. Goldstein K, Scheerer M: Abstract and concrete behavior: An experimental study with special tests. *Psychol Monogr* 43:1–151, 1941.
51. Walsh KW: *Neuropsychology: A Clinical Approach.* New York: Churchill Livingstone, 1987.
52. Luria AR: *Higher Cortical Functions in Man.* London: Tavistock, 1966.
53. Luria AR, Homskaya ED: Disturbance in the regulative role of speech with frontal lobe lesions, in Warren JM, Akert K (eds): *The Frontal Granular Cortex and Behavior.* New York: McGraw-Hill, 1964, pp 353–371.
54. Duncan J: Disorganisation of behaviour after frontal lobe damage. *Cog Neuropsychol* 3:271–290, 1986.
55. Newell A, Simon HA: *Human Problem Solving.* Englewood Cliffs, NJ: Prentice Hall, 1972.
56. Diamond A: Developmental progression in human infants and infant monkeys, and the neural bases of inhibitory control of reaching, in Diamond A (ed): *The Development and Neural Bases of Higher Cognitive Functions.* New York: NY Academy of Science Press, 1989.
57. Dempster FN: The rise and fall of the inhibitory mechanism: Toward a unified theory of cognitive development and aging. *Dev Rev* 12:45–75, 1992.
58. Roberts RJ, Hager LD, Heron C: Prefrontal cognitive processes: Working memory and inhibition in the antisaccade task. *J Exp Psychol Gen* 123:374–393, 1994.
59. Shallice T: *From Neuropsychology to Mental Structure.* Cambridge, England: Cambridge University Press, 1988.
60. Shallice T, Burgess P: Higher-order cognitive impairments and frontal lobe lesions in man, in Levin HS, Eisenberg HM, Benton AL (eds): *Frontal Lobe*

Function and Dysfunction. New York: Oxford University Press, 1991.

61. Fuster JM: *The Prefrontal Cortex: Anatomy, Physiology, and Neuropsychology of the Frontal Lobe.* New York: Raven Press, 1980.

62. Fuster JM: The prefrontal cortex and temporal integration, in Jones EG, Peters A (eds): *Cerebral Cortex:* Vol 4. *Association and Auditory Cortices.* New York: Raven Press.

63. Goldman-Rakic PS: Circuitry of primate prefrontal cortex and regulation of behavior by representational memory, in Plum F, Mountcastle V (eds): *Handbook of Physiology, The Nervous System: V.* Bethesda, MD: American Physiological Society, 1987.

64. Funahashi S, Bruce CJ, Goldman-Rakic PS: Dorsolateral prefrontal lesions and oculomotor delayed-response performance: Evidence for mnemonic "scotomas." *J Neurosci* 13:1479–1497, 1993.

65. Cohen J, Forman S, Braver T, et al: Activation of prefrontal cortex in a nonspatial working memory task with functional MRI. *Hum Brain Mapping* 1:293–304, 1994.

66. D'Esposito M, Shin RK, Detre JA, et al: Object and spatial working memory activates dorsolateral prefrontal cortex: A functional MRI study. *Soc Neurosci Abstr* 21:1498, 1995.

67. D'Esposito M, Detre J, Alsop D, et al: The neural basis of the central executive system of working memory. *Nature* 378:279–281, 1995.

68. Jonides J, Smith E, Koeppe R, et al: Spatial working memory in humans as revealed by PET. *Nature* 363:623–625, 1993.

69. Cohen JD, Servan-Schreiber D: Context, cortex, and dopamine: A connectionist approach to behavior and biology in schizophrenia. *Psychol Rev* 99:45–77, 1992.

70. Kimberg DY, Farah MJ: A unified account of cognitive impairments following frontal lobe damage: The role of working memory in complex, organized behavior. *J Exp Psychol Gen* 122:411–428, 1993.

71. Smith E, Jonides J, Koeppe RA, et al: *J Cog Neurosci* 7:337–356, 1995.

72. Wilson F, Scalaidhe S, Goldman-Rakic P: Dissociation of object and spatial processing domains in prefrontal cortex. *Science* 260:1876, 1993.

Chapter 26

CALLOSAL DISCONNECTION

Kathleen Baynes
Michael S. Gazzaniga

BRIEF HISTORICAL BACKGROUND

Demonstration of Hemispheric Independence Requires Appropriate Techniques

Patients who have undergone cortical disconnection have been primary to the evolution of our
understanding of localized brain function. The hypothesis that disconnection of neural transmission
between the centers of comprehension and language production would cause problems with repetition was central to Wernicke's prediction that
conduction aphasia should exist. Callosal disconnection from naturally occurring lesions plays a
role in the explanation of a number of syndromes
including limb apraxia (Chap. 27), pure alexia
(Chap. 18), and unilateral agraphia (Chap. 20).
However, the most systematic investigation of
hemispheric specialization and hemispheric integration in cases of callosal disconnection has been
carried out with patients who have undergone callosotomy for control of intractible epilepsy. These
so-called split-brain patients are the focus of this
chapter.

In his early work with split-brain patients,
Akelaitis failed to discover cognitive sequelae of
the surgery using standard neuropsychological
procedures.[1,2] It was the Bogen group that recognized the importance of providing a nonverbal
means of response to demonstrate the presence of
two independent cognitive systems within the
same subject.[3,4] The presentation of stimuli to one
hemifield using brief (tachistoscopic) displays and

the use of manual responses (Fig. 26-1) opened
the way to exploration of each hemisphere's
unique properties. Initial studies confirmed neurologists' assertions that the left hemisphere was
dominant for language whereas the right could
neither name nor describe objects presented to it
visually or tactually, although it could perform
certain visuospatial tasks. Current techniques permit visual displays with extended durations, thus
allowing more precise observations. Further-
refined experiments continue to develop our understanding of perceptual, cognitive, mnemonic,
and linguistic processes and their integration into
coherent thought and behavior. Such techniques
continue to provide a unique means of testing
hemispheric hypotheses and enriching our understanding of neurological and neuropsychological
symptoms, from alexia to alien hand sign.

LANGUAGE

Variability of Right Hemispheric Language Representation

Perhaps the most striking observation regarding
split-brain subjects is the presence of complex,
generative language in only one hemisphere.
Nonetheless, the series of patients operated on by
Bogen demonstrated a well-developed right hemispheric lexicon in the majority of patients examined, although that lexicon appeared to be limited
to simple auditory and visual comprehension and
some written output.[4-6] The Wilson-Roberts

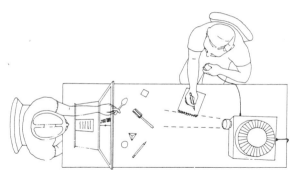

Figure 26-1

Visual information can be presented to one hemi-sphere at a time in split-brain patients by flashing the stimulus to one side or the other of a fixation point, for less time than is required to make an eye movement from the fixation point to the stimulus. Responses made with one hand favor the contralateral hemi-sphere, although some ipsilateral control is possible. (From Gazzaniga,[7] with permission.)

series, however, demonstrated much less frequent right hemispheric participation in even rudimentary language processing. By 1983, of the 28 completed callosotomies, only 3 patients had a documented right hemispheric lexicon.[7] Moreover, there was considerable variation in the quality and sophistication of the language available to the right hemisphere.[8]

In those patients with right hemispheric language capability, semantic and conceptual information appear to be more adequately represented in the right hemisphere than is phonologic and syntactic information. The visual and auditory lexicons of the right hemisphere (RH) appear to be similar to, albeit somewhat smaller than, the corresponding left hemispheric lexicons.[9] Both hemispheres can make a variety of semantic judgments, recognizing categorical, functional, and associative relations.[9] The ability to discriminate word from nonword letter strings is limited but possible,[10–12] which suggests that the visual word form is represented in the RH of these patients.

Limited Control of Speech and Grammar in the Isolated Right Hemisphere

Phonologic information is difficult for the RH to manipulate, although it may possess limited pho-

nologic competence and be able to produce speech. Sidtis[8] assessed discrimination of phonemes (such as "ba" versus "pa") in two callosotomy patients. The RH of one patient was able to discriminate but not identify phoneme contrasts and was also able to identify rhyming words. Not surprisingly, this patient was able to produce some verbal responses to left visual field (LVF) stimuli within a year of her completed surgery.[9] The other patient had more difficulty with the discrimination task and refused to respond to the identification task. His right hemisphere was also unable to identify rhyming words.[8] This patient's RH remained mute until more than 10 years after his surgery; he has now gained rudimentary control of speech within the RH.[13,14] Although he remained unable to make accurate judgments that require moving from letter to sound,[13] he was able to integrate visual and auditory phonologic information within his RH.[15] This remarkable development has implications for the limits of functional plasticity and for the role of the RH in long-term recovery from aphasia.

The linguistic prowess of the RH does not appear to extend to the use of grammatical rules for comprehension or the production of sentences. The ability to use grammatical information to guide comprehension is limited,[9,16] although the RH can distinguish between grammatical and ungrammatical sentences,[16] possibly on the basis of prosodic cues. In a left-handed patient with right hemispheric language dominance, comprehension of grammatical relations appears to be possible only for the RH.[17] Even when the RH is able to make a verbal response to a LVF word or picture, it appears to lose control of speech output rapidly as the LH takes over and expands in a confabulatory fashion on the RH's utterance,[14] perhaps because it lacks the ability to generate more complex, sentence-length responses.

Right Hemispheric Reading

Right hemispheric reading proceeds more slowly than left hemispheric reading and may use a different mode of processing,[12] as has been reported for some deep dyslexic patients. Likewise, a right hemispheric lexicon with more diffuse or associative organization than that of the left hemisphere has been suggested as the source of certain reading errors in deep dyslexic[18,19] and pure alexic patients[20] (Chap. 18). Although insensitivity to grammar and poor print-to-sound skills in the RH of these patients is consistent with some aspects of those claims, both hemispheres appear to be capable of generating the range of error types found in deep dyslexia.[13] The language profile seen in callosotomy patients is more consistent with the profile reported by Coslett and Saffran for the preserved reading of their pure alexic patient than with that reported for deep dyslexic patients.

MEMORY

Recall and Recognition Memory Following Callosotomy

Changes in mnemonic capacity after callosotomy may reflect discrete processing capacities in the isolated hemispheres. Loss of general memory capacity as measured by standardized tests has been reported for some patients,[21,22] while Clark and Geffen[23] suggested that discrepancies in memory function reported after callosotomy might be due to involvement of the hippocampal commissure. Phelps and coworkers[24] have observed a decrement in both visual and verbal recall following posterior callosal section, which may damage the hippocampal commissure, but preserved or even improved memory after anterior callosal section, which does not. Recognition memory was relatively intact in both groups. Kroll and colleagues[24a,b] reported that complete callosotomy interferes with the binding of visual and verbal material yielding error patterns similar to those of hippocampally lesioned patients.

There appear to be hemisphere-specific changes in the accuracy of memory processes that may be useful in understanding the behavior of some neurologically impaired patients. The left hemisphere (LH) appears to make greater use of general knowledge schemas to explain perceptions and experiences and to use them to "interpret" events[25] than does the RH, and this predilection has an impact on the accuracy of memory.[26]

When subjects were presented with a series of pictures that represented common events (i.e., getting up in the morning or making cookies) and were then asked, several hours later, to identify whether pictures in another series had appeared in the first, both hemispheres were equally accurate in recognizing the previously viewed pictures and rejecting unrelated ones. Only the RH, however, correctly rejected pictures in the second set that were not previously viewed but were semantically congruent with pictures from the first set. The LH incorrectly "recalled" significantly more of these pictures as having occurred in the first set, presumably because they fit into the schema it had constructed regarding the event. This finding is consistent with the view of a LH "interpreter" that constructs theories to assimilate perceived information into a comprehensible whole. In doing so, however, the elaborative processing involved has a deleterious effect on the accuracy of perceptual recognition. This result has been confirmed by Metcalfe and coworkers[27] and extended to include verbal material.

HEMISPHERIC DOMINANCE

The Left Hemisphere as Interpreter

The LH is considered to be the "dominant" hemisphere in most right-handed people. The term *dominant* is usually taken to mean language-dominant, but Gazzaniga[28] has suggested that the LH is not only superior in terms of language function but also in the ability to make simple inferences and to interpret its own behavior and emotions.[29] It is unclear whether these functions are dependent upon the development of generative language skills or if the two arise independently. Nonetheless, such observations strongly suggest that the LH is not only more able than the right to express itself verbally but that it plays a dominant role in interpreting behavior and providing a rationale for events in the world.

These observations can also yield insight regarding the confabulatory behavior seen in some amnesic patients who are unable to encode new information. Finding themselves in situations for which they cannot remember the antecedents, they may be compelled to explain them in the same way that the LH explains behavior motivated by the RH.

Visuospatial Functions

There are other areas that demonstrate differential hemispheric contributions. The expected right hemispheric superiority in visuospatial function has been demonstrated in callosotomy patients.[3,30] In contrast, superior use of visual imagery has been demonstrated in the LH, using a letter-based task.[31] The use of tactile information to build spatial representations of abstract shapes also appears to be better developed in the RH.[30] Tasks such as Block Design from the Wechsler Adult Intelligence Scale (WAIS), however, which are typically associated with the right parietal lobe, appear to require integration between the hemispheres in some patients.[32] Furthermore, while the RH is better able to analyze unfamiliar facial information than the LH[33,34] and the left is better able to generate voluntary expressions,[35] both hemispheres share in the management of facial expression when spontaneous emotions are expressed.

Although the RH demonstrates superior levels of performance on a variety of perceptual and spatial tasks, the LH appears to have at least some competence in most areas and in some cases is essential for the solution of complex visual problems. The LH is superior at all language tasks and in a variety of tasks that require inferences. Moreover, verbal IQ appears to be stable following callosotomy, although performance IQ may decline.[22] Gazzaniga[36] suggests that the LH is also dominant for intelligent behavior, although that conclusion assumes a contemporary concept of intelligence that rests heavily on verbal abilities.

INTERHEMISPHERIC INTEGRATION OF PERCEPTION AND ATTENTION

Hemispheric Isolation of Visual and Tactile Information

When appropriate lateralization procedures are followed (see Fig. 26-1), visual and tactile percep-

tion are isolated in each hemisphere. Although, subjects can independently report visual material that has been isolated to one hemisphere or the other, they cannot make comparisons between the two hemifields. Performance is at or near chance levels in simple same/different comparisons when items are presented in different visual fields.[13,37,38] Despite reports of integration of higher-order information following callosotomy,[39,40] such results have not always been replicated or have proved explicable through the patient's strategic maneuvers.[37,41,42] At present, it appears that if visual or tactile information is presented so that it is initially perceived by only one hemisphere, the perception remains isolated within that hemisphere.

The animal literature, however, has documented that information from areas close to the visual midline is shared by both hemispheres.[43,44] It appears that this observation is also true for the human species in an area no more than 2° from the vertical meridian.[45] Although represented, the visual information in this area has little utility, as neither detailed shape comparisons nor brief displays could be reliably compared across the meridian.[46]

Sharing of Attentional Control

Although both higher cognitive function and basic perceptual information appear to be isolated within each hemisphere, there is some evidence for sharing of control of visual attention. The hemispheres appear to share control of the "attentional spotlight" via their subcortical connections. That is, if attention is directed to a particular position in the visual field by a cue in one field, that information can be used by both hemispheres.[38,47] Nonetheless, explicit interfield comparisons of spatial location cannot be made accurately,[38] nor can attention be simultaneously directed to different points in each visual field.[48]

It also appears that attentional resources are limited despite the "splitting" of consciousness. Holtzman demonstrated that increasing processing demands in one hemisphere had a deleterious effect on performance in the other hemisphere.[49] Nonetheless, in comparison with normal subjects, there was less decrement in a dual-task condition for callosotomized subjects.[50] Thus, although the two hemispheres may compete for cognitive resources, there is evidence for independence of function. This latter finding is consistent with the observation of Luck and coworkers[51] that visual search is independently mediated by both hemispheres. Using a standard spatial cueing paradigm that incorporated a bilateral cue to assess the influence of information presented to one hemisphere on the performance of the other, Mangun and colleagues[52] demonstrated differential processing of spatial cues, with only the LVF (right-hand) trials yielding an advantage for validly cued trials. Although the failure to find a right visual field (RVF) advantage for valid trials is at odds with the other split-brain results,[47,53] it is consistent with a view of the RH as dominant in terms of spatial attention (Chap. 10).

SPECIFICITY OF CALLOSAL FIBERS

Observations regarding functional specificity come from two sources in human studies. First, sections are completed in two stages, usually anterior first, allowing for observation of functional differences. Second, development of improved imaging techniques such as magnetic resonance imaging (MRI) has allowed for verification and definition of the fibers resected during callosotomy.

It has long been noted that separating up to two-thirds of the anterior callosum leads to little if any change in ability.[54] If the anterior split continues far enough, disruption of the ability to transfer sensory and position information from hand to hand will be observed. In contrast, the section of the splenium disrupts the transfer of visual information between the hemispheres, which isolates lateralized visual input. After posterior section, although explicit identification and naming of LVF stimuli is not possible, some transfer of higher-order information may occur.[55]

In cases with inadvertent surgical sparing, very specific transfer of information has been found. Patient V. P. has sparing of fibers in the rostrum and splenium of the callosum. Although she cannot make explicit visual comparisons between fields, she was able to integrate visual and auditory information to make accurate between-field rhyme judgments when words both looked and sounded alike (i.e., between *boat* and *goat,* but not between *boat* and *note*).[56] Occasionally, strokes yield partial callosal lesions as well; one such patient with damage to the body of the corpus callosum demonstrates left-hand tactile anomia and agraphia[57] showing the importance of the fibers of the body of the callosum for the transfer of language information between the hemispheres.

CONCLUSIONS

Although the behaving being is remarkably intact following callosotomy, investigation reveals hemispheric capacities that refine and confirm hypotheses based on normal subjects and patients with focal lesions. The isolated RH usually cannot read, write, or speak, despite displaying a variety of conscious behaviors. Dissociations like left-handed tactile anomia or agraphia may be an indication of less language-competent right hemispheres. However, the ability to comprehend auditory and visual language may be present and can contribute to the presentation of aphasic and alexic patients. Recent observations indicate that the RH may participate in long-term recovery from aphasia. Perhaps of greater interest, however, is the study of callosotomy patients to investigate the hemispheric bases of cognition and the integration of diverse perceptual, sensory, and emotional information into a single behavioral plan. This population was the first in which independent function of the hemispheres was demonstrated as a result of which the important role played by the verbal left hemisphere in allowing the organism to observe and interpret its own actions and emotional states was recognized. Insights regarding the components of perception, memory, attention, and language continue to arise from this population and to inform models of normal perceptual and cognitive processing.

ACKNOWLEDGMENTS

Supported in part by NIH/NIDCD grant number R29 DC00811 to KB and NIH/NINDS grant number P01 NS17778 to MSG and the McDonnell-Pew Foundation.

REFERENCES

1. Akelaitis AJ: Studies on the corpus callosum: Higher visual functions in each homonymous field following complete section of corpus callosum. *Arch Neurol Psychiatry* 45:788–796, 1941.

2. Akelaitis AJ: A study of gnosis, praxis, and language following section of the corpus callosum and anterior commissure. *J Neurosurg* 7:94–102, 1944.

3. Bogen JE, Gazzaniga MS: Cerebral commissurotomy in man: Minor hemisphere dominance for certain visuospatial functions. *J Neurosurg* 23:394–399, 1965.

4. Sperry RW, Gazzaniga MS, Bogen JE: Interhemispheric relationships: The neocortical commissures: Syndromes of hemisphere disconnection, in Vinken PJ, Bruyn GW (eds): *Handbook of Clinical Neurology.* New York: Wiley, 1969, vol 4, pp 273–290.

5. Gazzaniga MS, Bogen JE, Sperry RW: Some functional effects of sectioning the cerebral commissures in man. *Proc Natl Acad Sci USA* 48:1765–1769, 1962.

6. Levy J, Nebes RB, Sperry RW: Expressive language in the surgically separated minor hemisphere. *Cortex* 7:49–58, 1971.

7. Gazzaniga MS: Right hemisphere language following brain bisection: A twenty year perspective. *Am Psychol* 38:525–549, 1983.

8. Sidtis JJ, Volpe BT, Wilson DH, et al: Variability in right hemisphere language function after callosal section: Evidence for a continuum of generative capacity. *J Neurosci* 1:323–331, 1981.

9. Gazzaniga MS, Smylie CS, Baynes K, et al: Profiles of right hemisphere language and speech following brain bisection. *Brain Lang* 22:206–220, 1984.

10. Eviatar Z, Zaidel E: The effects of word length and emotionality on hemispheric contribution to lexical decision. *Neuropsychologia* 29:415–428, 1991.

11. Baynes K, Tramo MJ, Gazzaniga MS: Reading with a limited lexicon in the right hemisphere of a callosotomy patient. *Neuropsychologia* 30:187–200, 1992.

12. Reuter-Lorenz PA, Baynes K: Modes of lexical access in the callosotomized brain. *J Cogn Neurosci* 4:155–164, 1992.

13. Baynes K, Wessinger CM, Fendrich R, Gazzaniga MS: The emergence of the capacity to name left visual field stimuli in a callosotomy patient: Implica-

14. Gazzaniga MS, Nisenson L, Eliassen JC, et al: Collaboration between the hemispheres of a callosotomy patient: Emerging right hemisphere speech and the left hemisphere interpreter. Submitted.

15. Baynes K, Funnell MG, Fowler CA: Hemispheric contributions to the integration of visual and auditory information in speech perception. *Percept Psychophys* 55:633–641, 1994.

16. Baynes K, Gazzaniga MS: Right hemisphere language: Insights into normal language mechanisms? in Plum F (ed): *Language, Communication, and the Brain.* New York: Raven Press, 1987, pp 117–126.

17. Lutsep HL, Wessinger CM, Gazzaniga MS: Cerebral and callosal organisation in a right hemisphere dominant "split-brain" subject. *J Neurol Neurosurg Psychiatry* 59:50–54, 1995.

18. Schweiger A, Zaidel E, Dobkin B: Right hemisphere contribution to lexical access in an aphasic with deep dyslexia. *Brain Lang* 37:73–89, 1989.

19. Coltheart M: Deep dyslexia: A right hemisphere hypothesis, in Coltheart M, Patterson KE, Marshall JC (eds): *Deep Dyslexia.* London: Routledge, 1980.

20. Coslett HB, Saffran EM: Evidence for preserved reading in "pure alexia." *Brain* 112:327–359, 1989.

21. Zaidel D, Sperry RW: Memory impairment after commissurotomy in man. *Brain* 97:263–272, 1974.

22. Zaidel E: Language functions in the two hemispheres following complete cerebral commissurotomy and hemispherectomy, in Boller F, Grafman G (eds): *Handbook of Neuropsychology.* New York: Elsevier, 1990, vol 4, pp 115–150.

23. Clark CR, Geffen GM: Corpus callosum surgery and recent memory. *Brain* 112:165–175, 1989.

24. Phelps EA, Hirst W, Gazzaniga MS: Deficits in recall following partial and complete commissurotomy. *Cereb Cortex* 1:492–498, 1991.

24a. Kroll NEA, Knight RT, Metcalfe J, et al: Cohesion failure as a source of memory illusions. *Memory and Language.* In press.

24b. Jha AP, Kroll NEA, Baynes K, Gazzaniga MS: Memory encoding following complete callosotomy. *J Cogn Neurosci.* In press.

25. Gazzaniga MS: *The Social Brain.* New York: Basic Books, 1985.

26. Phelps EA, Gazzaniga MS: Hemispheric differences in mnemonic processing: The effects of left hemisphere interpretation. *Neuropsychologia* 30:293–297, 1992.

27. Metcalfe J, Funnell M, Gazzaniga MS: Right hemi-

sphere memory superiority: Studies of a split-brain patient. *Psychol Sci* 6:157–164, 1995.

28. Gazzaniga MS: *Consciousness and the Cerebral Hemispheres. The Cognitive Neurosciences.* Cambridge, MA: MIT Press, 1995, pp 1391–1400.

29. Gazzaniga MS, Smylie CS: Dissociation of language and cognition. *Brain* 107:145–153, 1984.

30. Milner B, Taylor L: Right hemisphere superiority in tactile pattern recognition after cerebral commissurotomy: Evidence for non-verbal memory. *Neuropsychologia* 10:1–15, 1972.

31. Farah MJ, Gazzaniga MS, Holtzman JD, Kosslyn SM: A left hemisphere basis for visual mental imagery? *Neuropsychologia* 23:115–118, 1985.

32. Gazzaniga MS: Organization of the human brain. *Science* 245:947–952, 1989.

33. Levy J, Trevarthen CB, Sperry RW: Perception of bilateral chimeric figures following hemispheric deconnection. *Brain* 95:61–78, 1972.

34. Gazzaniga MS, Smylie CS: Facial recognition and brain asymmetries: Clues to underlying mechanisms. *Ann Neurol* 13:536–540, 1983.

35. Gazzaniga MS, Smylie CS: Hemispheric mechanisms controlling voluntary and spontaneous facial expressions. *J Cogn Neurosci* 2:239–245, 1990.

36. Gazzaniga MS: Principles of human brain organization derived from split-brain studies. *Neuron* 14:217–228, 1995.

37. Seymour S, Reuter-Lorenz PA, Gazzaniga MS: The disconnection syndrome: Basic findings reaffirmed. *Brain* 117:105–115, 1994.

38. Holtzman JD, Sidtis JJ, Volpe BT, et al: Dissociation of spatial information for stimulus localization and the control of attention. *Brain* 104:861–872, 1981.

39. Sergent J: Unified response to bilateral hemispheric stimulation by a split-brain patient. *Nature* 305:800–802, 1983.

40. Sergent J: Furtive incursions into bicameral minds. *Brain* 113:537–568, 1990.

41. Corballis MC: Can commissurotomized subjects compare digits between the visual fields? *Neuropsychologia* 32:1475–1486, 1994.

42. Kingstone A, Gazzaniga MS: Higher-order subcortical processing in the split-brain patient: More illusory than real? *Neuropsychologia* 9:321–328, 1995.

43. Stone J: The naso-temporal division of the monkey retina. *J Comp Neurol* 136:585–600, 1966.

44. Fukuda Y, Sawai H, Watanabe M, et al: Nasotemporal overlap of crossed and uncrossed retinal ganglion cell projections in the Japanese monkey (Macaca fuscata). *J Neurosci* 9:2353–2373, 1989.

45. Fendrich R, Wessinger CM, Gazzaniga MS: Nasotemporal overlap at the retinal vertical meridian: Investigations with a callosotomy patient. *Neuropsychologia.* In press.

46. Fendrich R, Gazzaniga MS: Evidence of foveal splitting in a commissurotomy patient. *Neuropsychologia* 27:273–281, 1989.

47. Holtzman JD, Volpe BT, Gazzaniga MS: Spatial orientation following commissural section, in Parasuraman R, Davies DR (eds): *Varieties of Attention.* New York: Academic Press, 1984, pp 375–394.

48. Holtzman JD: Interactions between cortical and subcortical visual areas: evidence from human commissurotomy patients. *Vision Res* 24:801–813, 1984.

49. Holtzman JD, Gazzaniga MS: Dual task interactions due exclusively to limits in processing resources. *Science* 218:1325–1327, 1982.

50. Holtzman JD, Gazzaniga MS: Enhanced dual task performance following callosal commissurotomy in humans. *Neuropsychologia* 23:315–321, 1985.

51. Luck SJ, Hillyard SA, Mangun GR, Gazzaniga MS: Independent hemispheric attentional systems mediate visual search in split-brain patients. *Nature* 342:543–545, 1989.

52. Mangun GR, Plager R, Loftus W, et al: Monitoring the visual world: Hemispheric asymmetries and subcortical processes in attention. *J Cogn Neurosci* 6:265–273, 1994.

53. Reuter-Lorenz P, Fendrich R: Orienting attention across the vertical meridian: Evidence from callosotomy patients. *J Cogn Neurosci* 2:232–238, 1990.

54. Risse GL, Gates J, Lund G, et al: Interhemispheric transfer in patients with incomplete section of the corpus callosum: Anatomic verification with magnetic resonance imaging. *Arch Neurol* 46:437–443, 1989.

55. Sidtis JJ, Volpe BT, Holtzman JD, et al: Cognitive interaction after staged callosal section: Evidence for transfer of semantic activation. *Science* 212:344–346, 1981.

56. Gazzaniga MS, Kutas M, Van Petten C, Fendrich R: Human callosal function: MRI-verified neuropsychological functions. *Neurology* 39:942–946, 1989.

57. Baynes K, Tramo MJ, Reeves AG, Gazzaniga MS: Isolation of a right hemisphere cognitive system in a patient with anarchic hand syndrome. Submitted.

Chapter 27

DISORDERS OF SKILLED MOVEMENTS

Kenneth M. Heilman
Robert T. Watson
Leslie J. Gonzalez Rothi

Apraxia is an inability to correctly perform learned skilled movements. In part, it is defined by what it is not.[1] Patients with impaired motor performance induced by weakness, sensory loss, tremors, dystonia, chorea, ballismus, athetosis, myoclonus, ataxia, and seizures are not considered apraxic. Patients with severe cognitive, memory, motivational, and attentional disorders may have difficulty performing skilled motor acts because they cannot comprehend, cooperate, remember, or attend, but these deficits are also not considered apraxic.

Limb apraxia may be the most frequently unrecognized behavioral disorder associated with cerebral disease. It is most often associated with strokes and degenerative dementia of the Alzheimer type but also occurs with a variety of other diseases. Apraxia may be the presenting symptom and sign in cortical basal ganglionic degeneration.

Apraxia may go unrecognized for several reasons. The apraxia associated with strokes is often accompanied by weakness of the preferred arm. In attempting to perform skilled acts with the nonpreferred arm, apraxic patients may recognize that they are not performing well, but they may attribute their difficulty in performing skilled acts to the inexperience of this nondominant arm or to premorbid clumsiness of the nonpreferred arm. However, even when using their dominant limb, apraxic patients may be anosognosic for their apraxia[2] and therefore will not complain of a problem in performing skilled movements. Fi-

nally, many physicians and other health professionals do not test for limb apraxia and are not aware of the nature of errors that are associated with it or that it may be a disabling disorder.

The subtypes of limb apraxia are defined by the nature of errors made by the patient and the means by which these errors are elicited. Liepmann[3] subdivided limb apraxic disorders into three types: melokinetic (or limb-kinetic), ideomotor, and ideational. In addition to discussing these forms of apraxia, we will also discuss three additional forms of apraxia we have called disassociation apraxia, conduction apraxia, and conceptual apraxia. The apraxias are differentiated by the types of errors made by the patient and the means by which these errors are elicited.

Apraxia Testing

The physician must perform a thorough neurologic examination to be certain that abnormal performance is not induced by the nonapraxic motor, sensory, or cognitive disorders mentioned above. The presence of elemental motor defects does not prohibit apraxia testing; however, the examiner must interpret the results with the knowledge gained from the neurologic examination.

Both the right and left arm and hands should be tested independently. Patients should be requested to pantomime to verbal command (e.g., "Show me how you would use a pair of scissors"). All patients should also be asked to imitate the examiner's motor acts. The examiner may want to perform both meaningful and meaningless gestures for the patient to imitate. Independent of the results of the pantomime and imitation tests, the patient should be given actual objects and tools and asked to demonstrate how to use the tool or object. One should test transitive movements (i.e., using a tool or instrument) and intransitive movements (i.e., communicative gestures not using tools, such as waving good-bye). When having a patient pantomime, in addition to giving verbal commands, the examiner may also want to show the patient a tool or a picture of the tool or object that the patient is required to pantomime. It may be valuable to see if the patient can recognize transitive and intransitive pantomimes performed by the examiner and discriminate between those that are well and poorly performed. The patient should be given a task that requires several motor acts in sequence. Last, one may want to learn if the patient knows what tools operate on what objects (e.g., hammer and nail), what action is associated with each tool or object, and how to fabricate tools to solve mechanical problems.

LIMB KINETIC APRAXIA

In limb kinetic apraxia, there is a loss of the ability to make finely graded, precise, individual finger movements. Limb kinetic apraxia occurs in the limb contralateral to a hemispheric lesion. Lawrence and Kuypers[4] demonstrated that monkeys with lesions confined to the corticospinal system show similar errors. Because limb kinetic apraxia may be an elemental motor disorder rather than a disorder of learned skilled movements, it will not be discussed in this chapter.

IDEOMOTOR APRAXIA

Clinical Findings

Typically, the patient with ideomotor apraxia (IMA) makes the most errors when asked to pantomime transitive acts, typically improves with imitation, and may perform the best when using actual objects.

We classify apraxic errors as errors of content or of production.[5] In order to be considered as having IMA, a patient should make primarily production errors. Content errors occur when a patient substitutes another recognizable pantomime for the target pantomime. For example, when asked to pantomime using scissors, a patient may demonstrate hammering movements. Occasionally, a patient's performance is so profoundly impaired that the examiner cannot recognize the movement. When patients with IMA pantomime, their pantomimes may be incorrectly produced, but the goal or intent of the act can usually be recognized as correct.

Patients with IMA make two major types of production errors: spatial and temporal. Spatial errors can be divided into several subtypes, including postural (or internal configuration), spatial movement, and spatial orientation errors. Regarding postural errors, Goodglass and Kaplan[6] note that when apraxic patients are asked to pantomime, they often use a body part as the tool. For example, when patients with IMA are asked to pantomime using a pair of scissors, they may use their fingers as if they were the blades. Many normal subjects may make a similar error; therefore, it is imperative that the patient be instructed not to use a body part as a tool. Patients with IMA may continue to make errors using body parts as tools in spite of these instructions. Patients with IMA will often fail to position their hands as if they were holding the tool or object they were requested to pantomime.

When normal subjects are asked to use a tool, they will orient that tool to the target of that tool action (whether real or imaginary). Patients with IMA often fail to orient their forelimbs to a real or imaginary target. For example, when asked to pantomime cutting a piece of paper in half with a scissor, rather than keeping the scissors oriented in the sagittal plane, the patient may orient the scissors laterally.[5]

When making spatial movement or trajectory errors, patients with IMA will often make the correct core movement (e.g., twisting, pounding, cutting) but will not move their limb correctly through space.[5,7] These spatial trajectory errors are associated with incorrect joint movements such that frequently the apraxic patients will stabilize a joint that should be moving and move joints that should be stabilized. For example, in pantomiming the use of a screwdriver, the patient with IMA may rotate his arm at the shoulder joint and fix his elbow. Shoulder rotation moves the hand in circles rather than rotating the hand on a fixed axis. When multiple joint movements must be coordinated, the patient may be unable to coordinate the movement to get the desired spatial trajectory. For example, in pantomiming the sawing of wood, the shoulder and elbow joints must be alternatively flexed and extended. When the joint movements are not well coordinated, the patient may make primarily chopping or stabbing movements.

Poizner and colleagues[7] have noted that patients with IMA may make timing errors, including a long delay before initiating a movement and brief multiple stops (stuttering movements). Patients with IMA often do not demonstrate a smooth sinusoidal hand speed when they perform cyclic movements, such as cutting with a knife.

Pathophysiology

Whereas in right-handed individuals, IMA is almost always associated with left-hemisphere lesions, in left-handers IMA is usually associated with right-hemisphere lesions. Ideomotor apraxia can be induced by lesions in a variety of structures, including the corpus callosum, the inferior parietal lobe, and the supplementary motor area. IMA has also been reported with subcortical lesions that involve basal ganglia and white matter. Below, each of these anatomic areas is discussed and an attempt is made to develop a model of how the brain mediates learned skilled motor activity of the limbs.

Corpus Callosum In 1907 Liepmann and Maas[8] described a patient with a right hemiparesis from a lesion of the pons and a lesion of the corpus callosum. This patient was unable to pantomime correctly to command with his left arm. Because this patient had a right hemiparesis, his right hand could not be tested. Since the work of Broca and Wernicke, we have known that right-handers' left hemisphere is dominant for language. Liepmann and Maas could have attributed their patient's inability to pantomime to a disconnection between language and motor areas, such that the left hemisphere, which mediates comprehension of the verbal command, could not influence the right hemisphere, which is responsible for controlling the left hand. However, this patient could also not imitate gestures or use actual objects correctly, and language-motor disconnection could not account for these findings. Liepmann and Maas therefore posited that the left hemisphere of right-handers contains movement formulas (or spatiotemporal representations of movements) and that the callosal lesion disconnects these movement formulas from the motor areas of the right hemisphere.

Geschwind and Kaplan[9] and Gazzaniga and coworkers[10] found that their patients with callosal disconnection, unlike the callosal patient of Liepmann and Maas, could not correctly pantomime to command with the left hand but could imitate and correctly use actual objects with this hand, suggesting that the apraxia of callosal disconnection in these patients was induced by a language-motor disconnection. In addition, many of the errors made by the patient of Liepmann and Maas appeared to be content errors. However, Watson and Heilman[11] described a patient with an infarction of the body of the corpus callosum. The patient reported by Watson and Heilman had no weakness in her right hand and performed all tasks flawlessly with that hand; with her left hand, however, she could not correctly pantomime to command, imitate, or use actual objects. Although early in her course she made content errors, she subsequently made spatial and temporal errors. Her performance indicated that not only language but also movement representations were stored in the left hemisphere and her callosal lesion disconnected these movement formulas from the right hemisphere.

Inferior Parietal Lobe Whereas Geschwind[1] proposed that the ideomotor apraxia associated with left-sided parietal lesions was inducing a language motor disconnection, Heilman and colleagues[12] and Rothi and coworkers[13] proposed that the movement representations or movement formulas were stored in the left parietal lobe of right-handers and that destruction of the left parietal lobe should induce not only a production deficit (apraxia) but also a gesture comprehension/discrimination disorder. Apraxia induced by premotor lesions, lesions of the pathways that connect premotor areas to motor areas, or the pathways that lead to the premotor areas from the parietal lobe may also cause a production deficit. In contrast to parietal lesions, however, these lesions should not induce gesture comprehension/discrimination disorders. Heilman and colleagues[12] and Rothi and associates[13] tested patients with anterior and posterior lesions and found that while both groups were apraxic, the patients with a damaged parietal lobe had comprehension-discrimination disturbances and those with more anterior lesions did not.

Liepmann proposed that handedness was related to the hemispheric laterality of the movement representation. It is not unusual, however, to see right-handed patients with left-hemisphere lesions who are not apraxic. Although it is possible that these patients' lesions did not destroy a critical left-hemisphere area, it is also possible that not all right-handers have movement formulas entirely represented in their left hemisphere. Some people may have either bilateral movement representations or even right-hemisphere representations. Apraxia from a right-hemisphere lesion in a right-hander is rare but has been reported, suggesting that hand preference is not entirely determined by the laterality of the movement representations and may be multifactorial. Whereas the laterality of the movement formula may be the most important factor, there are other factors including primary motor factors such as strength, speed, precision, attentional factors, and even environmental factors.

Supplementary Motor Area Muscles move joints, and motor nerves from the spinal cord activate these muscles. The motor nerves are activated by corticospinal neurons. The corticospinal tract neurons are, in turn, activated by the premotor areas.

For each specific skilled movement there is a set of spatial loci that must be traversed in a specific temporal pattern. We proposed that movement formulas that are represented in the inferior parietal lobe are stored in a three-dimensional supramodal code. Although Geschwind[1] thought that the convexity premotor cortex was important for praxis, apraxia has not been reported from a lesion limited to this cortex, and its function in the control of praxis remains unknown. The convexity premotor cortex may be important in motor learning or in adapting the program to environmental pertubations.

The medial premotor cortex or supplementary motor area (SMA), however, appears to play an important role in mediating skilled movements. Whereas electrical stimulation of the primary motor cortex induces simple movements, SMA stimulation induces complex movements of the fingers, arms, and hands. The SMA receives projections from parietal neurons and projects to motor neurons. The SMA neurons appear to discharge before neurons in the primary motor cortex. Studies of cerebral blood flow, an indicator of cerebral metabolism, have revealed that a single repetitive movement increases activation of the contralateral motor cortex, but complex movements increase flow in the contralateral motor cortex and bilaterally in the SMA. When subjects remain still and think about making complex movements, blood flow to the SMA but not to the motor cortex is increased. Watson and coworkers[14] reported several patients with left-sided medial frontal lesions that included the SMA who demonstrated an ideomotor apraxia when tested with either arm. Unlike patients with parietal lesions, these patients could both comprehend and discriminate pantomimes.

The model we have discussed so far is illustrated in Fig. 27-1. The praxicon is a theoretical store of the temporospatial representations of learned skill movements. When a skilled act is being performed, these representations are transcoded into innervatory patterns by the SMA.

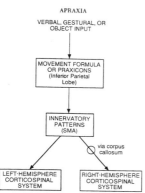

Figure 27-1

Diagrammatic model of ideomotor apraxia. SMA = supplementary motor area. (From Heilman and Rothi,[20] with permission.)

When the right-hand acts, the SMA programs the motor cortex (Brodmann's area 4) of the left hemisphere, and when the left hand acts, these innervatory patterns activate the motor regions of the right hemisphere via the corpus callosum.

DISASSOCIATION APRAXIAS

Clinical Findings

Heilman[15] described several patients who, when asked to pantomime to command, looked at their open hands or would slowly pronate and supinate their arms and hands but would not perform any recognizable action. Unlike the patients with ideomotor apraxia described above, these patients' imitations and use of objects were flawless. De Renzi and colleagues[16] reported patients similar to those reported by Heilman[15] and also other patients who had a similar defect in other modalities. For example, when asked to pantomime in response to visual or tactile stimuli, they may have been unable to do so, but they could pantomime to verbal command.

Pathophysiology

While callosal lesions may be associated with an ideomotor apraxia, callosal disconnection may also cause disassociation apraxia. The subjects of

Gazzaniga and associates and the patients described by Geschwind and Kaplan had disassociation apraxia. Whereas language in these patients was mediated by the left hemisphere, we posit that movement representations may have been bilaterally represented, and a callosal lesion induced a disassociation apraxia only of the left hand. Whereas the patient with callosal disassociation apraxia will not be able to correctly carry out skilled learned movements of the left arm to command, he or she will be able to imitate and use actual objects with the left hand. Patients with callosal disassociation apraxia will be unable to carry out movements to verbal command because the movement formulas in the right hemisphere have been disconnected from the left hemisphere, which mediates language. The patient with bilateral movement representation can imitate and use actual objects flawlessly with the left hand because these tasks do not require language and the patient's right hemisphere contains the movement formula and the other apparatus needed to transcode the time-space movement representations to motor acts.

Right-handed patients who have both language and movement formula represented in their left hemisphere may show a combination of disassociation and ideomotor apraxia with callosal lesions.[11] When asked to pantomime with their left hands, they may look at them and perform no recognizable movement (disassociation apraxia); but when imitating or using actual objects, they may demonstrate the spatial and temporal errors seen with ideomotor apraxia.

Left-handers may demonstrate an ideomotor apraxia with aphasia from a right-hemisphere lesion. These left-handers are apraxic because their movement representations were stored in their right hemispheres and their lesions destroyed these representations.[17,18] These left-handers were not aphasic because language was mediated by their left hemispheres (as is the case in the majority of left-handers). If these left-handers had a callosal lesion, they may have demonstrated a disassociation apraxia of the left arm and an ideomotor apraxia of the right arm.

The disassociation apraxia described by

Heilman[15] from left-hemisphere lesions was unfortunately incorrectly termed "ideational apraxia." The patients reported by Heilman[15] and those of De Renzi and associates[16] probably have an intrahemispheric language-movement formula, visual-movement formula, or somesthetic-movement formula disassociation. The locations of the lesions that cause these intrahemispheric disassociation apraxias are not known.

CONDUCTION APRAXIA

Clinical Findings

Ochipa and coworkers[19] reported a patient who, unlike patients with ideomotor apraxia who usually improve with imitation, was more impaired when imitating than when pantomiming to command.

Pathophysiology

Because this patient with conduction apraxia could comprehend the examiner's pantomime and gestures, we believe that the patient's visual system could access the movement representations, or what we have termed praxicons,[20] and that the activated movement representations could activate semantics. It is possible that decoding a gesture requires accessing different movement representations than does programming an action. Therefore, Ochipa and colleagues[19] and Rothi and coworkers[21] suggested that there may be two different stores of movement representations, an input praxicon and output praxicon. In the verbal domain, a disconnection of the hypothetical input and output lexicons induces conduction aphasia; in the praxis domain, a disconnection between the input and output praxicons could induce conduction apraxia.

Whereas the lesions that induce conduction aphasia are usually in the supramarginal gyrus or Wernicke's area, the location of lesions that induce conduction apraxia are unknown.

IDEATIONAL APRAXIA

Unfortunately, there has been much confusion about the meaning of the term *ideational apraxia*. The inability to carry out a series of acts, an ideational plan, has been called ideational apraxia.[22,23] In performing a task that requires a series of acts, these patients have difficulty sequencing the acts in the proper order (for example, instead of cleaning the pipe, putting tobacco in the bowl, lighting the tobacco, and smoking, the patient might attempt to light the empty bowl, put the tobacco in the bowl, and then clean it). Pick[23] noted that most of the patients with this type of ideational apraxia have a dementing disease.

Whereas most patients with ideational apraxia improve when they are using objects. De Renzi and colleagues[24] reported patients who made errors with the use of actual objects. Although the inability to use actual objects may be associated with a conceptual disorder, a severe production disorder may also impair object use.[25] However, as we will discuss in the next section, production and conceptual disorders may be associated with different types of errors.

CONCEPTUAL APRAXIA

Clinical Findings

To perform a skilled act, two types of knowledge are needed: conceptual knowledge and production knowledge. Dysfunction of the praxis production system induces ideomotor apraxia. Defects in the knowledge needed to successfully select and use the tools and objects we term conceptual apraxia. Whereas patients with ideomotor apraxia make production errrors (e.g., spatial and temporal errors), patients with conceptual apraxia make content and tool-selection errors. The patients with conceptual apraxia may not recall the types of actions associated with specific tools, utensils, or objects (tool-object action knowledge) and therefore make content errrors.[26,27] For example, when asked to demonstrate the use of a screwdriver, either pantomining or using the tool, the patient with the loss of tool-object action knowledge may pantomime a hammering movement or use the screwdrivers as if it were a hammer.

The patient with ideomotor apraxia may make production errors by moving the hand in circles rather than twisting the hand on its own axis. Although such patients make production errors by moving the hand in circles, they are demonstrating knowledge of the turning action of screwdrivers. Content errors (i.e., using a tool as if it were another tool) can also be induced by an object agnosia. However, Ochipa and associates[27] reported a patient who could name tools (and therefore was not agnosic) but often used them inappropriately.

Patients with conceptual apraxia may be unable to recall which specific tool is associated with a specific object (tool–object association knowledge). For example, when shown a partially driven nail, they may select a screwdriver rather than a hammer from an array of tools. This conceptual defect may also be in the verbal domain, such that when an actual tool is shown to a patient with conceptual apraxia, the patient may be able to name it (e.g., hammer); but when the patient is asked to name or point to a tool when its function is discussed, he or she cannot. The patient may also be unable to describe the functions of tools.

Patients with conceptual apraxia may also have impaired mechanical knowledge. For example, if they are attempting to drive a nail into a piece of wood and there is no hammer available, they may select a screwdriver rather than a wrench or pliers (which are hard, heavy, and good for pounding).[28] Mechanical knowledge is also important for tool development, and patients with ideational apraxia may be unable to develop tools correctly.[28]

Pathophysiology

Liepmann[3] thought that conceptual knowledge was located in the caudal parietal lobe, and De Renzi and Luccelli[26] placed it in the temporoparietal junction. The patient reported by Ochipa and coworkers[27] was left-handed and rendered conceptually apraxic by a lesion in the right hemisphere, suggesting that both production and conceptual knowledge have lateralized representations and that such representations are contralateral to the preferred hand. Further evidence that these conceptual representations are lateralized contralateral to the preferred hand comes from the observation of a patient who had a callosal disconnection and demonstrated conceptual apraxia of the nonpreferred (left) hand.[11] However, conceptual apraxia is perhaps most commonly seen in degenerative dementia of the Alzheimer type.[28] Ochipa and colleagues also noted that the severity of conceptual and ideomotor apraxia did not always correlate. The observation that patients with ideomotor apraxia may not demonstrate conceptual apraxia and patients with conceptual apraxia may not demonstrate ideomotor apraxia provides support for the postulate that the praxis production and praxis conceptual systems are independent. However, for normal function, these two systems must interact.

CONCLUSIONS

On the basis of material discussed in this chapter, it appears that movement representations (praxicons) are stored in the left inferior parietal lobe of right-handers. These representations code the spatial and temporal patterns of learned skilled movements. Injury to the parietal lobe induces a production deficit termed ideomotor apraxia. Patients with ideomotor apraxia make spatial and temporal errors. Patients with injury to these representations are not only impaired at pantomiming, imitating, and using actual objects but also cannot discriminate between well- and poorly performed gestures. These patients may also not be able to comprehend gestures.

There are patients who are more impaired at imitation of gestures than they are when gesturing to command (conduction apraxia), suggesting that movement representations (praxicons) may be divided into input and output subdivisions. In conduction apraxia, there is a dissociation between these input and output praxicons.

In order to perform learned skilled acts, these abstract movement representations have to be transcoded into motor programs. This transcoding appears to be performed by a premotor (supplementary motor area)–basal ganglia (putamen-globus pallidus-thalamus) system. Injuries to the brain that interrupt the connections between the movement representations stored in the parietal lobe and the portions of the brain that develop the innervatory patterns or the parts of the brain that allow the innervatory patterns to gain access to the motor system may also produce a praxis production deficit (ideomotor apraxia).

A patient may have intact representations of learned skilled movements but have modality-specific deficits in accessing these representations. For example, a patient with dissociation apraxia may be unable to pantomime to command but be able to pantomime correctly when seeing the tool.

Last, some patients, when pantomiming or using actual tools, may make content errors. Whereas spatial and temporal errors are related to deficits in the praxic production system, content errors are related to deficits in a hypothetical praxis conceptual system or action semantics. Dysfunction of this system, termed conceptual apraxia, may produce deficits of associative knowledge, such as tool-action or tool-object knowledge (i.e., knowing that a hammer is used to pound and that a hammer is associated with a nail). Defects in action semantics may also be associated with deficits in mechanical knowledge (i.e., knowing how to use alternative tools and how to fabricate tools).

REFERENCES

1. Geschwind N: Disconnection syndromes in animals and man. *Brain* 88:237–294, 585–644, 1965.
2. Rothi LJG, Mack L, Heilman KM: Unawareness of apraxic errors. *Neurology* 40(suppl 1):202, 1990.
3. Liepmann H: Apraxia. *Erbgn Ges Med* 1:516–543, 1920.
4. Lawrence DG, Kuypers HGJM: The functional organization of the motor system in the monkey. *Brain* 91:1–36, 1968.
5. Rothi LJG, Mack L, Verfaellie M, et al: Ideomotor apraxia: Error pattern analysis. *Aphasiology* 2:381–387, 1988.
6. Goodglass H, Kaplan E: Disturbance of gesture and pantomime in aphasia. *Brain* 86:703–720, 1963.
7. Poizner H, Mack L, Verfaellie M, et al: Three dimensional computer graphic analysis of apraxia. *Brain* 113:85–101, 1990.
8. Liepmann H, Mass O: Fall von linksseitiger Agraphie und Apraxie bei rechsseitiger Lahmung. *Z Psychol Neurol* 10:214–227, 1907.
9. Geschwind N, Kaplan E: A human cerebral disconnection syndrome. *Neurology* 12:675–685, 1962.
10. Gazzaniga M, Bogen J, Sperry R: Dyspraxia following diversion of the cerebral commisures. *Arch Neurol* 16:606–612, 1967.
11. Watson RT, Heilman KM: Callosal apraxia. *Brain* 106:391–403, 1983.
12. Heilman KM, Rothi LJ, Valenstein E: Two forms of ideomotor apraxia. *Neurology* 32:342–346, 1982.
13. Rothi LJG, Heilman KM, Watson RT: Pantomime comprehension and ideomotor apraxia. *J Neurol Neurosurg Psychiatry* 48:207–210, 1985.
14. Watson RT, Fleet WS, Rothi LJG, Heilman KM: Apraxia and the supplementary motor area. *Arch Neurol* 43:787–792, 1986.
15. Heilman KM: Ideational apraxia—A re-definition. *Brain* 96:861–864, 1973.
16. De Renzi E, Faglioni P, Sorgato P: Modality-specific and supramodal mechanisms of apraxia. *Brain* 105:301–312, 1982.
17. Heilman KM, Coyle JM, Gonyea EF, Geschwind N: Apraxia and agraphia in a left-hander. *Brain* 96:21–28, 1973.
18. Valenstein E, Heilman KM: Apraxic agraphia with neglect induced paragraphia. *Arch Neurol* 36:506–508, 1979.
19. Ochipa C, Rothi LJG, Heilman KM: Conduction apraxia. *J Clin Exp Neuropsychol* 12:89, 1990.
20. Heilman KM, Rothi LJG: Apraxia, in Heilman KM, Valenstein E (eds): *Clinical Neuropsychology,* 3d ed. New York: Oxford University Press, 1993.
21. Rothi LJG, Ochipa C, Heilman KM: A cognitive neuropsychological model of limb praxis. *Cogn Neuropsychol* 8:443–458, 1991.
22. Marcuse H: Apraktiscke Symotome bein linem Fall von seniler Demenz. *Zentralbl Mervheik Psychiatr* 27:737–751, 1904.
23. Pick A: *Studien über Motorische Apraxia und ihre Mahestenhende Erscheinungen.* Leipzig: Deuticke, 1905.
24. De Renzi E, Pieczuro A, Vignolo L: Ideational

apraxia: A quantitative study. *Neuropsychologia* 6:41–52, 1968.

25. Zangwell OL: L'apraxie ideatorie. *Nerve Neurol* 106:595–603, 1960.

26. De Renzi E, Lucchelli F: Ideational apraxia. *Brain* 113:1173–1188, 1988.

27. Ochipa C, Rothi LJG, Heilman KM: Ideational apraxia: A deficit in tool selection and use. *Ann Neurol* 25:190–193, 1989.

28. Ochipa C, Rothi LJG, Heilman KM: Conceptual apraxia in Alzheimer's disease. *Brain* 115:1061–1071, 1992.

Chapter 28

ACALCULIA

Jordan Grafman
Timothy Rickard

Acalculia is defined as an impairment of the ability to calculate. It is used interchangeably with the term *dyscalculia,* although some authors have suggested reserving the term *acalculia* for a complete inability to calculate and using the term *dyscalculia* in cases where some ability to calculate remains. In this chapter we use the term *acalculia* to refer to both forms of impairment.

Acalculia is a frequently appearing deficit following damage to the left posterior region of the brain, but it can occur following damage to other brain regions. It is a significant functional deficit for patients, since it may restrict their ability to use a checkbook, pay bills, exchange money, or plan activities. Acalculia is also an opportunity for clinical researchers interested in the organization of cognitive architectures, response execution, lexical-semantic stores, and the cooperation between fact-based and analogue-scaled cognitive processes to study these processes within the context of a relatively narrow domain of knowledge.

In this chapter, we review the contemporary cognitive neuropsychological approach to the study of calculation disorders, discuss current models of normal and abnormal calculation processing, and cautiously attempt to specify which aspects of numeric computation can be mapped to brain regions. These sections are followed by our suggestions for a comprehensive assessment of calculation and number processing disorders.

DESCRIPTION AND INCIDENCE OF ACALCULIA

There are a number of general classification schemes for describing forms of acalculia, which have divided acalculia into three broad types.[1] Type 1 is a secondary form of acalculia due to deficits in verbal processing. Type 2 is also a secondary form of acalculia and is due to deficits in visuospatial processing. Type 3 is the primary form of acalculia, which is independent of (but may coexist with) any other cognitive deficit. A *primary acalculia* has been described in individual cases and made up approximately 6 percent of acalculic patients with right-hemispheric lesions and 23 percent of acalculic patients with left-hemispheric lesions.

DEVELOPMENT OF NUMBER PROCESSING AND CALCULATION SKILLS

Some elements of calculation are preliterate and perhaps innate in origin. People without formal schooling can develop procedural skills related to counting, numerosity, and magnitude estimation. Numerical abilities at very young ages, however, appear to be limited to small numerical values.[2] An example is the ability to *subitize,* or quickly judge the number of a small group of items (e.g., dots on a page) without having to count them. This ability, which has been demonstrated in infants and monkeys as well as in adults, appears to be limited to set sizes of 4 or 5. Other elements of calculation—such as formal calculation procedures, number fact retrieval (e.g., $9 \times 9 = ?$), and estimation skills for large numbers—are generally learned with formal training. Children initially learn counting strategies for calculation, but these strategies are eventually replaced by fact retrieval skills.[3,4] Educators believe that extensive experience with procedural strategies and representational models of the calculation process is essential for the mastery of calculation. We refer the reader to papers by Dehaene,[5] Nesher,[6] Resnick,[7] and by Siegler and Shrager[8] for a comprehensive look at developmental changes in normal calculation ability, and to Gross and colleagues,[9] Lyytinen and coworkers,[10] Shalev and associates[11] for detailed discussions of developmental acalculia.

HISTORICAL SKETCH OF RESEARCH IN ACALCULIA

Brain-Behavior Correlates

Primary acalculia can take the form of either global or selective deficits in a large number of number processing and calculation abilities, including comprehension of numbers and numerical magnitude, performance on single-digit arithmetic operations, execution of procedures (such as carrying and borrowing, necessary for complex arithmetic), and solving of word problems. A large number of studies have implicated left posterior lesions in primary acalculia, most often in the vicinity of the left angular and supramarginal gyri.[12–15] In particular, the evidence suggests that arithmetic facts and calculation procedures are preferentially stored in that brain region.

Despite the strong association of acalculia and left posterior quadrant lesions, there are certain characteristics of acalculia that have led to the suggestion of a right-hemispheric contribution. The finding that acalculia can result from poor placement of digits in a multidigit problem suggests that right-hemispheric processes contribute to the spatial construction of a problem solution

if not its actual calculation.[15] Other work has suggested that magnitude estimation (e.g., which is larger, 3 or 4?) is a scaling process linked with the right hemisphere.[16] Estimation of magnitude is important in a number of real-world situations where a quick, approximate answer is adequate, and it appears also to provide a way to converge on the exact answer to simple and complex arithmetic problems, particularly when an answer has not been memorized. A contribution of magnitude processes to arithmetic may help explain results of a functional imaging study of Rueckert and colleagues in which a simple subtract-by-7's task activated not only the left angular gyrus and frontal cortex (the latter presumably reflecting a working memory component of the task, see Chaps. 22 and 25) but in most subjects the right parietal region as well.[17]

However, it appears that arithmetic facts and calculation procedures on one hand and spatial and magnitude processes on the other are not completely lateralized to the left and right hemispheres, respectively. Grafman and coworkers[15] found that patients with left-hemispheric lesions also made a large number of spatial errors (e.g., column misalignment). It has been claimed that magnitude estimation might be represented in the right cerebral cortex; however, in a functional neuroimaging study, magnitude estimation has been reported to activate left- as well as right-hemispheric brain regions.[18] To date, carefully controlled structural magnetic resonance imaging studies have not been done to demonstrate a clear effect of right posterior lesions on primary calculation ability.

In conclusion, the overwhelming evidence suggests that arithmetic facts and calculation procedures are stored in the left parietal cortex. However, a contribution of frontal lobe[19] and right parietal processes is also implicated. A more precise delineation of these contributions awaits further investigation.

Associated Deficits

Acalculia is often associated with other cognitive impairment by virtue of the location of the lesions that cause primary acalculia and because of the relationship of the domain-specific calculation procedures to other cognitive processes. Finger agnosia, agraphia, and right-left discrimination are frequently observed together with acalculia following left posterior cortical lesions, but each symptom may occur as frequently with other symptoms. This tetrad of symptoms is known collectively as the Gerstmann syndrome, and its appearance has been associated with lesions of the left angular gyrus.[20,21] Other symptoms associated with primary acalculia have included alexia, visuospatial deficits, and conduction aphasia. On-line serial calculations may involve working memory processes. Thus, a breakdown in serial calculation (as opposed to simple fact retrieval) may be associated with a general deficit in working memory, word fluency, or planning.

The Gerstmann syndrome symptom collection at first may seem like the odd quartet. Odd, that is, until it is remembered that preliterate calculation depended upon counting, numerosity, and magnitude estimation. Since counting often relied upon fingers, with fingers on different hands representing different quantities, it should not be completely surprising that calculation, finger recognition, left-right discrimination, and writing ability could all be impaired following an angular gyrus lesion.

Modular Aspects

Acalculia has been noted to be the initial symptom of degenerative dementias,[22] the outstanding symptom following a stroke, and the main symptom in several developmental disorders. These observations suggest that primary acalculia could be a result of a dysfunction in a modular system, that is, a system that is specialized for calculation. The modules impaired in these cases could be devoted to number fact storage (categorized perhaps by operation), and potentially to the actual calculation procedure (in the case of novel problems). Whether the procedure and the fact-retrieval stores are overlapping, adjacent, or distant remains to be adjudicated.

Numerous case studies indicate that selective fact retrieval for one or more of the basic operations is possible.[23–25] These selective deficits can appear independently of other cognitive impairment, suggesting that the modular approach applies even to the level of the individual arithmetic operation. Indeed, there is even a case study describing a more specific deficit for processing arithmetic problems involving only the numbers 7 or 9.[26] This deficit could not be attributed to a secondary acalculia (such as deficits in auditory lexicon or visual analysis) and were interpreted as reflecting a deficit in the semantic, or abstract, level of representation for those numbers. Whether these sorts of deficits are best understood as reflecting a very fine-grained modularity or as selective damage to parts of larger networks is still an open question. However, these and other data on number processing and calculation tasks do demonstrate, perhaps better than any other neuropsychological data to date, the hyperspecificity of function that can occur in at least some regions of the brain.

The evidence that argues for the modularity of various calculation skills was originally based on rather gross neuropsychological analyses. Over the last 15 years, however, a plethora of cognitive arithmetic models have been developed that offers the clinician and investigator exciting new hypotheses regarding the storage and retrieval of number facts and procedures. A few of these are described broadly in the next section.

CONTEMPORARY COGNITIVE MODELS AND THEIR FRACTIONATION IN ACALCULIA

The empirical research of many investigators, including Warrington, Deloche and Seron, and McCloskey, among others, has now established a solid empiric base on which to build functional cognitive models of number processing and calculation. In a seminal paper, Warrington[27] reported on a patient with a left parietal-occipital lobe lesion who was found to have an outstanding problem in calculation. Warrington noted that the patient had a particular deficit in arithmetic fact retrieval on all operations, even though his arithmetic knowledge—estimation and counting, number reading, and number writing—were all preserved.

At about the same time, Deloche and Seron[28] were conducting analyses of patients' ability to transcode between Arabic numerals and word numbers. Length of the number word but not Arabic numeral was an important factor in producing errors. Morphologic structure appeared to be maintained in the transcoding process. There was some regularity in patient lexical errors in that errors were often only one digit away from the answer. The main types of errors were "stack errors," which resulted in a distorted syntactic frame, such as "2" instead of "12," and "stack position" errors, which involved inappropriate lexical selection, such as "four" instead of "three." Anterior lesions tended to result in stack errors, whereas posterior lesions tended to result in stack position errors. Deloche and coworkers' results demonstrate the importance of evaluating the patient's ability to transcode as part of an overall acalculia test battery.

The work of McCloskey and colleagues has also stimulated much research in acalculia.[29,30] They have been primarily concerned with describing the components required to read, write, and pronounce numbers and to retrieve basic arithmetic facts from memory. In one study—using arithmetic fact verification, magnitude estimation, and matching tasks—they were able to demonstrate that some patients may have difficulty expressing number names even though the comprehension of numbers is intact. In another study, they argued that the word-number and Arabic-number systems could be dissociated. They have also shown that some patients may have more difficulty producing word numbers compared to Arabic numbers despite comprehension of both kinds of number symbols. Errors were similar for writing or speaking numbers. These and other results have led McCloskey and coworkers to argue for a common abstract syntactic frame for both verbal and written number production systems.

A few componential models of number processing and mental calculation now exist, and their underlying assumptions are based largely on the empiric research summarized above.[5,29,31] All models stress that certain operations in arithmetic resemble those processes required for comprehending symbols or information in other domains, such as reading words or understanding logic. For example, number processing probably has at least two routes to a fact lexicon, a direct visual route to a number lexicon and an indirect route that requires phonologic processing. Several other features would appear to be required in a complete model. Numbers, like letters and words, must be perceived as distinct meaningful entities and as orthographic or idiographic symbols. Working memory buffers and executive functioning must hold numeric information until it can be processed directly under an attentional spotlight. The representation of numbers and number facts should be independent of representations for the numeric computational procedures demanded by particular operational symbols. Output mechanisms servicing speech or graphomotor functions should be similar to those imagined for uttering or writing letters and words. In these types of cognitive architectures, a modular design assuming, among other things, a central abstract level of representation of numeric knowledge, is sometimes assumed.[29] On the other hand, based on their experimental paradigms, Campbell and colleagues[31] have argued that there is no abstract level of representation for numbers but rather that numeric cognition involves a *complex encoding* architecture that includes only interconnected, notation-dependent representations of numbers and of arithmetic problems, thus inextricably *linking* number perception and fact retrieval as well as interpenetration of number reading and fact retrieval processes (diminishing their modular characteristics). The issue of whether or not an abstract, semantic level of representation for numbers exists is a central one in this area of research and is an issue with potentially far-reaching implications for representation of knowledge more generally in the human brain.

These types of models, derived initially from empiric data, now make explicit predictions that can be tested in future research. This emerging interplay between theory and data promises to lead to rapid progress in understanding the architecture of number processing and calculation.

METHODOLOGIC ISSUES

Assessment of Acalculia

There are a number of clinical and experimental test batteries currently in use that can aid the clinician or researcher in determining the ability level and intactness of arithmetic cognitive processing of their subjects. These are discussed next.

Clinical Assessment Tools

The most common test used to assess calculation by clinical neuropsychologists has been the Wide Range Achievement Test (WRAT).[32] The arithmetic portion of this test allows for some sense of the subject's operational skills (addition, subtrac-

tion, etc.) but is limited in how it tests subjects and in the space provided for subjects to answer problems. The subtest itself does allow for a grade-equivalent score to be obtained, and results on this subtest can be compared to other language-based subtests from the WRAT. Much better tests, however, are available for the clinician, although many of these were originally designed for use with children. One commonly used test, the Key Math Test,[33] is commercially available; it has grade-equivalent and standardized scores. The test batteries generally sample all the standard arithmetic operations, including addition, subtraction, multiplication, division, fractions, percentages, quantification, algebra, geometric relations, practical use of quantities, etc. The advantage of using these test batteries is that they have been normed on children and adolescents and have all the psychometric and presentation advantages of commercial products. None of the commercially

Table 28-1

Suggested test battery for the evaluation of acalculia

Test	Description
1. Number recognition	Reading arabic numerals and and number words aloud
2. Number writing	Writing arabic numerals and number words to dictation
3. Number transcoding	Transcoding arabic numeral to number word and vice versa
4. Quantification	Estimating the quantity of collections of symbols or objects
5. Magnitude estimation	Deciding which of two arabic numerals or number words is the largest
6. Basic arithmetic operations	Addition, subtraction, multiplication, and division
7. Calculation fact verification	Computer-assisted presentation of calculation facts for response-time verification
8. Multicolumn calculation	All four operations—some problems should involve carry and borrow procedures
9. Magnitude comparison	Computer-assisted presentation of numeric quantities for response-time verification
10. Fractions	Computing percentages and fractions
11. Algebra	Algebraic computations
12. Numeric knowledge	Retrieving numeric knowledge such as "How many inches are there in one yard?"

Note: Single numbers and problems should be varied by the magnitude of the number, the numeric distance between component parts of the problem, the relationship of the error (e.g., test 7) to the correct answer, and by other important variables that can be found in the experimental literature.

available instruments, however, have norms for adults, nor were they specifically designed to test models of number processing and calculation.

Experimental Tasks

A few experimental batteries have been developed in the last 10 years that are based on cognitive models of calculation and number processing and include a variety of tasks not usually available in the clinical batteries referred to above.[34] Such supplemental experimental tasks include number transcoding, fact and operation verification tasks, and timed magnitude-estimation tasks. In addition, many authors have adapted error-analysis systems that may help isolate dysfunctional information-processing components in acalculia patients. Most of the experimental tasks alluded to above are easily programmed for response-time experiments using currently available test-authoring software and with designs that can be guided by articles appearing in experimental and cognitive psychology journals. Since there are a variety of error-analysis systems, we would recommend that readers peruse each author's rationale for his or her scoring system and then decide on the system that appears most convincing and practical to them. In Table 28-1 we suggest a set of tasks and an error-analysis approach that can be used in a general but comprehensive assessment of number processing and calculation.

CONCLUSIONS

Acalculia is a common developmental disorder and is a frequent concomitant of acute and progressive left posterior hemispheric lesions in children and adults. It can affect a patient's ability to balance a checkbook, make change, use a temperature gauge, etc. Clinically, it is important to assess number processing and calculation, and we have made suggestions for such an assessment in this chapter. Studying number processing and calculation in acalculic patients can also teach us about the cognitive architecture and computational demands of a relatively encap-

sulated cognitive function by revealing patterns of spared and impaired abilities across individual patients. Given that numbers and calculation represent a relatively closed information processing system with a limited number of rules and symbols, it makes for an ideal domain of study.

REFERENCES

1. Levin HS, Goldstein FC, Spiers PA: Acalculia, in Heilman K, Valenstein E (eds): *Clinical Neuropsychology.* New York, Oxford University Press, 1993, pp 91–118.
2. Gallistel CR, Gelman R: Preverbal and verbal counting and computation. *Cognition* 44(1–2):43–74, 1992.
3. Siegler RS: Strategy choice procedures and the development of multiplication skill. *J Exp Psychol General* 117:258–275, 1988.
4. Rickard TC, Bourne LE Jr: Some tests of an identical elements model of basic arithmetic skills. *J Exp Psychol Learn Mem Cog.* In press.
5. Dehaene S: Varieties of numerical abilities. *Cognition* 44(1–2):1–42, 1992.
6. Nesher P: Learning mathematics: A cognitive perspective. Special Issue: Psychological science and education. *Am Psychol* 41:1114–1122, 1986.
7. Resnick LB: Developing mathematical knowledge. Special issue: Children and their development: Knowledge base, research agenda, and social policy application. *Am Psychol* 44:162–169, 1989.
8. Siegler RS, Shrager EA: *How Children Discover New Strategies.* Hillsdale, NJ: Erlbaum, 1989.
9. Gross A, Tsur V, Manor O, Shalev RS: Developmental dyscalculia, gender, and the brain. *Arch Dis Child* 68:510–512, 1993.
10. Lyytinen H, Ahonen T, Rasanen P: Dyslexia and dyscalculia in children—Risks, early precursors, bottlenecks and cognitive mechanisms. *Acta Paedopsychiatr* 56:179–192, 1994.
11. Shalev RS, Weirtman R, Amir N: Developmental dyscalculia. *Cortex* 24:555–561, 1988.
12. Ashcraft MH, Yamashita TS, Aram DM: Mathematics performance in left and right brain-lesioned children and adolescents. *Brain Cog* 19:208–252, 1992.
13. Boller F, Grafman J: Acalculia: Historical develop-

ment and current significance. *Brain Cog* 2:205–223, 1983.

14. Rosselli M, Ardila A: Calculation deficits in patients with right and left hemisphere damage. *Neuropsychologia* 27:607–617, 1989.

15. Grafman J, Passafiume D, Faglioni P, Boller F: Calculation disturbances in adults with focal hemispheric damage. *Cortex* 18:37–49, 1982.

16. Dehaene S, Cohen L: Two mental calculation systems: A case study of severe acalculia with preserved approximation. *Neuropsychologia* 29:1045–1054, 1991.

17. Rueckert L, Lange N, Partiot A, et al: Visualizing cortical activation during mental calculation with functional MRI. 1996. Submitted.

18. Dehaene S, Tzourio N, Frak V, et al: Cerebral activations during number multiplications and comparison: A PET study. 1996. Submitted.

19. Tohgi H, Saitoh K, Takahashi S, et al: Agraphia and acalculia after a left prefrontal (F1, F2) infarction. *J Neurol Neurosurg Psychiatry* 58:629–632, 1995.

20. Mazzoni M, Pardossi L, Cantini R, et al: Gerstmann syndrome: A case report. *Cortex* 26:459–467, 1990.

21. Moore MR, Saver JL, Johnson KA, Romero JA: Right parietal stroke with Gerstmann's syndrome: Appearance on computed tomography, magnetic resonance imaging, and single-photon emission computed tomography. *Arch Neurol* 48:432–435, 1991.

22. Grafman J, Kampen D, Rosenberg J, et al: The progressive breakdown of number processing and calculation ability: A case study. *Cortex* 25:121–133, 1989.

23. Pesenti M, Seron X, Van Der Linden M: Selective impairment as evidence for mental organisation of arithmetic facts: BB, a case of preserved subtraction? *Cortex* 30:661–671, 1994.

24. Cipolotti L, Costello AD: Selective impairment for simple division. *Cortex.* In press.

25. Lampl Y, Eshel Y, Gilad R, Sarova-Pinhas I: Selective acalculia with sparing of the subtraction process in a patient with left parietotemporal hemorrhage. *Neurology* 44:1759–1761, 1994.

26. Weddell RA, Davidoff JB: A dyscalculic patient with selectively impaired processing of the numbers 7, 9, and 0. *Brain Cog* 17:240–271, 1991.

27. Warrington EK: The fractionation of arithmetic skills: A single case study. *Q J Exp Psychol* 34A:31–51, 1982.

28. Deloche G, Seron X: Some linguistic components of acalculia. *Adv Neurol* 42:215–222, 1984.

29. McCloskey M, Caramazza A, Basili A: Cognitive mechanisms in number processing and calculation: Evidence from dyscalculia. *Brain Cog* 4:171–196, 1985.

30. McCloskey M, Macaruso P: Representing and using numerical information. *Am Psychol* 50:351–363, 1995.

31. Campbell JI: Architectures for numerical cognition. *Cognition* 53(1):1–44, 1994.

32. Jastak S, Wilkinson GS: *Wide Range Achievement Test—Revised.* Wilmington, DE, Jastak Assessment Systems, 1984.

33. Connolly AJ, Nachtman W, Pritchett EM: *KeyMath Diagnostic Arithmetic Test.* Circle Pines, MN, American Guidance Services, 1976.

34. Deloche G, Seron X, Larroque C, et al: Calculation and number processing: Assessment battery; role of demographic factors. *J Clin Exp Neuropsychol* 16:195–208, 1994.

Part VI
DEMENTIA

Chapter 29

DEMENTIA: AN OVERVIEW

Daniel I. Kaufer
Jeffrey L. Cummings

INTRODUCTION

This overview of dementia syndromes will emphasize general principles of classification, etiology, pathophysiology, and management. A principal focus will be to elaborate a systematic and integrative approach to etiologic diagnosis based on recognizable constellations of brain-behavior relationships evident across a variety of conditions that impair cognition.

DEFINITION

The first widely applied standardized guidelines for the diagnosis of dementia were contained in DSM-III[1] The two essential diagnostic features of dementia as defined by DSM-III have been preserved in the current version (DSM-IV)[2] and include: 1) an impairment in social and occupational functioning and 2) memory and other cognitive deficits. Specific domains of cognitive disturbance embraced by the definition include aphasia, apraxia, agnosia, and disturbances in executive functions such as planning, organizing, and abstract thinking. Additional requirements include the exclusion of a delirium or inability to better account for the symptoms by an Axis I psychiatric disorder. Classification of dementia syndromes depends on evidence linking the clinical process to one or more medical etiologies (i.e., hypothyroidism), cerebrovascular disease (i.e., vascular

dementia), or excluding other medical conditions (i.e., Alzheimer's disease).

Cummings and Benson[3,4] proposed alternative criteria for dementia highlighting the clinical and topographic heterogeneity of dementia syndromes. These are contrasted with DSM-IV criteria in Table 29-1. They define dementia as an acquired and persistent impairment of intellectual function with compromise in at least three of the following spheres of mental activity: language, memory, visuospatial skills, emotion or personality, and cognition (e.g. abstraction, calculation, judgment, executive function).[3] In contrast to DSM-IV criteria, this definition allows for the possibility that memory disturbance may not be a presenting feature of a dementing illness, as is not infrequently the case with Pick's disease and other frontotemporal dementias (FTD).[4] The DSM-IV stipulation of a decline in social or occupational functioning provides a measure of ecological validity, but neurobiological sensitivity is lost due to the variable social and functional demands an individual may face. Emphasis placed by DSM-IV on the so-called "cortical" deficits of aphasia, apraxia, and agnosia may further diminish its sensitivity to other common manifestations of dementing illnesses including apathy, psychosis, and other neuropsychiatric symptoms.[5] Despite these differences, most patients meeting Cummings and Benson criteria for dementia would also be identified as demented using the DSM-IV approach.

Table 29-1

Comparison of DSM-IV criteria for dementia and Cummings and Benson definition of dementia (DSM-IV, APA, 1994; Cummings and Benson, 1980).

DSM-IV	Cummings and Benson
Multiple cognitive deficits including:	Acquired, persistent intellectual impairment involving at least three of the following domains:
Memory impairment and one or more of the following:	
Aphasia	Language
Apraxia	Memory
Agnosia	Visuospatial skills
	Emotion or personality
Executive dysfunction	Cognition/executive functions
Impairment in social or occupational functioning	
Decline from a previous level of functioning	
Clinical/laboratory evidence relating the disturbance to a general medical condition	
Deficits do not occur exclusively in the course of a delirium	

ETIOLOGIC CLASSIFICATION

Degenerative and Nondegenerative

Dementia refers to a clinical *syndrome* of acquired intellectual disturbances encompassing a large number of *disease* processes. The key features distinguishing dementia syndromes from delirium are the chronicity of the former and the primary attentional deficits associated with the latter. These distinctions are more relative than absolute. Virtually all etiologies producing delirium may also result in a dementia. Reversibility of either syndrome is principally determined by the specific etiology.

Dementias may result from a wide variety of disorders including degenerative, vascular, traumatic, demyelinating, neoplastic, infectious, inflammatory, hydrocephalic, systemic, and toxic conditions. Etiologies of dementia may be classified into two broad categories, degenerative and nondegenerative. Collectively, degenerative brain diseases are the most common etiology of dementia, with Alzheimer's disease (AD) accounting for about half of all cases.[4] Each degenerative dementia has a characteristic topography of involvement, although the nature of the underlying pathological alterations varies. Several degenerative brain diseases are associated with specific histopathological markers in affected regions: AD—cortical neuritic (senile) plaques and neurofibrillary tangles; Parkinson's disease (PD)—brain stem Lewy bodies progressive supranuclear palsy—subcortical neurofibrillary tangles (distinct from those of AD); and corticobasal ganglionic degeneration (CBGD)—cortical and subcortical achromatic inclusion bodies. Dementia with Lewy bodies (DLB) is a nosologically controversial degenerative condition exhibiting variable degrees of pathological features common to AD and Parkinson's disease.[6,7] Other degenerative conditions, such as Huntington's disease (HD) and spinocerebellar degeneration (SCD), have regionally selective but nonspecific pathological characteristics of neuronal loss and gliosis. Frontotemporal dementia (FTD) refers to a syndrome of selective frontal and anterior temporal lobe atrophy formerly known as Pick's disease; the presence of Pick bodies is a variable feature.[8] Hereditary forms or predisposing genetic factors have been identified in the majority of degenerative dementias; heritability is an uncommon feature of nondegenerative dementias. Wilson's disease, an autosomal recessive disorder of copper metabolism, and the most common forms of adult leukodystrophy, metachromatic (autosomal recessive) and adrenoleukodystrophy (X-linked), are metabolic-degenerative disorders usually expressed in youth or young adulthood. Similarly, autosomal dominant degenerative conditions, such as HD, some forms of SCD, and familial variants of AD and FTD, tend to have earlier ages of onset. The apolipoprotein E type 4 allele is a marker for earlier onset in sporadic forms and higher incidence in late-onset familial forms of AD.[9,10]

CLINICAL PATHOPHYSIOLOGY

Neuroimaging

Dementing processes usually entail selective involvement of CNS areas.[4] The differential nature and topography of involved neuronal systems results in distinctive patterns of intellectual and behavioral disturbances. The pathological processes in dementia are diverse, ranging from intrinsic molecular ultrastructural or metabolic defects to exogenous neuronal toxins to gross alterations in brain structure. From a clinical perspective, structural imaging techniques such as CT or MRI will often inform the evaluation and differential diagnosis of disorders with gross structural changes. Pertinent examples include mass lesions, cerebrovascular disease, demyelination, and

focal or regional atrophy as seen in HD (caudate), progressive supranuclear palsy (midbrain), and FTD (frontal and anterior temporal lobes). In the absence of radiographically demonstrable lesions, the underlying metabolic or cerebral perfusion derangements may, in some cases, be detectable by MRI spectroscopy, or with functional neuroimaging techniques such as single-photon emission tomography (SPECT) and positron emission tomography (PET).[11] Two burgeoning clinical applications of functional imaging in dementia are the identification of sympton-specific,[12,13] and disease-specific[14,15] patterns of altered cerebral perfusion (SPECT) or metabolism (PET). In the latter case, pre-clinical detection of genetically determined dementias may be possible.[16,17]

Neurochemistry

A broad range of neurochemical lesions may produce or contribute to dementia. Nutritional deficiencies of vitamin B_{12}, niacin, or, in the case of Wernicke's encephalopathy, thiamine, typically have systemic and CNS manifestations due to their widespread roles as essential cofactors in intermediate metabolism. Disturbances in thyroid and pituitary function may also have pervasive deleterious effects on both peripheral and CNS metabolic pathways. Chronic exposure to alcohol, illicit substances such as cocaine, or heavy metals such as lead, mercury, or aluminum (chronic renal dialysis) may produce characteristic syndromes of dementia. Prolonged episodes of hypoxia and carbon monoxide poisoning may result in dementia syndromes that reflect the inherent vulnerabilities of the hippocampus and globus pallidus, respectively. The basal ganglia is particularly susceptible to injury due to abnormal metabolism or toxic levels of metallic substances. In Wilson's disease, selective deposition of unbound copper in the putamen occurs due to a deficiency in the copper transport protein, ceruloplasmin. Hallervorden-Spatz disease, Fahr's disease, and manganese encephalopathy are associated with abnormal basal ganglia accumulations of iron, ferro-calcific aggregates, and manganese, respectively. Deficiency of the myelin synthetic enzyme arylsulfatase A underlies the dysmyelinating dementia of metachromatic leukodystrophy. In many cases, etiologically based treatments of dementing disorders produced by specific neurochemical or biochemical alterations effect a reversal, or retard the progression of the dementia.

Neurochemical deficits typically have a less well-defined etiological role in most degenerative dementias. However, a variety of central neurotransmitter abnormalities may contribute to the clinical manifestations of many degenerative conditions. There are two general types of central neurotransmitter systems: 1) local or intrinsic neurotransmitters, such as gamma-aminobutyric acid (GABA) and glutamate, and 2) projection or extrinsic neurotransmitters, including acetylcholine, dopamine, serotonin, and norepinephrine.[18] GABA and glutamate are the principal inhibitory and excitatory neurotransmitters of the CNS, respectively, and generally mediate neuronal information transfer along discrete channels in local cortical-cortical and cortical-subcortical circuits. The localized topography and channel-specificity of these amino acid neurotransmitters reflect their integral role in neocortically based intellectual functions but render them less susceptible to pharmacological manipulation.

Projection neurotransmitter systems arise from subcortical and brain stem nuclei and primarily exert a modulatory influence on widely distributed neuronal networks.[18,19] Cholinergic projections from the brain stem reticular system (lateral dorsal tegmentum and pedunculopontine nucleus) terminate in nonspecific thalamic nuclei and basal forebrain regions, activating cortical arousal and attentional mechanisms. Basal forebrain cholinergic nuclei have diffuse projections to neocortical and limbic areas such as the amygdala and hippocampus; disruption of these cholinergic efferents are implicated in the pathogenesis of memory and other intellectual disturbances seen in AD.

Dopaminergic projections from the substantia nigra to the putamen are disrupted in PD, producing the characteristic motor disturbances of tremor, rigidity, and bradykinesia. Dopaminergic efferents from the ventral tegmental area to the nucleus accumbens, septal area, amygdala (mesolimbic pathway), and anterior cingulate, medial temporal, and frontal lobe regions (mesocortical pathway) are affiliated with cognitive functioning and neuropsychiatric disturbances such as depression, mania, and psychosis.[20,21] Locus ceruleus is the origin of two primary ascending noradrenergic projections—a dorsal pathway arising from midbrain nuclei and terminating in neocortical, thalamic, basal forebrain, and medial temporal regions, and a ventral pathway arising from lower brain stem areas that project to the hypothalamus and midbrain reticular nuclei. These noradrenergic projections are thought to influence arousal, selective attention, and anxiety states.[19,22] Serotonergic projections arise from median and paramedian raphe nuclei in the brain stem and are widely distributed throughout the cerebral hemispheres. Serotonin principally acts as an inhibitor of diffuse neuronal systems; anxiety, disinhibition, and aggression are associated with altered serotonergic function.[22,23] Together, these diffusely projecting neurotransmitter systems regulate the excitatory and inhibitory tone of multiple, discrete neural circuits underlying specific domains of intellectual function. Regional variations in receptor density and receptor subtypes superimpose a response topography on these "diffuse" systems. Their generally indirect influence on cognition is paralleled by their integrated role in the modulation of behavioral states. Selective disturbances in this regulatory mosaic may produce characteristic patterns of neuropsychological and neuropsychiatric symptoms.

CLINICAL FEATURES

Cortical and Subcortical Syndromes

Dementia has many different etiologies, each with its own range of symptoms. In addition, a multitude of individual-specific factors including genetic predisposition, education, gender differences, age-related changes, preexisting brain disease, environmental exposures, and medical and psychiatric comorbidity may impinge on the expression of a dementing illness. Despite the etiologic and individual heterogeneity of dementing illnesses, two basic patterns of neurobehavioral features have been observed and named according to the predominant neuroanatomical regions involved.[4] One syndromic constellation includes *cortical* dementias such as AD. Cerebral cortical regions are the primary locus of involvement in AD, although restricted pathological alterations in subcortical regions are also present. *Subcortical* dementias—including extrapyramidal disorders such as Parkinson's disease, Huntington's disease, progressive supranuclear palsy, subcortical vascular disease, white matter diseases, and hydrocephalus—are distinguished by clinical symptoms principally referable to involvement of basal ganglia, limbic-related thalamic nuclei, and portions of the brain stem. From a functional anatomical perspective, striatum, globus pallidus, anterior and medial thalamus, and substantia nigral portion of the midbrain are interconnected with prefrontal cortical regions in a series of circuits with unique neurobehavioral affiliations.[24,25] Similar clinical deficits may result from lesions anywhere in these circuits or reflect circuit dysfunction at both cortical and subcortical levels, as in FTD. A third category, *mixed,* includes conditions such as dementia with Lewy bodies, corticobasal ganglionic degeneration, some vascular dementias, and slow virus infections, which typically produce symptoms attributable to dysfunction of both cortical and subcortical structures.

From a clinical viewpoint, distinguishing cortical and subcortical patterns of signs and symptoms facilitates a systematic approach to differential diagnosis. A classification of dementia based on degenerative vs. nondegenerative etiology and cortical-subcortical typology is presented in Table 29-2.

The clinical features of cortical and subcortical dementias arise from differential involvement of neural components underlying specific cognitive and behavioral functions. The neuropsychological and neurobehavioral concomitants of cortical dementias generally reflect the functional specificity of pathologically disturbed neocortical regions. Cerebral cortex can be viewed as consisting of functionally specialized domains that are linked together in serial and parallel modular networks for information processing.[19] Structural or functional disturbances in these cortically based networks may produce deficits in instrumental intellectual skills such as language, visuospatial functions, and mathematical abilities. Elementary sensory and motor functioning is typically preserved. Subcortical dementias, in contrast, are characterized by slowing and dilapidation of executive functions, affective and personality disturbances, forgetfulness, and movement disorders.[26,27] These features are attributable to disruption of one or more of the structures participating in the frontal-subcortical circuits, the nodes of which are less functionally specialized than neocortical neural regions. Some features of subcortical dementias are reminiscent of delirium. A comparison between the features of cortical and subcortical dementias are presented in Table 29-3.

DIFFERENTIAL DIAGNOSIS

Table 29-4 presents a summary of clinical-pathoanatomic profiles for the major causes of degenerative and other dementias. Attention to concomitant features such as extrapyramidal and focal or lateralizing neurological signs complements a systematic approach to the differential diagnosis of dementia syndromes based on the cortical-subcortical organizing principle. Identifying reversible or treatable etiologies of dementia is a preeminent concern.

Cortical Dementia

AD is the prototype cortical dementia syndrome. Deficits in short-term memory, visuospatial functions, naming, and verbal fluency are the common initial manifestations of AD. Apathetic indifference, diminished insight or lack of awareness of their deficits, and poor abstract thinking frequently accompany the core neuropsychological deficits. Insidious onset is the rule, although the initial clinical symptoms may be precipitated by a surgical procedure, infection, or minor head in-

Table 29-2

Etiological classification of dementias based on cortical and subcortical features

DEGENERATIVE	NONDEGENERATIVE
Cortical Dementias	
Alzheimer's disease	Multiple cortical infarcts
	Angular gyrus syndrome
Subcortical Dementias	
Extrapyramidal syndromes:	Vascular dementias:
Parkinson's disease	Binswanger's disease
Progressive supranuclear palsy	Lacunar state
Striatonigral degeneration	Infectious dementia:
Shy-Drager syndrome	HIV dementia
Spinocerebellar degeneration	Whipple's disease
Idiopathic basal ganglia calcification	Neurosyphilis
Wilson's disease	Demyelinating dementia:
Huntington's disease	Multiple sclerosis
Neuroacanthocytosis	Miscellaneous dementias:
Hallervorden-Spatz	Symptomatic hydrocephalus
Progressive subcortical gliosis	Dementia syndrome of depression
Mixed Cortical/Subcortical Dementias	
Frontotemporal dementia (includes amyotrophic lateral sclerosis with dementia)	Multiple cerebral infarctions
	Toxic/metabolic disorders:
Dementia with Lewy bodies	Deficiencies (B_{12}, niacin, etc.)
Corticobasal ganglionic degeneration	Endocrinopathies (thyroid, etc.)
Leukodystrophies:	Chronic alcohol/drug abuse
Metachromatic leukodystrophy	Marchiafava-Bignami
Adrenoleukodystrophy	Industrial/environmental toxins
Prion diseases (also infectious)	Posttraumatic encephalopathy
	Vasculitides (systemic and CNS)

jury. Focal neurological signs are conspicuously absent early in the course; later on motor dysfunction, myoclonus, and seizures may develop.

The principal distinguishing features of AD are the nature of the memory deficits, the presence of other intellectual disturbances, and the absence of neurological signs. Primary attentional functions are initially preserved in AD, distinguishing it from toxic and systemic etiologies of delirium. More isolated disturbances in language or visuospatial functions may reflect cerebrovascular insults or focal cortical degenerative syndromes. The angular gyrus syndrome is a symp-tom complex of fluent aphasia, constructional disturbances, and elements of the Gerstmann syndrome (acalculia, finger agnosia, dysgraphia, and right-left disorientation).[28] It may result from left hemisphere cerebrovascular lesions in the distribution of the posterior branches of the middle cerebral artery and is distinguished from AD by its abrupt onset and the relative absence of nonverbal memory deficits. Focal degenerative conditions such as primary progressive aphasia and CBGD are also characterized by asymmetric hemispheric involvement and relatively preserved memory but, as with AD, have a more insidious

Table 29-3

Clinical features of cortical and subcortical dementias

Feature	Cortical Dementia	Subcortical Dementia
Onset	Insidious	Insidious
Duration	Months to years	Months to years
Course	Progressive	Progressive or constant
Attention	Normal	Normal (slow response time)
Speech	Normal	Hypophonic, dysarthric, mute
Language	Aphasic	Normal or anomic
Memory	Learning deficit (AD)	Retrieval deficit
Cognition	Acalculia, concrete (AD)	Slow, dilapidated
Awareness	Impaired	Usually preserved
Demeanor	Unconcerned, disinhibited	Apathetic, abulic
Psychosis	May be present	May be present
Motor signs	None	Tremor, chorea, rigidity, dystonia
EEG	Mild diffuse slowing	Normal or mild slowing (diffuse or focal)

onset and progressive course.[29,30] In CGBD, unilateral sensory and motor disturbances including apraxia, astereognosis, dystonia, myoclonus, and the alien hand syndrome are often present.

Subcortical Dementias

Extrapyramidal system involvement is a common feature of subcortical dementias. Parkinsonian features concurrent with a dementia syndrome characterized by retrieval memory deficits, cognitive slowing, and executive dysfunction have a wide differential diagnosis.[4] Parkinson's disease (PD), progressive supranuclear palsy, multiple system atrophies, the rigid form of Huntington's disease, and many secondary basal ganglia disorders produce parkinsonism with dementia. Most patients with idiopathic PD exhibit some degree of intellectual impairment; 20 to 30 percent will have deficits severe enough to meet criteria for dementia.[31] The subcortical dementias of PD and

progressive supranuclear palsy (PSP) exhibit overlapping executive deficits[32,33] and are both associated with reductions in frontal lobe metabolism or blood flow.[34,35] PSP is principally distinguished by the early features of gait imbalance and bulbar symptoms (dysarthria and pseudobulbar affect), axial rigidity, and a supranuclear vertical gaze palsy.[36]

Communicating or "normal pressure" hydrocephalus (NPH) is an uncommon but potentially reversible syndrome produced by impaired egress of cerebrospinal fluid via arachnoid granulations from the intracranial compartment. A subcortical dementia syndrome of apathy, psychomotor slowing, retrieval memory deficits, and executive dysfunction may develop over a period of months, and is typically preceded by a characteristic "magnetic" or "apraxic" gait.[37] Incontinence generally appears later, if at all. The rapidity of decline and prominent gait and balance disturbances help distinguish NPH from PD and

Table 29-4
Differential diagnostic profiles of clinico-pathoanatomic features of dementia

Etiology	Clinical Features	Pathoanatomical Correlates
Cortical dementias		
Alzheimer's disease	Memory deficit (learning) Aphasia, apraxia, agnosia Apathy/indifference	Hippocampus, nucleus basalis (cholinergic) Temporal and parietal neocortex Anterior cingulate, parietal neocortex
Mixed Dementias		
Frontotemporal dementia	Memory deficit (retrieval) Speech/language stereotypies Disinhibition Hyperorality (Kluver-Bucy)	Dorsolateral prefrontal cortex Frontal/temporal neocortex Orbitofrontal cortex Amygdala/anterior temporal cortex
Lewy body dementia	Memory deficit (learning) Aphasia, apraxia, agnosia Extrapyramidal signs Fluctuating attentional deficits Visual hallucinations, delusions	Nucleus basalis, hippocampal formation Temporal and parietal neocortex Substantia nigra (dopamine) Pedunculopontine nucleus (cholinergic)? Neocortex (serotonin/cholinergic imbalance)?
Corticobasal ganglionic degeneration	Unilateral limb signs (dystonia, clumsiness, myoclonus) Cortical sensory loss, apraxia, alien hand phenomena Rigidity Supranuclear gaze palsy (late)	Subthalamic nucleus, thalamus, globus pallidus Parietal and frontal neocortex (asymmetric) Substantia nigra (dopamine) Midbrain
Subcortical Dementias		
Progressive supranuclear palsy	Supranuclear gaze palsy Dysarthria/dysphagia Gait/balance disturbances, axial ridigity Pseudobulbar palsy	Midbrain Bulbar cranial nerves Globus pallidus, subthalamic nucleus, substantia nigra Brainstem, prefrontal cortex
Parkinson's disease	Memory deficit (retrieval) Executive dysfunction Tremor, rigidity, bradykinesia	Caudate; nucleus basalis (cholinergic) Caudate nucleus Substantia nigra, putamen (dopamine)

Table 29-4 (Continued)

Differential diagnostic profiles of clinico-pathoanatomic features of dementia

Etiology	Clinical Features	Pathoanatomical Correlates
Huntington's disease	Memory deficit (retrieval)	Caudate nucleus
	Executive dysfunction	Caudate nucleus
	Choreiform movements	Putamen, subthalamic nucleus, globus pallidum
Symptomatic hydrocephalus	Gait disturbance	Midline subcortical structures and connections
	Memory deficit (retrieval)	
	Executive dysfunction	
	Incontinence	
Dementia syndrome of depression	Memory deficit (retrieval)	Subcortical white or gray matter
	Impaired concentration/attention	
	Executive dysfunction	
	Parkinsonian features (except tremor)	
Vascular dementia (multiple lacunar strokes or Binswanger's disease)	Memory deficit (retrieval)	Thalamic or basal ganglia-prefrontal disconnection
	Executive dysfunction	Location-dependent
	Focal or asymmetric elementary neurological signs	

other extrapyramidal syndromes. CT or MRI often shows panventricular enlargement, particularly in the anterior ventricular regions, out of proportion to the degree of cortical gyral atrophy. However, these radiographic findings lack absolute specificity, emphasizing the diagnostic primacy of clinical features. Radionuclide cisternography may lend support to the diagnosis.

Depression may influence the symptomatic expression of dementia or may cause a syndrome of dementia (dementia of depression). About 40 percent of PD patients exhibit significant depressive symptoms; degree of memory impairment distinguishes them from PD patients without depression.[38,39] Depression is also common in HD, vascular dementia, and other subcortical syndromes. The dementia syndrome of depression is a reversible dementia most commonly seen in elderly patients with a history of severe or psychotic depression. Impaired attention and concentration, forgetfulness, psychomotor slowing, decreased

motivation, and impaired ability to grasp the meaning of situations are characteristic features.[40,41]

Vascular dementia (VaD) is a heterogeneous syndrome with multiple clinical presentations depending on lesion type and location. Whereas infarctions in the territory of large cerebral vessels produce characteristic syndromes of cortically based higher intellectual functions, diffuse or multifocal small vessel ischemic disease affecting periventricular white matter or basal ganglia and thalamic nuclei result in a classic subcortical dementia syndrome. Dementia arising from multiple lacunar infarcts is associated with a preponderance of lesion sites in the frontal lobe white matter, implicating disruption of frontal-subcortical circuit pathways as the relevant pathological mechanism.[42] More diffuse involvement of subcortical white matter secondary to small vessel ischemia (Binswanger's disease) also functionally disconnects cortical and subcortical regions.

Hypertension and other risk factors for vascular disease are commonly present. VaD syndromes are radiographically distinguishable by characteristic MRI findings on T2-weighted images.

Huntington's disease (HD) is a hyperkinetic extrapyramidal syndrome with choreiform movements and a subcortical dementia. The genetic defect in HD is an autosomal dominant trinucleotide repeat mutation on chromosome four. Severe atrophy of the caudate nuclei is the pathological feature accompanying the frequently prominent behavioral and mood disturbances, including depression, irritability, and impulsivity.

Human immunodeficiency virus (HIV) infection is the most common cause of infectious dementia. Typical manifestations reflect subcortical dysfunction—psychomotor slowing, memory and concentration impairment, and apathy—due to direct CNS invasion of the virus.[43] Gait, motor, and sensory disturbances may be present due to a vacuolizing myelopathy. Opportunistic infections such as toxoplasmosis and progressive multifocal leukoencephalopathy may produce superimposed deficits.

Mixed Cortical and Subcortical Dementias

DLB, or dementia with Lewy bodies, refers to one or more clinical syndromes with overlapping features of AD and PD.[16,17] A characteristic clinical profile including fluctuating cognitive impairments, prominent psychiatric features (hallucinations, delusions, and depression), gait and balance difficulties, and unexplained loss of consciousness has been suggested.[44] Neuropsychological disturbances are variable, but may reflect more severe deficits in attention, verbal fluency, and visuospatial processing compared to "pure" AD patients.[7] Extrapyramidal signs are common but not an invariable feature, and the presentation may be dominated by neuropsychiatric symptoms.[45] AD patients with either extrapyramidal signs or psychotic symptoms have been reported to have more rapid cognitive decline than AD patients without either feature.[46,47] As many patients with DLB meet research criteria for the diagnosis of

AD, the clinical distinction between AD with extrapyramidal signs and psychotic symptoms and DLB is presently unclear. Genetic, biochemical, and neuropathological variables may help discriminate the clinicopathological relationship of DLB to AD and to PD with dementia.[48,49]

FTD, or frontotemporal dementia, entails a dementia syndrome with variable pathological features involving selective frontal and anterior temporal degeneration. The core features of FTD are primarily neuropsychiatric and may include behavioral disinhibition, apathy, inappropriate behavior, lack of social awareness, distractibility, impulsivity, and stereotyped or perseverative behaviors.[8] Behavior and personality changes often appear many years before the appearance of frank neuropsychological deficits.[14] Memory function, calculations, and visuospatial skills are preserved early in the course, contrasting with the initial manifestations of AD. The presence of nonfluent speech and language disturbances, motor and verbal stereotypies, hyperorality or change in dietary habits, and earlier age of onset also may help distinguish FTD from AD.[50] Pathological involvement is concentrated in frontal lobe cortical areas, with differential involvement of limbic temporal cortex and subcortical basal ganglia structures, particularly the striatum. Gliosis and regional atrophy are typical features; the presence of Pick bodies and swollen neurons may be associated with more severe white matter involvement and more pronounced atrophic changes. Characteristic clinical and pathological features of FTD may occur with motor neuron disease, with additional degenerative changes in lower brain stem and spinal cord motor neurons.

TREATMENT AND MANAGEMENT OF DEMENTIA

Disease-Specific Therapy

Etiologically based treatment is not available for any of the degenerative dementias, although treatments informed by disease pathophysiology have recently become available. In AD, the profound reduction in basal forebrain and neocortical acetylcholine, together with evidence linking cholinergic deficits to memory dysfunction have motivated intensive efforts directed towards enhancing central cholinergic function.[51] To date, acetylcholinesterase inhibitors such as donepezil have been the most successful in ameliorating some of the cognitive deficits of AD.[52,53] Other cholinergic-enhancing agents, including direct muscarinic and nicotinic receptor agonists, are currently undergoing clinical trials. Alpha-tocopherol (vitamin E) at a dose of 2000 i. u. a day has been shown to slow the functional progression of AD.[54]

Therapeutic strategies in cerebrovascular disease are aimed at both limiting the acute damage of cerebral ischemia and secondary prevention. Excitotoxic mechanisms have been widely implicated in neuronal damage produced by acute ischemia and other neurological conditions and may prove amenable to intervention.[55] The progression of vascular dementia may be impeded by aggressive control of risk factors such as hypertension and by the use of platelet antiaggregating agents such as aspirin and ticlopidine.

Selegilene is a monoamine oxidase B inhibitor commonly used as an adjunctive treatment of PD. Selegilene has a modest impact on the symptoms of PD although it may also have a neuroprotective effect in delaying the progression of PD and AD.[56,54]

The dementia syndrome of depression is potentially reversible with standard antidepressant therapies, including tricyclic antidepressants and selective serotonin reuptake inhibitors. Refractory cases may benefit from electroconvulsive therapy.

Transient improvement in the symptoms of hydrocephalic dementia (particularly gait) following lumbar puncture helps to confirm the diagnosis and may have prognostic significance. The response to shunting in NPH is highly variable, but is usually beneficial if there is an identifiable cause and symptom duration has been brief.[57,58]

Toxic and metabolic dementias often respond to removal of the offending agent or reversal of the metabolic abnormality. Steroid and other immunosuppressive agents may ameliorate the cognitive and neuropsychiatric disturbances associated with vasculitis and other CNS inflammatory disorders. The dementia and movement disorders of Wilson's disease may be prevented or reversed with penicillamine treatment. Improved cognitive functioning in symtomatic HIV infection may accompany the use of zidovudine.[59] Evacuation of subdural hematomas and surgical resection of CNS neoplasms produce variable improvement, depending on the size, location, and nature of the mass lesion.

Nonspecific Therapy

Neuropsychiatric disturbances are a frequent accompaniment of dementia syndromes and are often a major source of distress to caregivers. Psychotic and agitated behaviors are commonly treated with antipsychotic agents such as haloperidol, although extrapyramidal side effects and the risk of tardive movement disorders limit their application and utility in elderly demented patients. Newer antipsychotic agents such as risperidone, olanzapine, and quetiapine offer advantages in terms of reduced parkinsonian side effects. In AD, there is evidence suggesting that cholinergic agents may ameliorate agitated and psychotic behaviors.[60] Trazodone, in doses up to 300 to 400 mg per day, may have a beneficial impact on insomnia and agitated symptoms. Propanolol and benzodiazepines may be useful for acute symptoms of anxiety and agitation, but are occasionally associated with behavioral complications—depression and paradoxical agitation, respectively. Antiepileptic drugs such as carbamazepine, valproate, and gabapentin are being investigated for their potential use in controlling agitation, mania, and behavioral disinhibition. Apathy may be a prominent feature of AD, FTD, PD, PSP, and HD,[61] but is generally poorly responsive to treatment. Preliminary evidence suggests that apathy may be the target symptom most responsive to cholinesterase-inhibitor therapy in AD.[62] Depressive symptoms and signs contribute to cognitive and functional morbidity and often respond to pharmacological treatments. Aggressive behaviors may respond to serotonergic-enhancing agents, or when sexual in nature, to estrogen or antitestosterone therapy. Supportive care for progressive dementias includes maintenance of nutritional needs, dietary modification when aspiration risk is present, surveillance for signs of intercurrent respiratory or urinary tract infections, mobilization when possible, and skin care when bedridden.

CONCLUSIONS AND FUTURE DIRECTIONS

Dementia syndromes may result from a large number of brain diseases. Degenerative dementing illnesses have selective and characteristic topographies of pathological involvement and associated biochemical lesions. Memory processes mediated by distributed cortical and subcortical networks are compromised in dementia, and two general clinical patterns of dementia can be distinguished on the basis of a cortical or subcortical locus of primary involvement. Cortical dementias such as AD produce impaired learning of new information and other deficits in intellectual domains associated with dysfunction of cortically based neural networks. Retrieval memory deficits characterize the subcortical dementia syndrome, which is associated with less discretely localized executive and neuropsychiatric disturbances. The subcortical dementia syndrome results from lesions disrupting the integrity of functional circuits linking prefrontal, basal ganglia, and thalamic areas. Distinguishing subcortical and cortical syndromes of dementia facilitates the etiologic differential diagnosis of dementing disorders and provides insight into functional clinicopathological relationships. Improved accuracy in the diagnosis of degenerative and other dementias will derive from a more precise understanding of how genetic determinants influence the appearance of pathological disturbances in brain function and lead to the associated clinical manifestations. Integrated knowledge of these relationships provides the basis for unraveling the mechanisms of dementing brain diseases and may help identity therapeutic targets to reverse or prevent these ravaging disorders.

ACKNOWLEDGMENTS

The project was supported by National Institute on Aging Core Center Grants (AG10123 and AG05133) and the Augustus Rose Fellowship of the John Douglas French Alzheimer's Foundation (DK).

REFERENCES

1. *Diagnostic and Statistical Manual of Mental Disorders,* 3d ed. Washington, DC: American Psychiatric Association, 1980.
2. *Diagnostic and Statistical Manual of Mental Disorders,* 4th ed. Washington, DC, American Psychiatric Association, 1994.
3. Cummings JL, Benson DF, LoVerme S Jr. Reversible dementia. *JAMA* 1980;243:2434–2439.
4. Cummings JL, Benson DF. *Dementia: A clinical approach,* 2d ed. Boston: Heinemann-Butterworths, 1992.
5. Cummings JL, Victoroff JI. Noncognitive neuropsychiatric syndromes in Alzheimer's disease. *Neuropsychiatry Neuropsychol Behav Neurol* 1990; 3: 140–158.
6. Perry R, Irving D, Blessed G, et al. Senile dementia of the Lewy body type: a clinically and neuropathologically distinct form of dementia in the elderly. *J Neurol Sci* 1990;95:119–139.
7. Hansen L, Salmon D, Galasko D, et al. The Lewy body variant of Alzheimer's disease: a clinical and pathological entity. *Neurology* 1990;40:1–8.
8. Lund and Manchester Groups. Clinical and neuropathological criteria for frontotemporal dementia. *J Neurol Neurosurg Psychiatry* 1994;57:416–418.
9. van Duijn CM, de Knijff P, Cruts A, et al. Apolipoprotein E4 allele in a population-based study of early-onset Alzheimer's disease. *Nat Genet* 1994;7: 74–78.
10. Strittmatter WJ, Saunders AM, Schmechel D, et al. Apolipoprotein E: high-avidity binding to beta-amyloid and increased frequency of type 4 allele in late-onset familial Alzheimer's disease. *Proc Natl Acad Sci* 1993;90:1977–1981.

11. Prichard JW, Brass LM. New anatomical and functional imaging methods. *Ann Neurol* 1992;32:395–400.

12. Mayberg HS. Neuro-imaging studies of depression in neurological diseases. In: Starkstein SE, Robinson RG, eds. *Depression in neurological diseases.* Baltimore: Johns Hopkins University Press, 1993:186–216.

13. Sultzer D, Levin HS, Mahler ME, et al. A comparison of psychiatric symptoms in vascular dementia and Alzheimer's disease. *Am J Psychiatry* 1993;150:1806–1812.

14. Miller BL, Cummings JL, Vilanueva-Meyer J, et al. Frontal lobe degeneration: clinical, neuropsychological, and SPECT characteristics. *Neurology* 1991;41:1374–1382.

15. Jagust WL, Eberling JL, Richardson BR, et al. The cortical topography of temporal lobe hypometabolism in early Alzheimer's disease. *Brain Res* 1993;629:189–198.

16. Grafton ST, Mazziota JC, Pahl JJ, et al. A comparison of neurological, metabolic, structural, and genetic evaluations in persons at risk for Huntington's disease. *Ann Neurol* 1990;28:614–621.

17. Small GW, Mazziota JC, Collins MT, et al. Apolipoprotein E type 4 allele and cerebral glucose metabolism in relatives at risk for familial Alzheimer's disease. *JAMA* 1995;273:942–947.

18. Cummings JL, Coffey CE. Neurobiological basis of behavior. In: Coffey CE, Cummings JL, eds. *Textbook of geriatric neuropsychiatry.* Washington DC: American Psychiatric Association Press, 1994:72–96.

19. Mesulam M-M. Large scale neurocognitive networks and distributed processing for attention, language, and memory. *Ann Neurol* 1990;28:597–613.

20. Wolfe N, Katz DI, Albert ML, et al. Neuropsycological profile linked to low dopamine: in Alzheimer's disease, major depression, and Parkinson's disease. *J Neurol Neurosurg Psychiatry* 1990;53:915–917.

21. Cummings JL. Behavioral complications of drug treatment of Parkinson's disease. *J Am Geriatr Soc* 1991;39:708–716.

22. Hoehn-Saric R. Neurotransmitters in anxiety. *Arch Gen Psychiatry* 1982;39:735–742.

23. Palmer AM, Stratmann GC, Procter AW, Bowen DM. Possible neurotransmitter basis of behavioral changes in Alzheimer's disease. *Ann Neurol* 1988;23:616–620.

24. Alexander GE, Delong MR, Strick PL. Parallel organization of functional circuits linking basal ganglia and cortex. *Annu Rev Neurosci* 1986;9:357–381.

25. Cummings JL. Frontal-subcortical circuits and human behavior. *Arch Neurol* 1993;50:873–880.

26. Albert ML, Feldman RG, Willis AL. The "subcortical dementia" of progressive supranuclear palsy. *J Neurol Neurosurg Psychiatry* 1974;37:121–130.

27. Cummings JL, Benson DF. Subcortical dementia. *Arch Neurol* 1984;41:874–879.

28. Benson DF, Cummings JL, Tsai SY. Angular gyrus syndrome simulating Alzheimer's disease. *Arch Neurol* 1982;39:616–620.

29. Mesulam M-M. Slowly progressive aphasia without generalized dementia. *Ann Neurol* 1982;11:592–598.

30. Gibb, WRG, Luthert, PJ, Marsden CD. Clinical and pathological features of corticobasal degeneration. In: Streifler MB, Korczyn AD, Melamed ED, Youdim MBH, eds. *Advances in neurology,* vol. 53: Parkinson's disease: Anatomy, pathology, and therapy. New York: Raven Press, 1990:51–54.

31. Cummings JL. Intellectual impairment in Parkinson's disease: clinical, pathological, and biochemical correlates. *J Ger Psychiatry Neurol* 1988;1:24–36.

32. Robbins TW, James M, Owen AM, et al. Cognitive deficits in progressive supranuclear palsy, Parkinson's disease, and multiple system atrophy in tests sensitive to frontal lobe dysfunction. *J Neurol Neurosurg Psychiatry* 1994;57:79–88.

33. Pillon B, Gouider-Khouja N, Deweer B, et al. Neuropsychological pattern of striatonigral degeneration: comparison with Parkinson's disease and progressive supranuclear palsy. *J Neurol Neurosurg Psychiatry* 1995;58:174–179.

34. Foster NL, Gilman S, Berent S, et al. Cerebral hypometabolism in progressive supranuclear palsy studied with positron emission tomography. *Ann Neurol* 1988;24:399–406.

35. Sawada H, Udaka F, Kameyama M, et al. SPECT findings in Parkinson's disease associated with dementia. *J Neurol Neurosurg Psychiatry* 1992;55:960–963.

36. Collins SJ, Ahlskog, Parisi JE, Maraganore DM. Progressive supranuclear palsy: neuropathologically based diagnostic clinical criteria. *J Neurol Neurosurg Psychiatry* 1995;58:167–173.

37. Benson DF. Hydrocephalic dementia. In: Fredericks JAM, ed. *Handbook of clinical neurology: Neu-*

robehavioral disorders. Vol. 2. New York: Elsevier Science, 1985:323–333.

38. Cummings JL. Depression and Parkinson's disease: a review. *Am J Psychiatry* 1992;149:443–445.

39. Tröster, AI, Paolo AM, Lyons KE, Glatt SL, Hubble JP, Koller WC. The influence of depression on cognition in Parkinson's disease: a pattern of impairment distinguishable from Alzheimer's disease. *Neurology* 1995;45:672–676.

40. Folstein MF, McHugh PR. Dementia syndrome of depression. In: Katzman R, Terry RD, Bick KI, eds. *Alzheimer's disease, senile dementia and related disorders.* Raven Press: New York, 1978:87–93.

41. Caine ED. Pseudodementia. Current concepts and future directions. *Arch Gen Psychiatry* 1981;38: 1359–1364.

42. Ishii N, Nishihara Y, Imamura T. Why do frontal lobe symptoms predominate in vascular dementia with lacunes? *Neurology* 1986;36:340–345.

43. Navia B, Jordan BJ, Price RW. The AIDS dementia complex: I. clinical features. *Ann Neurol* 1986; 19:517–514.

44. McKeith IG, Perry RH Fairbarn AF, Jabeen S, Perry EK. Operational criteria for senile dementia of the Lewy body type. *Psychol Med* 1992;22: 911–922.

45. McKeith IG, Fairbarn AF, Bothwell RA, et al. An evaluation of the predictive validity and inter-rater reliability of clinical diagnostic criteria for senile dementia of Lewy body type. *Neurology* 1994;44: 872–877.

46. Chui HC, Lyness SA, Sobel E, Schneider LS. Extrapyramidal signs and psychiatric symptoms predict faster cognitive decline in Alzheimer's disease. *Arch Neurol* 1994;51:676–681.

47. Stern Y, Albert M, Brandt, et al. Utility of extrapyramidal signs and psychosis as predictors of cognitive and functional decline, nursing home admission, and death in Alzheimer's disease: prospective analyses from the Predictors study. *Neurology* 1994; 44:2300–2307.

48. Harrington CR, Louwagie, J, Rossau R, et al. Influence of apolipoprotein E genotype on senile dementia of the Alzheimer's and Lewy body types. Significance for etiological heories of Alzheimer's disease. *Am J Pathol* 1994;145:1472–1484.

49. Perry EK, Morris CM, Court JA, et al. Alteration in nicotine binding sites in Parkinson's disease, Lewy body dementia and Alzheimer's disease: Possible index of early neuropathology. *Neuroscience* 1995;64:385–395.

50. Mendez MF, Selwood A, Mastri AR, Frey WH 2d. Pick's disease versus Alzheimer's disease: A comparison of clinical characteristics. *Neurology* 1993; 43:289–292.

51. Schneider LS. Clinical pharmacology of aminoacridines in Alzheimer's disease. *Neurology* 1993; 43(suppl 4):S64-S790).

52. Rogers SL, Friedhoff LT, and the Donepezil Study Group. The efficacy and safety of donepezil in patients with Alzheimer's disease: results of a multicentre, randomized, double-blind, placebo-controlled trial. *Dementia* 1996;7:292–303.

53. Rogers, SL, Farlow MR, Doody RS, et al. A double-blind, placebo-controlled trial of donepezil in patients with Alzheimer's disease. *Neurology* 1998; 50:136–145.

54. Sano M, Ernesto C, Thomas RG, et al. A controlled trial of selegilene, alphatocopherol, or both as treatment for Alzheimer's disease. *N Engl J Med* 1997;336:1216–1222.

55. Lipton SA, Rosenberg PA. Excitatory amino acids as a final common pathway for neurological disorders. *N Engl J Med* 1994;330:613–622.

56. Parkinson Study Group. Effects of tocopherol and deprenyl on the progression of disability in early Parkinson's disease. *N Engl J Med* 1993;328: 176–183.

57. Graff-Radford NR, Godersky JC, Jones MP. Variables predicting surgical outcome in symtomatic hydrocephalus in the elderly. *Neurology* 1989;39: 1601–1604.

58. Clarfield AM. Normal-pressure hydrocephalus: saga or swamp? *JAMA* 1989;262:2592–2593.

59. Sidtis JJ, Gatsonis C, Price RW, et al. Zidovudine treatment of the AIDS Dementia Complex: Results of a placebo-controlled trial. *Ann Neurol* 1993;33: 343–349.

60. Cummings JL, Kaufer DI. Neuropsychiatric aspects of Alzheimer's disease: The cholinergic hypothesis revisited. *Neurology* 1996;47:876–883.

61. Kaufer DI, Cummings JL. Personality alterations in degenerative brain disorders. In: J. Ratey, ed., *Neuropsychiatry of personality disorders.* Cambridge, MA: Blackwell Scientific Publications; 1995:172–209.

62. Kaufer DI. Beyond the cholinergic hypothesis: The effect of metrifonate and other cholinesterase-inhibitors on neuropsychiatric symptoms in Alzheimer's disease. *Demen Geriatr Cogn Disord* 1998;9 (suppl 2):8–14.

Chapter 30

THE COGNITIVE NEUROPSYCHOLOGY OF ALZHEIMER'S DISEASE

Robert D. Nebes

Much of the psychological research on Alzheimer's disease (AD) has had a clinical focus in that the main goal has been to discriminate AD from normal aging and from other conditions, such as depression, that are often confused with early stage AD. Since this approach is generally concerned with diagnosis, it necessarily uses tasks that are clinically validated and standardized. Recently, however, researchers have begun to apply the theories and methodologies of cognitive psychology to AD. The main goal of this approach is to understand the mechanisms underlying the cognitive dysfunctions present in AD. Thus, for example, rather than investigating which memory task best differentiates early AD from normal aging, the cognitive neuropsychology approach is more concerned with whether the memory loss in AD is due to an impairment in the initial encoding of information into memory, a loss of information from the memory store, or a retrieval deficit. It is this cognitive neuropsychology of AD that is briefly reviewed in this chapter.

Alzheimer's disease is a dementing condition that produces severe decrements in multiple areas of cognition, from visual perception to problem solving. Because the decrements are so diverse, most studies restrict themselves to examining relatively discrete aspects of cognition (e.g., short-term memory, syntax, etc.). This has produced a somewhat fragmented literature in which patients' performance in one cognitive domain is investigated without regard to possible interactive effects produced by concurrent problems in other cognitive

operations. Also, there has been little attempt to determine whether changes in one or more fundamental processing mechanisms may be responsible for the large number of apparently independent cognitive deficits seen in AD. That is, it is possible that most or all of the diverse deficits seen in AD patients may arise from a dysfunction in one basic mechanism. The present chapter briefly reviews what is known about the nature of the decrements produced by AD (see Ref. 1 for a more extensive review) in three areas of cognition: attention, memory, and language. From this review, it becomes clear that not all cognitive operations are equally disrupted by AD. The chapter then discusses several of the broader theoretical constructs that have recently been advanced to explain why some mental operations are grossly impaired by AD while others appear to be relatively spared.

ATTENTION

The term *attention* has been applied to a number of very different mental functions, some of which are severely impaired in AD while others remain intact.[2] One major sense of attention involves selection. Humans can process only a limited amount of information at any one time; thus they must select which information they will fully process. Limitations of selective attention are of two types: divided attention and focused attention. To the degree that persons cannot process multiple sources of information as efficiently as they can process one source, they show a limitation in divided attention. Similarly, to the extent that they find it difficult to ignore (i.e., not process) information they know is irrelevant, they show a limitation in focused attention.

Patients with AD have severe problems dividing their attention, but focused attention appears to be less disrupted. One study[3] examined AD patients' ability to divide and focus their attention within the same stimulus. The stimulus was a large digit made up of smaller digits (e.g., a large 1 made up of small 2s). In the focused-attention condition, subjects were told before each trial to direct their attention either to the large digit or to its smaller component digits and to decide whether a 1 or a 2 was present. In the divided-attention condition, they had to attend to both the large digit and its smaller component digits to see if a 1 or a 2 was present in either. In comparison to normals, AD patients were much more impaired in dividing than in focusing their attention. What might be the cause of this problem? In order to attend to multiple sources of information, it is necessary to disengage from one stimulus, shift to the next, and then refocus on this new stimulus. The AD patients' main difficulty appears to lie in disengaging from a currently attended stimulus. This was shown by a study[4] in which subjects were to respond to a stimulus that appeared on either the right or left side of a computer screen. Before each trial, subjects were given a cue that told them on which side the stimulus would appear, thus allowing them to shift the focus of their attention to the proper side of the screen before the stimulus appeared. On most trials this cue was valid (i.e., correct), but on certain trials it was invalid, leading them to shift their attention to the wrong side of the screen. Thus, when the stimulus appeared on those trials with invalid cues, subjects had to disengage their attention from the incorrect side of space and shift to the side on which the stimulus had actually appeared. This disengagement operation was dramatically slower in the AD patients. Therefore, AD patients appear able to focus attention but have trouble disengaging in order to flexibly redeploy their attentional focus.

The other major sense of the term *attention* is alertness—an individual's readiness to process external information and to respond. Fluctuations in alertness can be divided into (1) phasic changes—the rapid mobilization of resources to process an expected input and (2) tonic changes —the slow decline in performance across a long, repetitive task. Phasic changes in alertness are evident in the way a warning signal facilitates subjects' response time (RT) to a later stimulus by allowing them to maximize their alertness for the upcoming stimulus. Not only do AD patients respond faster to a stimulus when given a warning, but the time the patients need to reach maximal alertness (i.e., the optimal delay between the warning and stimulus) is no longer than that required by the normal old.[5] This suggests that AD does not grossly impair patients' ability to mobilize their attentional resources to prepare for an upcoming stimulus. Studies of tonic alertness have found that this component of alertness is also relatively preserved in AD. Tonic alertness is typically tested by giving subjects a long, unbroken period of repetitive testing. A decrease in tonic attention is evident as a decline in response accuracy or RT across time on task. Several studies[3,5] have shown that the performance of AD patients declines no more rapidly than does that of the normal old. Thus, the attentional deficit in AD is most evident in divided-attention situations. Focused attention and tonic and phasic alertness are much less impaired in these patients.

LANGUAGE

Language deficits are among the most prominent early symptoms of AD. However, not all aspects of language are disrupted.[6] AD causes only minimal deficits in syntax, as patients' speech generally remains grammatically correct. However, AD patients often perform badly on tests involving semantics—the production and comprehension of meaning. They have difficulty finding the appropriate word both in spontaneous speech and in formal tests such as object naming. Their speech is littered with indefinite terms such as "stuff" and "things" and thus often conveys little information.

Their comprehension of language, especially of complex sentences and stories, can be quite poor. These patients also have difficulty searching semantic categories and producing semantic associates to a given stimulus.

One explanation for these problems is that AD disrupts patients' knowledge of concept meaning (see Chap. 23). It has been suggested that AD patients no longer know the distinctive semantic attributes of concepts, such as their physical features and functions. A loss of basic perceptual and abstract knowledge about concepts could explain the problems AD patients have in finding the appropriate word or name, understanding and using language, dealing with abstract concepts, etc. It could even contribute to the patients' problems in a variety of other cognitive areas, since humans tend to use language and symbols extensively when storing and manipulating information. Many investigators feel that this semantic dysfunction is one of the core deficits of AD that differentiates it from other dementing diseases.[7]

It is still not clear, however, whether semantic information is actually lost in AD or whether the problems these patients have on semantic tasks spring from failures of more general-purpose cognitive operations such as those involved in accessing and evaluating information. This possibility is raised by studies that have found relatively normal performance by AD patients on some semantic tasks. For example, one recent study[8] presented AD patients with a target word (e.g., *fish*) followed by a stimulus word and measured how accurately and rapidly they could decide whether the stimulus was related to the target. On some of the trials, the stimulus was a semantic attribute of the target (e.g., *fins*), while on others it was not (e.g., *laces*).

In this study, AD patients were extremely accurate in their decisions about the relationship between a target and its attributes. This study also looked at how decision time varied as a function of the relative importance that the attribute had for the meaning of the target. Attribute importance reflects the likelihood that a particular attribute comes to mind when a target concept is presented. For example, when given "airplane" and asked to name its attributes, people are more likely to think of wings than of wheels, even though both are physical features of an airplane. In this study, the decision time of normals was inversely related to attribute importance—that is, the more important the attribute, the faster their decision. This same pattern was found in the AD patients. These results suggest that not only do AD patients retain knowledge of concept attributes, but they still know the relative importance that different attributes of a concept have for concept meaning.

Overall, investigations into AD patients' semantic abilities have produced a multitude of contradictory results. The underlying cause of their deficits on some semantic tasks—loss of semantic knowledge versus inability to use intact semantic knowledge—is one of the more controversial issues in the cognitive neuropsychology of AD.

MEMORY

While AD causes major deficits in most areas of cognition, the symptom that people commonly associate with this disease is a loss of memory. However, even memory is not uniformly impaired.[1,9] Memory has multiple components and processes, some of which are more disrupted by AD than others. Primary or short-term memory is viewed as a limited-capacity temporary store of information held in consciousness, while secondary or long-term memory is an unlimited-capacity permanent store. There is no question that AD severely disrupts secondary memory. Alzheimer patients have great difficulty recalling any substantial amount of information for more than a few minutes, especially if they engage in any interfering cognitive activity prior to recall. Even if the stimuli are repeated several times or memory cues or possible answers in the form of a recognition test are provided, AD patients still perform quite poorly[10] on tests of secondary memory. By contrast, primary memory seems less affected by AD, although it is not normal. For example, when given a list of words to remember, AD patients tend to recall only the last few items they heard—i.e., what they do recall appears to come from primary memory.

What might be the source of the secondary-memory problems in AD? In order to remember a stimulus, it must be encoded into memory, maintained in storage, and later retrieved. There is a great deal of evidence for a major dysfunction in AD patients' initial processing of information (i.e., encoding). Stimulus factors known to affect encoding in normals (e.g., word familiarity) do not influence encoding in AD patients. Also, in AD patients, unlike normals, semantic knowledge about the stimulus or the context in which the stimulus appears does not always facilitate memory encoding. As for storage, if the level of initial learning is equated in AD patients and normals (a difficult feat), the rate at which information is lost from secondary memory appears to be approximately the same in the two groups. That is, the rate of forgetting may be relatively normal in AD patients. The effect that AD has on memory retrieval is unclear due to the severity of the encoding deficit. One way of demonstrating that a retrieval defect contributes to memory problems is to show that the problems decrease when the demand on retrieval is minimized, either by giving memory cues or by using a recognition task. However, as stated above, such approaches do not help AD patients. But it is possible that memory encoding is so deficient in AD patients that the resultant memory trace is impoverished to the point that cues and recognition choices cannot activate it.

While secondary memory performance is very poor in AD, there are other constituents of memory that appear to be much less disrupted. One is memory for distant events (remote memory). The normal old tend to remember information from the remote past better than more recent events (i.e., their memory accuracy shows a temporal gradient). Remote memory has been assessed by such tests as memory for important public events (John F. Kennedy's death), famous faces from a particular era (e.g., Harry S. Truman), or personal events in an individual's life. While AD patients do not perform as well as normals in such tasks, their memory does show a temporal gradient in that they recall distant information better than more recent information, suggesting a relative preservation of remote memory.

A second aspect of memory that may be at least partially preserved in AD is implicit memory (see Chap. 22). Unlike the memory described up to this point (so-called explicit memory), implicit-memory tasks do not require intentional recollection of prior information. Rather, they measure the facilitation that prior experience has on a subject's performance. For example, if subjects are shown a series of stimulus words and later given the first few letters of those words (word stem), being asked to complete each stem with one of the previously presented stimulus words, this is a measure of explicit memory. By contrast, if, when given the word stem, they are just asked to complete the stem with the first word that comes to mind (no mention being made of any relationship to the prior stimulus words), this is a measure of implicit memory. In such an implicit-memory task, the subjects' previous experience with the stimulus words is evident as an increased likelihood that they will complete the stems with words from the stimulus list (in comparison to a baseline condition where they did not experience the stimuli). The effect of prior experience with the stimuli is thus evident implicitly as a change in the subjects' behavior rather than as explicit recall. This distinction between explicit and implicit memory has generated a great deal of interest because patients with organic amnesias (e.g., Korsakoff patients) can show normal implicit-memory performance despite a total inability to recall the stimuli explicitly. What about AD patients? At present the evidence is mixed. Some studies have shown the implicit memory of AD patients to be grossly defective. However, other researchers[11] argue that normal implicit memory can be demonstrated in AD if the study design ensures that the patients adequately attend to and encode the initial stimulus material. That is, if their initial processing of the stimuli is successful, it may be possible to demonstrate relatively normal implicit memory.

DISCUSSION

From this brief review it is clear that while AD patients have multiple deficits, not all aspects of cognition are equally impaired. Several theoretical mechanisms have been proposed to explain this variability. Some investigators have suggested that the attentional capacity of AD patients is severely diminished. If so, then AD patients should perform poorly on any task that makes a major demand on attentional capacity while performing relatively normally on tasks that require only automatic processes.[12] Attentional capacity has been conceptualized as the mental energy necessary for the active and intentional manipulation of information. By contrast, automatic processes require neither conscious awareness nor intention and place little demand on attentional capacity. For example, actively searching through your memory for a particular piece of information to answer a question is thought to require substantial attentional capacity. By contrast, retrieval of a word's phonology and meanings is thought to be automatic. Unfortunately, there is little direct evidence supporting this attractive hypothesis. One problem is that criteria for what constitutes an automatic process have been specifically defined in only a few experimental paradigms, and AD patients do not always perform normally in these paradigms. For example, the incidental encoding into memory of certain types of information (e.g., the sensory modality in which a stimulus was presented or its frequency of presentation) meets some investigators' criteria for automaticity. However, AD patients' memory for such information is quite poor.[13] Thus, a reduction in attentional capacity seems unlikely to be the sole explanation for the variability seen in AD patients' cognitive performance.

Recently, a variant of the attentional-capacity model has been suggested in which AD patients' deficits are hypothesized to arise from a failure of inhibitory processes.[14] It is argued that AD patients fail to inhibit partially activated but incorrect information. This would result in their processing capacity being swamped by unimportant information that normal individuals would suppress. Evidence for this hypothesis comes from a variety of sources. Alzheimer patients tend to make many intrusion errors (e.g., when remembering a story, they will incorporate information

from outside the story into their recall). They also have difficulty inhibiting the irrelevant meanings of ambiguous words. When normal individuals encounter a word with multiple distinct meanings in a sentence, those meanings that are irrelevant to that particular context are rapidly inhibited. For example, when normal individuals see the word *bank* in the context of a sentence about a river, both senses of the word (i.e., one relevant to money, the other to a river) are automatically activated. However, in normals, within a half second or so, the irrelevant sense of the word (i.e., a place that holds money) is inhibited. By contrast, in AD patients, both the relevant and irrelevant senses of *bank* tend to remain active.[15] Such a failure to inhibit contextually irrelevant information would not only overload AD patients' processing capacity but also interfere with their understanding of the sentence's meaning. A breakdown in inhibitory control in AD patients could contribute to many of their cognitive deficits, including memory, language, problem solving, etc. While the evidence for this model is still limited, it may turn out to be an important mechanism underlying the cognitive deficits of AD.

Another theoretical construct that shows promise for explaining the pattern of cognitive deficits in AD is the central executive system. The central executive system is conceived of as the mechanism that organizes and coordinates simultaneously active processing programs. It resolves scheduling conflicts and orchestrates the operation of concurrent processes. Any central executive system dysfunction would make it difficult for AD patients to intentionally manipulate and process stimulus information, especially in complex tasks where multiple mental operations must be carried out either simultaneously or in the proper sequence.[16] For example, in order to comprehend and remember a sentence, it is necessary to coordinate the decoding of language symbols with the encoding of this information into memory. At the present time, however, it is difficult to evaluate whether a central executive system dysfunction could account for the full array of deficits found in AD, because the nature of the central executive system has not been clearly defined, nor have comparatively pure measures of central executive system function been devised.

SUMMARY

While substantial progress has been made in characterizing the types of mental operations impaired in AD, the mechanisms underlying these deficits are still not clear. Are we dealing with an accumulation of many discrete deficits, such as would result from numerous focal brain lesions, or are only a few basic cognitive dysfunctions responsible for the total array of impairments in AD? To some extent the answer to this question may depend on future advances in cognitive psychology, as it is this area of research that has provided the theoretical frameworks and methodologies underlying the cognitive-neuropsychological approach to AD.

REFERENCES

1. Nebes RD: Cognitive dysfunction in Alzheimer's disease, in Craik FIM, Salthouse TA (eds): *The Handbook of Aging and Cognition.* Hillsdale, NJ, Erlbaum, 1992, pp 373–446.
2. Parasuraman R, Haxby JV: Attention and brain function in Alzheimer's disease: A review. *Neuropsychology* 7:242–272, 1993.
3. Filoteo JV, Delis DC, Massman PJ, et al: Directed and divided attention in Alzheimer's disease: Impairment in shifting attention to global and local stimuli. *J Clin Exp Neuropsychol* 14:871–883, 1992.
4. Parasuraman R, Greenwood PM, Haxby JV, Grady CL: Visuospatial attention in dementia of the Alzheimer type. *Brain* 115:711–733, 1992.
5. Nebes RD, Brady CB: Phasic and tonic alertness in Alzheimer's disease. *Cortex* 29:77–90, 1993.
6. Nebes RD: Semantic memory in Alzheimer's disease. *Psychol Bull* 106:377–394, 1989.
7. Martin A: Degraded knowledge representations in patients with Alzheimer's disease, in Squire LR, Butters N (eds): *Neuropsychology of Memory.* Amsterdam, North-Holland, 1992, pp 220–232.
8. Nebes RD, Brady CB: Preserved organization of semantic attributes in Alzheimer's disease. *Psychol Aging* 5:574–579, 1990.
9. Carlesimo GA, Oscar-Berman M: Memory deficits in Alzheimer's patients: A comprehensive review. *Neuropsychol Rev* 3:119–169, 1992.
10. Weingartner H, Kaye W, Smallberg SA, et al: Memory failures in progressive idiopathic dementia. *J Abnorm Psychol* 90:187–196, 1981.
11. Grosse DA, Wilson RS, Fox JH: Preserved word-stem-completion priming of semantically encoded information in Alzheimer's disease. *Psychol Aging* 5:304–306, 1990.
12. Jorm AF: Controlled and automatic information processing in senile dementia. *Psychol Med* 16:77–88, 1986.
13. Grafman J, Weingartner H, Lawlor B, et al: Automatic memory processes in patients with dementia—Alzheimer's type. *Cortex* 26:361–371, 1990.
14. Spieler DH, Balota DA, Faust ME: Stroop performance in younger adults, healthy older adults and individuals with senile dementia of the Alzheimer type. *J Exp Psychol: Hum Percept Perform.* In press.
15. Balota DA, Duchek JM: Semantic priming effects, lexical repetition effects and contextual disambiguation effects in healthy aged individuals and individuals with senile dementia of the Alzheimer type. *Brain Lang* 40:181–201, 1991.
16. Becker JT: Working memory and secondary memory deficits in Alzheimer's disease. *J Clin Exp Neuropsychol* 10:739–753, 1988.

Chapter 31

DEMENTIA IN PARKINSON DISEASE, HUNTINGTON DISEASE, AND OTHER DEGENERATIVE CONDITIONS

Diane M. Jacobs
Yaakov Stern
Richard Mayeux

PARKINSON DISEASE

Epidemiology

The idiopathic form of Parkinson disease is one of the most common neurologic disorders, affecting between 80 to 200 people per 100,000.[1] The prevalence of Parkinson disease increases with advancing age. Although the average age of onset is approximately 65 years, more than 1 percent of persons in the United States over age 80 have Parkinson disease. The annual incidence is 1 per 10,000 people.

Estimates of the prevalence of dementia among Parkinson patients vary widely, depending upon the population studied and the criteria used to diagnose dementia. Rajput and colleagues[2] found that only 9 percent of their patients were demented on the basis of clinical examination, while Pirozzolo and colleagues[3] reported dementia in 93 percent of their Parkinson patients based upon performance on formal neuropsychological measures. Estimates of dementia prevalence ranging from 30 to 50 percent have frequently been reported.[1,4,5] In a community-based study, Mayeux and associates[1] found an overall prevalence rate of Parkinson disease with dementia of 41.1 per 100,000, with prevalence increasing with age from 0 below age 50 to 787.1 per 100,000 above age 79.

The risk of incident dementia among patients with Parkinson disease is far greater than that expected among individuals of the same age without Parkinson disease. Rajput and colleagues[6] found a significantly higher cumulative probability of developing dementia among Parkinson patients (21 percent) than among age-referenced controls (5.7 percent). Similarly, in a population-based community study, Marder and colleagues[7] reported that the risk of dementia in Parkinson patients was nearly twice that of healthy elderly matched in age and gender. The identification of dementia in patients with Parkinson disease is of clinical significance, as dementia is the single most important factor limiting standard pharmacotherapy of Parkinson disease.[8] Dementia also increases the mortality rate for Parkinson patients.[9]

Among Parkinson patients, risk factors for developing dementia include advancing age and older age at onset of Parkinson disease; severity of motor symptoms; depression; poor tolerance of levodopa or other standard treatment for Parkinson disease, including serious side effects such as hallucinations, delusions, and delirium; and facial masking as a presenting sign.[10,11]

Characteristics of Dementia

The dementia associated with Parkinson disease is generally characterized by predominant impairment of executive functions (e.g., initiating responses, planning, set shifting), visuospatial skills, free-recall memory, and verbal fluency. Language functions other than verbal fluency are relatively preserved, as are orientation, cued recall, and recognition memory. The neuropsychological profile of dementia in Parkinson disease is similar to the pattern of impaired and preserved cognitive abilities associated with damage to the frontal lobes, particularly the prefrontal cortex[12,13] (see Chaps. 24 and 25).

Impairment of executive functions in Parkinson dementia may be disproportionately severe relative to deficits in other cognitive domains. Executive functions commonly affected by Parkinson disease include response initiation, planning, set-shifting, and ability to benefit from feedback. The neuropsychological measure most frequently used to evaluate executive dysfunction in Parkinson disease is the Wisconsin Card Sorting Test (WCST), a task in which the patient is asked to sort a deck of cards based upon three categorical sorting rules.[14] Because successful performance on the WCST requires the ability to form concepts, shift set, monitor one's responses, and benefit from feedback provided by the examiner, it is highly sensitive to the pattern of executive dysfunction often observed in patients with Parkinson disease.

Bowen and colleagues[15] were the first to examine the performance of Parkinson disease patients on the WCST, and their results have been replicated numerous times. In their original investigation, Bowen et al. found that Parkinson patients were impaired in their ability to form concepts, and had an increased number of total and nonperseverative errors. Further, patients were able to verbalize the correct response but failed to use this information to modify their behavior appropriately. This dissociation between thought and action had been observed previously in patients with frontal-lobe lesions[16,17] and thereby lent further support to the notion that dementia in Parkinson disease was due, at least in part, to frontal-lobe dysfunction.

The extent to which the neuropsychological profile of dementia in Parkinson disease differs from that associated with Alzheimer disease is controversial. Several extensive reviews of comparative studies have been written.[18–20] While some investigators have concluded that the two dementias differ in etiology and phenomenology,[21] others propose that the similarities between Parkinson and Alzheimer dementia far outweigh the differences.[19,22] Perhaps the most frequently replicated observed difference on neuropsychological testing between demented patients with Parkinson and Alzheimer disease is performance on delayed memory testing relative to immediate recall. In Alzheimer disease, delayed recall and recognition memory of recently learned information is severely impaired relative to normative data and to performance on immediate recall; that is, Alzheimer patients rapidly forget information that was recalled accurately on immediate memory testing.[23,24] In contrast, delayed recall and recognition memory in Parkinson disease may be impaired relative to normative data but often is commensurate with the level of recall on testing of immediate memory. Hence, Parkinson disease is associated with relatively good retention of newly acquired information over a delay interval. The memory impairment associated with Parkinson disease is considered primarily a retrieval deficit, while Alzheimer disease is characterized by deficient encoding or consolidation of information (Table 31-1).

Even in the absence of overt dementia, cognitive impairment occurs frequently in Parkinson disease. Common domains of relative impairment in nondemented Parkinson disease patients include attentional and executive functions, visuospatial skills, recall memory, and verbal fluency. Circumscribed cognitive impairments have been observed even in very high functioning Parkinson patients.[25] Nevertheless, the mild or relatively circumscribed cognitive dysfunction that is evident in many patients with Parkinson disease does not progress to frank dementia in all affected individuals. Jacobs and colleagues[26] found that the performance of nondemented patients with Parkinson disease on tests of letter and category fluency was a highly sensitive neuropsychological predictor of incident dementia. Stern and colleagues[23] concluded that although cognitive problems preceding dementia in Parkinson disease patients continue to worsen with the onset of dementia, there is also a qualitative shift in the pattern of cognitive

Table 31-1

Neuropsychological characteristics of dementia in Alzheimer, Parkinson, and Huntington diseases and progressive supranuclear palsy

	Alzheimer disease	Parkinson disease	Huntington disease	Progressive supranuclear palsy
Orientation	Impaired	Normal	Normal	Normal
Memory				
Immediate recall	Impaired	Impaired	Impaired	Normal–mildly impaired
Delayed recall	Severely impaired	Impaired	Impaired	Normal–mildly impaired
Delayed recognition	Severely impaired	Normal	Normal	Normal
Percent retained[a]	0–50	50–80+	50–80+	50–80+
Executive functions/ problem solving	Severely impaired	Severely impaired[b]	Severely impaired[b]	Severely impaired[b]
Language				
Naming	Severely impaired; anomia, paraphasia	Normal–mildly impaired; anomia	Normal; visual misperceptions	Normal; visual misperceptions
Verbal fluency	Impaired	Severely impaired	Severely impaired	Severely impaired
Visuospatial skills	Impaired	Impaired	Severely impaired	Impaired

[a]Percent retained = (immediate recall/delayed recall) × 100.

[b]Executive functions often are disproportionately impaired relative to other cognitive abilities.

deficits, with substantial broadening and worsening of memory dysfunction, as dementia emerges.

Depression is common in Parkinson disease, occurring in approximately 45 percent of patients.[27] The incidence rate of depression in Parkinson disease is 1.86 percent per year.[27] Depression has been found to coexist with dementia in some Parkinson patients[28] and has been identified as a risk factor for incident dementia in nondemented patients.[10,11]

Pathology

The pathologic hallmark of Parkinson disease is loss of pigmented cells in the substantia nigra and other pigmented nuclei. Lewy bodies are found within the neurons remaining in the affected areas.[29,30] The pattern of neuropsychologic deficit typical of dementia in Parkinson disease, includ-

ing prominent impairment on "frontal lobe" or executive tasks, has been attributed to degeneration of the medial substantia nigra, with associated loss of nigral projections of dopamine to the limbic and frontal areas,[31] and to cholinergic deficiency,[32] although numerous other neurotransmitter systems also have been implicated.[30,33] Other pathologic entities that have been proposed as the neuropathologic basis for dementia in Parkinson disease include coincident Alzheimer disease[34,35] and cortical Lewy bodies.[36,37]

HUNTINGTON DISEASE

Epidemiology

Huntington disease is an autosomal dominant disorder with complete penetrance that is characterized by progressive involuntary choreiform movements, psychiatric features, and dementia. The genetic mutation has been identified as an unstable trinucleotide repeat (CAG) on the short arm of chromosome 4.[38] Prevalence estimates of Huntington disease range from 4 to 10 per 100,000.[39]

Dementia is a ubiquitous feature of Huntington disease; however, the severity of cognitive impairment does vary from patient to patient. The juvenile-onset form is associated with severe and rapidly progressive dementia, while cognitive dysfunction is relatively mild and slowly progressive in patients with onset of motor symptoms after age 50.[40] The dementia associated with midlife onset of Huntington disease, the most frequent presentation, is intermediate between the juvenile and late onset in terms of severity and rapidity of course. Degree of dementia is closely associated with severity of motor involvement.[41]

Characteristics of Dementia

The neuropsychological profile of dementia associated with Huntington disease is similar to that observed in patients with Parkinson disease and is characterized by lack of initiative, impaired attention and executive functions, poor memory and visuospatial skills, but relatively preserved language functions with the exception of verbal fluency. Impairment on tests of visuospatial function may be partly attributable to abnormalities in eye movement that are common in patients with Huntington disease. Errors made on tests of visual confrontation naming are often visual misperceptions of the test stimuli rather than paraphasic or anomic errors, again suggesting that eye-movement abnormalities may contribute to these errors. Nevertheless, specific impairments manipulating egocentric space (i.e., perceiving an object with reference to its distance and direction from the observer) in Huntington disease have been described.[42,43]

The memory impairment of Huntington disease, like that of Parkinson disease, is characterized by poor performance on all memory measures (e.g., immediate and delayed free recall, cued recall) relative to normative data. Rates of retention from immediate to delayed testing, however, are relatively preserved,[24] and Huntington disease patients demonstrate significantly more improvement on testing of delayed recognition memory than do patients with Alzheimer disease.[44] As in Parkinson disease, the memory impairment of Huntington disease is characterized by severely impaired retrieval of stored information. Patients have difficulty initiating and organizing systematic retrieval strategies (see Table 31-1).

Personality changes and psychiatric disturbances are common and prominent features of Huntington disease, which may precede the onset of motor or cognitive symptoms by as much as 10 years.[45] Apathy, irritability, and poor impulse control are common. Major depression occurs at some time in nearly 40 percent of patients with Huntington disease.[46,47] Five to 10 percent of patients experience schizophrenia-like disorders, characterized by auditory and tactile hallucinations, paranoid delusions, and thought disorder.[48]

Pathology

The core pathologic feature of Huntington disease is atrophy of the caudate and putamen bilaterally. Bamford and colleagues[49] demonstrated that the cognitive impairment in 60 drug-free Huntington patients—including performance on tests of complex psychomotor skill, verbal memory, and visuospatial functioning—was closely linked to the extent of caudate atrophy as measured by computed tomography scan.

PROGRESSIVE SUPRANUCLEAR PALSY

Epidemiology

Clinical characteristics of progressive supranuclear palsy include supranuclear ophthalmoplegia primarily affecting vertical gaze, pseudobulbar palsy, dysarthria, and axial and nuchal rigidity.[50] The prevalence of progressive supranuclear palsy (PSP) has been estimated as 1.4 per 100,000, with an age-adjusted prevalence for the population over age 55 of 7 per 100,000.[51] It has, however, been suggested that the prevalence of progressive supranuclear palsy has been underestimated because it often is misdiagnosed as Parkinson disease.[52] The usual age of onset is between 60 and 70, but onset as early as the mid-40s has been reported.[51] Symptom onset is insidious, and the disease course is progressive, leading to death in 5 to 7 years. Dementia is a common although not ubiquitous feature of progressive supranuclear palsy. Cognitive or behavioral symptoms were reported in seven of the nine cases described by Steele and coworkers.[50] Subsequent estimates of the prevalence of dementia in progressive supranuclear palsy range from 20 to 60 percent.

Characteristics of Dementia

The neuropsychological profile of dementia in progressive supranuclear palsy is often considered prototypical of "subcortical" or "subcorticofrontal" dysfunction. Albert and colleagues[53] described forgetfulness, slowed thought processes, emotional or personality changes, and impaired ability to manipulate acquired knowledge as typical cognitive changes in progressive supranuclear palsy. Executive dysfunction is a prominent feature at all stages of the disease course.[54,55] Although performance on relatively simple attentional tasks may be normal, performance on more complex tasks—such as those requiring sequencing, mental flexibility, abstraction, and reasoning—is severely impaired. Slowness of information processing is pervasive and marked. Dubois and colleagues[56] found processing time in patients with progressive supranuclear palsy to be increased, even relative to patients with Parkinson disease. Albert and colleagues[53] reported that when patients were allowed additional time to respond (sometimes as long as 4 to 5 min for a single question), their performance improved by as much as 50 percent. Verbal fluency is generally very severely impaired; however, other language functions remain preserved. As in Huntington patients, erroneous responses on tests of visual confrontation naming are frequently visual misperceptions[57] and may be secondary to the oculomotor impair-

ments that characterize this disorder. Anomic and paraphasic errors are uncommon. Although language is relatively preserved, severe dysarthria often impairs communicative ability.[57] The memory disorder of progressive supranuclear palsy is generally mild.[58] Although PSP patients may be impaired on memory tasks requiring free recall, they are able to benefit from retrieval cues and perform normally on tests of cued recall (see Table 31-1).[59]

The most commonly reported personality changes in progressive supranuclear palsy are apathy and inertia.[53,60] These symptoms likely reflect the mental slowing that is typical of this disorder. Irritability and depression are also common. Emotional disinhibition (i.e., either laughing or crying excessively with preserved affect) has also been described.

Pathology

Cell loss and pathology in progressive supranuclear palsy occur in various regions of the basal ganglia, brainstem, and cerebellum, including the pallidum, subthalamic nucleus, red nucleus, substantia nigra, superior colliculi, nuclei cuneiformis and subcuneiformis, periaqueductal gray matter, pontine tegmentum, and the dentate nucleus. Consistent with the clinical picture of dementia in progressive supranuclear palsy, functional brain imaging shows subfrontal glucose hypometabolism.[61] Pillon and colleagues[54] interpreted the clinicopathologic association in progressive supranuclear palsy as "frontal deafferentation."

CORTICAL-BASAL GANGLIONIC DEGENERATION

Epidemiology

Cortical-basal ganglionic degeneration (CBGD) is a relatively rare condition characterized by rigidity, focal dystonias or myoclonus, supranuclear gaze palsy, "alien-limb" phenomena, cortical sensory loss, postural-action tremor, postural instability, and severe apraxia.[62,63] Muscle strength is generally preserved. Signs and symptoms are often strikingly asymmetric. Although many of the signs of CBGD are similar to those found in Parkinson disease, the alien-limb phenomena and marked apraxia are distinguishing features. Alien-limb signs often observed in CBGD include levitation and posturing of the arm, particularly when attention is diverted or the eyes are closed.

Prevalence estimates for CBGD are unavailable, and there are no known risk factors. Onset is typically between age 60 and 70, and the average duration of disease from onset to death is 6 to 8 years. Although dementia was not described as a prominent feature in the initial report of this disorder,[62] subsequent reports have found dementia to be common and in some cases severe.[64]

Characteristics of Dementia

The neuropsychological profile of dementia associated with CBGD is characterized by a prominent dysexecutive syndrome, similar to that of patients with PSP; deficient dynamic motor control (e.g., bimanual coordination, temporal organization); asymmetric praxis disorders; and poor free recall but intact cued recall and recognition memory.[59] The most notable and frequently reported feature is the presence of ideational and ideomotor apraxia. Often patients can accurately describe an action (e.g., using a key to open a door) that they are completely unable to perform. Other reported neuropsychological characteristics include "decreased intellectual efficiency"[62] or slowing of thought processes, aphasia (anomia, paraphasia),[63,65] acalculia,[65] right-left confusion,[63] and perseveration.[63] Rediess and Satran[66] reported a patient who was tested serially with a comprehensive neuropsychological battery. One year after onset of motor and personality changes, this patient had impairments of psychomotor speed, verbal fluency, visuoperceptual ability, and nonverbal memory. Verbal memory was strikingly preserved. Four years after symptom onset, however, the patient's dementia was global and severe.

Changes in personality that have been reported in association with CBGD include irritability[66] and increased aggression.[63]

Pathology

Cortical basal ganglionic degeneration is associated with atrophy of frontal and parietal cortex.[62,67] Convolutional atrophy is often greater in the cerebral hemisphere contralateral to the side of the body with pronounced motor involvement. Cortical cell loss, gliosis, and Pick cells are observed, as are nerve cell loss and gliosis in the substantia nigra, locus ceruleus, thalamus, lentiform nucleus, subthalamic nucleus, red nucleus, and midbrain tegmentum.[67] Pathology is generally absent in the temporal and hippocampal regions.[67]

MULTIPLE-SYSTEM ATROPHY AND CEREBELLAR DEGENERATION

The term *multiple-system atrophy* has been applied to several disorders of the motor system sometimes referred to as Parkinson-plus syndromes. These disorders include striatonigral degeneration, sporadic olivopontocerebellar atrophy, and Shy-Drager syndrome. Each of these disorders is characterized by parkinsonian motor signs plus a unique feature that distinguishes it from idiopathic Parkinson disease.[68] Tremor is absent in striatonigral degeneration, and the response to levodopa is limited, as striatal neurons containing dopamine receptors are lost. Olivopontocerebellar atrophy is characterized by parkinsonism plus ataxia and other cerebellar signs. Familial olivopontocerebellar atrophy is a dominantly inherited disorder that presents as a cerebellar syndrome. Finally, Shy-Drager syndrome is characterized by parkinsonism plus autonomic dysfunction, particularly progressive, primary orthostatic hypotension. Although striatonigral degeneration, sporadic olivopontocerebellar atrophy, and Shy-Drager syndrome had previously been considered to be distinct and separate entities, they are now felt to represent different manifestations of a single disease process.[69]

Although motor signs are the prominent and distinguishing features of multiple-system atrophy, changes in cognition may also be present. The profile of cognitive impairment is generally one of relatively preserved overall intellectual functioning but with poor performance on tests of executive function, especially those requiring sequencing and set shifting.[70] Thought processes may be slowed. Performance on tests of language and visual perception generally is within normal limits with the possible exception of verbal fluency.

Cognitive impairment may also be associated with pure cerebellar atrophy.[71-75] As in patients with multiple-system atrophy, overall intelligence is generally preserved in patients with pure cerebellar atrophy; however, performance on tests of executive function may be impaired. Reported areas of cognitive deficit include planning on a complex problem-solving task, response initiation, shifting of attention, and verbal fluency. Appollonio and colleagues[74] found patients with cerebellar degeneration to be impaired relative to normal subjects on "effort-demanding" tests of memory, but the poor memory performance of these subjects was felt to be secondary to their executive dysfunction.

ACKNOWLEDGMENTS

This work was supported by Federal grants AG07232, AG08702, RR00645, and the Parkinson's Disease Foundation.

REFERENCES

1. Mayeux R, Denaro J, Hemenegildo N, et al: A population-based investigation of Parkinson's disease with and without dementia: Relationship to age and gender. *Arch Neurol* 49:492–497, 1992.
2. Rajput AH, Offord K, Beard CM, Kurland LT: Epidemiological survey of dementia in parkinsonism and control population, in Hassler RG, Christ JF (eds): *Advances in Neurology. Parkinson-Specific Motor and Mental Disorders.* New York: Raven Press, 1986, vol 40, pp 229–234.
3. Pirozzolo FJ, Hansch EC, Mortimer JA, et al: Dementia in Parkinson disease: A neuropsychological analysis. *Brain Cogn* 1:71–83, 1982.
4. Lieberman A, Dziatolowski M, Kupersmith M, et al: Dementia in Parkinson disease. *Ann Neurol* 6:355–359, 1979.
5. Celesia GG, Wanamaker WM: Psychiatric disturbances in Parkinson's disease. *Dis Nerv Syst* 33:577–583, 1972.
6. Rajput AH, Offord KP, Beard CM, Kurland LT: A case-control study of smoking habits, dementia, and other illnesses in idiopathic Parkinson's disease. *Neurology* 37:226–232, 1987.
7. Marder K, Tang M-X, Cote LJ, et al: Predictors of dementia in community-dwelling elderly patients with Parkinson's disease. *Neurology* 43:S115, 1993.
8. Mayeux R: A current analysis of behavioral problems in patients with idiopathic Parkinson's disease (review). *Move Dis* 4(suppl 1):S48–S56, 1989.
9. Marder K, Leung D, Tang M, et al: Are demented patients with Parkinson's disease accurately reflected in prevalence surveys? A survival analysis. *Neurology* 41:1240–1243, 1991.
10. Stern Y, Marder K, Tang MX, Mayeux R: Antecedent clinical features associated with dementia in Parkinson's disease. *Neurology* 43:1690–1692, 1993.
11. Marder K, Tang M-X, Cote L, et al: The frequency and associated risk factors for dementia in patients with Parkinson's disease. *Arch Neurol* 52:695–701, 1995.
12. Bondi MW, Kaszniak AW, Bayles KA, Vance KT: Contributions of frontal system dysfunction to memory and perceptual abilities in Parkinson's disease. *Neuropsychology* 7:89–102, 1993.
13. Taylor AE, Saint-Cyr JA, Lang AE, Kenny FF: Frontal lobe dysfunction in Parkinson's disease: The cortical focus of neostriatal outflow. *Brain* 109:845–883, 1986.
14. Berg EA: A simple objective test for measuring flexibility in thinking. *J Gen Psychol* 39:15–22, 1948.
15. Bowen FP: Behavioral alterations in patients with basal ganglia lesions, in Yahr MD (ed): *The Basal Ganglia.* New York: Raven Press, 1976, pp 169–180.
16. Milner B: Effects of different brain lesions on card sorting: The role of the frontal lobes. *Arch Neurol* 9:90, 1963.
17. Teuber HL: The frontal lobes and their functions: Further observations in carnivores, subhuman primates and man. *Int J Neurol* 5:282–300, 1966.
18. Dubois B, Boller F, Pillon B, Agid Y: Cognitive deficits in Parkinson's disease, in Boller F, Grafman J (eds): *Handbook of Neuropsychology.* Amsterdam: Elsevier, 1991, vol 5, pp 195–240.
19. Brown RG, Marsden CD: "Subcortical dementia": The neuropsychological evidence. *Neuroscience* 25:363–387, 1988.
20. Mahler ME, Cummings JL: Alzheimer's disease

and the dementia of PD: Comparative investigations. *Alz Dis Assoc Disord* 4:133–149, 1990.

21. Cummings JL: Subcortical dementia. Neuropsychology, neuropsychiatry and pathophysiology. *Br J Psychiatr* 149:682–697, 1986.

22. Whitehouse PJ: The concept of subcortical dementia: Another look. *Ann Neurol* 19:1–6, 1986.

23. Stern Y, Richards M, Sano M, Mayeux R: Comparison of cognitive changes in patients with Alzheimer's and Parkinson's disease. *Arch Neurol* 50:1040–1045, 1993.

24. Troster AI, Butters N, Salmon DP, et al: The diagnostic utility of savings scores: Differentiating Alzheimer's and Huntington's diseases with the Logical Memory and Visual Reproduction tests. *J Clin Exp Neuropsychol* 15:773–788, 1993.

25. Mohr E, Juncos J, Cox C, et al: Selective deficits in cognition and memory in high functioning Parkinson's patients. *J Neurol Neurosurg Psychiatr* 53:603–606, 1990.

26. Jacobs DM, Marder K, Cote LJ, et al: Neuropsychological characteristics of preclinical dementia in Parkinson's disease. *Neurology* 45:1691–1696, 1995.

27. Dooneief G, Mirabello E, Bell K, et al: An estimate of the incidence of depression in idiopathic Parkinson's disease. *Arch Neurol* 49:305–307, 1992.

28. Sano M, Stern Y, Williams J, et al: Coexisting dementia and depression in Parkinson's disease. *Arch Neurol* 46:1284–1286, 1989.

29. Gibb WRG, Scott T, Lees AJ: Neuronal inclusions of Parkinson's disease. *Move Disord* 6:2–11, 1991.

30. Jellinger K: New developments in the pathology of Parkinson's disease, in Streifler MB, Korczyn AD, Melamed E, Youdim MBH (eds): *Advances in Neurology: Parkinson's Disease: Anatomy, Pathology, and Therapy.* New York: Raven Press, 1991, vol 53, pp 1–16.

31. Rinne JO, Rummukainen J, Paljarvi L, Rinne UK: Dementia in Parkinson's disease is related to neuronal loss in the medial substantia nigra. *Ann Neurol* 26:47–50, 1989.

32. Dubois B, Pillon B, Lhermitte F, Agid Y: Cholinergic deficiency and frontal dysfunction in Parkinson's disease. *Ann Neurol* 28:117–121, 1990.

33. Hornykiewicz O: Movement disorders, in Marsden CD, Fanh S (eds): *Brain Neurotransmitter Changes in Parkinson's Disease.* London: Butterworth, 1982, pp 41–58.

34. Hakim AM, Mathieson G: Dementia in Parkinson's disease: A neuropathologic study. *Neurology* 29:1209–1214, 1979.

35. Paulus W, Jellinger K: The neuropathologic basis of different clinical subgroups of Parkinson's disease. *J Neuropathol Exp Neurol* 50:743–755, 1991.

36. Kosaka K, Tsuchiya K, Yoshimura M: Lewy body disease with and without dementia: A clinicopathological study of 35 cases. *Clin Neuropathol* 7:299–305, 1988.

37. Byrne EJ, Lennox GG, Godwin-Austin RB, et al: Dementia associated with cortical Lewy bodies: Proposed clinical diagnostic criteria. *Dementia* 2:283–284, 1991.

38. Huntington's Disease Collaborative Research Group: A novel gene containing a trinucleotide repeat that is expanded and unstable on Huntington's disease chromosomes. *Cell* 72:971–983, 1993.

39. Harper PS: The epidemiology of Huntington's disease. *Hum Genet* 89:365–376, 1992.

40. Bird ED: The brain in Huntington's chorea. *Psychol Med* 8:357–360, 1978.

41. Brandt J, Strauss ME, Larus J, et al: Clinical correlates of dementia and disability in Huntington's disease. *J Clin Neuropsychol* 6:401–412, 1984.

42. Potegal M: A note on spatial-motor deficits in patients with Huntington's disease: A test of hypothesis. *Neuropsychologia* 9:233–235, 1971.

43. Fedio P, Cox CS, Neophytides A, et al: Neuropsychological profile of Huntington's disease: Patients and those at risk, in Chase TN, Wexler NS, Barbeau A (eds): *Advances in Neurology.* New York: Raven Press, 1979, vol 23, 239–271.

44. Delis DC, Massman PJ, Butters N, et al: Profiles of demented and amnesic patients on the California Verbal Learning Test: Implications for the assessment of memory disorders. *Psychol Assess* 3:19–26, 1991.

45. Martin JB: Huntington's disease: New approaches to an old problem. *Neurology* 34:1059–1072, 1984.

46. Caine E, Shoulson I: Psychiatric syndromes in Huntington's disease. *Am J Psychiatry* 140:728–733, 1983.

47. Folstein SE: *Huntington's Disease.* Baltimore: Johns Hopkins University Press, 1989.

48. Shoulson I. Huntington's disease: Cognitive and psychiatric features. *Neuropsychiatry Neuropsychol Behav Neurol* 3:15–22, 1990.

49. Bamford KA, Caine ED, Kido DK, et al: Clinical-pathologic correlation in Huntington's disease: A neuropsychological and computed tomography study. *Neurology* 39:796–801, 1989.

50. Steele JC, Richardson JC, Olszewski J: Progressive supranuclear palsy. *Arch Neurol* 10:333–358, 1964.

51. Golbe LI, Davis PH, Schoenberg BS, Duvoisin RC: Prevalence and natural history of progressive supranuclear palsy. *Neurology* 38:1031–1034, 1988.

52. Lees AJ: Progressive supranuclear palsy (Steele-Richardson-Olszewski syndrome), in Cummings JL (ed): *Subcortical Dementia.* New York: Oxford University Press, 1990.

53. Albert ML, Feldman RG, Willis AL: The "subcortical dementia" of progressive supranuclear palsy. *J Neurol Neurosurg Psychiatry* 37:121–130, 1974.

54. Pillon B, Dubois B, Ploska A, Agid Y: Severity and specificity of cognitive impairment in Alzheimer's, Huntington's, and Parkinson's diseases and progressive supranuclear palsy. *Neurology* 41:634–643, 1991.

55. Litvan I: Cognitive disturbances in progressive supranuclear palsy. *J Neural Trans* 42:69–78, 1994.

56. Dubois B, Pillon B, Legault F, et al: Slowing of cognitive processing in progressive supranuclear palsy. *Arch Neurol* 45:1194–1199, 1988.

57. Podoll K, Schwarz M, Noth J: Language functions in progressive supranuclear palsy. *Brain* 114:1457–1472, 1991.

58. Milberg W, Albert M: Cognitive differences between patients with progressive supranuclear palsy and Alzheimer's disease. *J Clin Exp Neuropsychol* 11:605–614, 1989.

59. Pillon B, Blin J, Vidailhet M, et al: The neuropsychological pattern of corticobasal degeneration: comparison with progressive supranuclear palsy and Alzheimer's disease. *Neurology* 45:1477–1483, 1995.

60. Janati A, Appell AR: Psychiatric aspects of progressive supranuclear palsy. *J Nerv Ment Dis* 172:85–89, 1984.

61. Foster NL, Gilman S, Berent S, et al: Cerebral hypometabolism in progressive supranuclear palsy studied with positron emission tomography. *Ann Neurol* 24:399–406, 1988.

62. Rebeiz JJ, Kolodny EH, Richardson EP: Cortico-dentatonigral degeneration with neuronal achromasia. *Arch Neurol* 18:20–33, 1968.

63. Riley DE, Lang AE, Lewis A, et al: Cortical-basal ganglionic degeneration. *Neurology* 40:1203–1212, 1990.

64. Watts RL, Williams RS, Growdon JD, et al: Corticobasal ganglionic degeneration (abstr). *Neurology* 35(suppl 1):178, 1985.

65. Case records of the Massachusetts General Hospital. *N Engl J Med* 313:739–748, 1985.

66. Rediess S, Satran R: Corticobasal degeneration: Serial neuropsychological examination of a case (abstr). *J Int Neuropsychol Soc* 1:147, 1995.

67. Gibb RG, Luthert PJ, Marsden CD: Corticobasal degeneration. *Brain* 112:1171–1192, 1989.

68. Fahn S: Parkinsonism, in Rowland LP (ed): *Merritt's Textbook of Neurology,* 9th ed. Baltimore, MD: Williams & Wilkins, 1995, pp 713–730.

69. Penney JB: Multiple systems atrophy and nonfamilial olivopontocerebellar atrophy are the same disease. *Ann Neurol* 37:553–554, 1995.

70. Robbins TW, James M, Lange KW, et al: Cognitive performance in multiple system atrophy. *Brain* 115:271–291, 1992.

71. Grafman J, Litvan I, Massaquoi S, et al: Cognitive planning deficit in patients with cerebellar atrophy. *Neurology* 42:1493–1496, 1992.

72. Akshoomoff NA, Courchesne E, Press GA, Iragui V: Contribution of the cerebellum to neuropsychological functioning: Evidence from a case of cerebellar degenerative disorder. *Neuropsychologia* 30:315–328, 1992.

73. Fiez JA, Petersen SE, Cheney MK, Raichle ME: Impaired non-motor learning and error detection associated with cerebellar damage. *Brain* 115:155–178, 1992.

74. Appollonio IM, Grafman J, Schwartz V, et al: Memory in patients with cerebellar degeneration. *Neurology* 43:1536–1544, 1993.

75. Akshoomoff NA, Courchesne E: A new role for the cerebellum in cognitive operations. *Behav Neurosci* 106:731–738, 1992.

CONTRIBUTORS

Michael P. Alexander, M.D.
Director, Stroke Rehabilitation program
Braintree Hospital
Braintree, Massachusetts
Department of Neurology
Boston University School of Medicine
Boston, Massachusetts

Russell M. Bauer, Ph.D., A.B.P.P./A.B.C.N.
Associate Professor
Center for Neuropsychological Studies
Departments of Clinical and Health Psychology and
  Neurology
University of Florida
Gainesville, Florida

Kathleen Baynes, Ph.D.
Assistant Professor of Neurology
Center for Neuroscience
University of California at Davis
Davis, California

D. Frank Benson, M.D.
late of Neurology Department
UCLA School of Medicine
Los Angeles, California

H. Branch Coslett, M.D.
Professor of Neurology
Temple University School of Medicine
Director, Memory Disorders Research Center
Department of Veterans Affairs Medical Center
Boston, Massachusetts

Jeffrey L. Cummings, M.D.
Professor of Neurology and Psychology
UCLA School of Medicine
Los Angeles, California

Tim Curran, Ph.D.
Assistant Professor of Psychology
Department of Psychology
Case Western Reserve University
Cleveland, Ohio

Maureen Dennis, Ph.D.
Senior Scientist
Department of Psychology and Research Institute
The Hospital for Sick Children
Associate Professor
Department of Surgery, Faculty of Medicine
University of Toronto
Toronto, Ontario, Canada

Hanna Damasio, M.D.
Professor of Neurology
Director of the Human Neuroanatomy
University of Iowa College of Medicine
Iowa City, Iowa
Adjunct Professor for Biological Studies, The Salk
  Institute
La Jolla, California

Antonio R. Damasio, M.D., Ph.D.
M. W. Van Allen Professor and Head of Neurology
University of Iowa College of Medicine
Iowa City, Iowa
Adjunct Professor
Salk Institute for Biological Studies
La Jolla, California

Ennio De Renzi, M.D.
Professor of Neurology
Chief, Neurological Department
University of Moderna
Moderna, Italy

Mark D'Esposito, Ph.D, M.D.
Associate Professor of Neurology
University of Pennsylvania Medical Center
Philadelphia, Pennsylvania

Martha J. Farah, Ph.D.
Director, Center for Cognitive Neuroscience
Professor of Psychology
University of Pennsylvania
Philadelphia, Pennsylvania

Todd E. Feinberg, M.D.
Chief
Betty and Morton Yarmon Division of Neurobehavior
    and Alzheimer's Disease
Associate Attending, Psychiatry and Neurology
Beth Israel Medical Center
New York, New York
Associate Professor, Neurology and Psychiatry
Albert Einstein College of Medicine
Bronx, New York

Michael S. Gazzaniga, Ph.D.
Director, Program in Cognitive Neuroscience
Dartmouth University
Hanover, New Hampshire

Georg Goldenberg, M.D.
Neuropsychological Department
Krankenhaus München Bogenhausen
Munich, Germany

Jordon Grafman, Ph.D.
Chief, Cognitive Neuroscience Section
National Institutes of Neurological Disorders and
    Stroke
National Institutes of Health
Bethesda, Maryland

Murray Grossman, M.D.
Associate Professor
Department of Neurology
University of Pennsylvania Medical Center
Philadelphia, Pennsylvania

Kenneth M. Heilman, M.D.
James E. Rooks, Jr., Professor of Neurology
College of Medicine
University of Florida
Gainesville, Florida

Diane M. Jacobs, Ph.D.
Assistant Professor of Neuropsychology
Department of Neurology
Gertrude H. Sergievsky Center
Columbia University College of Physicians and
    Surgeons
New York, New York

Daniel I. Kaufer, M.D.
Assistant Professor of Psychiatry and Neurology
University of Pittsburgh Medical Center
Pittsburgh, Pennsylvania

Daniel Y. Kimberg, Ph.D.
Research Associate
Center for Cognitive Neuroscience
University of Pennsylvania
Philadelphia, Pennsylvania

Maureen W. Lovett, Ph.D.
Senior Scientist, Research Institute
The Hospital for Sick Children
Associate Professor
Departments of Pediatrics and Psychology
University of Toronto
Toronto, Ontario, Canada

Richard Mayeux, M. D., M.S.E.
Gertrude E. Sergievsky Professor of Neurology,
    Psychiatry, and Public Health (Epidemiology)
Sergievsky Center
Columbia University
New York, New York

M.-Marsel Mesulam, M.D.
Ruth and Evelyn Dunbar Professor of Neurology and
    Psychiatry
Northwestern University Medical Center
Chicago, Illinois

Bruce L. Miller, M.D.
Professor of Neurology
UCLA School of Medicine
Reed Neurological Research Institute
Los Angeles, California

Robert D. Nebes, Ph.D.
Professor of Psychiatry
University of Pittsburgh Medical School
Pittsburgh, Pennsylvania

Robert D. Rafal, M.D.
Professor of Neurology
University of Bangor
Bangor, Wales

Marcus E. Raichle, M.D.
Co-Director of Radiological Sciences
Professor of Radiology, Neurology, Anatomy, and
  Neurobiology
Washington University School of Medicine
St. Louis, Missouri

Timothy Rickard, Ph.D.
Postdoctoral Fellow
Cognitive Neuroscience Section
National Institutes of Neurological Disorders and
  Stroke
National Institutes of Health
Bethesda, Maryland

David M. Roane, M.D.
Assistant Professor of Psychiatry
Beth Israel Medical Center
New York, New York

David P. Roeltgen, M.D.
Neurologist
Williamsport Hospital
Williamsport, Pennsylvania
Adjunct Associate Professor of Neurology
Hahemann University
Philadelphia, Pennsylvania

Leslie J. Gonzalez Rothi, Ph.D.
Associate Professor of Neurology
University of Florida
Speech Pathology Services
VA Medical Center
Gainesville, Florida

Eleanor M. Saffran, Ph.D.
Professor of Communication Sciences and Neurology
Temple University School of Medicine
Philadelphia, Pennsylvania

Daniel L. Schacter, Ph.D.
Professor of Psychology
Harvard University
Cambridge, Massachusetts

Yaakov Stern, Ph.D.
Associate Professor of Clinical Neuropsychology
Columbia University
New York, New York

Karin Stromswold, M. D., Ph.D.
Assistant Professor of Psychology and Cognitive
  Science
Rutgers University
New Brunswick, New Jersey

Edward Valenstein, M.D.
Professor of Neurology
University of Florida
Gainesville, Florida

Robert T. Watson, M.D.
Professor of Neurology and Clinical and Health
  Psychology
University of Florida
Gainesville, FL

Tricia Zawacki, B.A.
Graduate Student
Center for Neuropsychological Studies
Department of Clinical and Health Psychology
University of Florida
Gainesville, Florida

Stuart Zola, Ph.D.
Research Career Scientist
Veterans Administration Medical Center
Professor in Residence
Departments of Psychiatry and Neurosciences
University of California San Diego School of
  Medicine
La Jolla, California

INDEX